Nutrition and Diabetes

Nutrition and Diabetes

Pathophysiology and Management

Second Edition

Edited by

Emmanuel C. Opara

Sam Dagogo-Jack

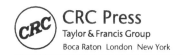

CRC Press is an imprint of the
Taylor & Francis Group, an **informa** business

CRC Press
Taylor & Francis Group
6000 Broken Sound Parkway NW, Suite 300
Boca Raton, FL 33487-2742

First issued in paperback 2021

© 2019 by Taylor & Francis Group, LLC
CRC Press is an imprint of Taylor & Francis Group, an Informa business

No claim to original U.S. Government works

ISBN 13: 978-1-03-209400-7 (pbk)
ISBN 13: 978-1-138-71000-9 (hbk)

Visit the Taylor & Francis Web site at
http://www.taylorandfrancis.com

and the CRC Press Web site at
http://www.crcpress.com

Publisher's Note
The publisher has gone to great lengths to ensure the quality of this reprint but points out that some imperfections in the original copies may be apparent.

Contents

SECTION I Pathophysiology and Treatment of Obesity

SECTION II   Pathophysiology and Treatment of Diabetes

Foreword

There has been no let-up in the acquisition of knowledge regarding the epidemiology, pathogenesis, and treatment of diabetes and obesity since the first edition of this book was published more than a decade ago. The resulting change in the way many people think about them makes a new edition timely.

The idea that overweight and (moderate) obesity is unhealthy, even in physically fit people, has been challenged. It is, they contend, not the overweight itself that is unhealthy but its associated morbid conditions—namely diabetes, hypertension, and cardiovascular disease. In support of this notion, there is some evidence that they are linked in a Mendelian fashion. Others—the majority—still believe the link is causal and that obesity is often the primary abnormality. The distinction is important, for, if the former view is correct, there is no need to treat overweight people providing they are happy and do not also suffer from diabetes, hypertension, or cardiovascular disease, whereas, if the latter view is correct, even modest overweight is clinically relevant.

Contrary to what Malthus would have had us believe, population growth has not yet outgrown humankind's ability to supply itself with food. Distribution and the wherewithal to purchase food do, however, remain problems that are beyond medicine's ability to resolve, and undernutrition in the midst of plenty is still with us.

While the general principles of good nutrition were established almost a century ago, the details are still poorly understood. The key role of energy supply and its relationship to body weight, and the importance of vitamins and trace elements and quality of dietary proteins to health, have long been recognized, but much remains to be learned. The relevance of differences in the nature of dietary carbohydrates and whether they are associated with dietary fiber has, however, a much shorter history—as has recognition of subtle differences in the nature and origin of dietary fats.

There is some evidence, for example, to suggest that the incidence of type 2 diabetes can be reduced by substituting camel's for cow's milk in the diet. But even after decades of anecdotal evidence and 20 or so years of scientific study—mostly outside the United States and Western Europe—the matter is undecided. This reflects just how difficult the truly scientific study of even comparatively minor changes in dietary practice on population health is to resolve—not least because of the logistics involved in conducting long-term research on human beings.

Since the last edition of the book, there has been more understanding of the part played by the gastrointestinal tract as an endocrine organ in the control of appetite and metabolic processes.

The desire and ability to eat is, and presumably always has been, controlled by a number of factors, one of which—namely, the availability and affordability of food, regardless of quality—is no longer a consideration in the developed, and increasingly the developing, world. This leaves physiological and societal factors as major determinants of the distribution and prevalence of obesity in and between nation states. That genetic considerations play an important role has long been recognized, but exactly how they manifest themselves is only slowly being elucidated.

Undoubtedly one of the most important advances in our understanding and treatment of type 2 diabetes has been the growth of bariatric surgery. Once reserved solely for treating diet-resistant, life-threatening obesity, it is now increasingly being used for the treatment of patients with type 2 diabetes who are only modestly overweight (body mass index [BMI] of at least 30). The resulting remarkable change in metabolism, leading in many cases to an immediate improvement or total remission of the diabetic diathesis, cannot be attributed to weight loss. It is thought largely to result from changes in the enteroinsular axis, most notably in the secretion of GIP and GLP-1(7-36) amide. How long the improvement, or cure in some cases, continues awaits lifelong follow-up studies.

Concurrently, developments in peptide synthesis have seen the introduction of GLP-1 analogues for the clinical treatment of type 2 diabetes and the experimental use of GIP analogues for the treatment of obesity. A similar approach using analogues with either agonistic or antagonistic actions to the hormones controlling appetite can confidently be expected.

Glucagon, whose role in the adverse manifestations of diabetes has largely been ignored, has recently come to share center stage with insulin deficiency in the pathogenesis of the diabetic syndrome. It is currently being investigated as the target for a therapeutic approach that involves either impeding glucagon secretion or blocking its receptors.

Vincent Marks
Clinical Biochemistry, University of Surrey,
Guildford, United Kingdom

Preface

Diabetes and obesity are two common disorders that have come to be appropriately recognized as enormous burdens both to the afflicted individuals and modern society in general. What is even more striking is the relationship between obesity and impaired glucose regulation that predominantly results in overt diabetes. Consequently, as the incidence of obesity has risen in virtually every population, so has that of type 2 diabetes. Perhaps more alarming is the increasing incidence of obesity and type 2 diabetes among children. Given the chronic nature of both conditions and their known associations with cardiovascular and other serious complications, the coexistence of obesity and diabetes in children portends a dire future for society.

The purpose of *Nutrition and Diabetes: Pathophysiology and Management* is to provide a unique forum that highlights the link between the problems of obesity and diabetes. The pathophysiological underpinnings and pertinent aspects of each disorder are discussed exhaustively in relevant sections of the book. Importantly, the inter-relationships in the pathobiology and manifestations of obesity and diabetes come into focus, and many areas of overlap become obvious in the various chapters of the book. Enormous efforts have been made by the different contributors to first provide an overview of each topic, then discuss the mechanistic aspects of the given problem, and finally link these pathophysiological processes to the rationale of therapeutic strategies. The second edition of this book has been reorganized and is divided into two sections: Pathophysiology and Treatment of Obesity, and Pathophysiology and Treatment of Diabetes. New topics have been added in each section, including the emerging roles of probiotics in the pathogenesis and treatment of both obesity and diabetes.

Nutrition and Diabetes: Pathophysiology & Management is intended to be a reference handbook for physicians, nutritionists, dietitians, and other healthcare workers who deal daily with the various problems associated with obesity and diabetes. Researchers who desire a deeper understanding of the current state of knowledge, as well as gaps in our knowledge, would find this volume a worthwhile companion. Furthermore, the book should be of interest to experts and officials involved in formulating health policies in both advanced economies and developing countries. Finally, members of the general literate public (especially individuals afflicted with obesity and/or diabetes) would find this book a valuable source of actionable information to augment advice provided by their healthcare team.

The editors would like to thank all the chapter authors for the generous gift of their time to discuss important aspects of diabetes and obesity and make this a unique book. Each of you has helped to make this second edition a worthwhile project, and we are greatly indebted to you.

Emmanuel C. Opara and Sam Dagogo-Jack

Editors

Emmanuel C. Opara, PhD, received his MSc degree in Clinical Biochemistry at the University of Surrey in England and a PhD in Medical Biochemistry from the University of London. After a World Health Organization–sponsored research fellowship at the Mayo Clinic in Rochester, Minnesota, he was a visiting fellow at the National Institute of Diabetes and Digestive and Kidney Diseases, National Institutes of Health in Bethesda, Maryland before spending 15 years on faculty at the Duke University Medical Center in Durham, North Carolina. He subsequently was research professor in the Biomedical Engineering program at the Illinois Institute of Technology, Chicago while serving as a senior investigator in the Human Islet Transplant program at the University of Chicago. He accepted his present position as a professor at the Wake Forest Institute for Regenerative Medicine in 2009 while also serving as a professor in the Center on Obesity, Diabetes & Metabolism at the Wake Forest School of Medicine. He also serves as professor and graduate program director at the Wake Forest University campus of the joint Virginia Tech-Wake Forest School of Biomedical Engineering & Sciences.

Dr. Opara is a member of many professional organizations, including the American Diabetes Association, Endocrine Society, American Federation for Medical Research, American Pancreatic Association, and Biomedical Engineering Society. He was honored by the Society of Black Academic Surgeons with a distinguished service award in 2007.

Sam Dagogo-Jack, MD, is Professor of Medicine and Chief of the Division of Endocrinology, Diabetes and Metabolism at the University of Tennessee Health Science Center (UTHSC), Memphis, Tennessee, where he holds the A. C. Mullins Endowed Chair in Translational Research. He is also Director of the General Clinical Research Center at UTHSC. Dr. Dagogo-Jack has studied, practiced, researched, and taught medicine and diabetology in Africa, Asia, Australia, Europe, North and South America, the Caribbean countries, and the Middle-East. His current research focuses on the interaction of genetic and environmental factors in the prediction and prevention of prediabetes and diabetes. Dr. Dagogo-Jack is a recipient of the *Banting Medal for Leadership* from the American Diabetes Association and the *Distinction in Endocrinology Award* from the American College of Endocrinology. He served as the 2015 President, Medicine & Science, of the American Diabetes Association.

Contributors

Zhenzhong Bai
Research Center for High Altitude Medicine
Qinghai University Medical School
Xining, People's Republic of China

Connie W. Bales
Duke University Medical Center
Durham VA Medical Center
Durham, North Carolina

Robert Benjamin
Division of Pediatric Endocrinology and
    Diabetes
Duke University Medical Center
Durham, North Carolina

Khalil N. Bitar
Professor of Regenerative Medicine
Director of GI Research
Wake Forest Institute of Regenerative Medicine
Professor of Gastroenterology, Physiology and
    Biomedical Engineering and Sciences
Wake Forest School of Medicine
Winston-Salem, North Carolina

Schafer Boeder
Division of Endocrinology and Metabolism
University of California
San Diego, California

R. Brandt
Department of Chemical and Biological
    Engineering
Illinois Institute of Technology
Chicago, Illinois

A. Cinar
Department of Chemical and Biological
    Engineering
Illinois Institute of Technology
Chicago, Illinois

Sam Dagogo-Jack
A.C. Mullins Endowed Chair in Translational
    Research
Professor of Medicine and Director
Division of Endocrinology, Diabetes &
    Metabolism
Department of Medicine
University of Tennessee Health Science Center
Memphis, Tennessee

Danae A. Delivanis
Division of Endocrinology, Diabetes, Nutrition,
    and Metabolism
Mayo Clinic
Rochester, Minnesota

Shaun P. Deveshwar
Wake Forest Institute for Regenerative
    Medicine
Winston-Salem, North Carolina

Ayotunde O. Dokun
Division of Endocrinology
Department of Medicine
University of Tennessee Health Sciences
    Center
Memphis, Tennessee

Steven Edelman
Division of Endocrinology and Metabolism
University of California
San Diego, California

Olufemi A. Fasanmade
Associate Professor of Medicine
Department of Medicine, College of
    Medicine, University of Lagos
Honorary Consultant Physician and
    Endocrinologist
Lagos University Teaching Hospital
Lagos, Nigeria

Mark N. Feinglos
Division of Endocrinology, Metabolism and
   Nutrition
Department of Medicine
Duke University Medical Center
Durham, North Carolina

J. Feng
Department of Chemical and Biological
   Engineering
Illinois Institute of Technology
Chicago, Illinois

Adolfo Z. Fernandez, Jr.
Wake Forest Baptist Health
Associate Professor of Surgery
Chief, Division of Bariatric and Minimally
   Invasive Surgery
Wake Forest University School of Medicine
Medical Center Boulevard
Winston-Salem, North Carolina

Peter R. Flatt
SAAD Centre for Pharmacy and Diabetes
School of Biomedical Sciences
University of Ulster
Coleraine, United Kingdom

I. Hajizadeh
Department of Chemical and Biological
   Engineering
Illinois Institute of Technology
Chicago, Illinois

N. Hobbs
Department of Chemical and Biological
   Engineering
Illinois Institute of Technology
Chicago, Illinois

Nigel Irwin
SAAD Centre for Pharmacy and Diabetes
School of Biomedical Sciences
University of Ulster
Coleraine, United Kingdom

Michael D. Jensen
Division of Endocrinology, Diabetes, Nutrition,
   and Metabolism
Mayo Clinic
Rochester, Minnesota

William F. Kendall, Jr.
Department of Surgery
Halifax Health, Center for Transplant Services
University of Florida College of Medicine
Daytona Beach, Florida

J. Kilkus
Department of Chemical and Biological
   Engineering
Illinois Institute of Technology
Chicago, Illinois

Kenneth L. Koch
Professor of Internal Medicine
Chief, Section on Gastroenterology
Wake Forest School of Medicine
Winston-Salem, North Carolina

William E. Kraus
Division of Cardiology
Department of Medicine
Duke Molecular Physiology Institute
Duke University Medical Center
Durham, North Carolina

Wanda C. Lakey
Division of Endocrinology, Metabolism and
   Nutrition
Department of Medicine
Duke University Medical Center
and
Durham VA Medical Center
Durham, North Carolina

C. Lazaro
Department of Chemical and Biological
   Engineering
Illinois Institute of Technology
Chicago, Illinois

Lillian F. Lien
Division Chief of Endocrinology, Metabolism,
   and Diabetes
University of Mississippi Medical Center
Jackson, Mississippi

E. Littlejohn
Department of Chemical and Biological
   Engineering
Illinois Institute of Technology
Chicago, Illinois

Donald A. McClain
Center on Diabetes, Obesity and Metabolism
Wake Forest School of Medicine
Winston-Salem, North Carolina

and

VA Medical Center
Salisbury, North Carolina

Robert W. McGarrah
Division of Cardiology
Department of Medicine
Duke Molecular Physiology Institute
Duke University Medical Center
Durham, North Carolina

Gary D. Miller
Department of Health and Exercise Science
Wake Forest University
Winston-Salem, North Carolina

Amie A. Ogunsakin
Division of Endocrinology, Diabetes and
    Metabolism
Department of Medicine
University of Tennessee Health Sciences Center
Memphis, Tennessee

Emmanuel C. Opara
Wake Forest Institute for Regenerative Medicine
and
Center on Diabetes, Obesity & Metabolism
and
Virginia Tech-Wake Forest School of
    Biomedical Engineering & Sciences
Wake Forest School of Medicine
Winston-Salem, North Carolina

Nicholette D. Palmer
Department of Biochemistry
Wake Forest School of Medicine
Winston-Salem, North Carolina

Gabrielle Page-Wilson
Division of Endocrinology
Department of Medicine
Vagelos College of Physicians & Surgeons
Columbia University
New York, New York

Puja B. Patel
Wake Forest Institute for Regenerative
    Medicine
Winston-Salem, North Carolina

Varun Pathak
SAAD Centre for Pharmacy and Diabetes
School of Biomedical Sciences
University of Ulster
Coleraine, United Kingdom

Kathryn N. Porter Starr
Duke University Medical Center
Durham VA Medical Center
Durham, North Carolina

Lipika Salaye
Center on Diabetes, Obesity and Metabolism
Wake Forest School of Medicine
Winston-Salem, North Carolina

S. Samadi
Department of Chemical and Biological
    Engineering
Illinois Institute of Technology
Chicago, Illinois

Jacques E. Samson
Assistant Professor
Maternal Fetal Medicine
Department of Obstetrics and Gynecology
University of Tennessee Health Science Center
Memphis, Tennessee

M. Sevil
Department of Chemical and Biological
    Engineering
Illinois Institute of Technology
Chicago, Illinois

Natascha Thompson
Associate Professor of Internal Medicine
    and Pediatrics
Program Director Medicine-Pediatrics
    Residency Program
University of Tennessee Health Science
    Center
Memphis, Tennessee

K. Turksoy
Department of Chemical and Biological
  Engineering
Illinois Institute of Technology
Chicago, Illinois

Stephen J. Walker
Wake Forest Institute for Regenerative
  Medicine
Winston-Salem, North Carolina

Kenlyn R. Young
Duke University Medical Center
Durham, North Carolina

Section I

Pathophysiology and Treatment
of Obesity

1 Central and Peripheral Modulators of Appetite and Satiety

Gabrielle Page-Wilson and Sam Dagogo-Jack

CONTENTS

1.1 INTRODUCTION

Regulation of energy homeostasis is critical to the survival of any species. Therefore, intricate behavioral, metabolic, and neuroendocrine mechanisms have evolved to integrate energy intake and dissipation. A delicate balance between intake and expenditure of energy is required to maintain healthy weight. Perhaps for teleological reasons, the mechanisms that regulate energy homeostasis are biased in favor of net positive energy and are geared toward defense of weight loss rather than prevention of obesity. Hence, spontaneous weight loss in the absence of disease is rare, and the experience of progressive weight gain in free-living humans is common.

The adaptations that defend against weight loss eventually become maladaptive when obesity and its related metabolic and cardiovascular complications supervene, as in the present era (Bray 1996, Flegal et al. 2002). At its core, obesity signifies chronic disequilibrium between food consumption and energy expenditure. Total energy expenditure (TEE) comprises basal or resting energy expenditure (REE), thermic effect of food (TEF), mandatory physical activities of daily living (ADL), and volitional physical activity or exercise (Macdonald 1998). The contributions of TEF and ADL to TEE are rather modest, and the rate of voluntary physical activity is universally low among humans, leaving REE the energy-expenditure mode of choice for most people.

REE declines with age, which explains the tendency to positive energy balance and obesity in older persons. The TEE also is correlated positively with body surface area and is higher in obese than lean individuals. However, the REE compensation for obesity is ineffective in inducing weight loss or restoring normal weight. Therefore, REE, the major component of energy expenditure for most sedentary persons, is a practically nonmodifiable factor in energy homeostasis. This leaves restriction of food intake and volitional exercise as the main strategies for effective weight control.

1.2   APPETITE AND SATIETY

The "afferent" limb of the energy homeostasis loop is food consumption. Food intake is driven by appetite and terminated by satiety. Hunger is the physiological response to appetite, whereas meal termination occurs in response to satiety signals. The exact mechanisms controlling the primal instincts of appetite and hunger are incompletely understood. It is known, however, that a host of behavioral, environmental, cognitive, and situational influences can modify responses to hunger. Thus, appetite triggers hunger, but the latter can be overridden or suppressed to enable delay of food intake to a more appropriate time. Similarly, several organic and psychiatric disorders are associated with perturbations of appetite. The present review focuses on the neuro-hormonal regulation of food intake and attempts to integrate seminal experimental findings in rodents with current and future directions in human metabolic research and antiobesity drug development.

1.3   CENTRAL NERVOUS SYSTEM LOCALIZATION OF FEEDING CONTROL

The hypothalamus integrates diverse signals, including brain neurotransmitters, peripheral neuro-humoral afferents, adipocyte-derived signals, gastrointestinal peptides, and other afferent inputs, to regulate energy homeostasis. The medial basal hypothalamus (MBH), which includes the ventromedial and arcuate nuclei, plays a critical role in the regulation of energy balance. The arcuate nucleus (ARC), situated at the base of the hypothalamus, houses two well-described neuronal populations, including proopiomelanocortin (POMC) and neuropeptide Y (NPY)/agouti-related peptide (AgRP) neurons that are important regulators of feeding. These neurons express receptors for hormones and neuropeptides and respond to peripheral changes in energy balance (Schwartz et al. 2000). The paraventricular nucleus (PVN) in the anterior hypothalamus, the major site of corticotropin-releasing hormone (CRH) and thyrotropin-releasing hormone (TRH) secretion, receives rich projections from the ARC. The PVN is involved in the integration of paracrine and endocrine metabolic signals, with classical neuroendocrine pathways mediated through the thyroid and hypothalamic-pituitary-adrenal axes. In addition to these nuclei, the brainstem also plays a role in appetite regulation, processing satiety signals that are conveyed following meal ingestion by vagal afferent projections that converge in the nucleus tractus solitarius (NTS) of the hindbrain (Williams et al. 2001). Neuronal projections from the NTS to the PVN and lateral hypothalamus link the brainstem with the hypothalamus (Grill and Hayes 2012). However, studies in decerebrate rats, in which the hindbrain and forebrain are disconnected, demonstrate that the brainstem can independently control meal size in response to satiety signals like cholecystokinin (CCK), showing that the hindbrain and forebrain may both contribute to energy balance (Grill and Smith 1988).

1.4 HYPOTHALAMIC NEUROPEPTIDES THAT STIMULATE FOOD INTAKE

The hypothalamic orexigenic signals include NPY, AgRP, and the hypocretins/orexins.

1.4.1 NEUROPEPTIDE Y

NPY is a 36-amino acid polypeptide that rapidly stimulates food intake following intracerebroventricular (ICV) injection in rodents. The appetite-stimulating effects of NPY lead to sustained hyperphagia and weight gain in mice receiving chronic ICV administration. The specificity of NPY's effect has been established in studies that employed co-administration of NPY antagonists or its antibodies, both of which inhibited food intake in rats (Kalra et al. 1999). The role of NPY as a central physiological trigger of meal initiation is suggested by studies showing a rapid increase in hypothalamic NPY expression in the PVN before meal times, and persistence of NPY gene expression throughout the period of enforced hunger. The orexigenic action of NPY is mediated by interactions with Y1 and Y5 receptors (Henry et al. 2005). NPY also has diverse actions that enhance activation of the HPA axis, amplify the stress response, and alter seizure threshold (Beck 2006), which are obvious limitations to a direct deployment of NPY for treatment of cachexia and eating disorders. Interestingly, NPY expression in the arcuate nucleus is potently antagonized by the anorexigenic hormone leptin, as well as by insulin. Furthermore, activation of the Y2 receptor subtype on NPY neurons triggers inhibitory presynaptic signals. Consequently, central administration of PYY3-36 (a Y2 receptor agonist secreted by intestinal endocrine L cells) into the arcuate elicits a marked inhibition of food intake. Also, Y2 receptor knock-out mice lose their responsiveness to the anorectic effect of PYY3-36 (Batterham et al. 2002). The longstanding interest in the therapeutic potential of NPY antagonism was revived by the discovery of Y2R and Y4R receptor agonists and Y5R antagonists. To date, the success of these small molecules has been limited in clinical trials in humans by side effects or lack of efficacy (Brothers and Wahlestedt 2010).

1.4.2 AGOUTI-RELATED PROTEIN

AgRP is expressed exclusively in the arcuate nucleus of the hypothalamus and co-localizes to the same neurons that secrete NPY (Goldstone et al. 2002). Several reports have confirmed that administration of AgRP potently enhances appetite in rodents, with central administration of AgRP increasing food intake for up to 7 days (Rossi et al. 1998). In contrast to the potent but relatively short-lived effect of NPY, chronic administration of AgRP results in sustained hyperphagia and obesity (Small et al. 2001). AgRP exerts its orexigenic effect by antagonizing the effect of POMC-derived peptide α-MSH at MC3 and MC4 receptors, increasing food intake and decreasing energy expenditure. The arcuate neurons that co-secrete NPY/AgRP are stimulated by fasting and potently inhibited by leptin and insulin (Breen et al. 2005). Several other important regulators of AgRP expression have been identified. Glucocorticoids impact AgRP expression, as illustrated by rodent studies demonstrating a decline in AgRP expression following adrenalectomy that is reversed by glucocorticoid replacement (Savontaus et al. 2002). The gut hormone ghrelin has also been shown to stimulate AgRP gene expression in the ARC, and ghrelin orexigenic effects have been shown to be partially mediated by NPY/AgRP (Chen et al. 2004).

1.4.3 HYPOCRETINS/OREXINS

The hypothalamic peptides hypocretins-1 and hypocretins-2 were discovered in 1998 by subtractive polymerase chain reaction (de Lecea et al. 1998). In the same year, homologous hypothalamic peptides named orexins 1 and 2 were discovered by Sakurai et al. (Sakurai et al. 1998) and shown to potently stimulate food intake in rats (Sakurai et al. 1998). The hypocretins/orexins stimulate food intake in rodents, an effect that is blocked by neutralizing antibodies to endogenous hypocretins (Willie et al. 2001).

In addition to directly stimulating food intake, the hypocretins/orexins may also influence energy homeostasis in other ways. For example, hypocretin levels increase in response to exercise, neuroglycopenia, and enforced wakefulness (Nishino 2003). Hypocretin-secreting neurons localize exclusively to the lateral hypothalamus, the region of the brain long known to integrate appetite signals. Although intriguing as modulators of food intake, interest in the hypocretins/orexins shifted to their role in sleep regulation when the genes for hypocretins/orexins were found to be the loci for narcolepsy (Chemelli et al. 1999, Lin et al. 1999). Documented mutations in the human hypocretin/orexin genes are rare among patients with sleep disorders, but nearly 90% of patients with narcolepsy-cataplexy have subnormal cerebrospinal fluid hypocretin levels (Nishino et al. 2001).

The latter finding is inconsistent with a primary orexigenic role of the hypocretins/orexins as the mechanism for the increased prevalence of obesity, insulin resistance, and type 2 diabetes among patients with narcolepsy (Nishino et al. 2001). These metabolic disorders are more likely the result of the physical hypoactivity associated with narcolepsy. It must be noted, however, that the hypocretin/orexin system functions centrally as the major integrator of excitatory impulses from monoaminergic (dopamine, norepinephrine, serotonin, histamine) and cholinergic fibers that maintain wakefulness and vigilance (Taheri et al. 2002). Thus, besides a direct orexigenic effect, the hypocretins/orexins could exert metabolic effects through modulation of central autonomic outflow. However, the hypocretins/orexins are less attractive candidates for drug development, because their reported effects on food intake are less robust and consistent compared with the orexigenic effects of NPY.

1.5 ANOREXIGENIC NEUROPEPTIDES

As a central integrator of energy homeostasis, the hypothalamus also is a source of neuropeptides that inhibit food intake or induce satiety. The hypothalamic anorexigenic agents include the melanocortins, cocaine- and amphetamine-regulated transcript (CART), and serotonin.

1.5.1 MELANOCORTINS

The melanocortins are derived from site-specific post-translational cleavage of the precursor parent molecule POMC. Cleavage of POMC within the anterior pituitary gives rise to adrenocorticotropic hormone (ACTH), which acts through the melanocortin 2 (MC2) receptor to stimulate adrenal steroidogenesis. Elsewhere in the brain, POMC is cleaved to another melanocortin α-MSH, which is an agonist for the MC3 and MC4 receptors. Administration of α-MSH (ICV) in rodents results in weight loss through inhibition of food intake and stimulation of energy expenditure (Neary et al. 2004). These actions are mediated through activation of two neuronal melanocortin receptor subtypes (MC3r and MC4r) and antagonized by an adjacent subset of hypothalamic neurons that express AgRP and NPY. Thus, the MC4 receptor plays a critical role on body-weight regulation. The NPY/AgRP neurons are inhibited by leptin and insulin.

The integrated physiology of the interactions of these opposing neuropeptides is evident from their weight-related alterations. Following weight loss, the decreasing levels of insulin and leptin lead to activation of NPY/AgRP neurons and inhibition of POMC neurons (Flier 1998, Schwartz et al. 2000). These counterregulatory changes induce accelerated food intake and accumulation of fat. Defects along the melanocortin signaling pathway, such as those seen in transgenic mice with targeted disruption of the MC4 receptor (knock-outs), result in hyperphagia and obesity (Huszar et al. 1997). Recently, fairly widespread functional mutations of the human MC4 receptor has been demonstrated to patients with severe childhood obesity (Farooqi et al. 2000). It should be noted, however, that the majority of obese patients have no demonstrable mutations in MC4, yet such persons may possibly benefit from future therapies targeting activation of MC4 pathways. While intranasal administration of a melanocortin fragment (MSH/ACTH 4–10) initially looked promising in that regard, MSH/ACTH 4–10 failed to have an anorexigenic effect in obese males, despite its inducing modest weight loss in individuals of normal weight (Fehm et al. 2001, Hallschmid et al. 2006). Similarly, the use of a more selective MC4R agonist (MK-0493) did not result in weight loss in obese humans (Krishna et al. 2009). However, a newly developed MC4R agonist (RM-493) may prove more promising, as recent data suggests that it effectively increases REE in obese adults (Chen et al. 2015).

1.5.2 Cocaine- and Amphetamine-Regulated Transcript

CART is widely expressed in the brain, especially in the hypothalamic nuclei and in the anterior pituitary. Within the arcuate nucleus, POMC co-localizes to neurons that also express CART. Injection of CART (1–100 pmol, ICV) resulted in dose-dependent inhibition of food intake in rats. The effect was observed within 20 minutes and lasted approximately 4 hours. The decrease in food intake following treatment with CART was accompanied by inhibition of gastric emptying and reduction of oxygen consumption. The arcuate POMC/CART neurons act as downstream effectors of the anorexigenic action of leptin and are markedly stimulated by ICV injection of leptin (Cowley et al. 2001). Interactions between CART and the endogenous opioid, serotoninergic (Rothman et al. 2003), and cannabinoid (Cota et al. 2003) systems provide additional mechanisms for the anorexigenic effects of CART.

1.5.3 Serotonin

The amino acid derivative 5-hydroxytryptamine (serotonin, 5-HT) has ubiquitous neurotransmitter functions on numerous central nervous system (CNS) targets (Blundell 1984). Receptors for 5-HT are widely expressed in regions including the limbic system, raphe nucleus, and the hypothalamus. Activation of 5-HT receptors (especially the 5-HT2c subtype) is associated with inhibition of food intake. A similar anorexigenic effect is observed following augmentation of serotonin abundance through inhibition of its re-uptake. Conversely, studies in rodents have shown that deletion of the serotonin 5-HT2c gene results in marked hyperphagia (Tecott et al. 1995). Unfortunately, clinical experience with selective serotonin reuptake inhibitors shows modest and inconsistent effects on body weight, which indicates that the serotonergic pathway is overridden by more powerful orexigenic impulses under normal physiological conditions. Nonetheless, sibutramine, a selective agonist of the serotonin 2C receptor, is an effective weight-loss medication. (Sibutramine was withdrawn from use in 2010 because of increase risk of cardiovascular events.)

While serotoninergic effects on food intake were once thought to be mediated primarily by central 5-HT pathways, recent studies utilizing genetic mouse models have underscored the importance of the melanocortin system in mediating the anorexigenic effect of 5-HT. Serotonin has been shown to impact satiety by inhibiting AgRP neuronal activity and decreasing inhibition of POMC neurons via 5-HT1B receptor activation (Heisler et al. 2006). 5-HT2cRs on POMC neurons have also been shown to play a role in mediating serotonin's capacity to suppress food intake (Xu et al. 2008). Lorcaserin, a 5-HT2c agonist, was approved by the FDA in 2012 for treatment of obesity.

1.5.4 Brain-Derived Neurotrophic Factor

Brain-derived neurotrophic factor (BDNF) is a member of the neurotrophin family of secreted peptides that acts at the tropomysin-related kinase B (TrkB) receptor to activate phospholipase C gamma, mitogen-activated protein kinase, and phosphatidylinositol-3 kinase (PI3-K) intracellular

TABLE 1.1

Selected Central Neuropeptides That Modulate Food Intake

Orexigenic	Anorexigenic
Neuropeptide Y	α-Melanocyte stimulating hormone
Agouti-related protein	Corticotropin-releasing hormone
Orexin a	Cocaine-amphetamine regulated transcript
Orexin b	Serotonin

signaling pathways (Reichardt 2006). While neurotrophins are most well-known for their impact on neuronal survival and differentiation (Chao 2003), there is evidence to support an important role for BDNF in energy homeostasis. Central administration of BDNF has been shown to reduce body weight in rodents (Lapchak and Hefti 1992), and reduced BDNF levels in heterozygous BDNF mice have been associated with increased food intake and obesity (Lyons et al. 1999). Similarly, decreased BDNF signalling, resulting from loss of a functional BDNF allele (Gray et al. 2006) or a de novo mutation in TrkB (Yeo et al. 2004), has been associated with hyperphagia and obesity in humans. Moreover, large-scale, genome-wide association studies of single nucleotide polymorphisms in BDNF genes have been associated with obesity (Hotta et al. 2009, Thorleifsson et al. 2009). BDNF's role as an anorexigenic factor is further supported by studies in rodents demonstrating reduced hypothalamic BDNF expression with fasting and increased BDNF gene expression following the administration of either glucose or melanocortin agonists (Xu et al. 2003, Unger et al. 2007). Continued studies designed to elucidate the role of BDNF in energy balance may lead to mechanistic insights that can be harnessed for developing novel treatment strategies for obesity in the future. Table 1.1 shows a list of orexigenic and anorexigenic central neuropeptides.

1.6 PERIPHERAL SIGNALS IN THE REGULATION OF FOOD INTAKE

The peripheral hormones that regulate food intake include several gastrointestinal, pancreatic, and adipocyte-derived peptides (Table 1.2). Based on extensive studies in rodents and limited human data, these peptides can be classified as having orexigenic (e.g., ghrelin) or anorexigenic (e.g., insulin, peptide YY, glucagon-like polypeptide, cholecystokinin, leptin) effects.

TABLE 1.2

Selected Peripheral Modulators of Food Intake

Signal	Main Targets
Anorexigenic	
Leptin	Hypothalamus
Peptide YY	Hypothalamus
Pancreatic polypeptide	Hypothalamus
Insulin	Hypothalamus
Cholecystokinin	Brainstem/vagus
GLP-1	Local GI/diverse
Oxyntomodulin	Local GI/diverse
Orexigenic	
Ghrelin	Hypothalamus

GI, gastrointestinal; GLP-1, glucagon-like peptide 1.

1.6.1 Adipocyte-Derived Signals

There is a mature and growing body of literature on the roles of several adipocyte products (including nonesterified fatty acids, adipocytokines, and leptin) in the regulation of metabolic fuel economy, energy balance, glucoregulation, food intake, and body weight. Products such as nonesterified fatty acids have long been proposed as mediators of obesity-associated insulin resistance and glucose dysregulation (Randle et al. 1988, Paolisso et al. 1998, Unger 1995, Laaksonen et al. 2002), as discussed elsewhere in this book.

1.6.2 Adipocytokines

The adipocytokine TNF-α (also known as *cachectin*, for its association with cachexia or wasting) is a mediator of insulin resistance and is secreted in higher amounts by adipocytes from obese subjects (Hotamisligil et al. 1993, 1994, 1996, Kern et al. 1995, Norman et al. 1995, Moller 2000). Other circulating and adipose-derived proinflammatory cytokines also have been implicated in the pathogenesis of obesity-associated insulin resistance and diabetes (Grimble 2002, Freeman et al. 2002). On the other hand, adiponectin is secreted in abundant amounts by fat cells from insulin-sensitive persons and is deficient in persons with obesity or insulin resistance (Stefan et al. 2002). Thus, numerous adipose tissue products serve as markers, signals, or modulators of energy balance, fuel economy, intermediary metabolism, glucoregulation, and other metabolic events that intersect with food intake and body-weight homeostasis. Of these numerous adipose tissue products, leptin is perhaps the best characterized in terms of its role in the regulation of food intake and related mechanisms.

1.6.3 Leptin

The positional cloning of the mouse (*ob*) gene and its human homologue (Zhang et al. 1994) represents a major milestone in obesity research. Two separate mutations of the *ob* gene result in either a premature stop codon or complete absence of *ob* mRNA in the *ob/ob* mouse (Zhang et al. 1994). The resultant absence of a normal *ob* gene product leads to overfeeding, massive obesity, delayed sexual maturation (Chehab et al. 1996), and immune defects (Matarese 2000) in *ob/ob* mice. The human *ob* or *lep* gene is transcribed and translated into a secreted protein mainly in white adipose tissue, but activity can also be reported in brown adipose tissue, gastric epithelium, and placental tissue (Masuzaki et al. 1997, Bado et al. 1998). Circulating leptin levels are increased by feeding, decreased during fasting or following weight loss, and altered by a variety of hormonal and physiological factors (Krempler et al. 2000, Page-Wilson et al. 2017).

A pedigree with severe childhood obesity associated with deletion of a guanine nucleotide in codon 133 of the human *lep* gene was the first human example of congenital leptin deficiency to be identified (Montague et al. 1997). A missense *lep* mutation in codon 105 has also been identified in a Turkish pedigree (Strobel et al. 1998). Three individuals (two female, one male) homozygous for this mutation have the phenotype of hypoleptinemia, marked hyperphagia, massive obesity, and hypothalamic hypogonadism. Excluding these rare reports, common forms of human obesity do not appear to be caused by discernible *lep* mutations (Considine et al. 1995, Maffei et al. 1996). Treatment with recombinant leptin results in a marked reduction in food intake and profound weight loss in *ob/ob* mice (Halaas et al. 1995, Pelleymounter et al. 1995, Campfield et al. 1995, Weigle et al. 1995, Chehab et al. 1996, Matarese 2000). Leptin therapy is also remarkably effective in correcting obesity in humans with congenital leptin deficiency (Pelleymounter et al. 1995, Farooqi et al. 1999, 2002, Licinio et al. 2004).

1.6.3.1 Mechanism of Action

Leptin exerts its effects through interaction with cognate cell membrane receptors (lep-r) (Tartaglia et al. 1995). One full length (isoform-b) and several alternatively spliced forms (a, c, d, e, f) of lep-r have been identified in brain and peripheral tissues (Takaya et al. 1996, Lee et al. 1996). Lep-r is a member of the class 1 cytokine receptor family (Vaisse et al. 1996, Baumann et al. 1996, Wang et al. 1997). This receptor family mediates gene transcription via activation of the *jak-stat* pathway (Ghilardi and Skoda 1997). The long isoform, lep-r (b), expressed in the hypothalamus, mediates the central effects of leptin. Intracellular signaling pathways arising from activated lep-r (b) include the phosphorylation and activation of the signal transducer and activator of transcription (STAT) pathways mediated by STAT3 and STAT5, the SOCS3-mediated feedback inhibition pathway, and the extracellular regulated kinase (ERK) pathway (Bjorbaek et al. 1999, Robertson et al. 2008). The shorter isoforms of the leptin receptor are truncated in the cytoplasmic domain but can bind leptin and probably mediate some peripheral actions (Takaya et al. 1996, Lee et al. 1996, Kieffer et al. 1996).

Leptin-receptor activation results in decreased expression of NPY, thereby inhibiting the powerful orexigenic effects of NPY (Ghilardi and Skoda 1997). Leptin's action to suppress food intake is mediated through an elaborate neuronal circuitry that involves suppression of orexigenic signals (NPY, AgRP, MCH, hypocretins 1 and 2/orexins a and b) and activation of anorexigenic (α-MSH, MC4, CRH, CART) neuronal pathways (Schwartz et al. 2000). Mutations in the lep-r gene result in obesity and leptin resistance in *db/db* mice (Chen et al. 1996) and *fa/fa* rats (Phillips et al. 1996), respectively. Human lep-r mutations associated with morbid obesity have been described in a French kindred (Clement et al. 1998). Adipose tissue *lep* mRNA (Lonnqvist et al. 1995, Hamilton et al. 1995) and circulating leptin (Considine et al. 1996, Dagogo-Jack et al. 1996) levels are elevated in obese subjects, suggesting that obese persons are not responding optimally to the weight-regulating effects of leptin. The basis of this "leptin resistance" is unclear but may be related to alterations in circulating leptin-binding proteins (Lou et al. 2010), impaired blood-to-brain leptin delivery (Schwartz et al. 1996), or defects in leptin receptor signaling (Tartaglia et al. 1995, Bjorbaek et al. 1999, Ozcan et al. 2009, Myers et al. 2012).

1.6.3.2   Leptin and Insulin Action

Replacement doses of recombinant leptin, administered systemically, normalized plasma glucose and insulin levels in hyperglycemic, hyperinsulinemic *ob/ob* mice (Halaas et al. 1995, Weigle et al. 1995) and in leptin-deficient subjects with diabetes and insulin resistance (Licinio et al. 2004). Low doses of leptin administered intravenously or into the cerebral ventricles increased glucose utilization and decreased hepatic glycogen storage in wild-type mice (Kamohara et al. 1997). Furthermore, leptin therapy selectively depletes visceral fat stores and stimulates insulin sensitivity in rats (Barzilai and Gupta 1999). These findings indicate that leptin may be a naturally occurring insulin sensitizer. Indeed, addition of leptin to cultured human hepatocytes stimulates signaling along the phosphatidyl inositol 3′ kinase pathway, one of the mediators of insulin action (Cohen et al. 1996). Reversal of lipotoxicity may be another mechanism for the insulin-sensitizing effects of leptin (Bai et al. 1996, Shimabukuro et al. 1997). There is a marked variability in plasma leptin levels (even among persons of comparable adiposity), which may be partially related to differences in insulin sensitivity (Dagogo-Jack et al. 1997, Askari et al. 2010).

Basal (fasting) plasma leptin levels are similar in patients with diabetes compared with body mass index (BMI)- and gender-matched nondiabetic subjects (Sinha et al. 1996, Liu et al. 1999), but dynamic leptin response to secretagogues is attenuated in patients with diabetes (Liu et al. 1999, Dagogo-Jack et al. 2000). We have postulated that the increased leptin secretory response to food (as well as insulin and glucocorticoids) represents a counterregulatory attempt to limit hyperphagia and weight gain (Dallman et al. 1993, Dagogo-Jack et al. 1997) (Figure 1.1). This adaptation may be of physiological relevance, because feeding stimulates the secretion of insulin and cortisol (Rosmond et al. 2000), which in turn stimulate secretion of the satiety hormone leptin. Theoretically, a defect in leptin secretion could permit hyperphagia, promote weight gain, and aggravate insulin resistance. If impaired leptin secretion is confirmed as a general feature of diabetes, such diabetic dyslepti-nemia may provide a rationale for evaluation of leptin therapy. Indeed, patients with lipodystrophic

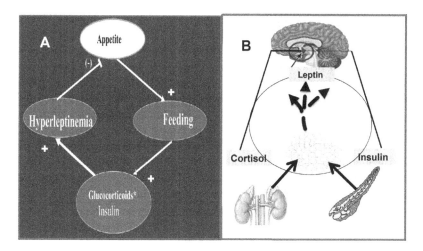

FIGURE 1.1 Increased appetite and consequent feeding induce postprandial plasma insulin and cortisol levels; glucocorticoids and insulin stimulate leptin secretion by adipocytes, which can induce satiety and prevent hunger between meals and during sleep (*A*). Leptin, glucocorticoids, and insulin have central effects on hypothalamic hunger and satiety centers (*B, small circle*), in part, by altering neuropeptide Y expression. Peripherally, a feedback loop (*B, wider circle*) involving direct suppression of glucocorticoid and insulin secretion by leptin ensures homeostasis. Impaired insulin- and glucocorticoid-stimulated leptin secretion in patients with diabetes would be permissive of increased caloric intake, weight gain, insulin resistance and hyperglycemia. (Adapted from Dagogo-Jack S. 2015. Dynamic leptin secretion in obesity and diabetes. In *Leptin: Regulation and Clinical Applications*. Edited by S. Dagogo-Jack, 189-202. New York: Springer.)

diabetes and leptin deficiency respond remarkably well to leptin replacement and often achieve independence from insulin and oral hypoglycemic agents (Oral et al. 2002).

1.6.3.3 Exogenous Leptin Therapy for Human Obesity

Administration of low physiological doses of recombinant methionyl-human-leptin (0.01–0.04 mg/kg) produced dramatic results in morbidly obese, leptin-deficient patients (Montague et al. 1997, Farooqi et al. 1999, 2002, Licinio et al. 2004). Following daily subcutaneous injection of recombinant leptin, significant weight loss was reported within 2 weeks. The weight loss was maintained at a rate of approximately 1–2 kg per month, without evidence of tachyphylaxis, throughout 12–18 months of treatment (Farooqi et al. 1999, Licinio et al. 2004). Analysis of body composition indicated that selective fat depletion accounted for approximately 95% of the total weight loss. Daily food consumption (and food-seeking behavior) decreased within 1 week of initiation of leptin replacement, and 95% of the total weight loss was accounted for by selective body fat depletion (Farooqi et al. 1999). Basal energy expenditure decreased (due to weight loss), but dynamic energy expenditure increased by approximately the same amount during leptin treatment, the latter being due to increased physical activity (Farooqi et al. 1999). The stimulatory effect of recombinant leptin on physical activity was first noted in ob/ob mice and is probably mediated by activation of the sympathetic nervous system (Haynes et al. 1997). Similar but less dramatic benefits on weight reduction were observed following leptin augmentation in a cohort of 54 lean and 73 obese men and women with normal leptin genotype (as indicated by baseline serum leptin levels > 10 ng/mL) (Heymsfield et al. 1999). The subjects were randomized to daily self-injection with placebo or different doses (0.01, 0.03, 0.10, or 0.30 mg/kg) of recombinant methionyl human leptin. The mean weight changes at 24 weeks ranged from -0.7 ± 5.4 kg for the 0.01 mg/kg dose, to -7.1 ± 8.5 kg for the 0.3 mg/kg dose.

As in patients with congenital leptin deficiency, loss of fat mass accounted for most of the weight loss following leptin treatment (Heymsfield et al. 1999). Notably, there was marked individual variability in the response to recombinant leptin among subjects with normal leptin genotypes. Subsequent studies of leptin treatment in obese individuals and post-Roux-en-Y gastric bypass (RYGB) patients failed to demonstrate weight loss (Zelissen et al. 2005, Korner et al. 2013). Similarly, leptin treatment did not influence body weight in obese individuals with type 2 diabetes (Moon et al. 2011). Leptin-deficient patients are clearly more sensitive to leptin treatment than patients with common forms of obesity.

The enthusiasm surrounding leptin's therapeutic potential for reversing obesity has waned due to its lack of consistent efficacy in obese populations. Nonetheless, the possibility of restoring leptin responsiveness by using it in conjunction with agents like exendin-4 has shown promise in rodents and is a strategy worthy of exploration in human obesity (Muller et al. 2012). Notably, recombinant methionyl human leptin (metreleptin) was recently approved by the U.S. Food and Drug Administration for the treatment of congenital or acquired general lipodystrophy. The currently known metabolic and behavioral effects of leptin are summarized in Table 1.3.

1.6.4 PANCREATIC SIGNALS

1.6.4.1 Insulin

Insulin was the first peripheral signal shown to regulate food intake through interaction with central hypothalamic neurons (Kennedy 1953). Protagonists of popular diets have claimed in the lay press that limitation of insulin secretion is the mechanism for hunger control in subjects fed low-carbohydrate, ketotic diets, yet the scientific evidence strongly disputes that claim. Insulin fulfills the role (shared by leptin) of serving as a marker of adipose tissue mass and is secreted in direct proportion to fat mass. Insulin secretion also serves as an acute response to caloric influx: Increased secretion begins within minutes of initiation of feeding, is maintained for the duration of food intake, and returns to basal secretory rate in the post-absorptive period. If insulin were an appetite stimulant (like ghrelin), its secretion would have preceded, not followed, ingestion of food.

The timing and pattern of postprandial insulin secretion suggest a role in the regulation of satiety and meal termination. Indeed, direct administration of insulin to the CNS suppresses food intake in rodents (Baura et al. 1993). Because circulating insulin reaches the CNS via receptor-mediated transport across the blood-brain barrier, it is possible that peak insulin levels attained

---

TABLE 1.3
Behavioral and Metabolic Effects of Leptin

Behavioral
- Inhibition of food intake
- Stimulation of physical activity

Body Composition
- Induction of fat-mass loss
- Preservation of lean-muscle mass
- Preservation of bone mass

Glucose and Fat Metabolism
- Improvement in insulin sensitivity
- Improvement in glucose tolerance
- Partitioning of triglycerides to adipocytes
- Increased fat oxidation
- Reduction of hepatic steatosis

---

during feeding trigger central mechanisms that mediate satiety. Postprandial insulin secretion also is a potent signal for leptin secretion (Bado et al. 1998). Thus, in addition to a direct effect, insulin could exert anorectic effects via a leptin-mediated mechanism. Paradoxically, patients with diabetes who are treated with exogenous insulin or medications that increase insulin secretion or sensitivity tend to gain weight. Although several mechanisms explain the weight gain during intensive diabetes therapy, additional putative mechanisms include "central" insulin resistance and diabetic dyslepti-nemia (Liu et al. 1999, Dagogo-Jack et al. 2000, 2008).

1.6.4.2 Pancreatic Polypeptide

Pancreatic polypeptide (PP) is secreted by specialized endocrine cells within the pancreatic islets of Langerhans. PP is also sparsely expressed in the endocrine cells of the small and large intestine (Cox 2007). PP is secreted post-prandially in proportion to meal size, and during insulin-induced hypogly-cemia. The release of PP and its biologic effects on food intake are mediated primarily by Y4 receptors and require parasympathetic activation (Havel et al. 1992, Field et al. 2010). Postprandial PP levels probably add to the physiological satiety signaling cascade that limits hyperphagia and helps main-tain interprandial intervals. Indeed, systemic administration of PP has been shown to reduce food intake in rodents (McLaughlin 1982), and reductions in energy intake ranging from 11% to 25% have been observed following intravenous infusions of PP in nonobese humans (Batterham et al. 2003b, Jesudason et al. 2007). Similarly, reductions in food intake have been observed following PP infusions in obese patients with Prader-Willi syndrome (Berntson et al. 1993). Furthermore, the administration of PP in patients with chronic pancreatitis has been shown to improve glucose tolerance (Brunicardi et al. 1996). Pharmacologic attempts to harvest PP's anorectic potential have been explored. However, to date, Y4 receptor agonists have not progressed beyond phase II studies (Valentino et al. 2010).

1.6.5 Gastrointestinal Peptides

1.6.5.1 Ghrelin

The polypeptide ghrelin was initially described and characterized as the endogenous ligand for the growth hormone secretagogue receptor in 1999 (Kojima et al. 1999). The ghrelin molecule contains 28 amino acids and an acyl radical, the latter being essential for biologic effect. The post-translational acylation of ghrelin is mediated by the enzyme gastric O-acyl transferase (GOAT) (Yang et al. 2008). Ghrelin is synthesized and secreted by the stomach, reaches the anterior pituitary via the circulation, and stimulates growth hormone secretion by the somatotrophs. The nutritional effects of ghrelin became evident when it was shown that central (ICV) administration potently increased food intake in rodents (Wren et al. 2000). A similar effect on food intake was observed following peripheral (IV) injection of ghrelin in rats (Wren et al. 2000). In humans, intravenous administration of ghrelin stimu-lates food intake by approximately 30% (Wren et al. 2001). Interestingly, ghrelin is the only metabo-tropic peptide thus far identified that stimulates food intake directly when administered peripherally.

Physiologic studies have indicated that ghrelin serves as a peripheral signal for hunger and meal initiation; blood levels peak sharply just before feeding and fall rapidly following food intake (Cummings et al. 2001). Prolonged administration of ghrelin in rodents leads to chronic hyper-phagia and weight gain, yet obese individuals typically exhibit high plasma leptin and low ghrelin levels (Tschop et al. 2001), with peak levels in the morning and the nadir at night. The mechanism of action of ghrelin involves stimulation of hypothalamic neurons (Nakazato et al. 2001) and inhibi-tion of gastric vagal afferent signals (Date et al. 2002). Based on the foregoing, it is plausible that ghrelin or its analogues could be candidates for future therapy for primary anorexia, as well as the anorexia and cachexia often seen in patients with HIV-AIDS, systemic disorders, and malignant diseases. Conversely, ghrelin antagonism is an attractive idea for drug development for obesity and hyperphagic disorders. Ghrelin O-acyltransferase (GOAT) is another potential therapeutic target, given that inhibition of its enzymatic activity could decrease circulating concentrations of active acyl ghrelin and decrease hunger (Gardiner and Bloom 2008).

1.6.5.2 Peptide YY

The gut-derived peptideYY (PYY) is a member of the neuropeptide Y family that includes PP and NPY (Larhammar 1996, Kalra et al. 1999, Wynne et al. 2004). PYY is synthesized by the mucosal endocrine L cells located in the small intestine and large bowel. PYY3-36 is the major isoform secreted into the circulation (Grandt et al. 1994). Feeding is a major stimulus for the release of PYY, which then serves as an anorectic/satiety signal from the intestinal cells. The potent anorectic effect of PYY3-36 has been demonstrated in rodent studies involving direct administration of PYY3-36 into the arcuate nucleus (Batterham et al., 2002). Similarly, the peripheral administration of PYY3-36 reduces appetite and food intake in both lean and obese humans inhibited food intake by approximately 30% compared with placebo (Batterham et al. 2003a).

PYY3-36 appears to exert its anorectic effect through coordinate inhibition of orexigenic NPY neurons and stimulation of POMC neurons in the arcuate nucleus. These molecular changes are observed following peripheral administration of PYY3-36 (Batterham et al. 2002). PYY3-36 is thought to exert its effect through interaction with high-affinity Y2 receptors in the hypothalamus, gaining direct access via an incomplete blood-brain barrier in the median eminence. Activation of the Y2 receptor subtype on NPY neurons triggers inhibitory presynaptic signals. Consonant with this mechanism, Y2 receptor knock-out mice lose their responsiveness to the anorectic effect of PYY3-36 (Batterham et al. 2002). Thus, circulating PYY3-36 appears to exert its anorectic effect by directly inhibiting orexigenic NPY neurons in the arcuate nucleus. Notably, the NPY neurons in the arcuate nucleus are the central integrating sites for numerous peripheral signals (including leptin, insulin, PYY3-36, and ghrelin) that regulate food intake. Studies indicate that PYY3-36 effectively suppresses appetite over the short term in lean and obese humans (Batterham et al. 2003a, Sloth et al. 2007), and modulates brain activity in hypothalamic appetite centers when administered intravenously (Batterham et al. 2007). However, nausea has been a dose-limiting effect of intravenous, intranasal, and oral administration (Sloth et al. 2007, Gantz et al. 2007, le Roux et al. 2008, Beglinger et al. 2008). Nonetheless, the anorectic effect of PYY3-36 is noteworthy, and this peptide and its analogues remain candidates of interest for obesity drug development.

1.6.5.3 Glucagon-Like Peptide 1

Glucagon-like peptide 1 (GLP-1) is derived from the precursor molecule prepro-glucagon. Site-specific cleavage of prepro-glucagon in the pancreas results in glucagon, whereas in the intestinal endocrine L cells, the result is GLP-1. Both GLP-1 and PYY are co-secreted by the intestinal L cells in response to the arrival of nutrients in the gut. Like PYY, GLP-1 also appears to serve as a gut-derived satiety signal. While GLP-1 has a short half-life and is rapidly degraded by the enzyme dipeptidyl peptidase-4 (DPP-4), central and peripheral administration of GLP-1 results in marked inhibition of feeding in rodents (Turton et al. 1996, Abbott et al. 2005). GLP-1 is often described as an incretin because of its effect in boosting postprandial insulin secretion. Additional glucoregulatory actions of GLP-1 include suppression of glucagon secretion and prolongation of gastric emptying (Kreymann et al. 1987). GLP-1 can induce modest weight loss by delaying gastric emptying, inducing satiety, and inhibiting food intake; the latter effect is likely mediated by direct GLP-1 stimulation of POMC/CART cells in the arcuate nucleus (Verdich et al. 2001, Secher et al. 2014). Accordingly, GLP-1's glycemic and anorectic properties have been harnessed therapeutically. Synthetic GLP-1 receptor agonists, which are resistant to degradation by the enzyme DPP-4, have been shown to effectively improve glycemic control in type 2 diabetes (Shyangdan et al. 2011). Exenatide, a long-acting GLP-1 receptor agonist that is approved for treatment of type 2 diabetes in patients inadequately controlled on oral agents, has been associated with dose-dependent weight loss (Kolterman et al. 2003, DeFronzo et al. 2005). A 20-week, randomized, double-blind, placebo-controlled trial of liraglutide, another long-acting GLP-1 analogue, as compared to an open-label orlistat arm, demonstrated weight loss of more than 5% of baseline weight in 61% of patients treated with liraglutide, as compared to 29.6% of placebo- and 44.2% of orlistat-treated patients (Astrup et al. 2009). While gastrointestinal side effects are common with liraglutide across the dose spectrum, the medication was approved by the U.S. Food and Drug Administration for the treatment of obesity in 2014. In the pivotal 56-week randomized, controlled trial, treatment with liraglutide 3.0 mg resulted in a mean weight loss of 8.4 kg, compared to 2.8 kg in the placebo group, in patients with a BMI of 30 or higher, or 27 kg/m^2 or more, with dyslipidemia and/or hypertension (Pi-Sunyer et al. 2015).

Endogenous GLP-1 abundance can be augmented by inhibition of DPP4. Although oral DPP-4 inhibitors have been shown to improve glycemic control and are approved for the treatment of type 2 diabetes, their effects on body weight are neutral (Amori et al. 2007, Dicker 2011). Recently, efforts have been made to establish GLP-1 and glucagon receptor co-agonists for the treatment of obesity. These compounds harness the lipolytic and thermogenic effects of glucagon, while counteracting glucagon-induced hyperglycemia by the co-administration of GLP-1 (Sanchez-Garrido et al. 2017). In response to promising animal data, showing PEGylated GLP-1 and glucagon receptor co-agonism results in weight loss and improved glucose tolerance in diet-induced obese mice (Day et al. 2009, Clemmensen et al. 2014), early clinical trials in humans are now underway (Sanchez-Garrido et al. 2017).

1.6.5.4 Oxyntomodulin

Oxyntomodulin (OXM) is produced from prepro-glucagon, mainly in the endocrine L-cells of the gut, and is secreted with GLP-1 following nutrient ingestion (Drucker 2005). This peptide hormone is composed of 37 amino acids, with sequence homology to GLP-1 and glucagon (Holst 1983). OXM has an affinity for GLP-1 and the glucagon receptor (Gros et al. 1993, Holst 1997) and, in addition to acutely inhibiting gastric emptying and gastric and pancreatic exocrine secretion, OXM has been shown to inhibit food intake and increase energy expenditure in both rodents and humans (Schjoldager et al. 1988, Dakin et al. 2001, Wynne et al. 2005, 2006, Bagger et al. 2015). In a randomized, controlled trial, an average weight loss of 2.3 kg was observed in overweight and obese subjects treated with subcutaneous OXM for 4 weeks, as compared to a 0.5-kg weight loss with placebo. Additionally, OXM infusions have been shown to improve glucose metabolism in type 2 diabetes (Shankar 2013). Given the therapeutic potential for native OXM to promote weight loss and glucose control, the therapeutic possibilities of stimulating endogenous OXM secretion, or synthesizing analogues, are currently receiving attention (Pocai 2014).

1.6.5.5 Cholecystokinin

CCK is best known for its role in food digestion, namely stimulation of pancreatic enzyme secretion and gallbladder contraction. However, CCK has been recognized as a potent satiety factor for more than 3 decades (Gibbs et al. 1973). Peripheral and central mechanisms appear to mediate the anorectic/satiety effects of CCK. Peripherally, activation of CCK$_A$ receptors on vagal nerve endings and on the pyloric sphincter reduces food intake (Moran 2000).

Centrally, interactions between CCK and leptin pathways elicit synergistic anorectic effects (Matson et al. 1997). An additional mechanism of action of CCK might also involve activation of brainstem neurons that regulate portion size. The effect of peripheral administration of CCK is transient and more consistent with a modulatory effect on satiety/meal termination than primary inhibition of meal initiation (West et al. 1987, Moran 2000). To induce durable inhibition of food intake, high doses and prolonged administration of CCK have been tried, but success has been limited by rapid development of tolerance (Crawley and Beinfeld 1983).

1.7 CONCLUSIONS

An elaborate network of central and peripheral neuro-hormonal signals (Figure 1.2) has evolved to regulate feeding, one of the primal activities necessary for survival and self-preservation. Despite decades of animal and human research, the full extent of the processes and humors involved in the

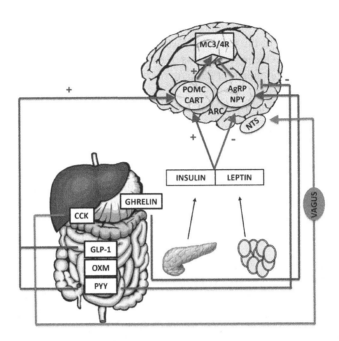

FIGURE 1.2 The hypothalamus and brainstem are critical regulators of appetite, integrating diverse hormonal signals from adipocytes (leptin), the pancreas (insulin), and the gastrointestinal tract (GLP-1, PYY, OXM, CCK, ghrelin) to regulate energy balance. Both insulin and the adipocyte-derived hormone leptin decrease food intake by acting in the arcuate nucleus (ARC) of the hypothalamus to stimulate POMC neurons and inhibit AgRP neurons, resulting in increased melanocortin receptor signaling (MC3/4R). GLP-1 and OXM are released from the L cells of the gut following nutrient ingestion and reduce food intake. GLP-1 directly stimulates POMC/CART neurons to suppress appetite. PYY decreases appetite by both inhibiting AgRP and stimulating POMC neurons. The gut hormone CCK, released primarily from the enteroendocrine cells of the duodenum, in response to nutrients and visceral stretch, stimulate satiety by way of the vagal afferent input to the nucleus tractus solitarius (NTS) of the hindbrain.

regulation of food intake remains to be elucidated. Current understanding indicates that energy homeostasis in health is predicated upon a balance between orexigenic and anorexigenic factors, both centrally and peripherally. Virtually all of the peripheral signals (e.g., insulin, PYY, leptin, CCK) are triggered by food ingestion and attenuated by fasting or starvation, indicating a response system that is tailored at satiety and meal termination. Ghrelin, the only peripheral signal that is activated pre-prandially, is unique in its role as a rare peripheral signal for hunger and meal initiation.

The rarity of peripheral hormonal signals that trigger meal initiation may be a reflection of the incompleteness of current understanding. However, a more plausible explanation is that appetite and hunger are under predominantly central control and are orchestrated by neuronal projections from various brain centers to POMC and AgRP/NPY expressing arcuate neurons. The central control of feeding is organized into an integrated neuroendocrine system that either stimulates or inhibits food intake. The orexigenic (e.g., NPY, AgRP) and anorexigenic (e.g., melanocortins) components of this system receive afferent neuroendocrine and metabolic signals from the periphery but may also be subject to local and paracrine influences, as well as inputs from higher brain centers. The coordinate regulation of these various opposing mechanisms leads to energy homeostasis that is physiologically skewed toward positive balance. An increased understanding of these mechanisms is a pre-requisite for the discovery of drug interventions that can dependably modulate food intake and prevent or treat obesity.

ACKNOWLEDGMENTS

Dr. Dagogo-Jack is supported in part by NIH grants R01 DK067269, DK62203 and DK 48411. Dr. Page-Wilson is supported in part by Robert Wood Johnson Foundation's Harold Amos Medical Faculty Development Program.

REFERENCES

Abbott, C. R., M. Monteiro, C. J. Small, A. Sajedi, K. L. Smith, J. R. Parkinson, M. A. Ghatei et al., 2005. The inhibitory effects of peripheral administration of peptide YY(3–36) and glucagon-like peptide-1 on food intake are attenuated by ablation of the vagal-brainstem-hypothalamic pathway. *Brain Res* 1044 (1):127–31. doi:10.1016/j.brainres.2005.03.011.

Amori, R. E., J. Lau, and A. G. Pittas. 2007. Efficacy and safety of incretin therapy in type 2 diabetes: Systematic review and meta-analysis. *JAMA* 298 (2):194–206. doi:10.1001/jama.298.2.194.

Askari, H., G. Tykodi, J. Liu, and S. Dagogo-Jack. 2010. Fasting plasma leptin level is a surrogate measure of insulin sensitivity. *J Clin Endocrinol Metab* 95 (8):3836–43. doi:10.1210/jc.2010-0296.

Astrup, A., S. Rossner, L. Van Gaal, A. Rissanen, L. Niskanen, M. Al Hakim, J. Madsen, M. F.Rasmussen, M. E. Lean, and N. N. Study Group. 2009. Effects of liraglutide in the treatment of obesity: A randomised, double-blind, placebo-controlled study. *Lancet* 374 (9701):1606–16. doi:10.1016/S0140-6736(09)61375-1.

Bado, A., S. Levasseur, S. Attoub, S. Kermorgant, J. P. Laigneau, M. N. Bortoluzzi, L. Moizo et al., 1998. The stomach is a source of leptin. *Nature* 394 (6695):790–3. doi:10.1038/29547.

Bagger, J. I., J. J. Holst, B. Hartmann, B. Andersen, F. K. Knop, and T. Vilsboll. 2015. Effect of oxyntomodulin, Glucagon, GLP-1, and combined Glucagon +GLP-1 infusion on food intake, appetite, and resting energy expenditure. *J Clin Endocrinol Metab* 100 (12):4541–52. doi:10.1210/jc.2015-2335.

Bai, Y., S. Zhang, K. S. Kim, J. K. Lee, and K. H. Kim. 1996. Obese gene expression alters the ability of 30A5 preadipocytes to respond to lipogenic hormones. *J Biol Chem* 271 (24):13939–42.

Barzilai, N., and G. Gupta. 1999. Interaction between aging and syndrome X: New insights on the pathophysiology of fat distribution. *Ann N Y Acad Sci* 892:58–72.

Batterham, R. L., M. A. Cohen, S. M. Ellis, C. W. Le Roux, D. J. Withers, G. S. Frost, M. A. Ghatei, and S. R. Bloom. 2003a. Inhibition of food intake in obese subjects by peptide YY3-36. *N Engl J Med* 349 (10):941–8. doi:10.1056/NEJMoa030204.

Batterham, R. L., M. A. Cowley, C. J. Small, H. Herzog, M. A. Cohen, C. L. Dakin, A. M. Wren, A. E. et al., 2002. Gut hormone PYY(3–36) physiologically inhibits food intake. *Nature* 418 (6898):650–4. doi:10.1038/nature02666.

Batterham, R. L., J. M. Rosenthal, F. O. Zelaya, G. J. Barker, D. J. Withers, and S. C. Williams. 2007. PYY modulation of cortical and hypothalamic brain areas predicts feeding behaviour in humans. *Nature* 450 (7166):106–9. doi:10.1038/nature06212.

Batterham, R. L., C. W. Le Roux, M. A. Cohen, A. J. Park, S. M. Ellis, M. Patterson, G. S. Frost, M. A. Ghatei, and S. R. Bloom. 2003b. Pancreatic polypeptide reduces appetite and food intake in humans. *J Clin Endocrinol Metab* 88 (8):3989–92. doi:10.1210/jc.2003-030630.

Baumann, H., K. K. Morella, D. W. White, M. Dembski, P. S. Bailon, H. Kim, C. F. Lai, and L. A. Tartaglia. 1996. The full-length leptin receptor has signaling capabilities of interleukin 6-type cytokine receptors. *Proc Natl Acad Sci U S A* 93 (16):8374–8.

Baura, G. D., D. M. Foster, D. Porte, Jr., S. E. Kahn, R. N. Bergman, C. Cobelli, and M. W. Schwartz. 1993. Saturable transport of insulin from plasma into the central nervous system of dogs in vivo. A mechanism for regulated insulin delivery to the brain. *J Clin Invest* 92 (4):1824–30. doi:10.1172/JCI116773.

Beck, B. 2006. Neuropeptide Y in normal eating and in genetic and dietary-induced obesity. *Philos Trans R Soc Lond B Biol Sci* 361 (1471):1159–85. doi:10.1098/rstb.2006.1855.

Beglinger, C., B. Poller, E. Arbit, C. Ganzoni, S. Gass, I. Gomez-Orellana, and J. Drewe. 2008. Pharmacokinetics and pharmacodynamic effects of oral GLP-1 and PYY3-36: A proof-of-concept study in healthy subjects. *Clin Pharmacol Ther* 84 (4):468–74.

Berntson, G. G., W. B. Zipf, T. M. O'Dorisio, J. A. Hoffman, and R. E. Chance. 1993. Pancreatic polypeptide infusions reduce food intake in Prader-Willi syndrome. *Peptides* 14 (3):497–503.

Bjorbaek, C., K. El-Haschimi, J. D. Frantz, and J. S. Flier. 1999. The role of SOCS-3 in leptin signaling and leptin resistance. *J Biol Chem* 274 (42):30059–65.

Blundell, J. E. 1984. Serotonin and appetite. *Neuropharmacology* 23 (12B):1537–51.

Bray, G. A. 1996. Health hazards of obesity. *Endocrinol Metab Clin North Am* 25 (4):907–19.

Breen, T. L., I. M. Conwell, and S. L. Wardlaw. 2005. Effects of fasting, leptin, and insulin on AGRP and POMC peptide release in the hypothalamus. *Brain Res* 1032 (1–2):141–8. doi:10.1016/j.brainres.2004.11.008.

Brothers, S. P., and C. Wahlestedt. 2010. Therapeutic potential of neuropeptide Y (NPY) receptor ligands. *EMBO Mol Med* 2 (11):429–39. doi:10.1002/emmm.201000100.

Brunicardi, F. C., R. L. Chaiken, A. S. Ryan, N. E. Seymour, J. A. Hoffmann, H. E. Lebovitz, R. E. Chance, R. L. Gingerich, D. K. Andersen, and D. Elahi. 1996. Pancreatic polypeptide administration improves abnormal glucose metabolism in patients with chronic pancreatitis. *J Clin Endocrinol Metab* 81 (10):3566–72. doi:10.1210/jcem.81.10.8855802.

Campfield, L. A., F. J. Smith, Y. Guisez, R. Devos, and P. Burn. 1995. Recombinant mouse OB protein: Evidence for a peripheral signal linking adiposity and central neural networks. *Science* 269 (5223):546–9.

Chao, M. V. 2003. Neurotrophins and their receptors: A convergence point for many signalling pathways. *Nat Rev Neurosci* 4 (4):299–309. doi:10.1038/nrn1078.

Chehab, F. F., M. E. Lim, and R. Lu. 1996. Correction of the sterility defect in homozygous obese female mice by treatment with the human recombinant leptin. *Nat Genet* 12 (3):318–20. doi:10.1038/ng0396-318.

Chemelli, R. M., J. T. Willie, C. M. Sinton, J. K. Elmquist, T. Scammell, C. Lee, J. A. Richardson, S. C. et al., 1999. Narcolepsy in orexin knockout mice: Molecular genetics of sleep regulation. *Cell* 98 (4):437–51.

Chen, H., O. Charlat, L. A. Tartaglia, E. A. Woolf, X. Weng, S. J. Ellis, N. D. Lakey, J. et al., 1996. Evidence that the diabetes gene encodes the leptin receptor: Identification of a mutation in the leptin receptor gene in db/db mice. *Cell* 84 (3):491–5.

Chen, H. Y., M. E. Trumbauer, A. S. Chen, D. T. Weingarth, J. R. Adams, E. G. Frazier, Z. Shen, D. J. et al., 2004. Orexigenic action of peripheral ghrelin is mediated by neuropeptide Y and agouti-related protein. *Endocrinology* 145 (6):2607–12. doi:10.1210/en.2003-1596.

Chen, K. Y., R. Muniyappa, B. S. Abel, K. P. Mullins, P. Staker, R. J. Brychta, X. Zhao, M. et al., 2015. RM-493, a melanocortin-4 receptor (MC4R) agonist, increases resting energy expenditure in obese individuals. *J Clin Endocrinol Metab* 100 (4):1639–45. doi:10.1210/jc.2014-4024.

Clement, K., C. Vaisse, N. Lahlou, S. Cabrol, V. Pelloux, D. Cassuto, M. Gourmelen, C. et al., 1998. A mutation in the human leptin receptor gene causes obesity and pituitary dysfunction. *Nature* 392 (6674):398–401. doi:10.1038/32911.

Clemmensen, C., J. Chabenne, B. Finan, L. Sullivan, K. Fischer, D. Kuchler, L. Sehrer et al., 2014. GLP-1/glucagon coagonism restores leptin responsiveness in obese mice chronically maintained on an obesogenic diet. *Diabetes* 63 (4):1422–7. doi:10.2337/db13-1609.

Cohen, B., D. Novick, and M. Rubinstein. 1996. Modulation of insulin activities by leptin. *Science* 274 (5290):1185–8.

Considine, R. V., E. L. Considine, C. J. Williams, M. R. Nyce, S. A. Magosin, T. L. Bauer, E. L. Rosato, J. Colberg, and J. F. Caro. 1995. Evidence against either a premature stop codon or the absence of obese gene mRNA in human obesity. *J Clin Invest* 95 (6):2986–8. doi:10.1172/JCI118007.

Considine, R. V., M. K. Sinha, M. L. Heiman, A. Kriauciunas, T. W. Stephens, M. R. Nyce, J. P. Ohannesian et al., 1996. Serum immunoreactive-leptin concentrations in normal-weight and obese humans. *N Engl J Med* 334 (5):292–5. doi:10.1056/NEJM199602013340503.

Cota, D., G. Marsicano, M. Tschop, Y. Grubler, C. Flachskamm, M. Schubert, D. Auer et al., 2003. The endogenous cannabinoid system affects energy balance via central orexigenic drive and peripheral lipogenesis. *J Clin Invest* 112 (3):423–31. doi:10.1172/JCI17725.

Cowley, M. A., J. L. Smart, M. Rubinstein, M. G. Cerdan, S. Diano, T. L. Horvath, R. D. Cone, and M. J. Low. 2001. Leptin activates anorexigenic POMC neurons through a neural network in the arcuate nucleus. *Nature* 411 (6836):480–4. doi:10.1038/35078085.

Cox, H. M. 2007. Neuropeptide Y receptors; antisecretory control of intestinal epithelial function. *Auton Neurosci* 133 (1):76–85. doi:10.1016/j.autneu.2006.10.005.

Crawley, J. N., and M. C. Beinfeld. 1983. Rapid development of tolerance to the behavioural actions of cholecystokinin. *Nature* 302 (5910):703–6.

Cummings, D. E., J. Q. Purnell, R. S. Frayo, K. Schmidova, B. E. Wisse, and D. S. Weigle. 2001. A preprandial rise in plasma ghrelin levels suggests a role in meal initiation in humans. *Diabetes* 50 (8):1714–9.

Dagogo-Jack, S., H. Askari, G. Tykodi, J. Liu, and I. Umamaheswaran. 2008. Dynamic responses to leptin secretagogues in lean, obese, and massively obese men and women. *Horm Res* 70 (3):174–81. doi:10.1159/000145018.

Dagogo-Jack, S., C. Fanelli, D. Paramore, J. Brothers, and M. Landt. 1996. Plasma leptin and insulin relationships in obese and nonobese humans. *Diabetes* 45 (5):695–8.

Dagogo-Jack, S., J. Liu, H. Askari, G. Tykodi, and I. Umamaheswaran. 2000. Impaired leptin response to glucocorticoid as a chronic complication of diabetes. *J Diabetes Complications* 14 (6):327–32.

Dagogo-Jack, S., G. Selke, A. K. Melson, and J. W. Newcomer. 1997. Robust leptin secretory responses to dexamethasone in obese subjects. *J Clin Endocrinol Metab* 82 (10):3230–3. doi:10.1210/jcem.82.10.4154.

Dakin, C. L., I. Gunn, C. J. Small, C. M. Edwards, D. L. Hay, D. M. Smith, M. A. Ghatei et al., 2001. Oxyntomodulin inhibits food intake in the rat. *Endocrinology* 142 (10):4244–50. doi:10.1210/endo.142.10.8430.

Dallman, M. F., A. M. Strack, S. F. Akana, M. J. Bradbury, E. S. Hanson, K. A. Scribner, and M. Smith. 1993. Feast and famine: Critical role of glucocorticoids with insulin in daily energy flow. *Front Neuroendocrinol* 14 (4):303–47. doi:10.1006/frne.1993.1010.

Date, Y., N. Murakami, K. Toshinai, S. Matsukura, A. Niijima, H. Matsuo, K. Kangawa, and M. Nakazato. 2002. The role of the gastric afferent vagal nerve in ghrelin-induced feeding and growth hormone secretion in rats. *Gastroenterology* 123 (4):1120–8.

Day, J. W., N. Ottaway, J. T. Patterson, V. Gelfanov, D. Smiley, J. Gidda, H. Findeisen et al., 2009. A new glucagon and GLP-1 co-agonist eliminates obesity in rodents. *Nat Chem Biol* 5 (10):749–57. doi:10.1038/nchembio.209.

de Lecea, L., T. S. Kilduff, C. Peyron, X. Gao, P. E. Foye, P. E. Danielson, C. Fukuhara et al., 1998. The hypocretins: Hypothalamus-specific peptides with neuroexcitatory activity. *Proc Natl Acad Sci U S A* 95 (1):322–7.

DeFronzo, R. A., R. E. Ratner, J. Han, D. D. Kim, M. S. Fineman, and A. D. Baron. 2005. Effects of exenatide (exendin-4) on glycemic control and weight over 30 weeks in metformin-treated patients with type 2 diabetes. *Diabetes Care* 28 (5):1092–100.

Dicker, D. 2011. DPP-4 inhibitors: Impact on glycemic control and cardiovascular risk factors. *Diabetes Care* 34 Suppl 2:S276–8. doi:10.2337/dc11-s229.

Drucker, D. J. 2005. Biologic actions and therapeutic potential of the proglucagon-derived peptides. *Nat Clin Pract Endocrinol Metab* 1 (1):22–31. doi:10.1038/ncpendmet0017.

Farooqi, I. S., S. A. Jebb, G. Langmack, E. Lawrence, C. H. Cheetham, A. M. Prentice, I. A. Hughes et al., 1999. Effects of recombinant leptin therapy in a child with congenital leptin deficiency. *N Engl J Med* 341 (12):879–84. doi:10.1056/NEJM199909163411204.

Farooqi, I. S., G. Matarese, G. M. Lord, J. M. Keogh, E. Lawrence, C. Agwu et al., 2002. Beneficial effects of leptin on obesity, T cell hyporesponsiveness, and neuroendocrine/metabolic dysfunction of human congenital leptin deficiency. *J Clin Invest* 110 (8):1093–103. doi:10.1172/JCI15693.

Farooqi, I. S., G. S. Yeo, J. M. Keogh, S. Aminian, S. A. Jebb, G. Butler, T. Cheetham, and S. O'Rahilly. 2000. Dominant and recessive inheritance of morbid obesity associated with melanocortin 4 receptor deficiency. *J Clin Invest* 106 (2):271–9. doi:10.1172/JCI9397.

Fehm, H. L., R. Smolnik, W. Kern, G. P. McGregor, U. Bickel, and J. Born. 2001. The melanocortin melanocyte-stimulating hormone/adrenocorticotropin(4–10) decreases body fat in humans. *J Clin Endocrinol Metab* 86 (3):1144–8. doi:10.1210/jcem.86.3.7298.

Field, B. C., O. B. Chaudhri, and S. R. Bloom. 2010. Bowels control brain: Gut hormones and obesity. *Nat Rev Endocrinol* 6 (8):444–53. doi:10.1038/nrendo.2010.93.

Flegal, K. M., M. D. Carroll, C. L. Ogden, and C. L. Johnson. 2002. Prevalence and trends in obesity among US adults, 1999–2000. *JAMA* 288 (14):1723–7.

Flier, J. S. 1998. Clinical review 94: What's in a name? In search of leptin's physiologic role. *J Clin Endocrinol Metab* 83 (5):1407–13. doi:10.1210/jcem.83.5.4779.

Freeman, D. J., J. Norrie, M. J. Caslake, A. Gaw, I. Ford, G. D. Lowe, D. S. O'Reilly, C. J. Packard, N. Sattar, and Study West of Scotland Coronary Prevention. 2002. C-reactive protein is an independent predictor of risk for the development of diabetes in the West of Scotland coronary prevention study. *Diabetes* 51 (5):1596–600.

Gantz, I., N. Erondu, M. Mallick, B. Musser, R. Krishna, W. K. Tanaka, K. Snyder et al., 2007. Efficacy and safety of intranasal peptide YY3-36 for weight reduction in obese adults. *J Clin Endocrinol Metab* 92 (5):1754–7. doi:10.1210/jc.2006-1806.

Gardiner, J., and S. Bloom. 2008. Ghrelin gets its GOAT. *Cell Metab* 7 (3):193–4. doi:10.1016/j.cmet.2008.02.009.

Ghilardi, N., and R. C. Skoda. 1997. The leptin receptor activates janus kinase 2 and signals for proliferation in a factor-dependent cell line. *Mol Endocrinol* 11 (4):393–9. doi:10.1210/mend.11.4.9907.

Gibbs, J., R. C. Young, and G. P. Smith. 1973. Cholecystokinin decreases food intake in rats. *J Comp Physiol Psychol* 84 (3):488–95.

Goldstone, A. P., U. A. Unmehopa, S. R. Bloom, and D. F. Swaab. 2002. Hypothalamic NPY and agouti-related protein are increased in human illness but not in Prader-Willi syndrome and other obese subjects. *J Clin Endocrinol Metab* 87 (2):927–37. doi:10.1210/jcem.87.2.8230.

Grandt, D., M. Schimiczek, C. Beglinger, P. Layer, H. Goebell, V. E. Eysselein, and J. R. Reeve, Jr. 1994. Two molecular forms of peptide YY (PYY) are abundant in human blood: Characterization of a radioimmunoassay recognizing PYY 1-36 and PYY 3-36. *Regul Pept* 51 (2):151–9.

Gray, J., G. S. Yeo, J. J. Cox, J. Morton, A. L. Adlam, J. M. Keogh, J. A. Yanovski et al., 2006. Hyperphagia, severe obesity, impaired cognitive function, and hyperactivity associated with functional loss of one copy of the brain-derived neurotrophic factor (BDNF) gene. *Diabetes* 55 (12):3366–71. doi:10.2337/db06-0550.

Grill, H. J., and M. R. Hayes. 2012. Hindbrain neurons as an essential hub in the neuroanatomically distributed control of energy balance. *Cell Metab* 16 (3):296–309. doi:10.1016/j.cmet.2012.06.015.

Grill, H. J., and G. P. Smith. 1988. Cholecystokinin decreases sucrose intake in chronic decerebrate rats. *Am J Physiol* 254 (6 Pt 2):R853–6.

Grimble, R. F. 2002. Inflammatory status and insulin resistance. *Curr Opin Clin Nutr Metab Care* 5 (5):551–9.

Gros, L., B. Thorens, D. Bataille, and A. Kervran. 1993. Glucagon-like peptide-1-(7-36) amide, oxyntomodulin, and glucagon interact with a common receptor in a somatostatin-secreting cell line. *Endocrinology* 133 (2):631–8. doi:10.1210/endo.133.2.8102095.

Halaas, J. L., K. S. Gajiwala, M. Maffei, S. L. Cohen, B. T. Chait, D. Rabinowitz, R. L. Lallone, S. K. Burley, and J. M. Friedman. 1995. Weight-reducing effects of the plasma protein encoded by the obese gene. *Science* 269 (5223):543–6.

Hallschmid, M., R. Smolnik, G. McGregor, J. Born, and H. L. Fehm. 2006. Overweight humans are resistant to the weight-reducing effects of melanocortin4-10. *J Clin Endocrinol Metab* 91 (2):522–5. doi:10.1210/jc.2005-0906.

Hamilton, B. S., D. Paglia, A. Y. Kwan, and M. Deitel. 1995. Increased obese mRNA expression in omental fat cells from massively obese humans. *Nat Med* 1 (9):953–6.

Havel, P. J., S. J. Parry, D. L. Curry, J. S. Stern, J. O. Akpan, and R. L. Gingerich. 1992. Autonomic nervous system mediation of the pancreatic polypeptide response to insulin-induced hypoglycemia in conscious rats. *Endocrinology* 130 (4):2225–9. doi:10.1210/endo.130.4.1347741.

Haynes, W. G., D. A. Morgan, S. A. Walsh, A. L. Mark, and W. I. Sivitz. 1997. Receptor-mediated regional sympathetic nerve activation by leptin. *J Clin Invest* 100 (2):270–8. doi:10.1172/JCI119532.

Heisler, L. K., E. E. Jobst, G. M. Sutton, L. Zhou, E. Borok, Z. Thornton-Jones, H. Y. Liu et al., 2006. Serotonin reciprocally regulates melanocortin neurons to modulate food intake. *Neuron* 51 (2):239–49. doi:10.1016/j.neuron.2006.06.004.

Henry, M., L. Ghibaudi, J. Gao, and J. J. Hwa. 2005. Energy metabolic profile of mice after chronic activation of central NPY Y1, Y2, or Y5 receptors. *Obes Res* 13 (1):36–47. doi:10.1038/oby.2005.6.

Heymsfield, S. B., A. S. Greenberg, K. Fujioka, R. M. Dixon, R. Kushner, T. Hunt, J. A. Lubina et al., 1999. Recombinant leptin for weight loss in obese and lean adults: A randomized, controlled, dose-escalation trial. *JAMA* 282 (16):1568–75.

Holst, J. J. 1983. Gut glucagon, enteroglucagon, gut glucagonlike immunoreactivity, glicentin—current status. *Gastroenterology* 84 (6):1602–13.

Holst, J. J. 1997. Enteroglucagon. *Annu Rev Physiol* 59:257–71. doi:10.1146/annurev.physiol.59.1.257.

Hotamisligil, G. S., A. Budavari, D. Murray, and B. M. Spiegelman. 1994. Reduced tyrosine kinase activity of the insulin receptor in obesity-diabetes. Central role of tumor necrosis factor-alpha. *J Clin Invest* 94 (4):1543–9. doi:10.1172/JCI117495.

Hotamisligil, G. S., P. Peraldi, A. Budavari, R. Ellis, M. F. White, and B. M. Spiegelman. 1996. IRS-1-mediated inhibition of insulin receptor tyrosine kinase activity in TNF-alpha- and obesity-induced insulin resistance. *Science* 271 (5249):665–8.

Hotamisligil, G. S., N. S. Shargill, and B. M. Spiegelman. 1993. Adipose expression of tumor necrosis factor-alpha: Direct role in obesity-linked insulin resistance. *Science* 259 (5091):87–91.

Hotta, K., M. Nakamura, T. Nakamura, T. Matsuo, Y. Nakata, S. Kamohara, N. Miyatake et al., 2009. Association between obesity and polymorphisms in SEC16B, TMEM18, GNPDA2, BDNF, FAIM2 and MC4R in a Japanese population. *J Hum Genet* 54 (12):727–31. doi:10.1038/jhg.2009.106.

Huszar, D., C. A. Lynch, V. Fairchild-Huntress, J. H. Dunmore, Q. Fang, L. R. Berkemeier, W. Gu et al., 1997. Targeted disruption of the melanocortin-4 receptor results in obesity in mice. *Cell* 88 (1):131–41.

Jesudason, D. R., M. P. Monteiro, B. M. McGowan, N. M. Neary, A. J. Park, E. Philippou, C. J. Small, G. S. Frost, M. A. Ghatei, and S. R. Bloom. 2007. Low-dose pancreatic polypeptide inhibits food intake in man. *Br J Nutr* 97 (3):426–9. doi:10.1017/S0007114507336799.

Kalra, S. P., M. G. Dube, S. Pu, B. Xu, T. L. Horvath, and P. S. Kalra. 1999. Interacting appetite-regulating pathways in the hypothalamic regulation of body weight. *Endocr Rev* 20 (1):68–100. doi:10.1210/edrv.20.1.0357.

Kamohara, S., R. Burcelin, J. L. Halaas, J. M. Friedman, and M. J. Charron. 1997. Acute stimulation of glucose metabolism in mice by leptin treatment. *Nature* 389 (6649):374–77. doi:10.1038/38717.

Kennedy, G. C. 1953. The role of depot fat in the hypothalamic control of food intake in the rat. *Proc R Soc Lond B Biol Sci* 140 (901):578–96.

Kern, P. A., M. Saghizadeh, J. M. Ong, R. J. Bosch, R. Deem, and R. B. Simsolo. 1995. The expression of tumor necrosis factor in human adipose tissue. Regulation by obesity, weight loss, and relationship to lipoprotein lipase. *J Clin Invest* 95 (5):2111–9. doi:10.1172/JCI117899.

Kieffer, T. J., R. S. Heller, and J. F. Habener. 1996. Leptin receptors expressed on pancreatic beta-cells. *Biochem Biophys Res Commun* 224 (2):522–7. doi:10.1006/bbrc.1996.1059.

Kojima, M., H. Hosoda, Y. Date, M. Nakazato, H. Matsuo, and K. Kangawa. 1999. Ghrelin is a growth-hormone-releasing acylated peptide from stomach. *Nature* 402 (6762):656–60. doi:10.1038/45230.

Kolterman, O. G., J. B. Buse, M. S. Fineman, E. Gaines, S. Heintz, T. A. Bicsak, K. Taylor et al., 2003. Synthetic exendin-4 (exenatide) significantly reduces postprandial and fasting plasma glucose in subjects with type 2 diabetes. *J Clin Endocrinol Metab* 88 (7):3082–9. doi:10.1210/jc.2002-021545.

Korner, J., R. Conroy, G. Febres, D. J. McMahon, I. Conwell, W. Karmally, and L. J. Aronne. 2013. Randomized double-blind placebo-controlled study of leptin administration after gastric bypass. *Obesity (Silver Spring)* 21 (5):951–6. doi:10.1002/oby.20433.

Krempler, F., D. Breban, H. Oberkofler, H. Esterbauer, E. Hell, B. Paulweber, and W. Patsch. 2000. Leptin, peroxisome proliferator-activated receptor-gamma, and CCAAT/enhancer binding protein-alpha mRNA expression in adipose tissue of humans and their relation to cardiovascular risk factors. *Arterioscler Thromb Vasc Biol* 20 (2):443–9.

Kreymann, B., G. Williams, M. A. Ghatei, and S. R. Bloom. 1987. Glucagon-like peptide-1 7-36: A physiological incretin in man. *Lancet* 2 (8571):1300–4.

Krishna, R., B. Gumbiner, C. Stevens, B. Musser, M. Mallick, S. Suryawanshi, L. Maganti et al., 2009. Potent and selective agonism of the melanocortin receptor 4 with MK-0493 does not induce weight loss in obese human subjects: Energy intake predicts lack of weight loss efficacy. *Clin Pharmacol Ther* 86 (6):659–66. doi:10.1038/clpt.2009.167.

Laaksonen, D. E., T. A. Lakka, H. M. Lakka, K. Nyyssonen, T. Rissanen, L. K. Niskanen, and J. T. Salonen. 2002. Serum fatty acid composition predicts development of impaired fasting glycaemia and diabetes in middle-aged men. *Diabet Med* 19 (6):456–64.

Lapchak, P. A., and F. Hefti. 1992. BDNF and NGF treatment in lesioned rats: Effects on cholinergic function and weight gain. *Neuroreport* 3 (5):405–8.

Larhammar, D. 1996. Structural diversity of receptors for neuropeptide Y, peptide YY and pancreatic polypeptide. *Regul Pept* 65 (3):165–74.

le Roux, C. W., C. M. Borg, K. G. Murphy, R. P. Vincent, M. A. Ghatei, and S. R. Bloom. 2008. Supraphysiological doses of intravenous PYY3-36 cause nausea, but no additional reduction in food intake. *Ann Clin Biochem* 45 (Pt 1):93–5. doi:10.1258/acb.2007.007068.

Lee, G. H., R. Proenca, J. M. Montez, K. M. Carroll, J. G. Darvishzadeh, J. I. Lee, and J. M. Friedman. 1996. Abnormal splicing of the leptin receptor in diabetic mice. *Nature* 379 (6566):632–5. doi:10.1038/379632a0.

Licinio, J., S. Caglayan, M. Ozata, B. O. Yildiz, P. B. de Miranda, F. O'Kirwan, R. Whitby et al., 2004. Phenotypic effects of leptin replacement on morbid obesity, diabetes mellitus, hypogonadism, and behavior in leptin-deficient adults. *Proc Natl Acad Sci U S A* 101 (13):4531–6. doi:10.1073/pnas.0308767101.

Lin, L., J. Faraco, R. Li, H. Kadotani, W. Rogers, X. Lin, X. Qiu, P. J. de Jong, S. Nishino, and E. Mignot. 1999. The sleep disorder canine narcolepsy is caused by a mutation in the hypocretin (orexin) receptor 2 gene. *Cell* 98 (3):365–76.

Liu, J., H. Askari, and S. Dagogo-Jack. 1999. Basal and stimulated plasma leptin in diabetic subjects. *Obes Res* 7 (6):537–44.

Lonnqvist, F., P. Arner, L. Nordfors, and M. Schalling. 1995. Overexpression of the obese (ob) gene in adipose tissue of human obese subjects. *Nat Med* 1 (9):950–3.

Lou, P. H., G. Yang, L. Huang, Y. Cui, T. Pourbahrami, G. K. Radda, C. Li, and W. Han. 2010. Reduced body weight and increased energy expenditure in transgenic mice over-expressing soluble leptin receptor. *PLoS One* 5 (7):e11669. doi:10.1371/journal.pone.0011669.

Lyons, W. E., L. A. Mamounas, G. A. Ricaurte, V. Coppola, S. W. Reid, S. H. Bora, C. Wihler, V. E. Koliatsos, and L. Tessarollo. 1999. Brain-derived neurotrophic factor-deficient mice develop aggressiveness and hyperphagia in conjunction with brain serotonergic abnormalities. *Proc Natl Acad Sci U S A* 96 (26):15239–44.

Macdonald, I. A. 1998. Energy expenditure in humans: The influence of activity, diet and sympathetic nervous system. In *Clinical Obesity*, edited by PG. and Stock Kopelman, MJ., 112–128. Oxford, UK: Blackwell Science.

Maffei, M., M. Stoffel, M. Barone, B. Moon, M. Dammerman, E. Ravussin, C. Bogardus, D. S. Ludwig, J. S. Flier, M. Talley et al., 1996. Absence of mutations in the human OB gene in obese/diabetic subjects. *Diabetes* 45 (5):679–682.

Masuzaki, H., Y. Ogawa, N. Sagawa, K. Hosoda, T. Matsumoto, H. Mise, H. Nishimura et al., 1997. Nonadipose tissue production of leptin: Leptin as a novel placenta-derived hormone in humans. *Nat Med* 3 (9):1029–33.

Matarese, G. 2000. Leptin and the immune system: How nutritional status influences the immune response. *Eur Cytokine Netw* 11 (1):7–14.

Matson, C. A., M. F. Wiater, J. L. Kuijper, and D. S. Weigle. 1997. Synergy between leptin and cholecystokinin (CCK) to control daily caloric intake. *Peptides* 18 (8):1275–8.

McLaughlin, C. L. 1982. Role of peptides from gastrointestinal cells in food intake regulation. *J Anim Sci* 55 (6):1515–27.

Moller, D. E. 2000. Potential role of TNF-alpha in the pathogenesis of insulin resistance and type 2 diabetes. *Trends Endocrinol Metab* 11 (6):212–7.

Montague, C. T., I. S. Farooqi, J. P. Whitehead, M. A. Soos, H. Rau, N. J. Wareham, C. P. Sewter et al., 1997. Congenital leptin deficiency is associated with severe early-onset obesity in humans. *Nature* 387 (6636):903–8. doi:10.1038/43185.

Moon, H. S., G. Matarese, A. M. Brennan, J. P. Chamberland, X. Liu, C. G. Fiorenza, G. H. Mylvaganam et al., 2011. Efficacy of metreleptin in obese patients with type 2 diabetes: Cellular and molecular pathways underlying leptin tolerance. *Diabetes* 60 (6):1647–56. doi:10.2337/db10-1791.

Moran, T. H. 2000. Cholecystokinin and satiety: Current perspectives. *Nutrition* 16 (10):858–65.

Muller, T. D., L. M. Sullivan, K. Habegger, C. X. Yi, D. Kabra, E. Grant, N. Ottaway et al., 2012. Restoration of leptin responsiveness in diet-induced obese mice using an optimized leptin analog in combination with exendin-4 or FGF21. *J Pept Sci* 18 (6):383–93. doi:10.1002/psc.2408.

Myers, M. G., Jr., S. B. Heymsfield, C. Haft, B. B. Kahn, M. Laughlin, R. L. Leibel, M. H. Tschop, and J. A. Yanovski. 2012. Challenges and opportunities of defining clinical leptin resistance. *Cell Metab* 15 (2):150–6. doi:10.1016/j.cmet.2012.01.002.

Nakazato, M., N. Murakami, Y. Date, M. Kojima, H. Matsuo, K. Kangawa, and S. Matsukura. 2001. A role for ghrelin in the central regulation of feeding. *Nature* 409 (6817):194–8. doi:10.1038/35051587.

Neary, N. M., A. P. Goldstone, and S. R. Bloom. 2004. Appetite regulation: From the gut to the hypothalamus. *Clin Endocrinol (Oxf)* 60 (2):153–60.

Nishino, S. 2003. The hypocretin/orexin system in health and disease. *Biol Psychiatry* 54 (2):87–95.

Nishino, S., B. Ripley, S. Overeem, S. Nevsimalova, G. J. Lammers, J. Vankova, M. Okun, W. Rogers, S. Brooks, and E. Mignot. 2001. Low cerebrospinal fluid hypocretin (Orexin) and altered energy homeostasis in human narcolepsy. *Ann Neurol* 50 (3):381–388.

Norman, R. A., C. Bogardus, and E. Ravussin. 1995. Linkage between obesity and a marker near the tumor necrosis factor-alpha locus in Pima Indians. *J Clin Invest* 96 (1):158–162. doi:10.1172/JCI118016.

Oral, E. A., V. Simha, E. Ruiz, A. Andewelt, A. Premkumar, P. Snell, A. J. Wagner et al., 2002. Leptin-replacement therapy for lipodystrophy. *N Engl J Med* 346 (8):570–578. doi:10.1056/NEJMoa012437.

Ozcan, L., A. S. Ergin, A. Lu, J. Chung, S. Sarkar, D. Nie, M. G. Myers, Jr., and U. Ozcan. 2009. Endoplasmic reticulum stress plays a central role in development of leptin resistance. *Cell Metab* 9 (1):35–51. doi:10.1016/j.cmet.2008.12.004.

Page-Wilson, G., K. T. Nguyen, D. Atalayer, K. Meece, H. A. Bainbridge, J. Korner, R. J. Gordon et al., 2017. Evaluation of CSF and plasma biomarkers of brain melanocortin activity in response to caloric restriction in humans. *Am J Physiol Endocrinol Metab* 312 (1):E19–E26. doi:10.1152/ajpendo.00330.2016.

Paolisso, G., M. R. Tagliamonte, M. R. Rizzo, P. Gualdiero, F. Saccomanno, A. Gambardella, D. Giugliano, F. D'Onofrio, and B. V. Howard. 1998. Lowering fatty acids potentiates acute insulin response in first degree relatives of people with type II diabetes. *Diabetologia* 41 (10):1127–1132. doi:10.1007/s001250051041.

Pelleymounter, M. A., M. J. Cullen, M. B. Baker, R. Hecht, D. Winters, T. Boone, and F. Collins. 1995. Effects of the obese gene product on body weight regulation in ob/ob mice. *Science* 269 (5223):540–543.

Phillips, M. S., Q. Liu, H. A. Hammond, V. Dugan, P. J. Hey, C. J. Caskey, and J. F. Hess. 1996. Leptin receptor missense mutation in the fatty Zucker rat. *Nat Genet* 13 (1):18–19. doi:10.1038/ng0596-18.

Pi-Sunyer, X., A. Astrup, K. Fujioka, F. Greenway, A. Halpern, M. Krempf, D. C. Lau et al., 2015. A randomized, controlled trial of 3.0 mg of liraglutide in weight management. *N Engl J Med* 373 (1):11–22. doi:10.1056/NEJMoa1411892.

Pocai, A. 2014. Action and therapeutic potential of oxyntomodulin. *Mol Metab* 3 (3):241–251. doi:10.1016/j.molmet.2013.12.001.

Randle, P. J., A. L. Kerbey, and J. Espinal. 1988. Mechanisms decreasing glucose oxidation in diabetes and starvation: Role of lipid fuels and hormones. *Diabetes Metab Rev* 4 (7):623–638.

Reichardt, L. F. 2006. Neurotrophin-regulated signalling pathways. *Philos Trans R Soc Lond B Biol Sci* 361 (1473):1545–1564. doi:10.1098/rstb.2006.1894.

Robertson, S. A., G. M. Leinninger, and M. G. Myers, Jr. 2008. Molecular and neural mediators of leptin action. *Physiol Behav* 94 (5):637–642. doi:10.1016/j.physbeh.2008.04.005.

Rosmond, R., Y. C. Chagnon, G. Holm, M. Chagnon, L. Perusse, B. Lindell, B. Carlsson, C. Bouchard, and P. Bjorntorp. 2000. A glucocorticoid receptor gene marker is associated with abdominal obesity, leptin, and dysregulation of the hypothalamic-pituitary-adrenal axis. *Obes Res* 8 (3):211–218. doi:10.1038/oby.2000.24.

Rossi, M., M. S. Kim, D. G. Morgan, C. J. Small, C. M. Edwards, D. Sunter, S. Abusnana et al., 1998. A C-terminal fragment of Agouti-related protein increases feeding and antagonizes the effect of alpha-melanocyte stimulating hormone in vivo. *Endocrinology* 139 (10):4428–4431. doi:10.1210/endo.139.10.6332.

Rothman, R. B., N. Vu, X. Wang, and H. Xu. 2003. Endogenous CART peptide regulates mu opioid and serotonin 5-HT(2A) receptors. *Peptides* 24 (3):413–417.

Sakurai, T., A. Amemiya, M. Ishii, I. Matsuzaki, R. M. Chemelli, H. Tanaka, S. C. Williams et al., 1998. Orexins and orexin receptors: A family of hypothalamic neuropeptides and G protein-coupled receptors that regulate feeding behavior. *Cell* 92 (4):573–585.

Sanchez-Garrido, M. A., S. J. Brandt, C. Clemmensen, T. D. Muller, R. D. DiMarchi, and M. H. Tschop. 2017. GLP-1/glucagon receptor co-agonism for treatment of obesity. *Diabetologia*. doi:10.1007/s00125-017-4354-8.

Savontaus, E., I. M. Conwell, and S. L. Wardlaw. 2002. Effects of adrenalectomy on AGRP, POMC, NPY and CART gene expression in the basal hypothalamus of fed and fasted rats. *Brain Res* 958 (1):130–138.

Schjoldager, B. T., F. G. Baldissera, P. E. Mortensen, J. J. Holst, and J. Christiansen. 1988. Oxyntomodulin: A potential hormone from the distal gut. Pharmacokinetics and effects on gastric acid and insulin secretion in man. *Eur J Clin Invest* 18 (5):499–503.

Schwartz, M. W., E. Peskind, M. Raskind, E. J. Boyko, and D. Porte, Jr. 1996. Cerebrospinal fluid leptin levels: Relationship to plasma levels and to adiposity in humans. *Nat Med* 2 (5):589–593.

Schwartz, M. W., S. C. Woods, D. Porte, Jr., R. J. Seeley, and D. G. Baskin. 2000. Central nervous system control of food intake. *Nature* 404 (6778):661–671. doi:10.1038/35007534.

Secher, A., J. Jelsing, A. F. Baquero, J. Hecksher-Sorensen, M. A. Cowley, L. S. Dalboge, G. Hansen et al., 2014. The arcuate nucleus mediates GLP-1 receptor agonist liraglutide-dependent weight loss. *J Clin Invest* 124 (10):4473–4488. doi:10.1172/JCI75276.

Shankar, S. S., R. R. Shankar, L. Mixson, B. S. Pramanik, A. Stoch, and H. Steinberg. Oxyntomodulin has significant acute glucoregulatory effects comparable to liraglutide in subjecs with type 2 diabetes. *Diabetes* 62:A48.

Shimabukuro, M., K. Koyama, G. Chen, M. Y. Wang, F. Trieu, Y. Lee, C. B. Newgard, and R. H. Unger. 1997. Direct antidiabetic effect of leptin through triglyceride depletion of tissues. *Proc Natl Acad Sci U S A* 94 (9):4637–4641.

Shyangdan, D. S., P. Royle, C. Clar, P. Sharma, N. Waugh, and A. Snaith. 2011. Glucagon-like peptide analogues for type 2 diabetes mellitus. *Cochrane Database Syst Rev* (10):CD006423. doi:10.1002/14651858.CD006423.pub2.

Sinha, M. K., J. P. Ohannesian, M. L. Heiman, A. Kriauciunas, T. W. Stephens, S. Magosin, C. Marco, and J. F. Caro. 1996. Nocturnal rise of leptin in lean, obese, and non-insulin-dependent diabetes mellitus subjects. *J Clin Invest* 97 (5):1344–1347. doi:10.1172/JCI118551.

Sloth, B., J. J. Holst, A. Flint, N. T. Gregersen, and A. Astrup. 2007. Effects of PYY1-36 and PYY3-36 on appetite, energy intake, energy expenditure, glucose and fat metabolism in obese and lean subjects. *Am J Physiol Endocrinol Metab* 292 (4):E1062–E1068. doi:10.1152/ajpendo.00450.2006.

Small, C. J., M. S. Kim, S. A. Stanley, J. R. Mitchell, K. Murphy, D. G. Morgan, M. A. Ghatei, and S. R. Bloom. 2001. Effects of chronic central nervous system administration of agouti-related protein in pair-fed animals. *Diabetes* 50 (2):248–254.

Stefan, N., B. Vozarova, T. Funahashi, Y. Matsuzawa, C. Weyer, R. S. Lindsay, J. F. Youngren et al., 2002. Plasma adiponectin concentration is associated with skeletal muscle insulin receptor tyrosine phosphorylation, and low plasma concentration precedes a decrease in whole-body insulin sensitivity in humans. *Diabetes* 51 (6):1884–1888.

Strobel, A., T. Issad, L. Camoin, M. Ozata, and A. D. Strosberg. 1998. A leptin missense mutation associated with hypogonadism and morbid obesity. *Nat Genet* 18 (3):213–215. doi:10.1038/ng0398-213.

Taheri, S., J. M. Zeitzer, and E. Mignot. 2002. The role of hypocretins (orexins) in sleep regulation and narcolepsy. *Annu Rev Neurosci* 25:283–313. doi:10.1146/annurev.neuro.25.112701.142826.

Takaya, K., Y. Ogawa, N. Isse, T. Okazaki, N. Satoh, H. Masuzaki, K. Mori, N. Tamura, K. Hosoda, and K. Nakao. 1996. Molecular cloning of rat leptin receptor isoform complementary DNAs—identification of a missense mutation in Zucker fatty (fa/fa) rats. *Biochem Biophys Res Commun* 225 (1):75–83. doi:10.1006/bbrc.1996.1133.

Tartaglia, L. A., M. Dembski, X. Weng, N. Deng, J. Culpepper, R. Devos, G. J. Richards et al., 1995. Identification and expression cloning of a leptin receptor, OB-R. *Cell* 83 (7):1263–1271.

Tecott, L. H., L. M. Sun, S. F. Akana, A. M. Strack, D. H. Lowenstein, M. F. Dallman, and D. Julius. 1995. Eating disorder and epilepsy in mice lacking 5-HT2c serotonin receptors. *Nature* 374 (6522):542–546. doi:10.1038/374542a0.

Thorleifsson, G., G. B. Walters, D. F. Gudbjartsson, V. Steinthorsdottir, P. Sulem, A. Helgadottir, U. Styrkarsdottir et al., 2009. Genome-wide association yields new sequence variants at seven loci that associate with measures of obesity. *Nat Genet* 41 (1):18–24. doi:10.1038/ng.274.

Tschop, M., C. Weyer, P. A. Tataranni, V. Devanarayan, E. Ravussin, and M. L. Heiman. 2001. Circulating ghrelin levels are decreased in human obesity. *Diabetes* 50 (4):707–709.

Turton, M. D., D. O'Shea, I. Gunn, S. A. Beak, C. M. Edwards, K. Meeran, S. J. Choi et al., 1996. A role for glucagon-like peptide-1 in the central regulation of feeding. *Nature* 379 (6560):69–72. doi:10.1038/379069a0.

Unger, R. H. 1995. Lipotoxicity in the pathogenesis of obesity-dependent NIDDM. Genetic and clinical implications. *Diabetes* 44 (8):863–70.

Unger, T. J., G. A. Calderon, L. C. Bradley, M. Sena-Esteves, and M. Rios. 2007. Selective deletion of Bdnf in the ventromedial and dorsomedial hypothalamus of adult mice results in hyperphagic behavior and obesity. *J Neurosci* 27 (52):14265–74. doi:10.1523/JNEUROSCI.3308-07.2007.

Vaisse, C., J. L. Halaas, C. M. Horvath, J. E. Darnell, Jr., M. Stoffel, and J. M. Friedman. 1996. Leptin activation of State in the hypothalamus of wild-type and ob/ob mice but not db/db mice. *Nat Genet* 14 (1):95–7. doi:10.1038/ng0996-95.

Valentino, M. A., A. Terzic, and S. A. Waldman. 2010. Sizing up pharmacotherapy for obesity. *Clin Transl Sci* 3 (3):123–5. doi:10.1111/j.1752-8062.2010.00191.x.

Verdich, C., A. Flint, J. P. Gutzwiller, E. Naslund, C. Beglinger, P. M. Hellstrom, S. J. Long, L. M. Morgan, J. J. Holst, and A. Astrup. 2001. A meta-analysis of the effect of glucagon-like peptide-1 (7–36) amide on ad libitum energy intake in humans. *J Clin Endocrinol Metab* 86 (9):4382–9. doi:10.1210/jcem.86.9.7877.

Wang, Y., K. K. Kuropatwinski, D. W. White, T. S. Hawley, R. G. Hawley, L. A. Tartaglia, and H. Baumann. 1997. Leptin receptor action in hepatic cells. *J Biol Chem* 272 (26):16216–23.

Weigle, D. S., T. R. Bukowski, D. C. Foster, S. Holderman, J. M. Kramer, G. Lasser, C. E. Lofton-Day, D. E. Prunkard, C. Raymond, and J. L. Kuijper. 1995. Recombinant ob protein reduces feeding and body weight in the ob/ob mouse. *J Clin Invest* 96 (4):2065–70. doi:10.1172/JCI118254.

West, D. B., M. R. Greenwood, K. A. Marshall, and S. C. Woods. 1987. Lithium chloride, cholecystokinin and meal patterns: Evidence that cholecystokinin suppresses meal size in rats without causing malaise. *Appetite* 8 (3):221–7.

Williams, G., C. Bing, X. J. Cai, J. A. Harrold, P. J. King, and X. H. Liu. 2001. The hypothalamus and the control of energy homeostasis: Different circuits, different purposes. *Physiol Behav* 74 (4–5):683–701.

Willie, J. T., R. M. Chemelli, C. M. Sinton, and M. Yanagisawa. 2001. To eat or to sleep? Orexin in the regulation of feeding and wakefulness. *Annu Rev Neurosci* 24:429–58. doi:10.1146/annurev.neuro.24.1.429.

Wren, A. M., L. J. Seal, M. A. Cohen, A. E. Brynes, G. S. Frost, K. G. Murphy, W. S. Dhillo, M. A. Ghatei, and S. R. Bloom. 2001. Ghrelin enhances appetite and increases food intake in humans. *J Clin Endocrinol Metab* 86 (12):5992. doi:10.1210/jcem.86.12.8111.

Wren, A. M., C. J. Small, H. L. Ward, K. G. Murphy, C. L. Dakin, S. Taheri, A. R. Kennedy et al., 2000. The novel hypothalamic peptide ghrelin stimulates food intake and growth hormone secretion. *Endocrinology* 141 (11):4325–8. doi:10.1210/endo.141.11.7873.

Wynne, K., A. J. Park, C. J. Small, K. Meeran, M. A. Ghatei, G. S. Frost, and S. R. Bloom. 2006. Oxyntomodulin increases energy expenditure in addition to decreasing energy intake in overweight and obese humans: A randomised controlled trial. *Int J Obes (Lond)* 30 (12):1729–36. doi:10.1038/sj.ijo.0803344.

Wynne, K., A. J. Park, C. J. Small, M. Patterson, S. M. Ellis, K. G. Murphy, A. M. Wren et al., 2005. Subcutaneous oxyntomodulin reduces body weight in overweight and obese subjects: A double-blind, randomized, controlled trial. *Diabetes* 54 (8):2390–5.

Wynne, K., S. Stanley, and S. Bloom. 2004. The gut and regulation of body weight. *J Clin Endocrinol Metab* 89 (6):2576–82. doi:10.1210/jc.2004-0189.

Xu, B., E. H. Goulding, K. Zang, D. Cepoi, R. D. Cone, K. R. Jones, L. H. Tecott, and L. F. Reichardt. 2003. Brain-derived neurotrophic factor regulates energy balance downstream of melanocortin-4 receptor. *Nat Neurosci* 6 (7):736–742. doi:10.1038/nn1073.

Xu, Y., J. E. Jones, D. Kohno, K. W. Williams, C. E. Lee, M. J. Choi, J. G. Anderson et al., 2008. 5-HT2CRs expressed by pro-opiomelanocortin neurons regulate energy homeostasis. *Neuron* 60 (4):582–589. doi:10.1016/j.neuron.2008.09.033.

Yang, J., M. S. Brown, G. Liang, N. V. Grishin, and J. L. Goldstein. 2008. Identification of the acyltransferase that octanoylates ghrelin, an appetite-stimulating peptide hormone. *Cell* 132 (3):387–396. doi:10.1016/j.cell.2008.01.017.

Yeo, G. S., C. C. Connie Hung, J. Rochford, J. Keogh, J. Gray, S. Sivaramakrishnan, S. O'Rahilly, and I. S. Farooqi. 2004. A de novo mutation affecting human TrkB associated with severe obesity and developmental delay. *Nat Neurosci* 7 (11):1187–1189. doi:10.1038/nn1336.

Zelissen, P. M., K. Stenlof, M. E. Lean, J. Fogteloo, E. T. Keulen, J. Wilding, N. Finer et al., 2005. Effect of three treatment schedules of recombinant methionyl human leptin on body weight in obese adults: A randomized, placebo-controlled trial. *Diabetes Obes Metab* 7 (6):755–761. doi:10.1111/j.1463-1326.2005.00468.x.

Zhang, Y., R. Proenca, M. Maffei, M. Barone, L. Leopold, and J. M. Friedman. 1994. Positional cloning of the mouse obese gene and its human homologue. *Nature* 372 (6505):425–432. doi:10.1038/372425a0.

2 Genetic Determinants of Nutrient Processing

Nicholette D. Palmer

CONTENTS

2.1 INTRODUCTION

Success in the era of human genetic studies was first realized with the identification of rare variants underlying Mendelian forms of disease. Also termed *single-gene disorders*, these diseases are often the result of changes in DNA sequence (mutations) in one gene and have been observed to segregate within families. The first Mendelian disease for which the molecular basis was identified was sickle cell anemia [1]. Resulting from a nucleotide transversion (A→T), the codon at amino acid position 6 in the β-hemoglobin gene (*HBB*) is mutated from a glutamic acid to valine. The mutation produces a variant form of the β-chain of hemoglobin, termed *HbS*, which polymerizes in red blood cells after deoxygenation [2,3]. This aggregation of hemoglobin chains causes red blood cells to distort into a crescent or sickled shape. These defective red blood cells are unable to transport oxygen and cause obstructions in the vasculature, resulting in increased mortality. This discovery demonstrated a molecular basis for disease that has been successfully applied to many other Mendelian diseases (e.g., cystic fibrosis [4], Tay Sachs disease [5], and Huntington's disease [6].) The majority of Mendelian phenotypes identified to date result from protein coding mutations, with relatively few phenotypes attributed to variation outside the coding region [7]. As of November 2017, there were 5,132 Mendelian phenotypes with a known molecular basis, while 1,593 remain unknown, and many more Mendelian conditions have yet to be recognized [8].

In contrast to Mendelian disease, the genetic basis of common diseases including diabetes, obesity, and coronary artery disease are heterogeneous, with modest contributions from variants, inclusive of those that predispose to monogenic forms of disease [9,10]. In fact, many Mendelian diseases present as more phenotypically severe forms of common diseases [11]. For example, both type 2 diabetes (T2D) and maturity-onset diabetes of the young (MODY) share a common etiology (i.e., presence of hyperglycemia resulting from defective pancreatic beta-cell function). MODY is a Mendelian disease estimated to occur in 1/10,000 adults, with an observed autosomal-dominant inheritance pattern, and attributed to six known genes [12–17]. In contrast, T2D is a highly prevalent common disease in which the genetic variants identified explain a relatively small proportion of the heritability, while variants contributing to MODY have only a nominal impact on T2D [18].

Despite these shortcomings, studying the genes that cause related monogenic disorders has identified potential pathways involved in the molecular basis of common disease.

Great progress toward understanding the genetic basis of Mendelian and common disease has been enabled with the completion of the Human Genome Project. Launched in 1990, the Human Genome Project was an international effort to determine the nucleotide sequence of the human genome with identification and mapping of genes, the hereditary unit of the genome coding for proteins, and other molecules. Declared complete in 2003, the Human Genome Project identified approximately 30,000–40,000 protein-coding genes, a preponderance of segmental duplications in the euchromatic regions of the genome that make up 92% of the human genome—that is, heterochromatic regions, including centromeres and telomeres, were not sequenced as part of the Human Genome Project, and identified more than 1.4 million single-nucleotide polymorphisms (SNPs) [19].

Prior to the completion of the Human Genome Project, few genetic variants had been identified that were reproducibly associated with common diseases or quantitative phenotypes (e.g., lipid levels and blood pressure), limiting our insight into disease pathophysiology. Once completed, the catalog of genetic variation provided a basis for disease gene mapping. These advances paved the way for the first genome-wide association studies (GWAS), which allowed for a comprehensive and unbiased assessment of the contribution of common variation across the genome to diseases and related phenotypes. The first GWAS was reported in 2005, for age-related macular degeneration (AMD), and was conducted in 96 patients previously diagnosed with AMD and 130 age-matched control individuals who were AMD-free. Among the 103,611 SNPs examined, a single SNP in the promoter region of *HTRA1*, a serine protease gene, was identified as a major genetic risk factor for AMD [20].

Discovery has accelerated, with improvements in genotyping technologies and development of analytical methods. Today, genotyping arrays can simultaneously assess up to 4,284,426 SNPs (e.g., Illumina Omni5 array). A summation of work published to date is publicly available through the GWAS Catalog (www.ebi.ac.uk/gwas) and, as of the latest publication, includes 24,218 unique SNP-trait associations from 2,518 publications in 337 different journals [21]. Collectively, GWAS have identified thousands of genetic variants associated with disease and underlying complex traits, yet the majority of these variants make only nominal contributions to disease risk and explain only a small proportion of familial clustering. While this observation could suggest that cumulative variation could be more impactful, a sophisticated evaluation of environmental exposure has yet to be addressed [9].

Traditional epidemiologic studies documenting an increase in prevalence rates of common diseases also supports environmental contributions. As an example, in type 1 diabetes, a disease highly prevalent among European children, the number of prevalent cases is expected to increase by 70% by 2020 [22]. An increasing prevalence of obesity has also been observed in the United States, with rates rising from 15% in the late 1970s to 35% today [23,24]. Consistent with these increases are the increases in prevalence of T2D [24] and cardiovascular disease (CVD) [25]. Taken together, the nominal effect of genetic variation on disease risk and rapid increases in disease prevalence suggests the contribution of nongenetic factors.

2.2 NATURE VERSUS NURTURE DEBATE

The dichotomy of nature versus nurture was formally presented by Sir Francis Galton in 1874 with his publication of *English Men of Science: Their Nature and Nurture*. By historical definition, "nature is all that a man brings with himself into the world; nurture is every influence from without that affects him after his birth" [26]. Even early on, this subject area argued that a man's natural abilities (e.g., intelligence and character traits) were derived from hereditary factors. This assertion conflicted with the empiricist views of earlier scholars, such as Francis Bacon and John Locke, who argued that man's resemblance to "white paper, void of all characters," with "all the materials of reason and knowledge" derived from experience [27].

This debate continued into the twentieth century, with a noticeable shift toward nature resulting from rediscovery of Mendel's laws of heredity and initial insights into population genetics, and culminating with the Human Genome Project. Contemporary research now appreciates that nature and nurture domains are intertwined—that is, genes influence our response to environment, and our environment and experiences modulate the expression of genes. Although conceptually more complicated, the codependent nature of these domains argues for infinitely more finite time points at which the trajectory and progression toward disease are amenable to intervention.

2.3 NUTRITION, GENETICS, AND METABOLIC DISEASE

Metabolic syndrome is the designation of a group of interrelated risk factors that increase the incidence of CVD and T2D. Inclusive of central obesity, insulin resistance, dyslipidemia (i.e., increased triglycerides and reduced high-density lipoprotein), and hypertension, these perturbations promote the progression and pathogenesis of diet-related diseases. With the prevalence of obesity, diabetes, and hypertension increasing, the prevalence of metabolic syndrome has increased, with more than one-third of U.S. adults meeting disease criteria, thereby increasing morbidity and mortality [28].

The selective advantage of metabolic disease and its associated risk factors can be explained, in part, by the "thrifty gene" hypothesis [29]. Specific to the example of T2D and obesity, the "thrifty gene" hypothesis posits that there was evolutionary selection of genes related to energy storage and fat deposition that conferred benefit in times of food scarcity but which are associated with deleterious effects in a Westernized environment that is dominated by physical inactivity and excess caloric consumption. In support of this hypothesis is the finding that obesity and T2D have risen to epidemic proportions in certain ethnic groups living in a Westernized environment, compared to their native environment (e.g., Pima Indians) [30,31]. These gene-diet interactions describe the effect of dietary changes on genotype to produce a resultant phenotype or disease. This is supported by the interindividual variability observed in response to dietary modification (i.e., gene-nutrition interaction). A summary of relevant gene-nutrient interaction studies across a range of genes and dietary factors and their impact on metabolic disease is presented in Table 2.1.

TABLE 2.1
Gene-Nutrient Interactions and Their Effects on Metabolic Disease

Locus	Variant (Location)	Dietary Factor	Observation	References
Peroxisome proliferator-activated receptor delta (*PPARD*)	rs2016520 (5′ UTR)	Total fat	C allele carriers were protected from metabolic syndrome (OR = 0.62) with further reduced risk among low dietary fat consumers (OR = 0.42)	[44]
Acetyl-CoA carboxylase beta (*ACACB*)	rs4766587 (intronic)	n-6 polyunsaturated fatty acid (PUFA)	A allele carriers had increased risk of metabolic syndrome (OR = 1.29), which was exacerbated on a high-fat diet (OR = 1.62), particularly when rich in n-6 PUFA (OR = 1.82)	[83]
Nitric oxide synthase 3 (*NOS3*)	rs1799983 (E298D)	n-3 polyunsaturated fatty acid (PUFA)	A allele carriers had increased triacylglycerol (TAG) with low plasma n-3 PUFA	[84]

(Continued)

TABLE 2.1 (*Continued*)
Gene-Nutrient Interactions and Their Effects on Metabolic Disease

Locus	Variant (Location)	Dietary Factor	Observation	References
Apolipoprotein B (*APOB*)	rs512535 (intergenic)	Monounsaturated fat (MUFA)	G allele carriers had increased metabolic syndrome risk (OR = 1.65), which was exacerbated in habitual high-fat consumers (OR = 2.00) and high MUFA intake (OR = 1.89)	[85]
Apolipoprotein A-I (*APOA1*)	rs670 (intergenic)	Monounsaturated fat (MUFA)	G allele carriers had increased metabolic syndrome risk (OR = 1.42), which was exacerbated in habitual high-fat consumers (OR = 1.58) and high MUFA intake (OR = 1.57)	[85]
Transcription factor 7-like 2 (*TCF7L2*)	rs7903146	Total saturated fatty acids	T allele carriers on a high dietary saturated fat intake had increased risk of developing metabolic syndrome (OR = 2.35)	[86]

OR, odds ratio.

2.4 PEROXISOME PROLIFERATOR-ACTIVATED RECEPTOR-γ, OBESITY, AND TYPE 2 DIABETES

Most detailed studies of gene-diet interactions are the result of large epidemiological studies focusing on variants highlighted from candidate gene studies in which the gene being evaluated was selected *a priori* based on biological function. Peroxisome proliferator-activated receptor-γ (PPARγ) is a lipid-activated transcription factor involved in the regulation of glucose and lipid homeostasis, adipocyte differentiation and expression of adipocyte-specific genes, lipid storage, and insulin sensitization [32–34]. Two alternatively spliced isoforms of PPARγ, designated PPARγ1 and PPARγ2, are expressed among metabolic tissues including adipose, heart, muscle, and liver [35]. Present among both isoforms are ligand-dependent and -independent domains. Unique to PPARγ2 are an additional 28 amino acids, resulting in 5- to 10-times-higher ligand-independent activity, with activation via insulin stimulation, as compared with PPARγ1 [36].

Among the variants present in the peroxisome proliferator-activated receptor gamma gene (*PPARG*), the most intensively studied is an SNP in the coding region, resulting in a nonsynonymous amino acid change from proline to alanine at position 12 (i.e., Pro12Ala). This mutation varies in frequency across ethnic groups, with a 20% prevalence of Ala allele carriers among European populations as compared to limited observation in African populations (Figure 2.1). This amino acid substitution is located in the PPARγ2 domain, controlling the ligand-independent ability to activate target gene expression. Thus, presence of the Ala allele is related to a decrease in DNA-binding affinity among target gene promoters, thereby decreasing the expression of target genes [37]. In addition to transcriptional alterations, the Ala allele also possesses insulin-sensitizing effects in liver and skeletal muscle [37,38], which causes suppression of lipolysis in adipocytes and reduced release of free fatty acids [39]. Based on these physiological implications, this variant has been evaluated in the context of numerous common diseases, including obesity, T2D, and dyslipidemia.

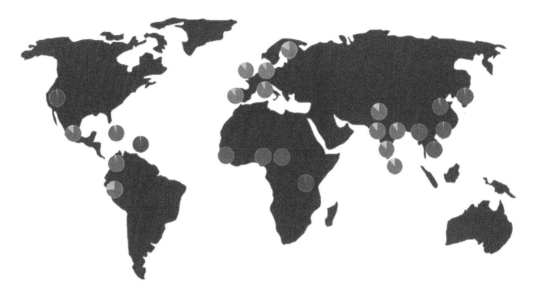

FIGURE 2.1 *PPARG* Pro12Ala allele frequency across representative 1000 Genomes Project populations. The 1000 Genomes Project (Phase 3) populations include African, American, Asian, European, and South Asian. For each pie chart, the darker color represents the frequency of the proline coding allele, and the lighter color represents the frequency of the alanine coding allele.

Several studies have investigated gene-diet interactions focusing on the *PPARG* Pro12Ala polymorphism and their impact on obesity (Table 2.2). Based on the observation that PPARγ is activated by fatty acids [40], four groups have examined the interaction of *PPARG* Pro12Ala with fatty acid intake on obesity-related traits. Luan et al. [41] detected an interaction between the *PPARG* Pro12Ala genotype and dietary polyunsaturated fatty acid to saturated fatty acid ratio. Carriers of the Ala allele had a higher body mass index (BMI) when the polyunsaturated fatty acid to saturated fatty acid ratio was low, and the converse was true when the polyunsaturated fatty acid to saturated fatty acid ratio was high (i.e., Ala allele carriers had lower BMI). Further examination of the polyunsaturated fatty acid species by Nieters et al. [42] revealed that Ala allele carriers who consumed high amounts of arachidonic acid had a significantly higher risk of obesity. Subsequent to this report, Memisoglu et al. [43] replicated these findings in a prospective cohort study of 2,141 nondiabetic women and also observed that total fat was correlated with plasma high-density lipoprotein cholesterol (HDL-C) among Ala allele carriers. Similar findings were reported by Garaulet et al., in which Ala allele carriers with high total fat intake had decreased weight loss. Exploration of the impact of genetic variation on components of the metabolic syndrome was further extended by Robitaille et al. [44], in which they observed only that variance in plasma HDL-C levels was attributed to the *PPARG* Pro12Ala genotype, dietary fat intake, and their interaction. Beyond population-based reports, these studies have been extended to randomized clinical trials. In a 1-year clinical trial for diabetes prevention in high-risk individuals using targeted drug therapy, Franks et al. [45] observed that while Ala allele carriers had higher waist circumference and subcutaneous fat tissue, Ala allele carriers in the metformin and lifestyle intervention arms had the greatest weight loss, with Ala12 allele carriers having a modifying effect on dietary polyunsaturated fatty acids and a reduction of visceral adipose tissue. In comparison, a randomized clinical trial examining a dietary intervention [46] found that, among diabetic individuals, there was a significant interaction of the Ala allele and the Mediterranean diet resulting in a reduction in waist circumference, which suggests that dietary modulation alone can reverse the negative effect associated with the Ala allele.

TABLE 2.2

PPARG Pro12Ala Gene-Diet Interaction Studies and Their Effects on Obesity

Study Design	Subjects	Observation	Reference
Population-based cohort study	592 adult nondiabetic patients	Ala allele carriers had a higher BMI when dietary polyunsaturated fat to saturated fat ratio was low; Ala allele carriers had a lower BMI when dietary polyunsaturated fat to saturated fat ratio was high	[41]
Case-control study	154 obese adults and 154 age- and sex-matched normal weight controls	Ala allele carriers who consumed high amounts of arachidonic acid were at increased risk to develop obesity	[42]
Prospective cohort study	2,141 nondiabetic women	Ala allele carriers decreased intake of MUFA was associated with increased BMI; among Ala allele carriers total fat was correlated with plasma HDL	[43]
Population-based cohort study	340 adults	Presence of the Pro12Ala variant, fat intake and their interaction contributed only to the variance of HDL among components of the metabolic syndrome	[44]
Randomized clinical trial	3,356 adults among 4 treatment groups	At baseline, Ala allele carriers had larger waists; Ala allele carriers in the metformin and lifestyle intervention arms had the greatest weight loss; Ala12 allele carriers had a modifying effect of dietary PUFA and a reduction of visceral adipose tissue	[45]
Randomized clinical trial	774 older adults	Ala allele carriers allocated to Mediterranean diet groups had decreased waist circumference, especially among patients with diabetes	[46]
Behavioral treatment program for obesity	1,465 adults	Ala allele carriers were less obese with high MUFA intake; Ala allele carriers with high total fat intake had decreased weight loss	[87]

BMI, body mass index; HDL, high-density lipoprotein; PPARG, peroxisome proliferator-activated receptor gamma; MUFA, monounsaturated fatty acid; PUFA, polyunsaturated fatty acid.

In summary, *PPARG* is one of the most well-studied genes linked to dietary interactions [41–43]. *PPARG* encodes a transcription factor that controls the expression of genes involved in adipocyte differentiation, lipid storage, and insulin sensitization. The most intensively studied variant at this locus is a Pro12Ala mutation that negatively impacts DNA-binding affinity and impairs transcriptional activity in target genes [37]. This variant has been widely associated with diabetes [47], with the Pro allele exhibiting deleterious effect. However, the Ala allele has been associated with increased adiposity [48,49]. These contrasting results suggest a role for environmental factors, inclusive of nutrient intake, particularly as this may impact membrane fatty acid composition, transcriptional regulation, and post-transcriptional processes.

2.5 FADS GENE CLUSTER AND POLYUNSATURATED FATTY ACIDS

Polyunsaturated fatty acid composition of phospholipids is associated with several common diseases, including the metabolic syndrome [50], CVD [51], psychiatric disorders [52,53], and immune-related disease [54]. Polyunsaturated fatty acid levels in phospholipids are determined by both nutrition and metabolism, with desaturases and elongases catalyzing their conversion. Human desaturases were first cloned and characterized in 1999, owing to their critical role in the availability of polyunsaturated fatty acids, which are important for a number of biological functions including brain development, inflammation, and hemostasis [55,56]. The fatty acid desaturase 1 gene (*FADS1*) encodes the Δ-5 desaturase, while the fatty acid desaturase 2 gene (*FADS2*) gene encodes the Δ-6 desaturase. Both the *FADS1* and *FADS2* genes are located on chromosome 11q12.2 in a head-to-head configuration. The Δ-5 desaturase is expressed at highest levels in the liver, with lower but comparable expression levels in the heart, brain, and lung, and low but detectable levels of expression in placenta, skeletal muscle, kidney, and pancreas. In comparison, the Δ-6 desaturase had a similar expression profile but with a greater overall abundance [55]. As depicted in Figure 2.2, these enzymes catalyze rate-limiting steps in the production of long chain fatty acids, including arachidonic acid (20:4(n-6)) and eicosapentaenoic acid (20:5(n-3)), which are precursors of eicosanoids, which mediate inflammatory processes [57,58].

Although this chromosomal region has been linked to multiple common diseases, including type 1 diabetes [59], osteoarthritis [60], bipolar disease [61], and asthma [62], the first study to examine the role of genetic variation on desaturase activity and its impact on fatty acid composition was a candidate gene study performed by Schaeffer et al. [63]. Using a population-based sample of 727 randomly selected, mainly Caucasian, participants, variants within the *FADS* gene cluster were found to be strongly associated with a subset of the n-6 and n-3 fatty acids—that is, the minor alleles were associated with increased levels of linoleic acid, eicosadienoic acid, dihomo-γ-linolenic acid, and α-linolenic acid, and decreased levels of γ-linolenic acid, arachidonic acid, adrenic acid, eicosapentaenoic acid, and docosapentaenoic acid. These findings were replicated and extended by Rzehak et al. [64], with evidence of association in erythrocyte membranes. Extension of genetic studies to genome-wide approaches (i.e., GWAS) likewise identified association of a variant in *FADS1*, rs174548, with several plasma glycerophospholipid concentrations, explaining up to 10% of the variance in certain species (e.g., arachidonic acid levels were significantly decreased among minor allele carriers) [65]. This observation was followed and corroborated in a larger study focused on identifying the genetic contributors of plasma polyunsaturated fatty acid concentrations wherein a significant association was also found near *FADS1* at rs174537 with arachidonic acid, which accounted for 18.6% of the additive variance in arachidonic acid concentrations [66]. Variants in this region are highly correlated, suggesting that any one of the associated variants could be the causal.

As with most GWAS conducted to date for common disease, the majority have been undertaken in populations of European ancestry. However, minority populations, particularly African American people, suffer a disproportionately higher prevalence of common diseases, including

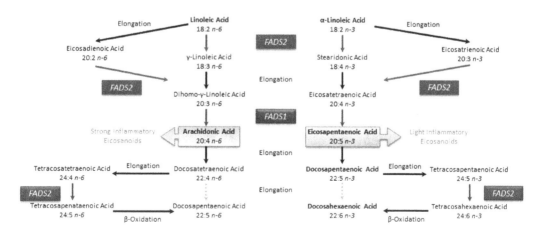

FIGURE 2.2 Polyunsaturated fatty acid (PUFA) biosynthetic pathway. Omega 3 (right) and Omega 6 (left) pathways are illustrated. Reaction catalyzed by *FADS1* and *FADS2* are highlighted. PUFAs derived from dietary sources are in bold.

T2D, hypertension, stroke, CVD, and certain types of cancer [67]. This observation raises the question of whether variable-frequency genetic variants could impact observed health disparities. To address this question, as it relates to polyunsaturated fatty acid metabolism, research efforts have focused on evaluating genetic variants and measuring circulating polyunsaturated fatty acid levels in ethnic minority samples and contrasting those with evidence derived from European populations.

Among studies focused on the differential impact of genetic variation on polyunsaturated fatty acid levels, studies examining the differences between European and African American populations have discovered profound differences among circulating levels of arachidonic acid and the frequency of variants in the *FADS* gene cluster [68–70]. Among African American, as compared with European-derived, populations, higher levels of arachidonic acid and ratios of arachidonic acid to precursors, including dihomo-γ-linolenic acid and linoleic acid, have been observed. These elevated fatty acid levels are associated with genetic variation in the *FADS* gene cluster. Specifically, variant rs174537, identified from GWAS as significantly associated with arachidonic acid levels [65,66], had an allele frequency of 0.65–0.67 in European Americans, and homozygous G allele carriers had increased levels of polyunsaturated fatty acids. In contrast, the same allele was more significantly associated with increased polyunsaturated fatty acids in African Americans for whom the minor allele frequency ranged from 0.89 to 0.91. A subsequent comparison of these frequencies across distinct geographic populations confirmed increased allele frequencies in admixed African-derived populations but found that the G allele was swept almost to fixation (i.e., approximately 99%), among representative populations from the African continent (Figure 2.3) [68].

Towards identification of the causal mechanism by which variation in the *FADS1* region gives rise to increased levels of polyunsaturated fatty acids, investigators have evaluated the impact of methylation status. Methylation is an epigenetic mechanism whereby methyl groups are added to a DNA molecule to change its activity without impacting the primary sequence. These additions can occur within multiple genomic contexts (i.e., transcription start sites, gene bodies, regulatory elements, or repeat sequences to silence gene expression) [71]. Under the hypothesis that variant rs174537 may serve as a genetic proxy for DNA methylation within the *FADS* gene cluster,

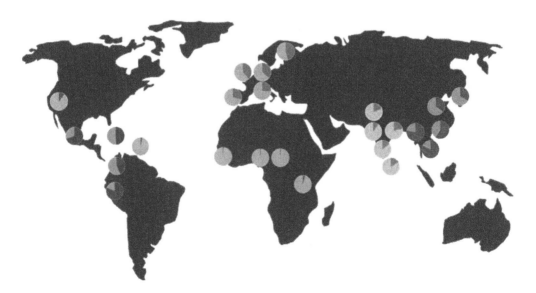

FIGURE 2.3 *FADS1* rs174537 allele frequency across representative 1000 Genomes Project populations. The 1000 Genomes Project (Phase 3) populations include African, American, Asian, European and South Asian. For each pie chart, the darker color represents the frequency of the T allele, and the lighter color represents the frequency of the G allele.

investigators performed whole-genome methylation profiling among 144 liver samples, liver being the primary organ involved in polyunsaturated fatty acid synthesis. Investigation of allele-specific methylation revealed significant results with CpG sites in the genomic region between *FADS1 and FADS2*, suggesting a role for methylation in transcriptional activity of these genes, with the primary effect observed at *FADS1* and, to a lesser extent, at *FADS2* [72]. These results were subsequently replicated and extended through the use of bisulfite sequencing to capture additional CpG sites [73].

In summary, *FADS1* and *FADS2* encode desaturases that are rate limiting in the conversion of linoleic acid to arachidonic acid and α-linolenic acid to eicosapentaenoic acid, respectively. Genetic variation within this region has been associated with increased levels of arachidonic acid, contributing to strong inflammatory eicosanoids. Therefore, it could be hypothesized that carriers of the G allele at variant rs174537 located in proximity to *FADS1*, or a highly correlated variant in the region, give rise to increased *FADS1* transcript levels or increased enzymatic efficiency of the FADS1 protein. This, combined with dramatic changes in the Western diet [74]—that is, increased consumption of linoleic acid that cannot be synthesized de novo and is deemed "essential"—could contribute to the disproportionate burden of complex disease observed in minority populations, especially inflammatory disorders, owing to higher levels of arachidonic acid.

2.6 CONCLUSIONS AND PERSPECTIVES

Susceptibility to common disease involves contributions from genetic, lifestyle, and environmental factors. These diseases, which include diabetes, obesity, CVD, and cancer, have high prevalence rates and associated public health burdens. An individual's genetic composition can define the nutrient state, metabolic response, and susceptibility to diet-dependent or related health disorders [75]. Through technological advances, the genetic basis of common disease has been systematically evaluated. In contrast to Mendelian disorders, in which a single gene exhibits a large effect, variants identified through GWAS have small to modest effect, suggesting only a fraction of the genetic contribution has been explained [9]. While this "missing heritability" is attributed, in part, to other types of genetic variation not currently captured by array-based technologies (e.g., rare variants, copy number variants, structural variants), the impact of environmental factors and their interaction with genetics has yet to be critically addressed and may provide insight into novel mechanisms of disease.

To critically assess the role of genetics and nutrition, the field of nutritional genomics is aimed at understanding the components of both nutrigenetics and nutrigenomics and how these impact human health [76]. While both are interrelated, nutrigenetics assesses how genetic variation impacts the interaction between dietary components and the health and disease potential of an individual. Nutrigenomics assesses the effects of dietary components on the genome—the genetic material, proteome—the total set of expressed proteins, and metabolome—the biochemical fingerprint of the cell [77]. In 2008, the International Society of Nutrigenetics/Nutrigenomics was formed to increase the understanding through research on the role of genetic variation and dietary response and the role of nutrients in gene expression [78].

The genetic landscape of an individual contributes to differential response to interventional strategies. In response to dietary interventions, variation can impact absorption, metabolism, and utilization [79]. Great progress has been made toward understanding the genetic composition of the human genome in its entirety with efforts such as the National Heart, Lung, and Blood Institute's Trans-Omics for Precision Medicine (TOPMed) Program, the Cohorts for Heart and Aging Research in Genomic Epidemiology (CHARGE) Consortium [80,81], and the Centers for Common Disease Genomics (CCDG) [82], which have focused on whole genome sequencing. However, a comprehensive assessment of lifestyle and environmental factors remains difficult to measure. To augment this potential shortcoming, multiple lines of investigation are now pursuing metabolomics. Metabolites are small molecule intermediates resulting from multiple cellular and biological processes that represent functional intermediate phenotypes proximal to the outcome of

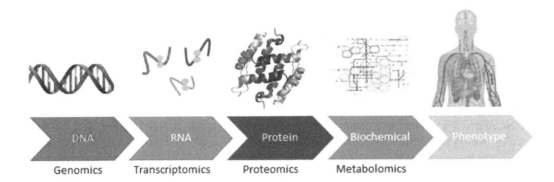

FIGURE 2.4   'Omics approaches to study common disease.

interest (Figure 2.4). Current technologies now allow for the routine measurement of metabolites that characterize pathways of amino acid, carbohydrate, vitamin, energy, lipid, nucleotide, peptide, and xenobiotic metabolism, which can be perturbed in response to diet, as exemplified by the *FADS* gene cluster example. Toward the future, identification of gene-diet interactions could elucidate novel disease pathways and mechanisms not readily apparent in a controlled setting. More broadly, a positive impact on public health may stem from personalized nutrition, whereby customized diets ascribed to an individual's genetic makeup may promote optimal metabolic health, thus mitigating the symptoms of existing diseases or preventing future illnesses.

REFERENCES

1. Pauling, L., H.A. Itano, et al. Sickle cell anemia, a molecular disease. *Science*, 1949. 109(2835): 443.
2. Ashley-Koch, A., Q. Yang, and R.S. Olney. Sickle hemoglobin (HbS) allele and sickle cell disease: A HuGE review. *Am J Epidemiol*, 2000. 151(9): 839–45.
3. Stuart, M.J. and R.L. Nagel. Sickle-cell disease. *Lancet*, 2004. 364(9442): 1343–60.
4. Tsui, L.C., et al. Cystic fibrosis locus defined by a genetically linked polymorphic DNA marker. *Science*, 1985. 230(4729): 1054–7.
5. Myerowitz, R. Tay-Sachs disease-causing mutations and neutral polymorphisms in the Hex A gene. *Hum Mutat*, 1997. 9(3): 195–208.
6. MacDonald, M.E., et al. A novel gene containing a trinucleotide repeat that is expanded and unstable on Huntington's disease chromosomes. *The Huntington's Disease Collaborative Research Group Cell*, 1993. 72(6): 971–83.
7. Makrythanasis, and S.E. Antonarakis. Pathogenic variants in non-protein-coding sequences. *Clin Genet*, 2013. 84(5): 422–8.
8. McKusick-Nathans Institute of Genetic Medicine, J.H.U. Online Mendelian Inheritance in Man. OMIM. 2017 November 15, 2017; Available from: https://www.omim.org/statistics/entry.
9. Manolio, T.A., et al. Finding the missing heritability of complex diseases. *Nature*, 2009. 461(7265): 747–53.
10. Eichler, E.E., et al. Missing heritability and strategies for finding the underlying causes of complex disease. *Nat Rev Genet*, 2010. 11(6): 446–50.
11. Scheuner, M.T., P.W. Yoon, and M.J. Khoury. Contribution of Mendelian disorders to common chronic disease: opportunities for recognition, intervention, and prevention. *Am J Med Genet C Semin Med Genet*, 2004. 125C(1): 50–65.
12. Yamagata, K., et al. Mutations in the hepatocyte nuclear factor-4alpha gene in maturity-onset diabetes of the young (MODY1). *Nature*, 1996. 384(6608): 458–60.
13. Yamagata, K., et al. Mutations in the hepatocyte nuclear factor-1alpha gene in maturity-onset diabetes of the young (MODY3). *Nature*, 1996. 384(6608): 455–8.
14. Vionnet, N., et al. Nonsense mutation in the glucokinase gene causes early-onset non-insulin-dependent diabetes mellitus. *Nature*, 1992. 356(6371): 721–2.
15. Malecki, M.T., et al. Mutations in NEUROD1 are associated with the development of type 2 diabetes mellitus. *Nat Genet*, 1999. 23(3): 323–8.

16. Stoffers, D.A., et al. Early-onset type-II diabetes mellitus (MODY4) linked to IPF1. *Nat Genet*, 1997. 17(2): 138–9.

17. Horikawa, Y., et al. Mutation in hepatocyte nuclear factor-1 beta gene (TCF2) associated with MODY. *Nat Genet*, 1997. 17(4): 384–5.

18. Winckler, W., et al. Evaluation of common variants in the six known maturity-onset diabetes of the young (MODY) genes for association with type 2 diabetes. *Diabetes*, 2007. 56(3): 685–93.

19. Lander, E.S., et al. Initial sequencing and analysis of the human genome. *Nature*, 2001. 409(6822): 860–921.

20. Klein, R.J., et al. Complement factor H polymorphism in age-related macular degeneration. *Science*, 2005. 308(5720): 385–9.

21. MacArthur, J., et al. The new NHGRI-EBI Catalog of published genome-wide association studies (GWAS Catalog). *Nucleic Acids Res*, 2017. 45(D1): D896–D901.

22. Patterson, C.C., et al. Incidence trends for childhood type 1 diabetes in Europe during 1989–2003 and predicted new cases 2005–20: a multicentre prospective registration study. *Lancet*, 2009. 373(9680): 2027–33.

23. Zhang, Q. and Y. Wang. Trends in the association between obesity and socioeconomic status in U.S. adults: 1971 to 2000. *Obes Res*, 2004. 12(10): 1622–32.

24. Mitchell, N.S., et al. Obesity: overview of an epidemic. *Psychiatr Clin North Am*, 2011. 34(4): 717–32.

25. Hennekens, C.H. Increasing burden of cardiovascular disease: current knowledge and future directions for research on risk factors. *Circulation*, 1998. 97(11): 1095–102.

26. Galton, F. *English Men Of Science: Their Nature And Nurture*. 1874, London, UK: Macmillan.

27. Locke, J. An essay concerning human understanding. 1690, London, UK: Thomas Bassett.

28. Moore, J.X., N. Chaudhary, and T. Akinyemiju. Metabolic syndrome prevalence by race/ethnicity and sex in the United States, national health and nutrition examination survey, 1988–2012. *Prev Chronic Dis*, 2017. 14: E24.

29. Neel, J.V. Diabetes mellitus: A 'thrifty' genotype rendered detrimental by 'progress'? *Am J Hum Genet*, 1962. 14: 353–62.

30. Esparza-Romero, J., et al. Differences in insulin resistance in Mexican and U.S. Pima Indians with normal glucose tolerance. *J Clin Endocrinol Metab*, 2010. 95(11): E358–62.

31. Schulz, L.O., et al. Effects of traditional and western environments on prevalence of type 2 diabetes in Pima Indians in Mexico and the U.S. *Diabetes Care*, 2006. 29(8): 1866–71.

32. Spiegelman, B.M. Peroxisome proliferator-activated receptor gamma: A key regulator of adipogenesis and systemic insulin sensitivity. *Eur J Med Res*, 1997. 2(11): 457–64.

33. Tontonoz, P., E. Hu, and B.M. Spiegelman. Stimulation of adipogenesis in fibroblasts by PPAR gamma 2, a lipid-activated transcription factor. *Cell*, 1994. 79(7): 1147–56.

34. Tontonoz, P., E. Hu, and B.M. Spiegelman. Regulation of adipocyte gene expression and differentiation by peroxisome proliferator activated receptor gamma. *Curr Opin Genet Dev*, 1995. 5(5): 571–6.

35. Vidal-Puig, A.J., et al. Peroxisome proliferator-activated receptor gene expression in human tissues. Effects of obesity, weight loss, and regulation by insulin and glucocorticoids. *J Clin Invest*, 1997. 99(10): 2416–22.

36. Werman, A., et al. Ligand-independent activation domain in the N terminus of peroxisome proliferator-activated receptor gamma (PPARgamma). Differential activity of PPARgamma1 and -2 isoforms and influence of insulin. *J Biol Chem*, 1997. 272(32): 20230–5.

37. Deeb, S.S., et al. A Pro12Ala substitution in PPARgamma2 associated with decreased receptor activity, lower body mass index and improved insulin sensitivity. *Nat Genet*, 1998. 20(3): 284–7.

38. Ek, J., et al. Studies of the Pro12Ala polymorphism of the peroxisome proliferator-activated receptor-gamma2 (PPAR-gamma2) gene in relation to insulin sensitivity among glucose tolerant caucasians. *Diabetologia*, 2001. 44(9): 1170–6.

39. Stumvoll, M., et al. Pro12Ala polymorphism in the peroxisome proliferator-activated receptor-gamma2 gene is associated with increased antilipolytic insulin sensitivity. *Diabetes*, 2001. 50(4): 876–81.

40. Xu, H.E., et al. Molecular recognition of fatty acids by peroxisome proliferator-activated receptors. *Mol Cell*, 1999. 3(3): 397–403.

41. Luan, J., et al. Evidence for gene-nutrient interaction at the PPARgamma locus. *Diabetes*, 2001. 50(3): 686–9.

42. Nieters, A., N. Becker, and J. Linseisen. Polymorphisms in candidate obesity genes and their interaction with dietary intake of n-6 polyunsaturated fatty acids affect obesity risk in a sub-sample of the EPIC-Heidelberg cohort. *Eur J Nutr*, 2002. 41(5): 210–21.

43. Memisoglu, A., et al. Interaction between a peroxisome proliferator-activated receptor gamma gene polymorphism and dietary fat intake in relation to body mass. *Hum Mol Genet*, 2003. 12(22): 2923–9.

44. Robitaille, J., et al. Features of the metabolic syndrome are modulated by an interaction between the peroxisome proliferator-activated receptor-delta -87T>C polymorphism and dietary fat in French-Canadians. *Int J Obes* (Lond), 2007. 31(3): 411–7.

45. Franks, P.W., et al. The Pro12Ala variant at the peroxisome proliferator-activated receptor gamma gene and change in obesity-related traits in the diabetes prevention program. *Diabetologia*, 2007. 50(12): 2451–60.

46. Razquin, C., et al. The Mediterranean diet protects against waist circumference enlargement in 12Ala carriers for the PPARgamma gene: 2 years' follow-up of 774 subjects at high cardiovascular risk. *Br J Nutr*, 2009. 102(5): 672–9.

47. Tonjes, A. and M. Stumvoll. The role of the Pro12Ala polymorphism in peroxisome proliferator-activated receptor gamma in diabetes risk. *Curr Opin Clin Nutr Metab Care*, 2007. 10(4): 410–4.

48. Ek, J., et al. Homozygosity of the Pro12Ala variant of the peroxisome proliferation-activated receptor-gamma2 (PPAR-gamma2): divergent modulating effects on body mass index in obese and lean Caucasian men. *Diabetologia*, 1999. 42(7): 892–5.

49. Masud, S., S. Ye, and S.A.S. Group. Effect of the peroxisome proliferator activated receptor-gamma gene Pro12Ala variant on body mass index: a meta-analysis. *J Med Genet*, 2003. 40(10): 773–80.

50. Vessby, B. Dietary fat, fatty acid composition in plasma and the metabolic syndrome. *Curr Opin Lipidol*, 2003. 14(1): 15–9.

51. Glew, R.H., et al. Abnormalities in the fatty-acid composition of the serum phospholipids of stroke patients. *J Natl Med Assoc*, 2004. 96(6): 826–32.

52. Maes, M., et al. Fatty acid composition in major depression: decreased omega 3 fractions in cholesteryl esters and increased C20: 4 omega 6/C20:5 omega 3 ratio in cholesteryl esters and phospholipids. *J Affect Disord*, 1996. 38(1): 35–46.

53. Nakada, T., I.L. Kwee, and W.G. Ellis. Membrane fatty acid composition shows delta-6-desaturase abnormalities in Alzheimer's disease. *Neuroreport*, 1990. 1(2): 153–5.

54. Goldring, M.B. and F. Berenbaum. The regulation of chondrocyte function by proinflammatory mediators: prostaglandins and nitric oxide. *Clin Orthop Relat Res*, 2004(427 Suppl): S37–46.

55. Cho, H.P., M. Nakamura, and S.D. Clarke. Cloning, expression, and fatty acid regulation of the human delta-5 desaturase. *J Biol Chem*, 1999. 274(52): 37335–9.

56. Cho, H.P., M.T. Nakamura, and S.D. Clarke. Cloning, expression, and nutritional regulation of the mammalian Delta-6 desaturase. *J Biol Chem*, 1999. 274(1): 471–7.

57. Calder, P.C. Polyunsaturated fatty acids, inflammatory processes and inflammatory bowel diseases. *Mol Nutr Food Res*, 2008. 52(8): 885–97.

58. Schmitz, G. and J. Ecker. The opposing effects of n-3 and n-6 fatty acids. *Prog Lipid Res*, 2008. 47(2): 147–55.

59. Nakagawa, Y., et al. Fine mapping of the diabetes-susceptibility locus, IDDM4, on chromosome 11q13. *Am J Hum Genet*, 1998. 63(2): 547–56.

60. Chapman, K., et al. Osteoarthritis-susceptibility locus on chromosome 11q, detected by linkage. *Am J Hum Genet*, 1999. 65(1): 167–74.

61. Fallin, M.D., et al. Genomewide linkage scan for bipolar-disorder susceptibility loci among Ashkenazi Jewish families. *Am J Hum Genet*, 2004. 75(2): 204–19.

62. Huang, J.L., et al. Sequence variants of the gene encoding chemoattractant receptor expressed on Th2 cells (CRTH2) are associated with asthma and differentially influence mRNA stability. *Hum Mol Genet*, 2004. 13(21): 2691–7.

63. Schaeffer, L., et al. Common genetic variants of the FADS1 FADS2 gene cluster and their reconstructed haplotypes are associated with the fatty acid composition in phospholipids. *Hum Mol Genet*, 2006. 15(11): 1745–56.

64. Rzehak, P., et al. Evidence for an association between genetic variants of the fatty acid desaturase 1 fatty acid desaturase 2 (FADS1 FADS2) gene cluster and the fatty acid composition of erythrocyte membranes. *Br J Nutr*, 2009. 101(1): 20–6.

65. Gieger, C., et al. Genetics meets metabolomics: a genome-wide association study of metabolite profiles in human serum. *PLoS Genet*, 2008. 4(11): e1000282.

66. Tanaka, T., et al. Genome-wide association study of plasma polyunsaturated fatty acids in the InCHIANTI Study. *PLoS Genet*, 2009. 5(1): e1000338.

67. Sankar, P., et al. Genetic research and health disparities. *JAMA*, 2004. 291(24): 2985–9.

68. Mathias, R.A., et al. The impact of FADS genetic variants on omega6 polyunsaturated fatty acid metabolism in African Americans. *BMC Genet*, 2011. 12: 50.

69. Sergeant, S., et al. Differences in arachidonic acid levels and fatty acid desaturase (FADS) gene variants in African Americans and European Americans with diabetes or the metabolic syndrome. *Br J Nutr*, 2012. 107(4): 547–55.

70. Mathias, R.A., et al. Adaptive evolution of the FADS gene cluster within Africa. *PLoS One*, 2012. 7(9): e44926.

71. Jones, P.A. Functions of DNA methylation: islands, start sites, gene bodies and beyond. *Nat Rev Genet*, 2012. 13(7): 484–92.

72. Howard, T.D., et al. DNA methylation in an enhancer region of the FADS cluster is associated with FADS activity in human liver. *PLoS One*, 2014. 9(5): e97510.

73. Rahbar, E., et al. Uncovering the DNA methylation landscape in key regulatory regions within the FADS cluster. *PLoS One*, 2017. 12(9): e0180903.

74. Cordain, L., et al. Origins and evolution of the Western diet: health implications for the 21st century. *Am J Clin Nutr*, 2005. 81(2): 341–54.

75. Fenech, M. Genome health nutrigenomics and nutrigenetics—diagnosis and nutritional treatment of genome damage on an individual basis. *Food Chem Toxicol*, 2008. 46(4): 1365–70.

76. Ordovas, J.M. and V. Mooser. Nutrigenomics and nutrigenetics. *Curr Opin Lipidol*, 2004. 15(2): 101–8.

77. DeBusk, R.M., et al. Nutritional genomics in practice: where do we begin?. *J Am Diet Assoc*, 2005. 105(4): 589–98.

78. Simopoulos, A.P. Editorial. *J Nutrigenet Nutrigenomics*, 2008. 1: 2–3.

79. Nielsen, D.E. and A. El-Sohemy. A randomized trial of genetic information for personalized nutrition. *Genes Nutr*, 2012. 7(4): 559–66.

80. Psaty, B.M., et al. Cohorts for Heart and Aging Research in Genomic Epidemiology (CHARGE) Consortium: Design of prospective meta-analyses of genome-wide association studies from 5 cohorts. *Circ Cardiovasc Genet*, 2009. 2(1): 73–80.

81. Morrison, A.C., et al. Whole-genome sequence-based analysis of high-density lipoprotein cholesterol. *Nat Genet*, 2013. 45(8): 899–901.

82. Fuchsberger, C., et al. The genetic architecture of type 2 diabetes. *Nature*, 2016. 536(7614): 41–47.

83. Phillips, C.M., et al. ACC2 gene polymorphisms, metabolic syndrome, and gene-nutrient interactions with dietary fat. *J Lipid Res*, 2010. 51(12): 3500–7.

84. Ferguson, J.F., et al. NOS3 gene polymorphisms are associated with risk markers of cardiovascular disease, and interact with omega-3 polyunsaturated fatty acids. *Atherosclerosis*, 2010. 211(2): 539–44.

85. Phillips, C.M., et al. Gene-nutrient interactions and gender may modulate the association between ApoA1 and ApoB gene polymorphisms and metabolic syndrome risk. *Atherosclerosis*, 2011. 214(2): 408–14.

86. Phillips, C.M., et al. Dietary saturated fat, gender and genetic variation at the TCF7L2 locus predict the development of metabolic syndrome. *J Nutr Biochem*, 2012. 23(3): 239–44.

87. Garaulet, M., et al. PPARgamma Pro12Ala interacts with fat intake for obesity and weight loss in a behavioural treatment based on the Mediterranean diet. *Mol Nutr Food Res*, 2011. 55(12): 1771–9.

3 The Enteroinsular Axis
Contribution to Obesity-Diabetes and Its Treatments

Varun Pathak, Nigel Irwin, and Peter R. Flatt

CONTENTS

3.1 INTRODUCTION

The global incidence of diabetes mellitus is rising exponentially, with an estimated 422 million confirmed cases worldwide in 2014, in comparison to 108 million in 1980 (WHO 2016). Unsurprisingly, this is becoming a significant financial burden for all nations, with healthcare costs for diabetes predicted to rise from the current £265 billion per year to £345 billion by 2030 (WHO 2016). There are two major forms of diabetes, type 1 diabetes mellitus (T1DM) and type 2 diabetes mellitus (T2DM), with the vast majority of cases being T2DM [1]. Although various environmental and genetic factors have been connected to the onset of T2DM, the most accepted cause is linked to over-nutrition and an inactive lifestyle [2]. Thus, one of the major contributing factors to T2DM is the co-existence of obesity [3]. Indeed, the initial treatment plan for almost all newly diagnosed T2DM patients includes key nutritional advice to balance the right amount of dietary carbohydrates, fat, protein, fiber, vitamins, and minerals with the view of maintaining a healthy lifestyle and reducing body weight [4]. Unfortunately, in many cases, diet and lifestyle changes are not sufficient to satisfactorily manage T2DM, and pharmacotherapy is required [5].

Although a large armory of clinically approved T2DM medications now exists [3], there is still an urgent need to develop novel, more effective drugs to help adequately control the disease and its related complications [3]. In this regard, gut hormones have shown promising therapeutic potential for the treatment of both obesity and T2DM. These peptide hormones are released from specialized cells in the gut, in response to nutrient ingestion, and include glucagon-like peptide 1 (GLP-1), glucose-dependent insulinotropic polypeptide (GIP), oxyntomodulin (OXM), cholecystokinin (CCK), and peptide YY (PYY) [6,7; Figure 3.1]. The idea that gut-derived hormones may have potential in the treatment of diabetes was first heralded by Unger and Eisentraut in 1969. As such, this early seminal work revealed that nutrient ingestion stimulates the secretion of gut-derived hormonal signals to control insulin release from pancreatic islets of Langherhans [8; Figure 3.1], a system now commonly termed the *enteroinsular axis*. It was not until 1979 that Creutzfeldt described the two fundamental biological characteristics that an enteroinsular axis–derived insulinotropic hormone,

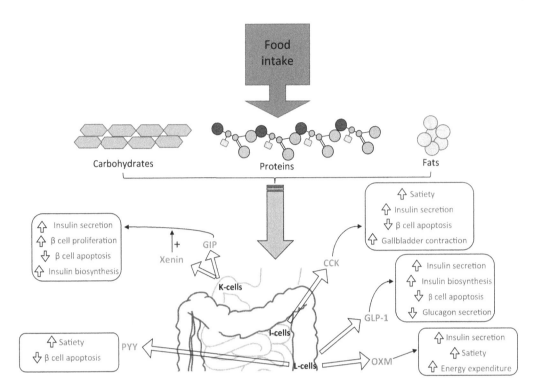

FIGURE 3.1   Nutrient stimulation of the major gut-derived hormones involved in metabolic control. Dietary nutrients activate G-protein–coupled receptors on the luminal side of enteroendocrine K-, I-, and L-cells to stimulate secretion of GIP, Xenin, cholecystokinin (CCK), glucagon-like peptide 1 (GLP-1), oxyntomodulin (OXM), and peptide YY (PYY). Major biological effects of each hormone are also displayed. Xenin, CCK, GLP-1, OXM, and PYY may also possess important centrally mediated physiological actions to regulate metabolism that are not shown here.

normally referred to as an *incretin hormone*, should possess [9]. Firstly, hormonal secretion from the gut must be induced by nutrient intake (Figure 3.1). Secondly, at physiological levels, the gut hormone should stimulate insulin secretion in a glucose-dependent manner.

Although various incretin hormone candidates have been proposed, only GLP-1 and GIP fulfill the criteria originally laid out by Crutzfeldt for a true incretin hormone. Indeed, a defect in the enteroinsular axis is believed to be fundamental in the pathogenesis of T2DM [10]. It is understood that T2DM patients present with reduced secretion of GLP-1 and impaired insulin-releasing action of GLP-1, and particularly GIP [11]. However, there are a number of other enteroendocrine hormones, such as OXM, CCK, and PYY, that are also released in response to nutrient intake and may have beneficial effects, alone or in combination, in obesity and diabetes [12; Table 3.1; Figure 3.1]. For instance, CCK, OXM, and PYY are known to activate anorexigenic pathways in the brain that positively regulate satiety and energy balance, as well as exert positive insulin-releasing effects at the level of the pancreas [13–17; Figure 3.1]. Therefore, as might be anticipated, a plethora of important research has been conducted to characterize the nutrient-induced secretion of these gut hormones, with a possible view to therapeutic application [18–21]. Although this work has been extremely informative, GLP-1, GIP, OXM, CCK, and PYY have extremely short biological half-lives [22], likely thwarting the potential use of a gut hormone secretagogue for the treatment of obesity-diabetes. In this respect, administration of stable, long-acting peptide forms may hold more promise. Therefore, this chapter will focus on the main advances in the area of stabilized forms of GLP-1, GIP, OXM, CCK, and PYY.

TABLE 3.1

Prominent Biological Actions of Selected Gut-Derived Peptide Hormones

Hormone	Release Site	Receptor	Biological Action
GLP-1	L-cells	GLP-1	Glucose-stimulated insulin secretion, inhibits beta-cell apoptosis, satiety, delays gastric emptying
GIP	K-cells	GIP	Glucose-stimulated insulin secretion, inhibits beta-cell apoptosis, insulin biosynthesis
OXM	L-cells	Glucagon/GLP-1	Glucose-stimulated insulin release, regulation of energy expenditure, satiety
CCK	I-cells	CCK_1/CCK_2	Satiety, gallbladder contraction, pancreatic enzyme secretion, insulin secretion
PYY	L-cells	Y_{1-5}	Satiety, inhibits beta-cell apoptosis

Note: Site of release, receptor interaction, and biological action of the major gut-derived hormones stimulated by nutrient intake.

CCK, cholecystokinin; GIP, glucose-dependent insulinotropic polypeptide; GLP-1, glucagon-like peptide 1; OXM, oxyntomodulin; PYY, peptide YY; CCK1, cholecystokinin receptor 1; CCK2, cholecystokinin receptor 2; Y1-5, Y receptors 1-5.

3.2 GLUCAGON-LIKE PEPTIDE 1

GLP-1 is synthesized post-translationally by the action of a prohormone convertase 1/3 (PC1/3) processing enzyme on the proglucagon gene product [23]. The bioactive forms of GLP-1, namely GLP-1(7–36)amide and GLP-1(7–37), are released from intestinal L-cells in response to feeding [24]. However, detectable levels of GLP-1 secretion have also been evidenced in the central nervous system (CNS) and pancreatic islets [25,26]. The biological effects of GLP-1 are mediated through interaction with a specific cell membrane–bound G-protein–coupled receptor (GPCR), appropriately named the GLP-1 receptor [27; Table 3.1]. The chief biological action of GLP-1 is recognized as an incretin hormone, stimulating glucose-dependent insulin release from pancreatic beta-cells in response to nutrient intake [7,28; Table 3.1; Figure 3.1]. Thus, activation of the GLP-1 receptor in pancreatic beta-cells induces downstream cAMP-dependent cell-signaling events that trigger classical insulin secretory pathways, and subsequent glucose-lowering effects [10]. In addition, GLP-1 also promotes islet cell neogenesis and beta-cell proliferation, while inhibiting beta-cell apoptosis and glucagon release from alpha-cells [29; Figure 3.1]. Notably, there is evidence that locally synthesized GLP-1 could be important for these positive islet actions [26,30], especially under conditions of beta-cell stress [31]. Besides expression in the pancreas, the GLP-1 receptor has been localized in many other tissues, including the heart, blood vessels, neurons, liver, skeletal muscle cells, and CNS, to name only a few [32]. Importantly, GLP-1 is also believed to induce satiety through interaction with hypothalamic GLP-1 receptors [33]. Based on these biological actions, which would be favorable in the treatment of obesity and T2DM, long-acting, enzyme-resistant GLP-1 mimetics are now available for clinical use in the United Kingdom (Table 3.2).

There are six clinically approved GLP-1 mimetics for T2DM (Table 3.2) and one for obesity [34], employing dosing regimens that vary from twice daily to once weekly [35]. The first drug to be approved in this class was exenatide, a synthetically produced peptide based on the structure of a substance originally found in the saliva secretions of the venomous Gila monster lizard [36]. Although only sharing approximately 50% sequence identity with human GLP-1, exenatide represents a potent, long-acting GLP-1 receptor agonist in humans [36]. All drugs in the GLP-1 mimetic class have essentially similar beneficial effects in T2DM, but small differences in efficacy, and particularly tolerability, have been noted [36]. This gives rise to the idea of possible patient stratification in relation to choice of GLP-1 based drugs [37]. In addition to this, there are continuing efforts to develop more potent and longer-acting GLP-1 analogues that can provide further pharmacokinetic

TABLE 3.2

Currently Available Glucagon-Like Peptide 1–Based Drugs

GLP-1 Mimetic	Developer	Dosage Frequency	Dose
Exenatide (Byetta)	AstraZeneca	Twice daily	5–10 µg
Exenatide (Bydureon)	AstraZeneca	Once a week	2 mg
Iraglutide (Victoza)	Novo Nordisk	Once daily	0.6–1.8 mg
Dulaglutide (Trulicity)	Eli Lilly	Once a week	0.75–1.5 mg
Lixisenatide (Lyxumia)	Sanofi	Once daily	10–20 µg
Albiglutide (Tanzeum)	GlaxoSmithKline	Once a week	30–50 mg

Note: There are currently six GLP-1 receptor agonists clinically approved for type 2 diabetes. These essentially belong to two major categories: shorter-acting drugs, including exenatide (Byetta; twice-daily dosing) and lixisenatide and liraglutide (both once-daily dosing), and longer-acting drugs that include exenatide (Bydureon), albiglutide, and dulaglutide (all once-weekly dosing).

GLP-1, glucagon-like peptide 1.

and pharmacodynamic advantages beyond what has already been achieved [36]. Notable examples currently undergoing clinical trials include HM11260C an exenatide-derived molecule covalently attached to the non-glycosylated Fc region of an antibody fragment via a short polyethylene glycol (PEG) linker [38; Figure 3.2]. PB1023 is a recombinant GLP-1 analogue genetically fused with an elastin-like protein with the repeated pentapeptide sequence VPGXG [39; Figure 3.2].

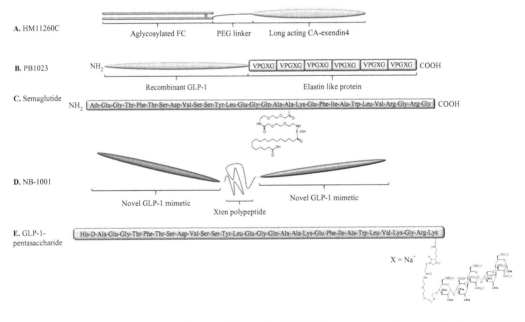

FIGURE 3.2   Structures of selected glucagon-like peptide 1 (GLP-1) receptor agonists currently in preclinical/clinical development, demonstrating distinct approaches to extend biological half-life. *A*, HM11260C (also known as langlenatide) is a modified exenatide analogue fused to the non-glycosylated Fc region of an antibody via a short-chain polyethyleneglycol (PEG) linker. *B*, PB1023 contains recombinant GLP-1 that is genetically fused with elastin like polypeptide. *C*, Semaglutide is based on the structure of liraglutide with amino acid replacements of Gly[8] for Aib[8] and Lys[34] for Arg[34], as well as conjugation to a C-18 fatty acid via a glutamyl linker. *D*, NB1001 is a genetically fused exenatide molecule to an Xten polymer-like protein. *E*, GLP-1 pentasaccharide with amino acid replacements of Gly[8] for Aib[8] coupled to a sulphated pentasaccharide at Lys[37] via a [gamma-maleimidobutyryl]-[3-(thio)propanoyl]-[1-aminoethyl-(2-(2-(2-ethoxy)ethoxy)ethyl linker (GMB-TP-TEG).

Semaglutide shares 94% sequence homology with human GLP-1, but has amino acid substitutions at position 8 (alpha-aminoisobutyric acid for alanine) and position 34 (arginine for lysine), with further C-18 acylation at Lys[26] via two 8-amino-3,6-dioxaoctanoic acid (ADO) linker moieties [40; Figure 3.2]. NB-1001 (Xten-GLP-1) is a novel GLP-1 mimetic covalently attached to a hydrophilic, biodegradable protein polymer called Xten [41; Figure 3.2]. In addition, a GLP-1-antithrombin III pentapeptide has been developed by conjugating a stabilized form of GLP-1 to an antithrombin III-binding pentasaccharide, and shown promising preclinical potential in T2DM [42; Figure 3.2]. Although potentially very interesting, all these novel GLP-1 derivatives, similar to the current clinically available drugs in this class, are peptidic in nature and therefore require parenteral delivery [43]. As such, of particular interest is the possible development of an orally available form of semaglutide [44], which could dramatically change the landscape of this specific field of therapeutics. Together, it is envisaged that the ongoing efforts to generate new GLP-1 compounds will ultimately enable clinicians to select the most appropriate GLP-1 drug according to an individual patient's needs [45]. Importantly, the previously reported safety concerns regarding sustained use of GLP-1 mimetics relating to pancreatitis, thyroid cancer, and emergence of neuroendocrine tumors [46,47], have now been fully allayed [48].

3.3 GLUCOSE-DEPENDENT INSULINOTROPIC POLYPEPTIDE

GIP was first incretin hormone to be discovered, although it was initially thought to principally inhibit gastric acid secretion [49], hence its original name *gastric inhibitory polypeptide* [50]. However, GIP is now considered as prominent insulinotropic agent, and the partner incretin hormone to GLP-1 [51; Figure 3.1]. The insulin-releasing actions of GIP are brought about by activation of specific GPCR GIP receptors on the surface of beta-cells that stimulate K_{ATP} channel and Ca^{+2}-dependent pathways, leading to insulin exocytosis [31]. GIP also acts as a prominent anti-apoptotic factor for beta-cells, encourages beta-cell growth, and promotes insulin biosynthesis [52–54; Table 3.1; Figure 3.1]. Given this favorable biological action profile, there has been significant interest in developing GIP-based compounds as antidiabetic therapies [55]. However, similar to GLP-1, GIP is an excellent substrate for the ubiquitous enzyme dipeptidyl peptidase-4 (DPP-4), meaning that the native hormone cannot be employed therapeutically due to a severely restricted pharmacokinetic profile [56]. Nonetheless, as has been the case for GLP-1, numerous structurally modified, enzyme-resistant, and long-acting analogues of GIP have been developed [55,57]. However, a second major barrier to the exploitation of GIP as an antidiabetic agent relates to the marked reduction in insulinotropic activity of GIP observed in T2DM patients [10].

To date, GIP unresponsiveness in T2DM has been attributed mostly to the downregulation of GIP receptors and/or GIP receptor desensitization in the face of persistent hyperglycemia [58,59]. Therefore, it has been advocated that reduced GIP action is a pathophysiological consequence of T2DM, rather than a specific contributor to the disease [53]. In full agreement, preclinical and clinical studies demonstrate that amelioration of hyperglycemia with insulin [60], phlorizin [61], sulfonylurea [62], or, more recently, sodium glucose transporter 2 (SGLT-2) inhibitor [63] treatment, can restore GIP effectiveness in T2DM. Interestingly, weight loss has also recently been shown to partially restore GIP activity within subcutaneous abdominal adipose tissue in obese subjects, and it would be interesting to establish if this effect also extends to GIP's action on pancreatic beta-cells [64]. In addition, studies have shown that a peptide hormone co-secreted with GIP from a subset of K-cells, namely xenin [65; Figure 3.1], can potentiate the biological actions of GIP [66]. In harmony with this, both GIP [67] and xenin [68] have been demonstrated to be produced locally within islet cells, suggesting possible positive intra-islet interactions. Encouragingly, numerous stable, long-acting xenin compounds have been characterized recently, and all have been shown to augment GIP action [66,69–72]. Moreover, an enzymatically stable GIP/xenin hybrid peptide that incorporates the key bioactive regions of GIP and xenin into a single molecule has recently been generated and revealed to restore GIP sensitivity and enhance beta-cell function following sustained administration in diabetic mice [66]. In a similar fashion, a novel dual GIP/GLP-1 receptor agonist hybrid has recently been shown to significantly improve glycemic control and reduce body weight in T2DM patients [73]. Thus, as-yet untapped therapeutic potential exists for various GIP-related molecules in the treatment of obesity and T2DM.

Another potentially interesting avenue for GIP in the treatment of obesity and T2DM centers on its actions outside of the pancreas. Indeed, GIP receptors are demonstrated on adipocytes [74], where GIP is known to increase lipoprotein lipase activity, fatty acid glucose uptake, as well as augmenting insulin-induced fatty acid incorporation into adipocytes and inhibiting lipolysis [55]. In addition to this, clinical findings have established that fat is a potent stimulus for GIP secretion [75] and that GIP levels are increased in obesity [76]. Thus, inhibition of GIP receptor signaling could represent a new treatment approach for obesity and related diabetes in humans, which is in part triggered by consumption of modern-day diets that are typically high in fat. This viewpoint is further strengthened through knowledge that genetic knockout of GIP receptor signaling, or chemical ablation of GIP-secreting K-cells, protects against the development of obesity in rodents [77,78]. With this in mind, various methods of GIP receptor antagonism have undergone preclinical testing in obesity and diabetes.

In terms of peptide-based GIP receptor antagonists, (Pro^3)GIP has received notable attention [79]. As such, (Pro^3)GIP has been shown to antagonize the biological activity of GIP in animals and related rodent-derived cell lines [79,80]. Prolonged administration of (Pro^3)GIP in various animal models of obesity and T2DM consistently improved metabolic state, which was linked to reduced adiposity, amelioration of insulin resistance, and marked improvements in glucose tolerance [81–84]. The favorable effects of (Pro^3)GIP in obesity and diabetes have been reviewed in detail elsewhere [55,85]. However, translation of (Pro^3)GIP effects toward the clinic could be hindered by recent knowledge regarding species-specific actions of this molecule. Thus, (Pro^3)GIP may actually function as a partial GIP receptor activator in humans [86], and very high concentrations induce slight agonist activity in Chinese hamster lung cells transfected with the human GIP receptor [87]. Such effects are not observed with recently reported second-generation GIP antagonists, including (Pro^3)GIP(3–30)Cex-K^{40}[Pal] and GIP(6–30)Cex-K^{40}[Pal] [87,88]. As such, N-terminal truncation of a shorter bioactive form of GIP, namely GIP(1–30) [89], has also yielded antagonists of the GIP receptor [90]. Indeed, recently GIP(3–30) has been characterized as a potent competitive antagonist of the human GIP receptor [91,92]. Whether the biological action profile of GIP(3–30) can be utilized in humans to mimic the clear metabolic benefits of (Pro^3)GIP in obese-diabetic rodents still remains to be answered.

Furthermore, active immunization against GIP is known to improve blood glucose control and metabolic status in mice with obesity-driven forms of diabetes [93–95]. In addition, administration of a monoclonal antibody directed against the C-terminus of GIP attenuated the development of obesity induced by high-fat feeding in mice [96]. In a similar fashion, monoclonal antibodies against the GIP receptor have also been generated that may be potentially useful therapeutic tools [97,98]. As well, a specific, non-peptidic, low-molecular-weight GIP receptor antagonist, SKL-14959, has been characterized [99], with pilot studies revealing that this compound can significantly reduce body weight in high-fat-fed mice [100]. Clearly, the safety, efficacy, and potential for inappropriate immunological responses still need to be established for these alternative methods of annulling GIP receptor signaling in humans. However, the overall concept is reinforced through recognition that the rapid cure of diabetes in obese subjects undergoing Roux-en-Y gastric bypass surgery is partly linked to surgical bypass of GIP-secreting K cells and subsequent reduction in circulating GIP concentrations [101].

3.3.1 Oxyntomodulin

OXM is a 37-amino acid peptide co-secreted with GLP-1 from enteroendocrine L-cells in response to feeding [102]. Similar to GLP-1, it is a PC1/3-derived, post-translational product of the proglucagon gene [12]. Interestingly, the amino acid sequence of OXM comprises the full sequence of glucagon with a C terminal octa-peptide extension [103]. To date, no specific OXM receptor(s) has been identified, and biological effects are attributed to interactions with GLP-1 and glucagon receptors [104]. As such, studies in rodents suggest that glucagon receptor activation by OXM increases energy expenditure, leading to reduced fat mass and improved metabolic control [104]. Thus, although T2DM is characterized by hyperglucagonemia [105], and glucagon antagonism has been suggested as a possible therapeutic avenue in this regard [106,107], centrally mediated actions of glucagon may actually help to improve metabolic control through modulation of energy balance [108]. In addition, simultaneous activation of GLP-1 receptors by OXM to induce well-characterized insulinotropic and body weight–lowering effects add to these beneficial anti-obesity and -diabetic actions [15]. Accordingly, rodent and clinical studies with OXM have demonstrated key advantages, such as reduced food intake and gastric emptying, as well as increased energy expenditure, with an overall lowering of body weight [3,109,110; Table 3.1; Figure 3.1].

Therefore, like the incretin peptides, OXM presents an exciting prospect for development of a novel class of obesity and diabetes drugs. However, native OXM also has a short half-life due to rapid enzymatic degradation by DPP-4, rendering OXM biologically inactive [111]. Structural modifications have been used to develop stable, longer-acting OXM derivatives. Some notable examples include D-Ser^{2}OXM[mPEG-PAL] [112] and D-Ser^{2}OXM(K-γ-glu-Pal) [113] that have N-terminal modifications to prevent DPP-4 action, and either fatty acid derivation and/or addition of a PEG residue to prolong the pharmacodynamic profile. In addition, a recent study has detailed the metabolic benefits of balanced co-agonism of GLP-1 and glucagon receptors in high-cholesterol-fed hamsters [114]. It is therefore unsurprising that major pharmaceutical companies are exploring options for developing novel dual GLP-1 and glucagon receptor–acting peptides for obesity and diabetes treatment [3]. Although some details in this regard are available, such as GLP-1/glucagon dual-receptor agonists currently being developed by Transition Therapeutics Inc., Merck, AstraZeneca, OPKO Biologics, Sanofi, Zealand Pharma, and Boehringer Ingelheim, details of the peptide structures and phases of development are somewhat vague [115,116]. In addition, G530L/NN9030 (NovoNordisk, Bagsværd, Denmark) has been developed as an enzymatically stable glucagon analogue that is intended to be used in combination with the long-acting GLP-1 mimetic, liraglutide, also owned by NovoNordisk [117]. Interestingly, a study in insulin-deficient T1DM mice has revealed a possible unexpected therapeutic role for OXM in T1DM, related to enhanced beta-cell mass [118].

One of the key challenges in progressing OXM derivatives toward the clinic is recognizing the most appropriate balance of GLP-1 and glucagon receptor activation to yield enhanced beneficial metabolic effects alongside reduced adverse effects. Nonetheless, novel hybrid molecules incorporating the structure of OXM along with structure of GIP have already been characterized and shown to exhibit weight-reducing and antidiabetic properties through positive modulation of glucagon, GLP-1, and GIP receptors [119]. Interestingly, this GIP-OXM hybrid was also revealed to improve bone strength and quality in an animal model of T2DM [120]. Thus, there appears to be a clear rationale for the clinical development of OXM-based therapeutics for the treatment of obesity and T2DM.

3.3.2 Cholecystokinin

CCK is an intestinal-derived hormone released by enteroendocrine I-cells in response to nutrient consumption [121]. CCK binds to specific GPCRs, namely CCK$_1$ receptors expressed in intestinal mucosa and vagal afferents, with activation leading to induction of gallbladder contraction, release of pancreatic juices, reduced gut motility, satiety, and control of energy turnover (Cummings and Overduin 2007; Table 3.1; Figure 3.1). However, CCK also binds CCK$_2$ receptors, which are confined to gastric mucosa and the CNS [122]. Based on the prominent satiety and energy regulation effects induced by CCK$_1$ receptor activation, therapeutic applicability of CCK for obesity and T2DM has long been suggested. This was first postulated by Gibbs and co-workers in 1973, where parenteral injection of biologically active CCK in rodents was shown to inhibit food intake in a dose-dependent manner [123]. Similar appetite-suppressive effects were later confirmed in pigs [124] and humans [125]. CCK has also been shown to stimulate insulin secretion in rodents [126] and humans [127]. Furthermore, evidence suggests that CCK plays an important role in inhibiting beta-cell apoptosis and preserving beta-cell mass [128], an effect that is closely linked to the beta-cell-sparing effects of GLP-1 [129]. The biological actions of CCK are therefore somewhat similar to the incretin hormones, giving further hope to the idea that CCK has promising potential as an anti-obesity and/or-diabetic therapy. However, like many other regulatory peptide hormones, CCK is rapidly cleaved and inactivated by circulating enzymes, most notably aminopeptidase A [130].

Preliminary studies have demonstrated that structural changes at the N terminal of CCK, or derivation with a covalently attached PEG or fatty acid molecule, can prevent enzymatic degradation and enhance the therapeutic potential of CCK [95,131,132]. Most recently, modification of the smallest bioactive form of CCK, namely CCK-8 [95], through addition of a pGlu-Gln dipeptide to the N-terminal, has yielded a peptide analogue with a significantly improved pharmacokinetic and pharmacodynamic profile, and clear obesity and diabetes therapeutic efficacy in preclinical studies [95,126]. Mechanistic studies reveal that (pGlu-Gln)-CCK-8 modulates hypothalamic neuropeptide Y and melanocortin pathways to induce significant appetite suppressive actions [14]. Interestingly, a novel (pGlu-Gln)-CCK-8/GLP-1 hybrid peptide has also been characterized that exhibits prominent insulinotropic, glucose-lowering, and satiety actions [133]. These beneficial effects are presumably related to the established additive and/or synergistic advantages of combining GLP-1 and CCK receptor signaling in obesity and diabetes [134–137]. Despite these positive observations, studies to establish the translational benefits of peptide-based, CCK-related therapies in humans are still missing. This represents a key area of future research for CCK-based therapeutics, with preclinical data suggesting likely positive outcomes.

3.3.3 PEPTIDE YY

PYY, named due to the characteristic Tyr (Y) residues found at N and C termini of the peptide [138], is a 36-amino acid peptide hormone co-secreted with GLP-1 and OXM from intestinal L-cells [139]. In addition, PYY release is also believed to be governed by a neuroendocrine reflex, whereby nutrient availability in the upper gut leads to neuronal stimulation of L-cells in the distal gut [140]. Moreover, similar to GIP, GLP-1, and CCK [26,67,141] PYY expression and secretion has been evidenced in pancreatic islet cells [68,142,143]. In the bloodstream, there are two biologically active forms of PYY, native PYY(1-36) and the DPP-4 metabolite PYY(3-36), with PYY(3-36) being the most abundant form [144]. PYY exerts its biological effects through interaction with the Y class of GPCRs, which are also activated by closely related ligands neuropeptide Y (NPY) and pancreatic polypeptide (PP) [12]. PYY(1-36) acts as a ligand for Y_1, Y_2, and Y_5 receptors; however, DPP-4 cleavage of the N-terminal Tyr^1-Pro^2 dipeptide, to yield PYY(3-36), results in the generation of a Y_2 receptor–specific ligand [145]. The biological action profile of PYY essentially includes inhibition of upper gastrointestinal motility, mucosal fluid and electrolyte secretion, as well as colonic transit that together promote satiety and modulate energy balance [12,146; Table 3.1; Figure 3.1]. In addition, PYY is believed to regulate energy intake centrally via Y_2 receptor activation and induction of the "ileal brake" mechanism, resulting in reduced gut motility [138,147]. Interestingly, a recent study in obese volunteers employing co-infusion of GLP-1, OXM, and PYY demonstrates impressive effects to suppress appetite [110], highlighting potentially exploitable therapeutic effects of simultaneous activation of numerous regulatory hormone receptors. Further to this, an important role for PYY in pancreatic beta-cell survival and function has also recently been revealed, which is considered to be a Y_1 receptor–dependent effect [68,148; Table 3.1; Figure 3.1]. However, to date, in terms of PYY therapies for obesity and diabetes, modulation of the effects of PYY(3-36) on Y_2 receptors has received the most attention [149].

Accordingly, studies in rodents and humans show that peripheral administration of PYY(3-36) induces a marked reduction in food intake [144,149] and enhanced energy expenditure [150]. To circumvent the need for parenteral administration of peptide therapies and therefore possibly improve patient compliance, small clinical studies with nasal delivery of PYY(3-36) have been conducted [16,151], as well as studies with oral delivery in rodents [152,153]. Although these approaches were relatively successful in terms of drug delivery, adverse effects have been observed following administration of PYY(3-36) in humans, including nausea, sweating, and abdominal discomfort, which may ultimately foil therapeutic realization of PYY(3-36) [16,154]. As noted earlier, Y_1 receptor activation has been shown to prevent beta-cell apoptosis [155], with obvious therapeutic benefits for diabetes. Indeed, the idea of a Y_1 receptor–specific PYY-based therapy for beta-cell replenishment in diabetes is further strengthened through knowledge that the remission of T2DM following certain types of bariatric surgery [156,157] is linked to enhanced PYY secretion and accompanying restoration of pancreatic islet survival [158,159]. Thus, while Y_2 receptor–specific drugs mimicking the action of PYY(3-36) have thus far failed to achieve clinical success for obesity and diabetes, a PYY compound specific for Y_1 receptors could hold real promise as a novel antidiabetic therapeutic.

3.4 FUTURE PERSPECTIVES

Given the complex nature of obesity and T2DM that involves multiple etiologies, the task of management of these diseases requires a diversified approach. In all cases, non-pharmacological lifestyle and nutritional advice to help reduce body weight is still of paramount importance in the management of obesity and related T2DM [160]. However, in the majority of T2DM cases, failure to achieve appropriate long-term glycemic control leads to the inevitable introduction of antidiabetic medication. Evidently, gut-derived regulatory peptides are attractive therapeutic candidates because they evoke physiological responses in a largely regulated and receptor-specific manner. The primary aim when developing peptide-based therapies has centered on enhancement of potency and durability of biological effects of the native peptide, which translates into dramatically improved therapeutic efficacy. This is clearly highlighted through the successful introduction of GLP-1 mimetics into the T2DM clinic [35], and, more recently, their approval for obesity management [34]. A similar avenue toward the clinic for GIP-, OXM-, CCK-, and PYY-based molecules can also be envisaged, given the notable benefits exerted by these peptides in obesity and diabetes. In addition, development of novel therapeutic compounds that can combine the biological actions of numerous regulatory gut hormones into a single compound—for instance, a hybrid molecule that incorporates a principally insulinotropic peptide with a hormone that exerts potent anorectic actions—appears a logical and achievable approach [117,133]. Moreover, through recent advances in peptide chemical engineering and medicinal chemistry, tri-agonist peptides have been successfully synthesized and characterized [38,117,119,161], with prominent metabolic and weight-lowering benefits noted. Clearly, our understanding of the physiology and therapeutic relevance of gut-derived hormones is rapidly advancing, which can be expected to lead to development of new and more effective therapeutic agents for both obesity and diabetes.

REFERENCES

1. DeFronzo, R. A., Ferrannini, E., Groop L. et al. 2015. Type 2 diabetes mellitus. *Nat Rev Dis Primers* 1: 15019.
2. Murea, M., Ma, L., Freedman, B. I. 2012. Genetic and environmental factors associated with type 2 diabetes and diabetic vascular complications. *Rev Diabet Stud* 9(1): 6–22.
3. Choudhury, S. M., Tan, T. M., Bloom, S. R. 2016. Gastrointestinal hormones and their role in obesity. *Curr Opin Endocrinol Diabetes Obes* 23(1): 18–22.
4. Ley, S. H., Hamdy, O., Mohan, V., Hu, F. B. 2014. Prevention and management of type 2 diabetes: Dietary components and nutritional strategies. *Lancet* 383(9933): 1999–2007.

5. Sami, W., Ansari, T., Butt, N. S., Hamid, M. R. 2017. Effect of diet on type 2 diabetes mellitus: A review. *Int J Health Sci (Qassim)* 11(2): 65–71.

6. Rehfeld, J. F. 1998. The new biology of gastrointestinal hormones. *Physiol Rev* 78(4): 1087–1108.

7. Drucker, D. J. 2007. The role of gut hormones in glucose homeostasis. *J Clin Invest* 117(1): 24–32.

8. Unger, R. H., and Eisentraut, A. M. 1969. Entero-insular axis. *Arch Intern Med* 123(3): 261–266.

9. Creutzfeldt, W. 1979. The incretin concept today. *Diabetologia* 16(2): 75–85.

10. Nauck, M. A., Heimesaat, M. M., Orskov, C., Holst, J. J., Ebert, R., Creutzfeldt, W. 1993. Preserved incretin activity of glucagon-like peptide 1 [7–36 amide] but not of synthetic human gastric inhibitory polypeptide in patients with type-2 diabetes mellitus. *Clin Invest* 91(1): 301–307.

11. Holst, J. J., Pedersen, J., Wewer Albrechtsen, N. J., Knop, F. K. 2017. The gut: A key to the pathogenesis of type 2 diabetes? *Metab Syndr Relat Disord* 15(6): 259–262.

12. Small, C. J., Bloom, S. R. 2004. Gut hormones as peripheral anti-obesity targets. *Curr Drug Targets CNS Neurol Disord* 3(5): 379–388.

13. Dakin, C. L., Small, C. J., Batterham, R. L. et al. 2004. Peripheral oxyntomodulin reduces food intake and body weight gain in rats. *Endocrinology* 145(6): 2687–2695.

14. Montgomery, I. A., Irwin, N., Flatt, P. R. 2013. Beneficial effects of (pGlu-Gln)-CCK-8 on energy intake and metabolism in high fat fed mice are associated with alterations of hypothalamic gene expression. *Horm Metab Res* 45(6): 471–473.

15. Kosinski, J. R., Hubert, J., Carrington, P. E. et al. 2012. The glucagon receptor is involved in mediating the body weight-lowering effects of oxyntomodulin. *Obesity (Silver Spring)*. 20(8): 1566–1571.

16. De Silva, A., and Bloom, S. R. 2012. Gut hormones and appetite control: A focus on PYY and GLP-1 as therapeutic targets in obesity. *Gut Liver* 6(1): 10–20.

17. Secher, A., Jelsing, J., Baquero, A. F. et al. 2014. The arcuate nucleus mediates GLP-1 receptor agonist liraglutide-dependent weight loss. *J Clin Invest* 124: 4473–4488.

18. Breen, D. M., Rasmussen, B. A., Côté, C. D., Jackson, V. M., Lam, T. K. 2013. Nutrient-sensing mechanisms in the gut as therapeutic targets for diabetes. *Diabetes* 62(9): 3005–3013.

19. Côté, C. D., Zadeh-Tahmasebi, M., Rasmussen, B. A., Duca, F. A., Lam, T. K. 2014. Hormonal signaling in the gut. *J Biol Chem* 289(17): 11642–11649.

20. Duca, F. A., Bauer, P. V., Hamr, S. C., Lam, T. K. 2015. Glucoregulatory relevance of small intestinal nutrient sensing in physiology, bariatric surgery, and pharmacology. *Cell Metab* 22(3): 367–380.

21. Reimann, F., Gribble, F. M. 2016. Mechanisms underlying glucose-dependent insulinotropic polypeptide and glucagon-like peptide-1 secretion. *J Diabetes Investig* 7(S1): 13–19.

22. Cuenco, J., Minnion, J., Tan, T. et al. 2017. Degradation paradigm of the gut hormone, pancreatic polypeptide, by hepatic and renal peptidases. *Endocrinology* 158(6): 1755–1765.

23. Brubaker, P. L., Schloos, J., Drucker, D. J. 1998. Regulation of glucagon-like peptide-1 synthesis and secretion in the GLUTag enteroendocrine cell line. *Endocrinology* 139(10): 4108–4114.

24. Elliott, R. M., Morgan, L. M., Tredger, J. A., Deacon, S., Wright, J., Marks, V. 1993. Glucagon-like peptide-1 (7–36) amide and glucose-dependent insulinotropic polypeptide secretion in response to nutrient ingestion in man: Acute post-prandial and 24-h secretion patterns. *J Endocrinol* 138(1): 159–166.

25. Trapp, S., Richards, J. E. 2013. The gut hormone glucagon-like peptide-1 produced in brain: Is this physiologically relevant? *Curr Opin Pharmacol* 13(6): 964–969.

26. Vasu, S., Moffett, R. C., Thorens, B., Flatt, P. R. 2014. Role of endogenous GLP-1 and GIP in beta cell compensatory responses to insulin resistance and cellular stress. *PLoS One* 9(6): e101005.

27. Drucker, D. J. 2005. Biologic actions and therapeutic potential of the proglucagon-derived peptides. *Nat Clin Pract Endocrinol Metab* 1(1): 22–31.

28. Gautier, J. F., Fetita, S., Sobngwi, E., Salaün-Martin, C. 2005. Biological actions of the incretins GIP and GLP-1 and therapeutic perspectives in patients with type 2 diabetes. *Diabetes Metab* 31(3): 233–242.

29. Vilsbøll, T. 2009. The effects of glucagon-like peptide-1 on the beta cell. *Diabetes Obes Metab* 11(3): 8–11.

30. Moffett, R. C., Vasu, S., Thorens, B., Drucker, D. J., Flatt, P. R. 2014. Incretin receptor null mice reveal key role of GLP-1 but not GIP in pancreatic beta cell adaptation to pregnancy. *PLoS One* 9(6): e96863.

31. Moffett, R. C., Vasu, S., Flatt, P. R. 2015. Functional GIP receptors play a major role in islet compensatory response to high fat feeding in mice. *Biochim Biophys Acta* 1850(6): 1206–1214.

32. Volz, A., Göke, R., Lankat-Buttgereit, B., Fehmann, H. C., Bode, H. P., Göke, B. 1995. Molecular cloning, functional expression, and signal transduction of the GIP-receptor cloned from a human insulinoma. *FEBS Lett* 373(1): 23–29.

33. Farr, O. M., Sofopoulos, M., Tsoukas, M. A. 2016. GLP-1 receptors exist in the parietal cortex, hypothalamus and medulla of human brains and the GLP-1 analogue liraglutide alters brain activity related to highly desirable food cues in individuals with diabetes: A crossover, randomised, placebo-controlled trial. *Diabetologia* 59(5): 954–965.

34. Mehta, A., Marso, S. P., Neeland, I. J. 2016. Liraglutide for weight management: A critical review of the evidence. *Obesity Science & Practice* 3(1): 1–14.

35. Htike, Z. Z., Zaccardi, F., Papamargaritis, D., Webb, D. R., Khunti, K., Davies, M. J. 2017. Efficacy and safety of glucagon-like peptide-1 receptor agonists in type 2 diabetes: A systematic review and mixed-treatment comparison analysis. *Diabetes Obes Metab* 19(4): 524–536

36. Trujillo, J. M., Nuffer, W., Ellis, S. L. 2015. GLP-1 receptor agonists: A review of head-to-head clinical studies. *Ther Adv Endocrinol Metab* 6(1): 19–28.

37. Jones, A. G., Lonergan, M., Henley, W. E., Pearson, E. R., Hattersley, A. T., Shields, B. M. 2016. Should studies of diabetes treatment stratification correct for baseline HbA1c? *PLoS One* 11(4): e0152428.

38. Lorenz, M., Evers. A, Wagner, M. 2013. Recent progress and future options in the development of GLP-1 receptor agonists for the treatment of diabesity. *Bioorg Med Chem Lett* 23(14): 4011–4018.

39. Arnold, S., Jowett, J., Balance, J. 2015. Synergistic action of PE0139, a super-long-acting basal insulin & PB1023 a weekly GLP1 receptor agonist. *Diabetes* 64(S1): A44.

40. Blundell, J., Finlayson, G., Axelsen, M. et al. 2017. Effects of once-weekly semaglutide on appetite, energy intake, control of eating, food preference and body weight in subjects with obesity. *Diabetes Obes Metab* 19(9): 1242–1251.

41. Manandhar, B., Ahn, J. M. 2015. Glucagon-like Peptide-1 (GLP-1) Analogs: Recent Advances, New Possibilities, and Therapeutic Implications. *J Med Chem* 58(3): 1020–1037.

42. Patterson, S., de Kort, M., Irwin, N. et al. 2015. Pharmacological characterization and antidiabetic activity of a long-acting glucagon-like peptide-1 analogue conjugated to an antithrombin III-binding pentasaccharide. *Diabetes Obes Metab* 17(8): 760–770.

43. Lee, C. Y. 2016. Glucagon-Like peptide-1 formulation–The present and future development in diabetes treatment. *Basic Clin Pharmacol Toxicol* 118(3): 173–180.

44. Jabbour, S., Pieber, T. R., Rosenstock, J., Hartoft-Nielsen, M. L., Højbjerg, O. K., Davies, M. 2016. Robust dose-dependent glucose lowering and body weight (BW) reductions with the novel oral formulation of semaglutide in patients with early type 2 diabetes (T2D). *Endocrine Reviews* 37(S2): OR15-3.

45. Kalra, S., Baruah, M. P., Sahay, R. K., Unnikrishnan, A. G., Uppal, S., Adetunji, O. 2016. Glucagon-like peptide-1 receptor agonists in the treatment of type 2 diabetes: Past, present, and future. *Indian J Endocrinol Metab* 20(2): 254–267.

46. Nauck, M. A., Friedrich, N. 2013. Do GLP-1–Based therapies increase cancer risk? *Diabetes Care* 36(2): S245–S252.

47. Elashoff, M., Matveyenko, A. V., Gier, B., Elashoff, R., Butler, P. C. 2015. Pancreatitis, pancreatic, and thyroid cancer with glucagon-like peptide-1–based therapies. *Gastrenterology* 141(1): 150–156.

48. Nauck, M. A., Meier, J. J. 2014. Studying pancreatic risks caused by incretin-based therapies is it a game? it's not a game! *Endocrinology* 8(4): 895–897.

49. Brown, J. C., Pederson, R. A. 1970. A multiparameter study on the action of preparations containing cholecystokinin-pancreozymin. *Scand J Gastroenterol* 5(6): 537–541.

50. Beck, B. 1989. Gastric inhibitory polypeptide: A gut hormone with anabolic functions. *J Mol Endocrinol* 2(3): 169–174.

51. Deacon, C. F., Ahrén, B. 2011. Physiology of Incretins in Health and Disease. *Rev Diabet Stud* 8(3): 293–306.

52. Trümper, A., Trümper, K., Hörsch, D. 2002. Mechanisms of mitogenic and anti-apoptotic signalling by glucose dependent insulinotropic polypeptide in beta (INS-1) cells. *J Endocrinol* 174(2): 233–246.

53. Kim, S. J., Nian, C., Tsuneoka, M., Koda, Y., Fosh, C. H. 2005. Glucose dependent insulinotropic polypeptide (GIP) stimulation of pancreatic beta cell survival is dependent upon phosphatidyl inositol 3 kinase (PI3K)/protein kinase B (PKB) signalling, inactivation of forkhead transcription factor Foxo1, and down regulation of bax expression. *J Biol Chem* 280(23): 22297–22307.

54. Renner, S., Fehlings, C., Herbach, N. et al. 2010. Glucose intolerance and reduced proliferation of pancreatic β-cells in transgenic pigs with impaired glucose-dependent insulinotropic polypeptide function. *Diabetes* 59(5): 1228–1238.

55. Irwin, N., Flatt, P. R. 2009. Therapeutic potential for GIP receptor agonists and antagonists. *Best Pract Res Clin Endocrinol Metab* 23(4): 499–512.

56. Mentlein, R., Gallwitz, B., Schmidt, W. E. 1993. Dipeptidyl-peptidase IV hydrolyses gastric inhibitory polypeptide, glucagon-like peptide-1(7–36)amide, peptide histidine methionine and is responsible for their degradation in human serum. *Eur J Biochem* 214(3): 829–835.

57. Gault, V. A., O'Harte, F. P., Flatt, P. R. 2003. Glucose-dependent insulinotropic polypeptide (GIP): Antidiabetic and anti-obesity potential? *Neuropeptides* 37(5): 253–263.

58. Shu, L., Matveyenko, A. V., Kerr-Conte, J., Cho, J. H., McIntosh, C. H., Maedler, K. 2009. Decreased TCF7L2 protein levels in type 2 diabetes mellitus correlate with downregulation of GIP- and GLP-1 receptors and impaired beta-cell function. *Hum Mol Genet* 18(13): 2388–2399.

59. Pathak, V., Vasu, S., Flatt, P. R., Irwin, N. 2014. Effects of chronic exposure of clonal β-cells to elevated glucose and free fatty acids on incretin receptor gene expression and secretory responses to GIP and GLP-1. *Diabetes Obes Metab* 16(4): 357–365.

60. Højberg, P. V., Vilsbøll, T., Rabøl, R. et al. 2009. Four weeks of near-normalisation of blood glucose improves the insulin response to glucagon-like peptide-1 and glucose-dependent insulinotropic polypeptide in patients with type 2 diabetes. *Diabetologia* 52(2): 199–207.

61. Piteau, S., Olver, A., Kim, S. J. et al. 2007. Reversal of islet GIP receptor down-regulation and resistance to GIP by reducing hyperglycemia in the Zucker rat. *Biochem Biophys Res Commun* 362(4): 1007–1012.

62. Fukase, N., Manaka, H., Sugiyama, K. et al. 1995. Response of truncated glucagon-like peptide-1 and gastric inhibitory polypeptide to glucose ingestion in non-insulin dependent diabetes mellitus. Effect of sulfonylurea therapy. *Acta Diabetol* 32(3): 465–469.

63. Millar, P. J., Pathak, V., Moffett, R. C. et al. 2016. Beneficial metabolic actions of a stable GIP agonist following pre-treatment with a SGLT2 inhibitor in high fat fed diabetic mice. *Mol Cell Endocrinol* 420: 37–45.

64. Asmar, M., Arngrim, N., Simonsen, L. et al. 2016. The blunted effect of glucose-dependent insulinotropic polypeptide in subcutaneous abdominal adipose tissue in obese subjects is partly reversed by weight loss. *Nutr Diabetes* 6(5): e208.

65. Taylor, A. I., Irwin, N., McKillop, A. M., Patterson, S., Flatt, P. R., Gault, V. A. 2010. Evaluation of the degradation and metabolic effects of the gut peptide xenin on insulin secretion, glycaemic control and satiety. *J Endocrinol* 207: 87–93.

66. Hasib, A., Ming, T. N., Gault, V. A. et al. 2017. An enzymatically stable GIP/xenin hybrid peptide restores GIP sensitivity, enhances beta cell function and improves glucose homeostasis in high-fat-fed mice. *Diabetologia* 30(3): 541–552.

67. Fujita, Y., Wideman, R. D., Asadi, A. et al. 2010. Glucose-dependent insulinotropic polypeptide is expressed in pancreatic islet alpha-cells and promotes insulin secretion. *Gastroenterology* 138(5): 1966–1975.

68. Khan, D., Vasu, S., Moffett, R. C., Irwin, N., Flatt, P. R. 2016. Islet distribution of Peptide YY and its regulatory role in primary mouse islets and immortalised rodent and human beta-cell function and survival. *Mol Cell Endocrinol* 436: 102–113.

69. Martin, C. M., Gault, V. A., McClean, S., Flatt, P. R., Irwin, N. 2012. Degradation, insulin secretion, glucose-lowering and GIP additive actions of a palmitate-derivatised analogue of xenin-25. *Biochem Pharmacol* 84(3): 312–319.

70. Martin, C. M., Parthsarathy, V., Pathak, V., Gault, V. A., Flatt, P. R., Irwin, N. 2014. Characterisation of the biological activity of xenin-25 degradation fragment peptides. *J Endocrinol* 221(2): 193–200.

71. Martin, C. M., Parthsarathy, V., Hasib, A. et al. 2016. Biological activity and antidiabetic potential of C-Terminal octapeptide fragments of the gut-Derived hormone xenin. *PLoS One* 11(3): e0152818.

72. Parthsarathy, V., Irwin, N., Hasib, A. et al. 2016. A novel chemically modified analogue of xenin-25 exhibits improved glucose-lowering and insulin-releasing properties. *Biochim Biophys Acta* 1860(4): 757–764.

73. Frias, J. P., Bastyr, E. J., Vignati, L. et al. 2017. The sustained effects of a dual GIP/GLP-1 receptor agonist, NNC0090-2746, in patients with type 2 diabetes. *Cell Metab* 26(2): 343–352.

74. Yip, R. G., Boylan, M. O., Kieffer, T. J., Wolfe, M. M. 1998. Functional GIP receptors are present on adipocytes. *Endocrinology* 139(9): 4004–4007.

75. Falko, J. M., Crockett, S. E., Cataland, S., Mazzaferri, E. L. 1975. Gastric inhibitory polypeptide (GIP) stimulated by fat ingestion in man. *J Clin Endocrinol Metab* 41(2): 260–565.

76. Salera, M., Giacomoni P., Pironi, L. et al. 1982. Gastric inhibitory polypeptide release after oral glucose: Relationship to glucose intolerance, diabetes mellitus, and obesity. *J Clin Endocrinol Metab* 55(2): 329–336.

77. Miyawaki, K., Yamada, Y., Ban, N. et al. 2002. Inhibition of gastric inhibitory polypeptide signaling prevents obesity. *Nat Med* 2002;8(7): 738–742.

78. Althage, M. C., Ford, E. L., Wang, S., Tso, P., Polonsky, K. S., Wice, B. M. 2008. Targeted ablation of glucose-dependent insulinotropic polypeptide-producing cells in transgenic mice reduces obesity and insulin resistance induced by a high fat diet. *J Biol Chem* 283: 18365–18376.

79. Gault, V. A., O'Harte, F. P. M., Harriott, P., Flatt, P. R. 2002. Characterization of the cellular and metabolic effects of a novel enzyme-resistant antagonist of glucose-dependent insulinotropic polypeptide. *Biochem Biophys Res Commun* 290: 1420–1426.

80. Irwin, N., Gault, V. A., Green, B. D. et al. 2004. Effects of short-term chemical ablation of the GIP receptor on insulin secretion, islet morphology and glucose homeostasis in mice. *Biol Chem* 385(9): 845–352.

81. Irwin, N., McClean, P. L., O'Harte, F. P. M., Gault, V. A., Harriott, P., Flatt, P. R. 2007. Early administration of the glucose-dependent insulinotropic polypeptide receptor antagonist, (Pro³)GIP, prevents the development of diabetes and related metabolic abnormalities associated with genetically-inherited obesity in *ob/ob* mice. *Diabetologia* 50: 1532–1540.

82. Gault, V. A., Hunter, K., Irwin, N. et al. 2007. Characterisation and glucoregulatory actions of a novel acylated form of the (Pro³)GIP receptor antagonist in type 2 diabetes. *Biol Chem* 388: 173–179.

83. McClean, P. L., Irwin, N., Cassidy, R. S., Holst, J. J., Gault, V. A., Flatt, P. R. 2007. GIP receptor antagonism reverses obesity, insulin resistance and associated metabolic disturbances induced in mice by prolonged consumption of high fat diet. *Am J Physiol Endocrinol Metab* 293: E1746–E1755.

84. McClean, P. L., Gault, V. A., Irwin, N., McCluskey, J. T., Flatt, P. R. 2008. Daily administration of the GIP-R antagonist (Pro3)GIP in streptozotocin-induced diabetes suggests that insulin-dependent mechanisms are critical to anti-obesity-diabetes actions of (Pro3)GIP. *Diabetes Obes Metab* 2008 10(4): 336–342.

85. Irwin, N., Gault, V., Flatt, P. R. 2010.Therapeutic potential of the original incretin hormone glucose-dependent insulinotropic polypeptide: Diabetes, obesity, osteoporosis and Alzheimer's disease? *Expert Opin Investig Drugs* 19(9): 1039–1048.

86. Sparre-Ulrich, A. H., Hansen, L. S., Svendsen, B. et al. 2016. Species-specific action of (Pro3)GIP–A full agonist at human GIP receptors, but a partial agonist and competitive antagonist at rat and mouse GIP receptors. *Br J Pharmacol* 173(1): 27–38.

87. Pathak, V., Gault, V. A., Flatt, P. R., Irwin, N. 2015. Antagonism of gastric inhibitory polypeptide (GIP) by palmitoylation of GIP analogues with N- and C-terminal modifications improves obesity and metabolic control in high fat fed mice. *Mol Cell Endocrinol* 401: 120–129.

88. Pathak, V., Vasu, S., Gault, V. A., Flatt, P. R., Irwin, N. 2015. Sequential induction of beta cell rest and stimulation using stable GIP inhibitor and GLP-1 mimetic peptides improves metabolic control in C57BL/KsJ db/db mice. *Diabetologia* 58(9): 2144–2153.

89. Alaña, I., Hewage, C. M., Malthouse, J. P., Parker, J. C., Gault, V. A., O'Harte, F. P. 2004. NMR structure of the glucose-dependent insulinotropic polypeptide fragment, GIP(1-30)amide. *Biochem Biophys Res Commun* 325(1): 281–286.

90. Hansen, L. S., Sparre-Ulrich, A. H., Christensen, M. et al. 2016. N-terminally and C-terminally truncated forms of glucose-dependent insulinotropic polypeptide are high-affinity competitive antagonists of the human GIP receptor. *Br J Pharmacol* 173(5): 826–838.

91. Gasbjerg, L. S., Christensen, M. B., Hartmann, B. et al. 2017. GIP(3-30)NH_2 is an efficacious GIP receptor antagonist in humans: A randomised, double-blinded, placebo-controlled, crossover study. *Diabetologia* 61(2): 413–423.

92. Sparre-Ulrich, A. H., Gabe, M. N., Gasbjerg, L. S. et al. 2017. GIP(3-30)NH_2 is a potent competitive antagonist of the GIP receptor and effectively inhibits GIP-mediated insulin, glucagon, and somatostatin release. *Biochem Pharmacol* 131: 78–88.

93. Irwin, N., McClean, P. L., Patterson, S., Hunter, K., Flatt, P. R. 2009. Active immunisation against gastric inhibitory polypeptide (GIP) improves blood glucose control in an animal model of obesity-diabetes. *Biol Chem* 390(1): 75–80.

94. Montgomery, I. A., Irwin, N., Flatt, P. R. 2010. Active immunization against (Pro(3))GIP improves metabolic status in high-fat-fed mice. *Diabetes Obes Metab* 12(9): 744–751.

95. Irwin, N., Montgomery, I. A., Flatt, P. R. 2012. Evaluation of the long-term effects of gastric inhibitory polypeptide-ovalbumin conjugates on insulin resistance, metabolic dysfunction, energy balance and cognition in high-fat-fed mice. *Br J Nutr* 108(1): 46–56.

96. Boylan, M. O., Glazebrook, P. A., Tatalovic, M., Wolfe, M. M. 2015. Gastric inhibitory polypeptide immunoneutralization attenuates development of obesity in mice. *Am J Physiol Endocrinol Metab* 309(12): E1008–E1018.

97. Ravn, P., Madhurantakam, C., Kunze, S. et al. 2013. Structural and pharmacological characterization of novel potent and selective monoclonal antibody antagonists of glucose-dependent insulinotropic polypeptide receptor. *J Biol Chem* 288(27): 19760–19772.

98. Könitzer, J. D., Pramanick, S., Pan, Q. 2017. Generation of a highly diverse panel of antagonistic chicken monoclonal antibodies against the GIP receptor. *MAbs* 9(3): 536–549.

99. Nakamura, T., Tanimoto, H., Mizuno, Y., Tsubamoto, Y., Noda, H. 2012. Biological and functional characteristics of a novel low-molecular weight antagonist of glucose-dependent insulinotropic polypeptide receptor, SKL-14959, in vitro and in vivo. *Diabetes Obes Metab* 14(6): 511–517.

100. Tsubamoto, Y., Nakamura, T., Kinoshita, H., Tanimoto, H., Noda, H. 2008. A novel low-molecular weight antagonist of glucose-dependent insulinotropic polypeptide receptor, SKL14959, prevents obesity and insulin resistance. *Diabetologia* 51: S373.

101. Meek, C. L., Lewis, H. B., Reimann, F., Gribble, F. M., Park, A. J. 2016. The effect of bariatric surgery on gastrointestinal and pancreatic peptide hormones. *Peptides* 77: 28–37.

102. Wynne, K., and Bloom, S. R. 2006. The role of oxyntomodulin and peptide tyrosine-tyrosine (PYY) in appetite control. *Nat Clin Pract Endocrinol Metab* 2(11): 612–620.

103. Ghatei, M. A., Uttenthal, L. O., Christofides, N. D., Bryant, M. G., Bloom, S. R. 1983. Molecular forms of human enteroglucagon in tissue and plasma: Plasma responses to nutrient stimuli in health and in disorders of the upper gastrointestinal tract. *J Clin Endocrinol Metab* 57: 488–495.

104. Pocai, A., Carrington, P. E., Adams, J. R. et al. 2009. Glucagon-like peptide 1/glucagon receptor dual agonism reverses obesity in mice. *Diabetes* 58(10): 2258–2266.

105. D'Alessio, D. 2011. The role of dysregulated glucagon secretion in type 2 diabetes. *Diabetes Obes Metab* 13(l): 126–132.

106. Irwin, N., Franklin, Z. J., O'Harte, F. P. 2013a. desHis¹Glu⁹-glucagon-[mPEG] and desHis¹Glu⁹(Lys³⁰PAL)-glucagon: Long-acting peptide-based PEGylated and acylated glucagon receptor antagonists with potential antidiabetic activity. *Eur J Pharmacol* 709(1–3): 43–51.

107. O'Harte, F. P., Franklin, Z. J., Irwin, N. 2014. Two novel glucagon receptor antagonists prove effective therapeutic agents in high-fat-fed and obese diabetic mice. *Diabetes Obes Metab* 16(12): 1214–1222.

108. Pocai, A. 2013. Action and therapeutic potential of oxyntomodulin. *Mol Metab* 3(3): 241–251.

109. Baggio, L. L., Huang, Q., Brown, T. J., Drucker, D. J. 2004. Oxyntomodulin and glucagon like peptide 1 differentially regulate murine food intake and energy expenditure. *Gastroenterology* 127(2): 546–558.

110. Tan, T., Behary, P., Tharakan, G. 2017. The effect of a subcutaneous infusion of GLP-1, OXM and PYY on energy intake and expenditure in obese volunteers. *J Clin Endocrinol Metab* 102(7): 2364–2372.

111. Pocai, A. 2012. Unraveling oxyntomodulin, GLP1's enigmatic brother. *J Endocrinol* 215(3): 335–346.

112. Kerr, B. D., Flatt, P. R., Gault, V. A. 2010. (D-Ser2)Oxm[mPEG-PAL]: A novel chemically modified analogue of oxyntomodulin with antihyperglycaemic, insulinotropic and anorexigenic actions. *Biochem Pharmacol* 80(11): 1727–1735.

113. Pathak, N. M., Pathak, V., Lynch, A. M., Irwin, N., Gault, V. A., Flatt, P. R. 2015. Stable oxyntomodulin analogues exert positive effects on hippocampal neurogenesis and gene expression as well as improving glucose homeostasis in high fat fed mice. *Mol Cell Endocrinol* 412: 95–103.

114. Patel, V., Joharapurkar, A., Kshirsagar, S. 2017. Balanced coagonist of GLP-1 and glucagon receptors corrects dyslipidemia by improving FGF21 sensitivity in hamster model. *Drug Res (Stuttg)* 67(12): 730–736. [Epub ahead of print].

115. Mittermayer, F., Caveney, E., Claudia, O. D. et al. 2015. Addressing unmet medical needs in type 2 diabetes: A narrative review of drugs under development. *Curr Diabetes Rev* 11(1): 17–31.

116. Sánchez-Garrido, M. A., Brandt, S. J., Clemmensen, C., Müller, T. D., DiMarchi, R. D., Tschöp, M. H. 2017 GLP-1/glucagon receptor co-agonism for treatment of obesity. *Diabetologia* 60(10): 1851–1861.

117. Finan, B., Clemmensen, C., Müller, T. D. 2015. Emerging opportunities for the treatment of metabolic diseases: Glucagon-like peptide-1 based multi-agonists. *Mol Cell Endocrinol* 15(418): 42–45.

118. Irwin, N., Pathak, V., Pathak, N. M., Gault, V. A., Flatt, P. R. 2015. Sustained treatment with a stable long-acting oxyntomodulin analogue improves metabolic control and islet morphology in an experimental model of type 1 diabetes. *Diabetes Obes Metab* 17(9): 887–895.

119. Bhat, V. K., Kerr, B. D., Flatt, P. R., Gault, V. A. 2013. A novel GIP-oxyntomodulin hybrid peptide acting through GIP, glucagon and GLP-1 receptors exhibits weight reducing and anti-diabetic properties. *Biochem Pharmacol* 85(11): 1655–1662.

120. Mansur, S. A., Mieczkowska, A., Flatt, P. R. et al. 2016. A new stable GIP-Oxyntomodulin hybrid peptide improved bone strength both at the organ and tissue levels in genetically-inherited type 2 diabetes mellitus. *Bone* 87: 102–113.

121. Koop, I., Schindler, M., Bosshammer, A., Scheibner, J., Stange, E., Koop, H. 1996. Physiological control of cholecystokinin release and pancreatic enzyme secretion by intraduodenal bile acids. *Gut* 39(5): 661–667.

122. Wank, S. A. 1995. Cholecystokinin receptors. *Am J Physiol* 269(5): G628–G646.

123. Gibbs, J., Young, R. C., Smith, G. P. 1997. Cholecystokinin decreases food intake in rats. *Obes Res* 5(3): 284–290.

124. Baldwin, B. A., Cooper, T. R., Parrot, R. F. 1982. Effect of cholecystokinin octapeptide on food intake in pigs. *Proc Nutr Soc* 41: 119.

125. Drewe, J., Gadient, A., Rovati, L. C., Beglinger, C. 1992. Role of circulating cholecystokinin in control of fat-induced inhibition of food intake in humans. *Gastroenterology* 102(5): 1654–1659.

126. Irwin, N., Frizelle, P., Montgomery, I. A., Moffett, R. C., O'Harte, F. P., Flatt, P. R. 2012. Beneficial effects of the novel cholecystokinin agonist (pGlu-Gln)-CCK-8 in mouse models of obesity/diabetes. *Diabetologia* 55(10): 2747–2758.

127. Ahrén, B., Pettersson, M., Uvnäs-Moberg, K., Gutniak, M., Efendic, S. 1991. Effects of cholecystokinin (CCK)-8, CCK-33, and gastric inhibitory polypeptide (GIP) on basal and meal-stimulated pancreatic hormone secretion in man. *Diabetes Res Clin Pract* 13: 153–161.

128. Lavine, J. A., Raess, P. W., Stapleton, D. S. et al. 2010. Cholecystokinin is up-regulated in obese mouse islets and expands beta-cell mass by increasing beta-cell survival. *Endocrinology* 151: 3577–3588.

129. Linnemann, A. K., Davis, D. B. 2016. Glucagon-like peptide-1 and cholecystokinin production and signaling in the pancreatic islet as an adaptive response to obesity. *J Diabetes Investig* 7(1): 44–49.

130. Migaud, M., Durieux, C., Viereck, J., Soroca-Lucas, E., Fournié-Zaluski, M. C., Roques, B. P. 1996. The in vivo metabolism of cholecystokinin (CCK-8) is essentially ensured by aminopeptidase A. *Peptides* 17(4): 601–607.

131. O'Harte, F. P., Mooney, M. H., Kelly, C. M., Flatt, P. R. 1998. Glycated cholecystokinin-8 has an enhanced satiating activity and is protected against enzymatic degradation. *Diabetes* 47: 1619–1624.

132. Irwin, N., Frizelle, P., O'Harte, F. P., Flatt, P. R. 2013. (pGlu-Gln)-CCK-8[mPEG]: A novel, long-acting, mini-PEGylated cholecystokinin (CCK) agonist that improves metabolic status in dietary-induced diabetes. *Biochim Biophys Acta* 1830(8): 4009–4016.

133. Pathak, V., Irwin, N., Flatt, P. R. 2015. A Novel CCK-8/GLP-1 hybrid peptide exhibiting prominent insulinotropic, glucose-lowering, and satiety actions with significant therapeutic potential in high-fat-fed mice. *Diabetes* 64(8): 2996–3009.

134. Brennan, I. M., Feltrin, K. L., Horowitz, M. et al. 2005. Evaluation of interaction between CCK and GLP-1 in their effects on appetite, energy intake, and antropyloroduodenal motility in healthy men. *Am J Physiol Regul Integr Comp Physiol* 288(6): 1477–1485.

135. Linnemann, A. K., Neuman, J. C., Battiola, T. J., Wisinski, J. A., Kimple, M. E., Davis, D. B. 2015. Glucagon-like peptide-1 regulates cholecystokinin production in β-Cells to protect from apoptosis. *Mol Endocrinol* 29(7): 978–987.

136. Trevaskis, J. L., Sun, C., Athanacio, J. et al. 2015. Synergistic metabolic benefits of an exenatide analogue and cholecystokinin in diet-induced obese and leptin-deficient rodents. *Diabetes Obes Metab* 17(1): 61–73.

137. Mhalhal, T. R., Washington, M. C., Newman, K., Heath, J. C., Sayegh, A. I. 2017. Exogenous glucagon-like peptide-1 reduces body weight and cholecystokinin-8 enhances this reduction in diet-induced obese male rats. *Physiol Behav* 179: 191–199.

138. Price, S. L., Bloom, S. R. 2014. Protein PYY and its role in metabolism. *Front Horm Res* 42: 147–154.

139. Pedersen-Bjergaard, U., Høst, U., Kelbaek, H. 1996. Influence of meal composition on postprandial peripheral plasma concentrations of vasoactive peptides in man. *Scand J Clin Lab Invest* 56(6): 497–503.

140. Lomax, A. E., Linden, D. R., Mawe, G. M., Sharkey, K. A. 2006. Effects of gastrointestinal inflammation on enteroendocrine cells and enteric neural reflex circuits. *Auton Neurosci* 250(7): 126–127.

141. Lavine, J. A., Kibbe, C. R., Baan, M. et al. 2015. Cholecystokinin expression in the β-cell leads to increased β-cell area in aged mice and protects from streptozotocin-induced diabetes and apoptosis. *Am J Physiol Endocrinol Metab* 309(10): E819–E828.

142. Upchurch, B. H., Aponte, G. W., Leiter, A. B. 1994. Expression of peptide YY in all four islet cell types in the developing mouse pancreas suggests a common peptide YY-producing progenitor. *Development* 120(2): 245–252.

143. Shi, Y. C., Loh, K., Bensellam, M. 2015. Pancreatic PYY is critical in the control of insulin secretion and glucose homeostasis in female mice. *Endocrinology* 156(9): 3122–3136.

144. Le Roux, C. W., Batterham, R. L., Aylwin, S. J. 2006. Attenuated peptide YY release in obese subjects is associated with reduced satiety. *Endocrinology* 147: 3–8.

145. Dumont, Y., Fournier, A., St-Pierre, S., Quirion, R. 1995. Characterization of neuropeptide Y binding sites in rat brain membrane preparations using [125I][Leu31,Pro34]peptide YY and [125I] peptide YY3-36 as selective Y1 and Y2 radioligands. *J Pharmacol Exp Ther* 272(2): 673–680.

146. Stadlbauer, U., Woods, S. C., Langhans, W., Meyer, U. 2015. PYY3-36: Beyond food intake. *Front Neuroendocrinol* 38: 1–11.

147. Fenske, W. K., Bueter, M., Miras, A. D., Ghatei, M. A., Bloom, S. R., le Roux, C. W. 2012. Exogenous peptide YY3-36 and Exendin-4 further decrease food intake, whereas octreotide increases food intake in rats after Roux-en-Y gastric bypass. *Int J Obes (Lond)*. 36(3): 379–384.

148. Persaud, S. J., Bewick, G. A. 2014. Peptide YY: More than just an appetite regulator. *Diabetologia* 57(9): 1762–1769.

149. Batterham, R. L., Bloom, S. R. 2003. The gut hormone peptide YY regulates appetite. *Ann N Y Acad Sci* 994: 162–168.

150. Sloth, B., Holst, J. J., Flint, A., Gregersen, N. T., Astrup A. 2007. Effects of PYY1-36 and PYY3-36 on appetite, energy intake, energy expenditure, glucose and fat metabolism in obese and lean subjects. *Am J Physiol Endocrinol Metab* 292: E1062–E1068.

151. Gantz I., Erondu, N., Mallick, M. et al. 2007. Efficacy and safety of intranasal peptide YY3-36 for weight reduction in obese adults. *J Clin Endocrinol Metab* 92(5): 1754–1757.

152. Acosta, A., Hurtado, M. D., Gorbatyuk, O. et al. 2011. Salivary PYY: A putative bypass to satiety. *PLoS One* 6(10): e26137.

153. Fazen, C., Valentin, D., Fairchild, T., Doyle, R. 2011. Oral delivery of the appetite suppressing peptide hPYY(3–36) through the vitamin B12 uptake pathway. *J Medicinal Chem* 54: 8707–8711.

154. Cegla, J., Cuenco, J., Minnion, J. et al. 2015. Pharmacokinetics and pharmacodynamics of subcutaneously administered PYY3-36 and its analogues in vivo. *Lancet* 385(1): S28.

155. Sam, A. H., Gunner, D. J., King, A. et al. 2012. Selective ablation of peptide YY cells in adult mice reveals their role in beta cell survival. *Gastroenterology* 143(2): 459–468.

156. Perugini, R. A., Malkani, S. 2011. Remission of type 2 diabetes mellitus following bariatric surgery: Review of mechanisms and presentation of the concept of 'reversibility'. *Curr Opin Endocrinol Diabetes Obes* 18(2): 119–128.

157. Ardestani, A., Rhoads, D., Tavakkoli A. 2015. Insulin cessation and diabetes remission after bariatric surgery in adults with insulin-treated type 2 diabetes. *Diabetes Care* 38(4): 659–664.

158. Ramracheya, R. D., McCulloch, L. J., Clark, A. 2016. PYY-Dependent restoration of impaired insulin and glucagon secretion in type 2 diabetes following Roux-En-Y gastric bypass surgery. *Cell Rep* 15(5): 944–950.

159. Guida, C., Stephen, S., Guitton, R., Ramracheya, R. D. 2017. The role of PYY in pancreatic islet physiology and surgical control of diabetes. *Trends Endocrinol Metab* 28(8): 626–636.

160. Van Gaal, L., and Dirinck, E. 2016. Pharmacological approaches in the treatment and maintenance of weight loss. *Diabetes Care* 39(2): S260–S267.

161. Gault, V. A., Bhat, V. K., Irwin, N., Flatt, P. R. 2013. A novel glucagon-like peptide-1 (GLP-1)/glucagon hybrid peptide with triple-acting agonist activity at glucose-dependent insulinotropic polypeptide, GLP-1, and glucagon receptors and therapeutic potential in high fat-fed mice. *J Biol Chem* 288(49): 35581–35591.

4 Metabolic Syndrome
Recognition, Etiology, and Physical Fitness as a Component

Robert W. McGarrah and William E. Kraus

CONTENTS

4.1 METABOLIC SYNDROME

The general concept of metabolic syndrome describes a clustering of metabolic abnormalities associated with increased risk of cardiovascular disease, diabetes, and hypertension.[1–4] Several definitions of metabolic syndrome exist,[5–9] with the most widely used coming from the National Cholesterol Education Program (NCEP) Adult Treatment Program-III (ATP III).[9,10] Using this definition, the prevalence of metabolic syndrome continues to increase in the United States, from 22% in 1994 to 34.5% in 2002.[7,11]

Several excellent reviews of metabolic syndrome exist.[12–15] Hence, rather than presenting another review of the topic, in this chapter, we will discuss several controversies continuing to plague the field and provide compelling lines of evidence establishing the strong relationship between metabolic syndrome, physical activity, and regular exercise. First, we will present evidence from cross-sectional studies consistently reporting significant inverse associations between levels of cardiorespiratory fitness or physical activity and the prevalence of metabolic syndrome (as defined in the ATP III report). Second, we will review studies investigating the effect of nutrition and exercise training on metabolic syndrome as currently defined. Third, we will briefly present evidence of the relationship between exercise and physical activity, and each of the five individual components of metabolic syndrome. In the course of this discussion, several areas of controversy will become apparent.

4.2 OVERVIEW OF CURRENT CONTROVERSIES WITH THE DEFINITION OF METABOLIC SYNDROME

The current diagnostic criteria for metabolic syndrome are detailed in Tables 4.1 through 4.3. As the various components of the condition are invariably associated with some degree of insulin resistance, most consider metabolic syndrome to be a prediabetic state. Studies over the past decade have consistently demonstrated a strong association of metabolic syndrome and the risk of future type 2 diabetes.[16–20] Additionally, metabolic syndrome increases the risk for incident cardiovascular disease and all-cause mortality,[21–23] fatty liver disease,[24–26] and chronic kidney disease.[27] One major area of uncertainty is whether metabolic syndrome *per se* confers risk for these clinical conditions beyond its individual components. That is, is metabolic syndrome truly a syndrome wherein the components act biologically together to lead to disease, or is it merely a convenient clustering of risk factors? To this point, although the ATP III guidelines provide a useful working definition, it is clear that the five diagnostic criteria are not independent. For example, low serum high-density lipoprotein (HDL) cholesterol and high serum triglycerides tend to track together in individuals. This makes the current scoring mechanism (i.e., the need to have three of the five diagnostic criteria) seem somewhat artificial and negatively impacts its predictive utility.

Thus, there is room for further refining the clinical definition of metabolic syndrome. One potential improvement would be to provide differential weighting of the individual diagnostic conditions by providing a scoring system that incorporates the relative predictive capacity of future events or conversion to diabetes of the various components. Another would be to refine the predictive capacity through inclusion of additional diagnostic criteria, such as elevated high-sensitivity C-reactive protein (hsCRP),[19] or, as we argue later, through an assessment of cardiorespiratory fitness.

There are other, less-obvious issues with the current definition. The ATP III and WHO (see Tables 4.1 and 4.2) include elevated blood pressure (BP) as part of the diagnostic criteria. Although most would agree that elevated waist circumference, fasting serum glucose, low serum HDL-cholesterol, and high serum triglycerides tend to all be a part of the same metabolic substrate for insulin resistance and diabetes mellitus, this is less clear for hypertension. More specifically, it is not apparent whether hypertension is another relatively common cardiovascular risk factor tending to occur more frequently than not with other relatively common risk factors (associated with the prediabetic state) or whether, in fact, it is part of a metabolic substrate that is characteristic of individuals on the path to developing diabetes. When all five criteria are considered, we and others

TABLE 4.1
Revised Adult Treatment Program-III Criteria
Metabolic syndrome is diagnosed when any three of the following are present

Risk Factor	Defining Level
Waist Circumference	
Men	> 102 cm (> 40 inches)
Women	> 88 cm (> 35 inches)
Triglycerides	≥ 150 mg/dL or treatment
HDL Cholesterol	
Men	< 40 mg/dL
Women	< 50 mg/dL
Blood pressure	≥ 130/ ≥ 85 mm Hg or treatment
Fasting glucose	≥ 100 mg/dL or treatment

TABLE 4.2

World Health Organization Criteria

Metabolic syndrome is diagnosed when the individual has: diabetes, IFG, IGT, or HOMA insulin resistance and at least two of the following:

Risk Factor	Defining Level
Waist-to-Hip Ratio	
Men	> 0.90
Women	> 0.85
Triglycerides	≥ 150 mg/dL or BMI > 30 kg/m^2 (men and women)
HDL	
Men	< 35 mg/dL
Women	< 39 mg/dL
Urinary albumin	
excretion rate	> 20 μg/min
Blood pressure	≥ 140/90 mm Hg

HDL, high-density lipoprotein; HOMA, homeostatic model assessment [resting determination of insulin sensitivity = (fasting glucose × 0.055551) × (fasting insulin/22.1)]; IFG, impaired fasting glucose; IGT, impaired glucose tolerance.

TABLE 4.3

IDF Criteria

Metabolic syndrome is diagnosed when the individual has: central obesity (waist circumference): ≥ 94 cm (men), ≥ 80 cm (women), and at least two of the following:

Risk Factor	Defining Level
Triglycerides	≥ 150 mg/dL or treatment
HDL	
Men	< 35 mg/dL
Women	< 39 mg/dL or treatment
Fasting glucose	≥ 100 mg/dL or previously diagnosed type 2 diabetes
Blood pressure	≥ 130/85 mm Hg or treatment

IDF, International Diabetes Federation.

have noticed that there are striking differences in the prevalence of qualifying criteria among individuals of difference ethnicities. For example, in African Americans, hypertension is more likely to be a qualifying criterion than it is in Caucasians. Conversely, in Caucasians, lipid abnormalities predominate (STRRIDE data; Table 4.4).[28,29]

Waist circumference measures, although attempting to account for differences in women and men, clearly do not account for other differences in body habitus that might influence the normalization of this measure. For example, should a waist circumference of 92 cm be equally applicable in a woman who is 152 cm (60 in) tall as it is in a woman who is 183 cm (72 in) tall? Further, sex differences can be striking in the contribution of waist circumference to metabolic abnormalities. We have observed that women have less visceral fat, lower triglycerides, and much lower serum concentrations of small, dense, atherogenic low-density LDL cholesterol than do men, even given similar waist circumferences

TABLE 4.4
Lipoprotein Subclass Distributions by Group and Gender/Race Statistical Comparisons

	Black Women	White Women	Black Men	White Men	Gender Difference		Race Difference	
	n = 40	n = 108	n = 29	n = 108				
Cholesterol (mg/dL)	195 ± 30.8	207 ± 31.9	187 ± 29.9	185 ± 30.5	< .0001	F > M	0.2466	
HDL-C (mg/dL)	53.0 ± 12.0	52.8 ± 12.4	42.4 ± 11.6	37.8 ± 11.9	< .0001	F > M	0.1855	
HDL size (nm)	9.17 ± 0.34	9.05 ± 0.36	8.90 ± 0.33	8.67 ± 0.34	< .0001	F > M	0.0004	B > W
Small HDL (mg/dL Chol)	17.3 ± 4.91	17.1 ± 5.09	19.3 ± 4.78	19.8 ± 4.87	< .0001	M > F	0.8559	
Large HDL (mg/dL Chol)	35.6 ± 13.0	35.7 ± 13.5	23.1 ± 12.6	18.0 ± 13.0	< .0001	F > M	0.2034	
LDL-C (mg/dL)	126 ± 24.4	131 ± 25.3	124 ± 23.8	121 ± 24.3	0.0074	F > M	0.7239	
LDL size (nm)	21.4 ± 0.75	21.2 ± 0.78	21.0 ± 0.73	20.5 ± 0.75	< .0001	F > M	0.0022	B > W
LDL particle (nmol/L)	1250 ± 314	1351 ± 326	1345 ± 305	1414 ± 312	0.0634	M > F	0.0557	W > B
Small LDL (mg/dL Chol)[a]	8.50 ± 30.1	14.3 ± 31.2	16.2 ± 29.3	34.7 ± 29.9	< .0001	M > F	0.0112	W > B
Medium LDL (mg/dL Chol)[a]	30.1 ± 33.5	35.0 ± 34.8	50.3 ± 32.6	41.9 ± 33.3	0.0034	M > F	0.5438	
Large LDL (mg/dL Chol)[a]	85.9 ± 43.4	78.1 ± 45.0	56.1 ± 42.2	40.1 ± 43.0	< .0001	F > M	0.0212	B > W
IDL(mg/dL Chol)[a]	1.08 ± 5.55	3.70 ± 5.75	1.59 ± 5.40	3.91 ± 5.51	0.9585		< .0001	W > B
Triglyceride (mg/dL)[a]	85.7 ± 77.9	143 ± 80.8	112 ± 75.8	176 ± 77.4	0.0002	M > F	< .0001	W > B
VLDL size (nm)	43.6 ± 10.7	49.8 ± 11.1	47.4 ± 10.4	53.9 ± 10.6	0.0019	M > F	< .0001	W > B
Small VLDL (mg/dL Tg)	17.4 ± 11.1	16.9 ± 11.5	20.0 ± 10.8	18.3 ± 11.0	0.2107		0.5084	
Medium VLDL (mg/dL Tg)	26.0 ± 28.0	42.3 ± 29.0	35.9 ± 27.2	50.5 ± 27.8	0.0121	M > F	0.0001	W > B
Large VLDL (mg/dL Tg)[a]	5.98 ± 62.5	46.0 ± 64.8	22.5 ± 60.7	71.2 ± 62.0	0.0006	M > F	< .0001	W > B

Data expressed as adjusted mean ± SD

Notes: Data determined by analysis of covariance adjusting for differences in age and BMI. No interactions between gender and race were observed.

[a] ANCOVA performed using ranked data.

ANCOVA, analysis of co-variance; HDL, high-density lipoprotein; HDL-C, high-density lipoprotein cholesterol; IDL, intermediate-density lipoprotein; LDL, low-density lipoprotein; SD, standard deviation; Tg, triglyceride; VLDL, very-low-density lipoprotein.

(STRRIDE data; Table 4.4).[28] Similar observations can be made for African Americans when compared with Caucasians (i.e., at nearly identical waist circumferences, African Americans have lower visceral fat and lower triglycerides compared to Caucasians). Thus, more precision may be achievable in the diagnosis of metabolic syndrome if the criteria were differentially weighted by height, sex, and ethnicity. Finally, as we will argue, there are likely other, relatively easily obtained, clinical measures contributing to the clinical picture of insulin resistance that may be mechanistically involved in its etiology. These include cardiorespiratory fitness (e.g., time to exhaustion on a maximal treadmill exercise test) and concentrations of specific lipoprotein subspecies, such as small dense LDL cholesterol.

4.3 DIETARY APPROACHES FOR THE TREATMENT OF METABOLIC SYNDROME

Several cross-sectional and prospective studies have attempted to define optimal dietary interventions to reduce the incidence of metabolic syndrome independent of weight loss.

The Mediterranean diet—which is high in fruits, vegetables, nuts, whole grains, and olive oil—has consistently been associated with improvements in both prevalent and incident metabolic syndrome. An Italian trial randomized 180 individuals with metabolic syndrome, as defined by the ATP III criteria, to a Mediterranean-style diet (n = 90) or a prudent diet (n = 90) composed of 50%–60% carbohydrates, 15%–20% proteins, and less than 30% total fat. The Mediterranean diet group received detailed advice about how to increase daily consumption of whole grains, fruits, vegetables, nuts, and olive oil. After 2 years, despite no difference in physical activity between the groups, the Mediterranean diet group lost more weight than the control group (–4 kg vs –1.2 kg, $P < .001$). Additionally, the Mediterranean diet group had significantly lower concentrations of the serum inflammation biomarkers hs-CRP, IL-6, IL-7 and IL-18; decreased insulin resistance; and improved endothelial function score as measured by BP and platelet aggregation response to l-arginine. Importantly, at the end of the study 40 patients in the Mediterranean diet group still had features of the metabolic syndrome, compared with 78 patients in the control group ($P < .001$).[30]

Another prospective study, called the Seguimiento Universidad de Navarra (SUN) Study, assessed the relationship of adherence to the Mediterranean diet and the development of metabolic syndrome in Spanish university graduate students over the course of 6 years. They identified 2,563 individuals free of metabolic syndrome or risk factors at baseline. Using self-reported dietary patterns, they found that those individuals with the highest adherence to the Mediterranean diet had lower incidence of metabolic syndrome than those with the lowest adherence, even after adjustment for age, sex, physical activity, smoking, and total energy intake.[31]

The PREDIMED study investigated the effect of the Mediterranean diet plus mixed nuts (30 g daily), Mediterranean diet plus extra virgin olive oil (EVOO, 1 L weekly), or advice on a low-fat diet, on metabolic syndrome prevalence and incidence. After 1 year of the intervention, the Mediterranean diet plus nuts group had a 13.7% decrease in prevalence of metabolic syndrome compared with a 2% decrease in the low-fat group ($P = .01$), while there was no difference in the Mediterranean diet plus EVOO group compared with the low-fat group (6.7% vs 2%, $P = .18$). There were no differences in incidence of metabolic syndrome among groups during this short-term follow-up period.[32] Thus the Mediterranean diet, especially when supplemented with nuts, may be an effective diet for metabolic syndrome treatment. Of note, this trial later demonstrated that both Mediterranean diet regimens reduced the risk of cardiovascular events compared to a low-fat diet.[33]

Most recently, in a large meta-analysis of approximately 535,000 individuals across 50 studies, adherence to the Mediterranean diet was associated with reduced risk of metabolic syndrome (log hazard ratio, –0.69; 95% confidence interval [CI], –1.24 to –1.16). Additionally, the Mediterranean diet demonstrated a protective role on components of metabolic syndrome, such as waist circumference, HDL cholesterol, triglycerides, systolic and diastolic BP, and glucose.[34]

The Dietary Approaches to Stop Hypertension (DASH) diet has also been studied as a dietary approach for the treatment of metabolic syndrome. A group in Iran randomized 116 individuals with metabolic syndrome, according to ATP III criteria, to one of three diets: a control diet, a weight-reduction diet (macronutrient composition similar to control but 500 kcal less per day), and the DASH diet (similar 500 kcal/day reduction to weight-reduction diet, but with increased consumption of fruit, vegetables, low-fat dairy, and whole grains, and decrease in saturated fat, total fat, and cholesterol, and a restriction to 2,400 mg sodium). They found that both the weight-reduction and DASH diets improved components of metabolic syndrome compared to the control diet, even after adjustment for degree of weight loss. Additionally, prevalence of metabolic syndrome decreased significantly ($P < .05$) in the DASH diet group compared with the weight-reduction and control diets (65% in DASH group compared with 81% in the weight-reducing and 100% in the control group after 6 months).[35]

The associations of vitamin D and calcium intake with the development of metabolic syndrome and outcomes in individuals with metabolic syndrome are also increasingly recognized. A study using the Third National Health and Nutrition Examination Survey (NHANES III) identified 8,421 men and women, 21.9% of whom had metabolic syndrome according to the ATP III definition. After adjustment for age, sex, race or ethnicity, education, smoking status, serum cotinine concentration, concentration of c-reactive protein (CRP), total cholesterol concentration, leisure time, physical activity, vitamin or mineral use during the previous 24 hours, alcohol use, intake of fruits and vegetables, and season of study participation, the odds of having metabolic syndrome decreased across increasing quintiles of serum concentration of 25-hydroxyvitamin D (25[OH]D).[36] In a study of more than 10,000 middle-aged and older US women participating in the Women's Health Study, the odds of having metabolic syndrome decreased for increasing quintiles of total calcium intake; although vitamin D intake was inversely associated with the presence of metabolic syndrome, it was not independent of total calcium intake.[37] Of note, the Women's Health Study only relied on dietary questionnaires and did not measure serum vitamin D concentrations, so these two results cannot be directly compared. Several observational studies have also investigated whether vitamin D concentrations predict incident metabolic syndrome. In a study of 4,164 individuals in Australia without metabolic syndrome at baseline, those with the highest quintile concentration of serum 25(OH)D had a significantly lower risk of metabolic syndrome over 5 years of follow-up compared with those in the lower two quintiles. These results persisted after adjustment for multiple clinical covariates.[38] Serum 25(OH)D concentrations are also associated with outcomes in individuals with metabolic syndrome. In a cohort of 1,801 individuals with metabolic syndrome referred for coronary angiography—after adjustment for age, sex, smoking, alcohol and physical activity, body mass index (BMI), waist circumference, diastolic BP, type 2 diabetes, total cholesterol, cystatin C, CRP, the New York Heart Association (NYHA) functional classification, cardiovascular medication, and month of blood sampling—those with optimal 25(OH)D concentrations had a significantly reduced risk of all-cause mortality compared with those with severe vitamin D deficiency.[39] Despite compelling cross-sectional and prospective observational data, randomized trials testing the effect of vitamin D and/or calcium supplementation on development of metabolic syndrome are necessary but, thus far, lacking.

Although evidence suggests that certain dietary habits decrease incidence, or even reverse, metabolic syndrome, a combination of lifestyle interventions is likely to provide the most benefit. In particular, diet combined with exercise has been shown to successfully improve metabolic syndrome and other markers of cardiometabolic health. A small, randomized trial in Norway assigned 137 middle-aged men with metabolic syndrome, according to International diabetes federation (IDF) criteria, to four groups: diet alone (n = 34), exercise alone (n = 34), the combination of diet and exercise (n = 43), or control (n = 26). After 1 year, both the diet (35% reduction) and exercise (23.5% reduction) groups had significantly less metabolic syndrome prevalence than the control group (11.5% reduction). The combined diet and exercise group had by far the largest reduction in metabolic syndrome (67.4% reduction), which may be attributable to the greater weight loss in this particular group.[40] Similar improvements in metabolic syndrome components, as well as serum markers of oxidative stress, were seen in 25 individuals who underwent a 6-month combined diet-and exercise-induced weight-loss program.[41]

4.4 CROSS-SECTIONAL STUDIES OF THE IMPORTANCE OF PHYSICAL FITNESS AND EXERCISE TO THE DIAGNOSIS AND ETIOLOGY OF METABOLIC SYNDROME

Cross-sectional studies have consistently found that higher levels of cardiorespiratory fitness or physical activity are associated with decreased risk of morbidity and/or mortality from diabetes,[42,43] cardiovascular disease,[44,45] hypertension,[46,47] cancer,[44] and metabolic syndrome.[48,49] In 1999, data from the Aerobics Center Longitudinal Study (ACLS) of the Cooper Clinic in Dallas, Texas, were analyzed for the relation between cardiorespiratory fitness and metabolic syndrome.[48] This study was published before the ATP III definition of metabolic syndrome was available, and, as a result, it used a slightly different definition of metabolic syndrome. In this study, the variables associated with insulin resistance identified by Kaplan[50] as part of the "deadly quartet" included systolic BP ($\geq$ 140 mm Hg), hypertriglyceridemia ($\geq$ 150 mg/dL), hyperglycemia (fasting glucose $\geq$ 110 mg/dL), and central adiposity (waist circumference $\geq$ 100 cm for both men and women). They did not include HDL cholesterol in this study due to its strong correlation with triglycerides (TG). A total of 15,534 men and 3,898 women were studied. Cardiorespiratory fitness was assessed by time-to-exhaustion on a treadmill exercise test; fitness categories were based on age and sex normative data. Finally, the association between fitness and clustering of metabolic abnormalities was assessed using proportional odds logit models. For the men, the age-adjusted cumulative odds ratio for abnormal markers of metabolic syndrome was 10.1 (confidence interval [CI], 9.1–11.2; $P < .0001$) when comparing the least-fit with the most-fit men, and 3.0 (95% CI, 2.7–3.4; $P < .0001$) when comparing the least-fit with the moderately fit. For women, the odds ratio was 4.9 (CI, 3.8–6.3; $P < .0001$) when comparing the least-fit to the most-fit women, and 2.7 (CI, 2.7–3.4; $P < .0001$) when comparing the least-fit to the moderately-fit. These data provide very strong evidence that a highly significant relation exists between cardiorespiratory fitness and clustering of factors of the metabolic syndrome.

In another study of the relationship between metabolic syndrome, physical activity, and fitness by Carroll et al.,[51] similar findings were reported. This study, only in men presenting for preventive assessment at a private hospital in the United Kingdom (n = 711), reported age-adjusted odds ratios for metabolic clustering of 0.28 (95% CI, 0.14–0.57) for moderate fitness versus low fitness and 0.12 (95% CI, 0.05–0.32) for high fitness versus low fitness ($P < .0001$). They also reported that, even after exclusion of obesity in the metabolic syndrome definition, the relationship between cardiorespiratory fitness and metabolic syndrome was still significant. Similar relationships were observed for physical activity measures obtained via recall questionnaire. The confidence level for a trend between physical activity and metabolic syndrome was less ($P < .05$) than it was for cardiorespiratory fitness and metabolic syndrome ($P < .0001$). This is likely due to the nature of the measure: Physical activity questionnaires are inherently less accurate than the more highly reproducible time-to-exhaustion result on an exercise test.

More recently, Irwin et al.[52] examined the relationship between fitness and metabolic syndrome in a smaller sample of women of three ethnicities (African American, n = 49; Native American, n = 46; and Caucasian, n = 51). In this study, the ATP III definition for metabolic syndrome was used. Physical activity was determined prospectively from detailed subject records that included all physical activity performed during two consecutive 4-day periods. Cardiorespiratory fitness was determined from maximal treadmill time during a graded exercise test. They reported significant inverse relations between metabolic syndrome and greater levels of moderate-intensity physical activity ($P < .01$), vigorous-intensity physical activity ($P < .01$) and maximal treadmill time ($P < .0004$) among an ethnically diverse population of women. This appears to be the first study of these relationships in minority women. Importantly, they found that, while all associations were statistically significant, the strongest association was between metabolic syndrome and maximal treadmill time. They suggested that cardiorespiratory fitness was a more objective, albeit indirect, measure of physical activity, and as such is a more accurate exposure variable. It is important to note that physical activity records are generally a reflection of recent activity levels, whereas cardiorespiratory fitness likely reflects a much longer-term effect of regular, habitual physical activity.

Highlighting the consistency and generalizability of the relationship between physical activity, cardiorespiratory fitness, and metabolic syndrome are similar data reported by Lakka et al.[53] in Finnish men and from Panagiotakos et al.[54] in Greek men and women. In the Lakka study, the relationships between physical activity and metabolic syndrome, and between cardiorespiratory fitness and metabolic syndrome were significant; and the magnitude and level of significance were much greater for the relation between cardiorespiratory fitness and metabolic syndrome than for physical activity and metabolic syndrome. In fact, total leisure-time physical activity was significantly related to metabolic syndrome when adjusted for age only, or for age and multiple other factors ($P < .03$). Neither low-intensity physical activity nor moderate and vigorous physical activity was significantly related with metabolic syndrome using either statistical model. However, cardiorespiratory fitness was inversely related to metabolic syndrome ($P < .001$) for both the age-adjusted model and for the model that adjusted for age, smoking, alcohol consumption, and socioeconomic status. They found that the least fit men were almost seven times more likely to have metabolic syndrome than the most fit men, even when major confounders were controlled.

Furthermore, Lakka found, even after controlling for BMI, that the least fit men had a nearly four-fold likelihood of having metabolic syndrome when compared with the most fit men, suggesting a strong independent relationship between cardiorespiratory fitness and prevalence of metabolic syndrome. The observation that cardiorespiratory fitness independent of BMI is a very strong predictor of metabolic risk, diabetes risk, and overall cardiovascular risk is supported by numerous studies from the Aerobics Center Longitudinal Study of Dallas.[55–58]

LaMonte et al. were one of the first groups to prospectively define the relationship between cardiorespiratory fitness and incidence of metabolic syndrome.[59] They defined a cohort of 9,007 men and 1,491 women free of metabolic syndrome, and quantified baseline cardiorespiratory fitness using a maximal treadmill test. They measured components of metabolic syndrome, defined with ATP-III criteria, at baseline and during follow-up examinations over a mean follow-up time of 5.7 years. After adjusting for multiple clinical covariables, there was a statistically significant stepwise decrease in risk of metabolic syndrome across incremental thirds of fitness levels in both men and women. Compared with individuals in the least third of fitness, the risk of developing metabolic syndrome was 20%–26% less among participants in the middle third and 53%–63% less among those in the highest third.

In aggregate, these findings imply that cardiorespiratory fitness should be included as a defining variable of metabolic syndrome. In fact, one of the conclusions of Lakka et al.[53] was that the measurement of peak oxygen consumption (VO_2) (a measure highly correlated with time to exhaustion in an exercise test) in sedentary men with cardiovascular risk factors might provide an efficient means of targeting individuals who would benefit from interventions to prevent metabolic syndrome and its consequences. Presumably, these relationships are as strong in women as in men, although the data are not as extensive in women.

4.5 METABOLIC SYNDROME AND EXERCISE TRAINING

Given the emergence of evidence over the past decade that cardiorespiratory fitness is associated with the prevalence and incidence of metabolic syndrome, several studies have tested whether improving cardiorespiratory fitness with exercise training affects the natural history of metabolic syndrome. One of the first studies to address this question is the Heritage Family Study.[60] The Heritage Family Study was a multi-center study, including a large number of individuals across a large age range (18–65 years) in African American and Caucasian men and women. Complete data were available on 621 subjects who completed the exercise training. Of these, 105 had metabolic syndrome as defined by ATP III. The race and gender distribution, coupled with the wide age range of study participants in this trial, make the findings likely generalizable to a large portion of the

US adult population. Furthermore, the research design emphasized close attention to the details of measurement and quality control within and between sites, strengthening the validity of the conclusions.[61] Of pertinence, exercise exposure was very carefully monitored and standardized; the data presented represented those individuals completing 95% or more of the prescribed exercise sessions.

Of the 105 subjects who had the ATP III definition of metabolic syndrome (waist circumference, fasting, triglycerides, HDL cholesterol and glucose, and BP), nearly one-third (30.5%, 32 of the 105) were no longer defined as having metabolic syndrome after the exercise training program of 20 weeks. This was a highly physiologically, clinically, and statistically significant effect. It is particularly impressive, given that the exercise stimulus was of a fairly modest weekly amount (likely a similar total amount of exercise as approximately 30 min of moderate-intensity exercise 6 days per week) and was of a relatively modest training duration. In Figure 4.1, the prevalence of individual risk factors and the prevalence of metabolic syndrome are shown, with both before and after prevalence rates. Of the five risk factors, all except the prevalence of low HDL cholesterol were significantly decreased with exercise training. In individuals with a clustering of metabolic syndrome risk factors (i.e., three or more risk factors), the prevalence of metabolic syndrome was even more substantially reduced with the exercise training intervention than any of the individual risk factors. In Table 4.5, the prevalence percentages for each of the five risk factors are shown individually for each subject subgroup (black men, white men, black women, and white women). The consistency of the exercise effects on metabolic syndrome across race and gender subgroups and over a large range of ages emphasizes the strong generalizability of these effects.

Since the Heritage Family Study, several other studies have demonstrated similar effects of exercise training on the metabolic syndrome. In our Studies of a Targeted Risk Reduction Intervention through Defined Exercise (STRRIDE), we sought to determine how much exercise is recommended to decrease the prevalence of metabolic syndrome.[62] Of the 227 individuals completing the study (out of 334 enrolled), 171 had complete data for all ATP-III defined criteria for metabolic syndrome. These individuals had been randomly assigned to a 6-month control or one of three 8-month exercise training groups: low amount/moderate intensity (equivalent to walking approximately 19 km/week), (2) low amount/vigorous intensity (equivalent to jogging approximately 19 km/week), or (3) high amount/vigorous intensity (equivalent to jogging approximately 32 km/week). Importantly, the exercise "amounts" were controlled for energy expenditure (i.e., the low-amount/moderate-intensity group expended the same kcal of energy as the low-amount/vigorous-intensity group). Metabolic

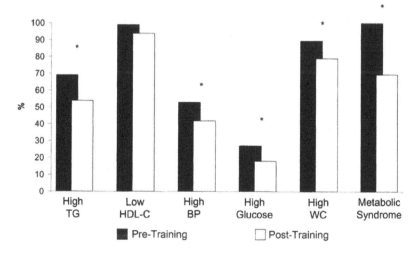

FIGURE 4.1 Prevalence of individual risk factors pre- and post-training among participants in the HERITAGE Family Study. *P < .05 pre- versus post-training. (BP, blood pressure; HDL-C, high-density lipoprotein cholesterol; WC, waist circumference; TG, triglycerides.)

TABLE 4.5

Prevalence (%) of Risk Factors Pre- and Post-Training Among Participants of the HERITAGE Family Study

	High TG	Low HDL	High BP	High Glucose	High WC
Black Men					
Pre	93	100	71	43	43
Post	79	100	43	29	43
White Men					
Pre	76	98	46	24	93
Post	63	93	42	7	76
Black Women					
Pre	26	100	87	35	100
Post	13	96	65	30	91
White Women					
Pre	81	100	26	15	100
Post	62	93	22	19	93

Source: Katzmarzyk, P.T. et al., *Med. Sci. Sport Exerc.*, 35, 1703–1709, 2003.

syndrome components, including blood samples for HDL and triglycerides, were measured pre- and post-intervention. The primary outcomes of interest were changes in the ATP-III score (the *sum* of ATP-III metabolic syndrome criteria) and the metabolic syndrome *z* score (a *continuous* score of the ATP-III metabolic syndrome criteria). Overall, as the high-amount/vigorous-intensity group improved metabolic syndrome compared to inactive controls and both low-amount exercise groups, there was a dose-dependent effect of exercise amount and improvement in metabolic syndrome. Surprisingly, however, the low-amount/moderate-intensity exercise improved metabolic syndrome compared to inactive controls, while the low-amount/vigorous-intensity exercise did not (Figure 4.2). These findings suggest that, at calorically equivalent amounts, moderate-intensity exercise may better improve metabolic syndrome and its variables than vigorous-intensity exercise.

In contrast to STRRIDE, Tjonna et al. studied the effect of aerobic interval training versus continuous, moderate-intensity exercise in 32 individuals with WHO-defined metabolic syndrome.[63] As in STRRIDE, the exercise regimens were matched for energy expenditure. After a 16-week intervention, while also better improving most metabolic syndrome criteria, aerobic interval training improved maximum oxygen consumption (VO_{2max}) comparably to continuous, moderate-intensity exercise.

We also examined the separate and combined effects of aerobic and resistance exercise on individuals with metabolic syndrome in our STRRIDE-AT/RT study.[64] In this 4-month study, resistance training (RT; 3 days/week, 3 sets/day of 8–12 repetitions of 8 different exercises targeting all major muscle groups) did not improve the metabolic syndrome *z* score, whereas aerobic training (AT; approximately 120 minutes/week at 75% of the VO_{2max}) and the combination of aerobic and resistance training did.

A recent meta-analysis of the effects of exercise on the metabolic syndrome included seven trials involving nine study groups and 206 participants.[65] This study found consistent improvements in most metabolic syndrome criteria in the exercise cohorts, including significant reductions in waist circumference of −3.4 cm (95% CI, −4.9 to −1.8), BP of −7.1 mm Hg (95% CI, −9.03 to −5.2) and an increase in HDL-C of +0.006 mmol/L (95% CI, 0.03–0.09). Mean plasma glucose and triglyceride

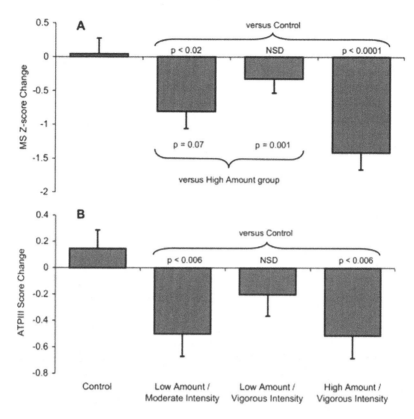

FIGURE 4.2 Effects of exercise amount and intensity on mean changes in (*A*) metabolic syndrome (MS) *z* score and (*B*) Adult Treatment Program-III (ATP III) score. NSD, no significant difference. (From Johnson, J.L. et al., *Am. J. Cardiol.*, 100, 1759–1766, 2007.)

concentrations showed no significant change after exercise training. Of note, the meta-analysis was not able to address the specific effects of certain exercise training programs on metabolic syndrome criteria.

In sum, although the ideal intensity and regimen of exercise training may be unclear, evidence consistently supports regular and routine exercise as an effective means to improve the metabolic syndrome and reduce metabolic syndrome incidence in a dose-dependent manner.

4.6 EXERCISE TRAINING AND INDIVIDUAL COMPONENTS OF METABOLIC SYNDROME

A discussion of the effects of individual exercise training studies on each of the five individual components of metabolic syndrome is beyond the scope of this review. Instead, we will summarize the effects by briefly discussing reviews and/or meta-analyses, and in some cases a few key exercise training studies.

4.6.1 BLOOD PRESSURE

Numerous meta-analyses of the effect of aerobic exercise on BP have been published, and the results have been consistent. Fagard[46] performed a meta-analysis on 44 randomized, controlled trials (RCTs) and concluded that aerobic exercise reduces BP; the lowering effect was greater in hypertensive (−7/−6 mm Hg) than normotensive (−3/−2 mm Hg) people. Furthermore, he concluded that the evidence in support of these findings achieved the highest level of confidence rating—a "Category A" level—indicating that the conclusion was based on a rich body of data from well-designed RCTs, providing a consistent pattern of results. In addition to this general finding, this report examined the effects of the individual components of exercise training: intensity, frequency, and individual session duration. The authors concluded that the beneficial aerobic exercise effect was not dependent on exercise intensity (between 40% and 70% of maximal exercise performance) and that the effect was similar for frequencies of 3–5 times per week and for session durations of 30–60 minutes.

In a somewhat larger and more recent meta-analysis, also on RCTs (N = 54), Whelton et al.[66] concluded that aerobic exercise decreased diastolic and systolic BP in both hypertensive and normotensive individuals. The effect was somewhat greater in the hypertensive (−5/−4 mm Hg) than the normotensive (−4/−2 mm Hg) participants. Additional analyses revealed that beneficial exercise effects occurred in Caucasians and Asians for both systolic and diastolic BP reductions. In African Americans, a significant beneficial effect was found for systolic, but not diastolic, BP. Importantly, only two studies meeting the analysis criteria included blacks, suggesting the need for additional studies in minorities. In spite of the finding of a consistent beneficial effect of exercise on BP in numerous meta-analyses,[67–70] important ethnic differences exist for health parameters in general, yet a relatively small number of studies of exercise and BP studied African Americans or Asians. While no analysis was presented for the separate effects of exercise on BP in women and men, 17 of the 51 trials studied predominantly women (≥ 80%), and only 10 studied predominantly men.

4.6.2 TRIGLYCERIDES

One of the more extensive reviews of the effects of exercise on lipids and lipoproteins was conducted by Durstine and Haskell.[71] First, in analyzing several cross-sectional studies comparing inactive controls to either endurance athletes, runners, cross-country skiers, tennis players, or individuals with longer treadmill test times, they concluded that generally active individuals have lower triglyceride concentrations. With regard to exercise training studies, they reported that training also generally reduced the triglyceride levels if the baseline levels were elevated. They also found that the degree of reduction in triglycerides was related to both the baseline amount of triglyceride elevation and to the volume of exercise training; however, in women, these findings were not as consistent.

In a meta-analysis of 51 studies, of which 28 were RCTs, Leon and Sanchez[72] reported an overall average decrease in triglycerides of 3.7% ($P < .05$). They also reported that men generally had a greater reduction than did women. However, confirming similar observations from previous reviews, they concluded that the blood lipid response to exercise, including the triglyceride response, was quite variable.

4.6.3 HIGH-DENSITY LIPOPROTEIN CHOLESTEROL

Durstine and Haskell[71] reported that in cross-sectional studies, endurance athletes have 20%–30% greater levels of HDL-cholesterol (HDL-C) when compared to inactive controls. Cross-sectional studies also suggest a dose-response relationship between amount of exercise and HDL-C concentrations. However, exercise-training studies have not been as consistent; many studies have reported a significant training benefit on HDL-C levels, while many other studies did not find a significant effect. Leon and Sanchez,[72] in their meta-analysis, reported a marked inconsistency of the effects of aerobic exercise training on blood lipids in general; they suggested the most frequent finding was a significant ($P < .05$) increase in HDL-C. However, this significant beneficial effect was reported in only 24 of the 51 studies (47%) included in the review. The exercise-induced change in HDL-C ranged from a decrease of 5.8% to an increase of 25%. Nevertheless, overall, there was an average increase of 4.6% across the studies ($P < .05$).

Some help in understanding the variability in the lipid response has been reported in an 8-month exercise training study by Kraus et al.[73] In the first randomized, controlled study of the effect of two different amounts of exercise training on HDL-C, the authors reported that only the greater amount of exercise (an amount of exercise calorically equivalent to approximately 17 miles of jogging per week), had a significant effect on increasing HDL-C, compared to an inactive control group. The two lower amounts of exercise training—both calorically equivalent to approximately 11 miles per week, one group at a moderate exercise intensity and the other group at a more vigorous exercise intensity—had small, nonsignificant, increases in HDL-C. Thus, the Kraus study confirmed the earlier analysis of Durstine and Haskell, in which cross-sectional studies suggest a dose-response effect of exercise training on HDL-C improvement.

4.6.4 Fasting Plasma Glucose

In a meta-analysis of controlled clinical trials (11 randomized and three nonrandomized) on the effects of exercise training on glycemic control in individuals with type 2 diabetes, Boule and colleagues[74] reported a significant ($P < .001$) beneficial exercise effect on glycosylated hemoglobin (HbA1c) (−0.66%) compared to the controls, a similar effect that has been observed in subsequent meta-analyses.[75,76] The difference found in this meta-analysis was close to the difference (−0.9%) between conventional and intensive glucose-lowering therapy reported in the United Kingdom Prospective Diabetes Study (UKPDS)[77,78]—an amount that was associated with significant improvement in clinical outcomes (development of microvascular and macrovascular complications of diabetes, including cardiovascular disease). The authors speculated that exercise might result in a greater reduction in cardiovascular complications than with insulin or sulfonylureas, since exercise has additional cardioprotective benefits and does not cause weight gain.

A comprehensive review by Ivy et al.[79] supports a key role of exercise and physical activity in prevention and treatment of diabetes. As diabetes is defined by fasting glucose, prevention of diabetes is, by definition, through the prevention of increases in fasting serum glucose. Ivy and colleagues reviewed numerous epidemiological studies (cross-sectional, retrospective, and prospective designs) providing strong support for the beneficial effect of physical activity in the prevention of type 2 diabetes. In Mauritians, the relationship between low levels of physical activity and increased prevalence of impaired fasting glucose and type 2 diabetes exists across both sexes and across the major ethnic groups on the island[80–82]; furthermore, total physical activity is a significant independent predictor, even after controlling for several major confounders. Mayer-Davies et al.[83] reported similar findings in a large, culturally and ethnically diverse sample of men and women. Kriska and colleagues reported the same relationship in Pima Indians.[84] Manson et al.,[85,86] in a prospective study, provided additional evidence of this relationship, including evidence of a dose-response effect of increased exercise frequency and reduced risk of type 2 diabetes. Ivy et al. presented additional evidence in reviews of bed-rest studies[87–89] and exercise-detraining studies[90–92]; together, they reveal a rapid deterioration in insulin action and glucose tolerance (if the individual/population was glucose intolerant) with even short periods of bed rest or detraining.

Does exercise training improve glucose tolerance and prevent development of type 2 diabetes? Exercise training reliably improves insulin action in all subjects but does not affect glucose tolerance in normal individuals. However, in glucose-intolerant individuals, exercise does result in improvements in glucose tolerance. In a 7-day exercise training study in 10 men with mild type 2 diabetes or impaired glucose tolerance, Holloszy et al.[93] found that two of three individuals with impaired glucose tolerance reverted to a normal oral glucose tolerance test after training, and, of seven men with type 2 diabetes, three had normal oral glucose tolerance tests after training, two had only impaired fasting glucose, and two still had diabetic oral glucose tolerance tests after 7 days of training. The two who still had diabetic oral glucose tolerance test had relative hypoinsulinemia, whereas the other eight who improved with exercise had mild to moderate hyperinsulinemia. The data suggest that when sufficient insulin reserve exists, exercise training has the potential to reverse glucose intolerance and even mild type 2 diabetes.

Results from cross-sectional studies of young and old endurance athletes compared to young and old (lean and not lean) untrained individuals show that untrained individuals have decreased insulin action and/or decreased glucose tolerance compared to young and old athletes.[94] The master athletes have essentially identical insulin and glucose responses to an oral glucose tolerance test, indicating that age need not result in impaired glucose tolerance. The authors suggest that earlier studies showing no improvement in insulin action and/or glucose tolerance generally used an insufficient exercise stimulus, waited too long after the final exercise bout, and/or used patients with relative insulin deficiency. When this group trained mildly diabetic individuals without insulin deficiency for 1 year and measured oral glucose tolerance test within 18 hours of the last bout of exercise, they found significantly improved glucose tolerance and insulin action and normalized fasting glucose levels.[95] Data from Reitman et al.[96] report that 6–10 weeks of intensive exercise lowers fasting glucose and improves glucose tolerance in obese type 2 diabetic individuals. Other studies in type 2 diabetic subjects support these findings.[97,98]

One cannot discuss the effects of exercise training on progression to diabetes in individuals without mention of the results of the seminal Diabetes Prevention Program.[99] In this study, the effects of pharmacologic therapy (metformin) and lifestyle interventions (exercise training at the level of American College of Sports Medicine/Centers for Disease Control and Prevention (ACSM/CDC) recommendations of 30 minutes per day most days of the week, diet, and 7% total loss of body weight) were compared with usual care. The results revealed that the lifestyle intervention reduced the risk of progression to diabetes in this population by 58% compared with usual care. The effects of metformin, although statistically and clinically significant, were less impressive in reducing rate of progression to diabetes by 31% compared to usual care. Similar results were observed with the lifestyle intervention arm (a combined weight-loss and exercise program) of the Finnish Diabetes Prevention Study.[100] Granted, these trials did not study the effects of exercise alone, but they point out the utility of lifestyle interventions in individuals with metabolic syndrome.

What type of exercise training best improves glycemic control in individuals with type 2 diabetes? Although systematic reviews and meta-analyses, including those mentioned previously, have found that structured aerobic exercise or RT can reduce HbA1c values, prospective studies have provided conflicting results. The earliest prospective study to address this question showed no improvement in HbA1c between AT and combined aerobic and RT in postmenopausal women with diabetes; however, some have attributed this negative finding to the relatively low baseline HbA1c among the groups (6.7%) and the small sample sizes (9–10 individuals per group).[101] This study also did not investigate the effect of RT alone. A more recent randomized trial examined the effect of AT, RT, or the combination in 251 male and female adults over a 22-week training period (the Diabetes Aerobic and Resistance Exercise [DARE] study).[102] Compared with sedentary controls, both the AT group (−0.51%; 95% CI, −0.87 to −0.14%) and RT group (−0.38%; 95% CI, −0.72 to −0.22%) had significant improvements in HbA1c values. However, the combined training program provided an additional change in HbA1c of −0.46% (95% CI, −0.83 to −0.09%) compared with AT alone and −0.59% (95% CI, −0.95 to −0.23%) compared with RT alone. A similar trend in HbA1c lowering was seen in the Health Benefits of Aerobic and Resistance Training in Individuals With Type 2 Diabetes (HART-D) study, in which combined aerobic and RT lowered HbA1c values more than aerobic or RT alone.[103] However, the degree of HbA1c lowering was less in HART-D than in DARE (−0.3% vs −1.0%). Additionally, no significant change in HbA1c was seen in either the AT or RT alone groups. The differences between these two studies might be explained by differences in diabetes duration (longer in HART-D) or differences in baseline diabetes medications. Overall, the results of these two prospective trials support the most recent (2008) physical activity guidelines that recommend combined aerobic and RT on a regular basis.

4.6.5 INSULIN SENSITIVITY

The metabolic syndrome is conceptually the same as the insulin resistance syndrome; the names are often interchangeable. That some prefer the term *insulin resistance syndrome* is due to the common understanding that an observable decrease in insulin sensitivity is the first detectable aberration in

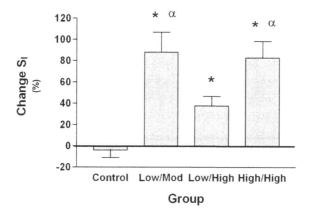

FIGURE 4.3 Relative changes (%) (after training/before training) in insulin sensitivity index derived from the intravenous glucose tolerance test (SI) in the control and exercise (low-volume/moderate-intensity [Low/Mod]; low-volume/high-intensity [Low/High]; high-volume/high-intensity [High/High]) groups. Line at 0.0 represents no change. (*, significant difference from control, $P \leq .05$; α, significant difference from the low-volume/high-intensity group, $P < .05$.) (From Houmard, J.A. et al., *J. Appl. Physiol.*, 96, 101–106, 2004.)

a course toward metabolic syndrome. In fact, some deterioration in insulin sensitivity is generally observed prior to elevations in triglycerides levels and decreases in HDL-C concentrations, which precede deterioration in fasting glucose and glucose tolerance measures, perhaps even before clinically significant increases in body weight, BMI, and waist circumference are apparent. In fact, as a reflection of this understanding, the World Health Organization includes a resting measure of insulin resistance in its definition of metabolic syndrome (refer to Table 4.2).

The relationship between exercise and insulin resistance is clear. In fact, one of the most consistent beneficial effects of exercise is a statistically and physiologically significant improvement in insulin action. This beneficial effect can be observed in a broad range of exercise conditions and models: after only a few bouts of acute exercise[93,104] or with longer-term exercise training,[105–108] with low-intensity or high-intensity exercise,[104,109] in exercising animals[108] and humans.[105–107] In a classic study, Seals et al.[94] observed that even young and lean, but sedentary individuals have nearly twice the insulin response after an oral glucose administration as young, lean, endurance athletes. Aging had no influence on this observation; the results were the same when the young, lean, sedentary individuals were compared to older (mean age, 60 years), lean, endurance athletes. This demonstrates an improved insulin action in endurance athletes when compared with sedentary controls. In a study from our group,[110] the data revealed that of the two groups performing the same amount of exercise (calorically equivalent to walking or jogging approximately 10 miles per week), the less-intensely exercising group had a greater improvement in insulin sensitivity (see Figure 4.3). This may be due specifically to a beneficial effect of low-intensity exercise—which is known to oxidize more fat than the same amount of more vigorous exercise—or, alternatively, this may be due to the higher exercise frequency and/or total time of weekly exercise required by the low-amount/moderate-intensity group to expend the same amount of calories through exercise. Whether this same observation holds for individuals with frank diabetes remains an open question and a potential area for future investigation.

4.6.6 Waist Circumference

In RCTs, providing a significant increase in exercise volume, either through a large weekly amount of exercise for a short time period (4,900 kcal/week for 12 weeks[111]) or a smaller weekly amount over a long time period (980 kcal/week for 48 weeks[112]), or both (2,000 kcal/week for 36 weeks[110]), statistically and physiologically significant decreases in waist circumference result. In the randomized, controlled exercise training study from the Kraus group,[110] two amounts of exercise (low dose,

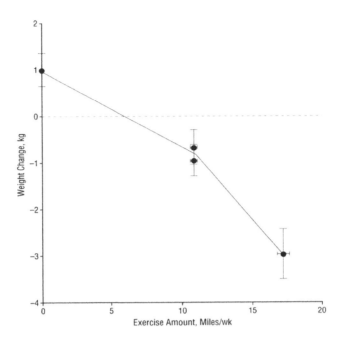

FIGURE 4.4 The relationship between mean amount of weight change and amount of exercise. (From Slentz, C.A. et al., *Arch. Intern. Med.*, 164, 31–39, 2004.)

approximately 1,200 kcal/week, and high dose, approximately 2,000 kcal/week) combined with a control (no extra kcal/week through exercise) revealed a clear, strong volume of exercise effect on reductions in abdominal obesity as measured by waist circumference (Figure 4.4). In this study, even the low-dose exercise groups had significantly less waist circumference compared to the inactive control group. Clearly, when a significant exercise training stimulus is provided, waist circumference and abdominal obesity are reduced.

4.7 RATIONALE FOR INCLUDING CARDIORESPIRATORY FITNESS IN METABOLIC SYNDROME

Lakka et al. suggested that a sedentary lifestyle and especially poor cardiorespiratory fitness are not only associated with metabolic syndrome, but also could be considered central defining features of metabolic syndrome.[53] Furthermore, they suggested that measurement of peak VO_2 in sedentary men with risk factors could provide a means of identifying those who would most benefit from interventions—especially lifestyle interventions—in individuals at risk of developing diabetes mellitus.

Numerous studies have revealed a clear, independent relationship between exercise capacity (cardiorespiratory fitness) and cardiovascular events and/or all-cause deaths in men and women.[44,45,56,113–120] Furthermore, Weinsier et al.,[121] using US data, and Prentice and Jeb,[122] using UK data, reviewed extensively the data concerning the question of whether the obesity and diabetes epidemic is primarily due to overeating or lack of physical activity (the "Gluttony vs Sloth" debate). Both have cautiously concluded that, even given the difficulty in measuring changes in caloric consumption or physical activity over the past decades, it is clear that physical inactivity is a major culprit in the obesity epidemic. They go on to suggest that perhaps physical inactivity is *the* major culprit.

This concept is supported by studies from the 1950s, in carefully performed studies in animals[123] and humans.[124] Mayer et al. observed that, at significant physical activity levels, increases or decreases in physical activity are matched with increases or decreases in food intake. However, below certain minimal levels of physical activity, further decreases in physical activity are not met by further decreases in food intake, but rather by increases in food intake and consequent body weight. They interpreted the data to suggest that a minimal level of physical activity might be necessary for appropriate appetite control. Data from our group provides support for this theory. In our study,[110] inactive controls gained weight over a 6-month period, whereas two different low-dose exercise training groups (equivalent to approximately 12 miles/week of walking or jogging) lost weight, and a higher dose (equivalent to approximately 17 miles/week) lost even more body mass. The data suggest that, below a certain level, appetite control is not appropriately balanced and weight gain occurs. If the Mayer hypothesis is correct, then the extreme levels of physical inactivity present in today's society may be at the root of the obesity and diabetes epidemic: These levels of inactivity may directly lead to the inability to balance food intake with decreasing physical activity levels, resulting in continuous weight gain and progression from metabolic syndrome to diabetes.

4.8   CONCLUSION

As mentioned previously, physical activity levels are poorly measured, whereas cardiorespiratory fitness is a relatively easily measured, reliable, and accurate clinical assessment that is a reasonable surrogate for physical activity. Studies show that both moderate and vigorous intensity activity can lead to increases in cardiorespiratory fitness.[73,125]

In a particularly compelling article titled "Exercise capacity: the prognostic variable that doesn't get enough respect," Mark and Lauer discuss what they refer to as "one of the most potent prognostic variables"[126]—exercise capacity/cardiorespiratory fitness. The article is precipitated by the Gulati et al.[120] study (see discussion above) reported in the same issue, along with numerous studies that have come before. Mark and Lauer argue that the overwhelming amount of data support the role of exercise capacity as a potent prognostic indicator of future health for both men and women, and for both symptomatic and asymptomatic individuals.

We believe the accumulated evidence provides a strong rationale for including cardiorespiratory fitness as one of the major defining diagnostic components of metabolic syndrome. Furthermore, by including cardiorespiratory fitness in the definition of metabolic syndrome, individuals and physicians would more likely focus directly on physical activity and fitness as measures of health. This would also demand attention to methods for increasing physical activity and cardiorespiratory fitness as an effective therapeutic intervention for metabolic syndrome and the prevention of progression to type 2 diabetes. A direct emphasis on physical activity and cardiorespiratory fitness certainly will have significant consequences on the prevalence of metabolic syndrome, obesity, progression to type 2 diabetes, and cardiovascular disease in the US population.

4.8.1   FUTURE DIRECTIONS FOR RESEARCH

It seems clear that regular exercise/physical activity has beneficial effects both for preventing and treating type 2 diabetes and metabolic syndrome. Two particularly promising areas of research involve studying the most effective amounts and intensities of exercise leading to such benefits in individuals with diabetes; investigating the unique role that RT exercise may have on insulin sensitivity and metabolic syndrome; and studies of the interactions among exercise, nutrition, environment, medical therapies, and genetics. We anticipate that such lines of investigation hold great promise for improving our effectiveness in diagnosing individuals with metabolic syndrome on the road to type 2 diabetes, and in ultimately preventing its development in susceptible individuals.

REFERENCES

1. Reaven GM. Banting Lecture: Role of insulin resistance in human disease (Review). *Diabetes.* 1988;37:1595–1607.
2. Bjorntorp P. Visceral obesity: A "civilization syndrome." *Obes Res.* 1993;1:206–222.

3. Vague J. The degree of masculine differentiation of obesities: A factor determining predisposition to diabetes, atherosclerosis, gout, and uric calculous disease. *Am J Clin Nutr.* 1956;4:20–34.

4. Kissebah AH. Relation of body fat distribution to metabolic complications of obesity. *J Clin Endo Metab.* 1982;54:254–260.

5. Alberti K, Zimmet PZ. World Health Organization (WHO) consultation: Definition, diagnosis and classification of diabetes mellitus and its complications. Part I: Diagnosis and classification of diabetes mellitus: Provisional report of a WHO consultation. *Diabet Med.* 1998;15:539–553.

6. Panel E. Executive Summary of the Third Report of the National Cholesterol Education Program (NCEP) Expert Panel on Detection, Evaluation, and Treatment of High Blood Cholesterol in Adults (Adult Treatment Panel III). *JAMA.* 2001;285:2486–2497.

7. Grundy SM, Cleeman JI, Daniels SR, Donato KA, Eckel RH, Franklin BA, Gordon DJ, et al., American Heart Association, National Heart, Lung, and Blood Institute. Diagnosis and management of the metabolic syndrome: An American Heart Association/National Heart, Lung, and Blood Institute Scientific Statement. *Circulation.* 2005;112:2735–2752.

8. Alberti KGMM, Zimmet P, Shaw J, IDF Epidemiology Task Force Consensus Group. The metabolic syndrome—a new worldwide definition. *Lancet (London, England).* 2005;366:1059–1062.

9. Alberti K, Eckel RH, Grundy SM, Zimmet PZ, Cleeman JI, Donato KA, Fruchart J-C, Philip James WT, Loria CM, Smith SC. Harmonizing the metabolic syndrome A joint interim statement of the International Diabetes Federation Task Force on Epidemiology and Prevention for the Study of Obesity. *Circulation.* 2009;120:1640–1645.

10. Expert Panel on Detection, Evaluation, and Treatment of High Blood Cholesterol in Adults. Executive Summary of The Third Report of The National Cholesterol Education Program (NCEP) Expert Panel on Detection, Evaluation, And Treatment of High Blood Cholesterol In Adults (Adult Treatment Panel III). *JAMA.* 2001;285:2486–2497.

11. Ford ES, Giles WH, Dietz WH. Prevalence of the metabolic syndrome among US adults: Findings from the third National Health and Nutrition Examination Survey. *JAMA.* 2002;287:356–359.

12. Eckel RH, Grundy SM, Zimmet PZ. The metabolic syndrome. *Lancet (London, England).* 2005;365:1415–1428.

13. Kahn R, Buse J, Ferrannini E, Stern M, American Diabetes Association, European Association for the Study of Diabetes. The metabolic syndrome: Time for a critical appraisal: Joint statement from the American Diabetes Association and the European Association for the Study of Diabetes. *Diabetes Care.* 2005;28:2289–2304.

14. Ferrannini E. Metabolic syndrome: A solution in search of a problem. *J Clin Endocrinol Metab.* 2007;92:396–398.

15. Grundy SM. Metabolic syndrome: A multiplex cardiovascular risk factor. *J Clin Endocrinol Metab.* 2007;92:399–404.

16. Hanson RL, Imperatore G, Bennett PH, Knowler WC. Components of the "metabolic syndrome" and incidence of type 2 diabetes. *Diabetes.* 2002;51:3120–3127.

17. Resnick HE, Jones K, Ruotolo G, Jain AK, Henderson J, Lu W, Howard BV, Strong Heart Study. Insulin resistance, the metabolic syndrome, and risk of incident cardiovascular disease in nondiabetic american indians: The Strong Heart Study. *Diabetes Care.* 2003;26:861–867.

18. Klein BEK, Klein R, Lee KE. Components of the metabolic syndrome and risk of cardiovascular disease and diabetes in Beaver Dam. *Diabetes Care.* 2002;25:1790–1794.

19. Sattar N, Gaw A, Scherbakova O, Ford I, O'Reilly DSJ, Haffner SM, Isles C, Macfarlane PW, Packard CJ, Cobbe SM, Shepherd J. Metabolic syndrome with and without C-reactive protein as a predictor of coronary heart disease and diabetes in the West of Scotland Coronary Prevention Study. *Circulation.* 2003;108:414–419.

20. Sattar N, McConnachie A, Shaper AG, Blauw GJ, Buckley BM, de Craen AJ, Ford I, et al. Can metabolic syndrome usefully predict cardiovascular disease and diabetes? Outcome data from two prospective studies. *Lancet (London, England).* 2008;371:1927–1935.

21. Ford ES. Risks for all-cause mortality, cardiovascular disease, and diabetes associated with the metabolic syndrome: A summary of the evidence. *Diabetes Care.* 2005;28:1769–1778.

22. Galassi A, Reynolds K, He J. Metabolic syndrome and risk of cardiovascular disease: A meta-analysis. *Am J Med.* 2006;119:812–819.

23. Gami AS, Witt BJ, Howard DE, Erwin PJ, Gami LA, Somers VK, Montori VM. Metabolic syndrome and risk of incident cardiovascular events and death. *J Am Coll Cardiol.* 2007;49:403–414.

24. Marceau P, Biron S, Hould F-S, Marceau S, Simard S, Thung SN, Kral JG. Liver pathology and the metabolic syndrome X in severe obesity. *J Clin Endocrinol Metab.* 1999;84:1513–1517.

25. Hamaguchi M, Kojima T, Takeda N, Nakagawa T, Taniguchi H, Fujii K, Omatsu T, et al. The metabolic syndrome as a predictor of nonalcoholic fatty liver disease. *Ann Intern Med.* 2005;143:722–728.

26. Hanley AJG, Williams K, Festa A, Wagenknecht LE, D'Agostino RB, Haffner SM. Liver markers and development of the metabolic syndrome: The insulin resistance atherosclerosis study. *Diabetes.* 2005;54:3140–3147.

27. Chen J, Muntner P, Hamm LL, Jones DW, Batuman V, Fonseca V, Whelton PK, He J. The metabolic syndrome and chronic kidney disease in U.S. adults. *Ann Intern Med.* 2004;140:167–174.

28. Johnson JL, Slentz CA, Duscha BD, McCartney J, Samsa GP, Houmard JA, Kraus WE. Gender and racial differences in lipoprotein subclass distribution; The STRRIDE study. *Atherosclerosis.* 2004;176:371–377.

29. Despres JP, Couillard C, Gagnon J, Bergeron J, Leon AL, Rao DC, Skinner JS, Wilmore JH, Bouchard C. Race, visceral adipose tissue, plasma lipids and lipoprotein lipase activity in men and women: The HERITAGE family study. *Arter Thromb Vasc Biol.* 2000;20:1932–1938.

30. Esposito K, Marfella R, Ciotola M, Di Palo C, Giugliano F, Giugliano G, D'Armiento M, D'Andrea F, Giugliano D. Effect of a mediterranean-style diet on endothelial dysfunction and markers of vascular inflammation in the metabolic syndrome. *JAMA.* 2004;292:1440.

31. Tortosa A, Bes-Rastrollo M, Sanchez-Villegas A, Basterra-Gortari FJ, Nuñez-Cordoba JM, Martinez-Gonzalez MA. Mediterranean diet inversely associated with the incidence of metabolic syndrome: The SUN prospective cohort. *Diabetes Care.* 2007;30:2957–2959.

32. Salas-Salvadó J, Fernández-Ballart J, Ros E, Martínez-González M-A, Fitó M, Estruch R, Corella D, et al., PREDIMED Study Investigators. Effect of a mediterranean diet supplemented with nuts on metabolic syndrome status. *Arch Intern Med.* 2008;168:2449.

33. Estruch R, Ros E, Salas-Salvadó J, Covas M-I, Corella D, Arós F, Gómez-Gracia E, et al. Primary prevention of cardiovascular disease with a mediterranean diet. *N Engl J Med.* 2013;368:1279–1290.

34. Kastorini C-M, Milionis HJ, Esposito K, Giugliano D, Goudevenos JA, Panagiotakos DB. The effect of mediterranean diet on metabolic syndrome and its components. *J Am Coll Cardiol.* 2011;57:1299–1313.

35. Azadbakht L, Mirmiran P, Esmaillzadeh A, Azizi T, Azizi F. Beneficial effects of a Dietary Approaches to Stop Hypertension eating plan on features of the metabolic syndrome. *Diabetes Care.* 2005;28:2823–2831.

36. Ford ES, Ajani UA, McGuire LC, Liu S. Concentrations of serum vitamin D and the metabolic syndrome among U.S. adults. *Diabetes Care.* 2005;28:1228–1230.

37. Liu S, Song Y, Ford ES, Manson JE, Buring JE, Ridker PM. Dietary calcium, vitamin D, and the preva-lence of metabolic syndrome in middle-aged and older U.S. women. *Diabetes Care.* 2005;28:2926–2932.

38. Gagnon C, Lu ZX, Magliano DJ, Dunstan DW, Shaw JE, Zimmet PZ, Sikaris K, Ebeling PR, Daly RM. Low serum 25-hydroxyvitamin D is associated with increased risk of the development of the metabolic syndrome at five years: Results from a National, Population-Based Prospective Study (The Australian Diabetes, Obesity and Lifestyle Study: AusDiab). *J Clin Endocrinol Metab.* 2012;97:1953–1961.

39. Thomas GN, ó Hartaigh B, Bosch JA, Pilz S, Loerbroks A, Kleber ME, Fischer JE, Grammer TB, Böhm BO, März W. Vitamin D levels predict all-cause and cardiovascular disease mortality in subjects with the metabolic syndrome: The Ludwigshafen Risk and Cardiovascular Health (LURIC) Study. *Diabetes Care.* 2012;35:1158–1164.

40. Anderssen SA, Carroll S, Urdal P, Holme I. Combined diet and exercise intervention reverses the meta-bolic syndrome in middle-aged males: Results from the Oslo Diet and Exercise Study. *Scand J Med Sci Sports.* 2007;17:687–695.

41. Rector RS, Warner SO, Liu Y, Hinton PS, Sun GY, Cox RH, Stump CS, Laughlin MH, Dellsperger KC, Thomas TR. Exercise and diet induced weight loss improves measures of oxidative stress and insulin sensitivity in adults with characteristics of the metabolic syndrome. *Am J Physiol Metab.* 2007;293:E500–E506.

42. Wei M, Gibbons LW, Mitchell TL, Kampert JB, Lee CD, Blair SN. The association between cardio-respiratory fitness and impaired fasting glucose and type 2 diabetes mellitus in men. *Ann Intern Med.* 1999;130:89–96.

43. Wei M, Gibbons LW, Kampert JB, Nichaman MZ, Blair SN. Low cardiorespiratory fitness and physical inactivity as predictors of mortality in men with type 2 diabetes. *Ann Intern Med.* 2000;132:605–611.

44. Blair SN, Kohl HWIII, Paffenbarger RSJ, Clark DG, Cooper KH, Gibbons LW. Physical Fitness and all-cause mortality. A prospective study of healthy men and women. *JAMA.* 1989;262:2395–2401.

45. Blair SN, Kohl HWIII, Barlow CE, Paffenbarger RSJ, Gibbons LW, Macera CA. Changes in physi-cal fitness and all-cause mortality. A prospective study of healthy and unhealthy men. *JAMA.* 1995;273:1093–1098.

46. Fagard RH. Exercise characteristics and the blood pressure response to dynamic physical training. *Med Sci Sport Exerc*. 2001;33:S484–492.

47. Blair SN, Kohl HWIII, Barlow CE, Gibbons LW. Physical fitness and all-cause mortality in hypertensive men. *Ann Med*. 1991;23:307–312.

48. Whaley MH, Kampert JB, Kohl HW III, Blair SN. Physical fitness and clustering of risk factors associated with the metabolic syndrome. *Med Sci Sport Exerc*. 1999;31:287–293.

49. Katzmarzyk PT, Church TS, Blair SN. Cardiorespiratory fitness attenuates the effects of metabolic syndrome on all-cause and cardiovascular disease mortality in men. *Arch Intern Med*. 2004;164:1092–1097.

50. Kaplan NM. The deadly quartet: Upper body obesity, glucose intolerance, hypertriglyceridemia and hypertension. *Arch Intern Med*. 1989;149:1514–1520.

51. Carroll S, Cooke CB, Butterly RJ. Metabolic clustering, physical acitivity and fitness in nonsmoking, middle-aged men. *Med Sci Sport Exerc*. 2000;32:2079–2086.

52. Irwin ML, Ainsworth BE, Mayer-Davis EJ, Addy CL, Pate RR, Durstine JL. Physical activity and the metabolic syndrome in a tri-ethnic sample of women. *Obes Res*. 2002;10:1030–1037.

53. Lakka TA, Laaksonen DE, Lakka H, Mannikko N, Niskanen LK, Rauramaa R, Salonen JT. Sedentary lifestyle, poor cardiorespiratory fitness, and the metabolic syndrome. *Med Sci Sport Exerc*. 2003;35:1279–1286.

54. Panagiotakos DB, Pitsavos C, Chrysohoou C, Skoumas J, Tousoulis D, Toutouza M, Toutouzas P, Stefanadis C. Impact of lifestyle habits on the prevalence of the metabolic syndrome amoung Greek adults from the ATTICA study. *Am Hear J*. 2004;147:106–112.

55. Lee CD, Jackson AS, Blair SN. US weight guidelines: Is it also important to consider cardiorespiratory fitness? *Intern J Obes Relat Metab Disord*. 1998;22:2–7.

56. Wei M, Kampert JB, Barlow CE, Nichaman MZ, Gibbons LW, Paffenbarger RSJ, Blair SN. Relationship between low cardiorespiratory fitness and mortality in normal-weight, overweight, and obese men. *JAMA*. 1999;282:1547–1553.

57. Farrell SW, Braun L, Barlow CE, Cheng YJ, Blair SN. Ther relation of body mass index, cardiorespiratory fitness and all-cause mortality in women. *Obes Res*. 2002;10:417–423.

58. Lee CD, Blair SN, Jackson AS. Cardiorespiratory fitness, body composition, and all-cause and cardiovascular disease mortality in men. *Am J Clin Nutr*. 1999;69:373–380.

59. LaMonte MJ, Barlow CE, Jurca R, Kampert JB, Church TS, Blair SN. Cardiorespiratory fitness is inversely associated with the incidence of metabolic syndrome: A prospective study of men and women. *Circulation*. 2005;112:505–512.

60. Katzmarzyk PT, Leon AL, Wilmore JH, Skinner JS, Rao DC, Rankinen T, Bouchard C. Targeting the metabolic syndrome with exercise: Evidence from the Heritage Family Study. *Med Sci Sport Exerc*. 2003;35:1703–1709.

61. Gagnon J, Province MA, Bouchard C. The HERITAGE Family study: Quality assurance and quality control. *Ann Epidemiol*. 1996;6:520–529.

62. Johnson JL, Slentz CA, Houmard JA, Samsa GP, Duscha BD, Aiken LB, McCartney JS, Tanner CJ, Kraus WE. Exercise training amount and intensity effects on metabolic syndrome (from Studies of a Targeted Risk Reduction Intervention through Defined Exercise). *Am J Cardiol*. 2007;100:1759–1766.

63. Tjønna AE, Lee SJ, Rognmo Ø, Stølen TO, Bye A, Haram PM, Loennechen JP, et al. Aerobic interval training versus continuous moderate exercise as a treatment for the metabolic syndrome: A pilot study. *Circulation*. 2008;118:346–354.

64. Bateman LA, Slentz CA, Willis LH, Shields AT, Piner LW, Bales CW, Houmard JA, Kraus WE. Comparison of aerobic versus resistance exercise training effects on metabolic syndrome (from the Studies of a Targeted Risk Reduction Intervention Through Defined Exercise - STRRIDE-AT/RT). *Am J Cardiol*. 2011;108:838–844.

65. Pattyn N, Cornelissen VA, Eshghi SRT, Vanhees L. The effect of exercise on the cardiovascular risk factors constituting the metabolic syndrome: A meta-analysis of controlled trials. *Sports Med*. 2013;43:121–133.

66. Whelton SP, Chin A, Xin X, He J. Effect of aerobic exercise on blood pressure: A meta-analysis of randomized, controlled trials. *Ann Intern Med*. 2002;136:493–503.

67. Halber JA, Silagy CA, Finucane P, Withers RT, Hamdorf PA, Andresw GR. The effectiveness of exercise training in lowering blood pressure: A meta-analysis of randomised controlled trials of 4 weeks or longer. *J Hum Hypertens*. 1997;11:641–649.

68. Kelley GA. Aerobic exercise and resting blood pressure among women: A meta-analysis. *Prev Med*. 1999;28:264–275.

69. Kelley GA, Sharpe KK. Aerobic exercise and resting blood pressure in older adults: A meta-analytic review of RCT's. *J Gerontol Ser A-Bio Sci Med Sci*. 2001;56:298–303.
70. Cornelissen VA, Buys R, Smart NA. Endurance exercise beneficially affects ambulatory blood pressure: A systematic review and meta-analysis. *J Hypertens*. 2013;31:639–648.
71. Durstine JL, Haskell WL. Effects of exercise training on plasma lipids and lipoproteins. *Exerc Sport Sci Rev*. 1994;22:477–524.
72. Leon AL, Sanchez OA. Response of blood lipids to exercise training alone or combined with dietary intervention. *Med Sci Sport Exerc*. 2001;33:S502–515.
73. Kraus WE, Houmard JA, Duscha BD, Knetgzer KJ, Wharton MB, McCartney J, Bales CW, et al. Effects of the amount and intensity of exercise on plasma lipoproteins. *New Engl J Med*. 2002;347:1483–1492.
74. Boule NG, Haddad E, Kenney GP, Wells GA, Sigal RJ. Effects of exercise on glycemic control and body mass in Type 2 Diabetes mellitus. *JAMA*. 2001;286:1218–1227.
75. Snowling NJ, Hopkins WG. Effects of different modes of exercise training on glucose control and risk factors for complications in type 2 diabetic patients: A meta-analysis. *Diabetes Care*. 2006;29:2518–2527.
76. Chudyk A, Petrella RJ. Effects of exercise on cardiovascular risk factors in type 2 diabetes: A meta-analysis. *Diabetes Care*. 2011;34:1228–1237.
77. Group UKPDS. Intensive blood-glucose control with sulphonylureas or insulin compared with conventional treatment and risk of complications in patients with type 2 diabetes. *Lancet*. 1998;352:837–853.
78. Group UKPDS. Effect of intensive blood-glucose control with metformin on complications in overweight patients with type 2 diabetes. *Lancet*. 1998;352:854–865.
79. Ivy JL, Zderic TW, Donovan FL. Prevention and treatment of non-insulin-dependent diabetes mellitus. *Exerc Sport Sci Rev*. 1999;27:1–35.
80. Dowse GK, Zimmet PZ, Gareeboo H, Alberti K, Tuomilehto CF, Finch PC, et al. Abdominal obesity and physical inactivity as risk factors for NIDDM and impaired glucose tolerance in Indian, Creole, and Chinese Mauritians. *Diabetes Care*. 1991;14:271–282.
81. Pereira MA, Kriska AM, Joswiak ML, Dowse GK, Collins VR, Zimmet PZ, Gareeboo H, et al. Physical inactivity and glucose tolerance in the multiethnic island of mauritius. *Med Sci Sport Exerc*. 1995;27:1626–1634.
82. Zimmet PZ, Collins VR, Dowse GK, Alberti K, Tuomilehto J, Gareeboo H, Chitson P. The relation of physical activity to cardiovascular disease risk factors in Mauritians. *Am J Epidemiol*. 1991;134:862–875.
83. Mayer-Davis EJ, D'Agostino R, Karter AJ, Haffner S, Rewers MJ, Saad M, Bergman RN. Intensity and amount of physical activity in relation to insulin sensitivity: The Insulin Resistance Atherolsclerosis Study. *JAMA*. 1998;279.
84. Kriska AM, LaPorte RE, Pettitt DJ, Charles MA, Nelson RG, Kuller LH, Bennett PH, et al. The association of physical activity with obesity, fat distribtution and glucose intolerance in Pima Indians. *Diabetologia*. 1993;36: 863–869.
85. Manson JE, Nathan DM, Krolewski AS, Stampfer JM, Willett WC, Hennekens CH. A prospective study of exercise and incidence of diabetes amoung U.S. male physicians. *JAMA*. 1992;268: 63–67.
86. Manson JE, Rimm EB, Stampfer JM, Colditz GA, Willett WC, Krolewski AS, Rosner B, et al. Physical activity and incidence of NIDDM in women. *Lancet*. 1991;338: 774–778.
87. Lipman RL, Schnure JJ, Bradley EM, Lecocq FR. Impairment of peripheral glucose utilization in normal subjects by prolonged bed rest. *J Lab Clin Med*. 1970;76:221–230.
88. Misbin RI, Moffa AM, Kappy MS. Insulin binding to monocytes in obese patients treated with carbohydrate restriction and changes in physical activity. *J Clin Endo Metab*. 1983;56:273–278.
89. Stuart CA, Shamgraw RE, Prince MJ, Peters EJ, Wolfe RR. Bed-rest-induced insulin resistance occurs primarily in muscle. *Metabolism*. 1988;37:802–806.
90. Heath GW, Gavin JR, Hinderliter JM, Hagberg JM, Bloomfield SA, Holloszy JO. Effects of exercise and lack of exercise on glucose tolerance and insulin sensitivity. *J Appl Physiol*. 1983;55:512–517.
91. King DS, Dalsky GP, Clutter W, Young DA, Staten MA, Cryer PE, Holloszy JO. Effects of exercise and lack of exercise on insulin sensitivity and responsiveness. *J Appl Physiol*. 1988;64:1942–1946.
92. Mikines KJ, Sonne B, Tronier B, Galbo H. Effects of training and detraining on insulin action in trained men. *J Appl Physiol*. 1989;66:704–711.
93. Rogers MA, Yamamoto c, King DS, Hagberg JM, Ehsani AA, Holloszy JO. Improvement in glucose tolerance after 1 wk of exercise in patients with mild NIDDM. *Diabetes Care*. 1988;11:613–618.
94. Seals DR, Hagberg JM, Allen WK, Hurley BF, Dalsky GP, Ehsani AA, Holloszy JO. Glucose tolerance in young and older athletes and sedentary men. *J Appl Physiol*. 1984;56:1521–1525.
95. Holloszy JO, Schultz J, Kusnierkiewicz J, Hagberg JM, Eshani AA. Effects of exercise on glucose tolerance and insulin resistance: Brief review and preliminary results. *Acta Med Scand*. 1986;711:55–65.

96. Reitman JS, Vasquez B, Klimes I, Nagulesparan M. Improvement of glucose homeostasis after exercise training in NIDDM. *Diabetes Care.* 1984;7:434–441.

97. Schneider SH, Amorosa AK, Khachadurian AK, Ruderman NB. Studies on the mechanism of improved glucose control during regular exercise in type 2 (non-insulin-dependent) diabetes. *Diabetologia.* 1984;26:355–360.

98. Dela F, Larsen JJ, Mikines KJ, Ploug T, Petersen LN, Galbo H. Insulin-stimulated muscle glucose clearance in patients with NIDDM: Effects of one-legged physical training. *Diabetes.* 1995;44:1010–1020.

99. Knowler WC, Barrett-Connor E, Fowler SE, Hamman RF, Lachin JM, Walker EA, Nathan DM, Diabetes Prevention Program Research Group. Reduction in the incidence of type 2 diabetes with lifestyle intervention or metformin. *N Engl J Med.* 2002;346:393–403.

100. Tuomilehto J, Lindström J, Eriksson JG, Valle TT, Hämäläinen H, Ilanne-Parikka P, Keinänen-Kiukaanniemi S, et al. Prevention of type 2 diabetes mellitus by changes in lifestyle among subjects with impaired glucose tolerance. *N Engl J Med.* 2001;344:1343–1350.

101. Cuff DJ, Meneilly GS, Martin A, Ignaszewski A, Tildesley HD, Frohlich JJ. Effective exercise modality to reduce insulin resistance in women with type 2 diabetes. *Diabetes Care.* 2003;26:2977–2982.

102. Sigal RJ, Kenny GP, Boulé NG, Wells GA, Prud'homme D, Fortier M, Reid RD, et al. Effects of aerobic training, resistance training, or both on glycemic control in type 2 diabetes: A randomized trial. *Ann Intern Med.* 2007;147:357–369.

103. Church TS, Blair SN, Cocreham S, Johannsen N, Johnson W, Kramer K, Mikus CR, et al. Effects of aerobic and resistance training on hemoglobin A1c levels in patients with type 2 diabetes: A randomized controlled trial. *JAMA.* 2010;304:2253–2262.

104. Braun B, Zimmermann B, Kretchmer N. Effects of exercise intensity on insulin sensitivity in women with NIDDM. *J Appl Physiol.* 1995;78:300–306.

105. Hawley JA, Houmard JA. Introduction - Preventing insulin resistance throught exercise: A cellular approach. *Med Sci Sport Exerc.* 2004;36:1187–1190.

106. Berggren JR, Hulver MW, Dohm GL, Houmard JA. Weight loss and exercise: Implications for muscle lipid metabolism and insulin action. *Med Sci Sport Exerc.* 2004;36:1191–1195.

107. Bruce CR, Hawley JA. Improvements in insulin resistance with aerobic exercise training: A lipocentric approach. *Med Sci Sport Exerc.* 2004;36:1196–1201.

108. Ivy JL. Muscle insulin resistance amended with exercise training: Role of GLUT4 expression. *Med Sci Sport Exerc.* 2004;36:1207–1211.

109. Houmard JA, Tanner CJ, Slentz CA, Duscha BD, McCartney JS, Kraus WE. Effect of the volume and intensity of exercise training on insulin sensitivity. *J Appl Physiol.* 2004;96:101–106.

110. Slentz CA, Duscha BD, Johnson JL, Ketchum K, Aiken LB, Samsa GP, Houmard JA, Bales CW, Kraus WE. Effects of the amount of exercise on body weight, body composition, and measures of central obesity: STRRIDE--a randomized controlled study. *Arch Intern Med.* 2004;164:31–39.

111. Ross R, Dagnone D, Jones PJH, Smith H, Paddags A, Hudson R, Janssen I. Reduction in obesity and related comorbid conditions after diet-induced weight loss or exercise-induced weight loss in men: A randomized, controlled trial. *Ann Intern Med.* 2000;133:92–103.

112. Binder EF, Birge SJ, Kohrt WM. Effects of endurance exercise and hormone replacement therapy on serum lipids in older women. *J Am Geriatr Soc.* 1996;44:231–236.

113. Ekelund LG, Haskell WL, Johnson JL, et al. Physical fitness as a predictor of cardiovascular mortality in asymptomatic North American men: The Lipid Research Clincis Mortality Follow-up study. *New Engl J Med.* 1988;319:1379–1384.

114. Meyers J, Prakash M, Froelicher V, Do D, Partington S, Atwood JE. Exercise capacity and mortality amount men referred for exercise testing. *New Engl J Med.* 2002;346:793–801.

115. Weiner DA, Ryan TJ, Parsons L, et al. Long-term prognostic value of exercise testing in men and women from the Coronary Artery Surgery Study (CASS) registry. *Am J Card.* 1995;75:865–870.

116. Slattery ML, Jacobs DRJ. Physical fitness and CVD mortality: The US Railroad Study. *Am J Epidemiol.* 1988;127:571–580.

117. Peters RK, Cady LDJ, Bischoff DP, et al. Physical fitness and subsequent myocardial infarction in healthy workes. *JAMA.* 1993;249:3052–3056.

118. Wyns W, Musschaert-Beauthier E, van Domburg R, et al. Prognostice value of symptom limited exercise testing in men with a high prevalence of coronary artery disease. *Eur Hear J.* 1985;6:939–945.

119. Roger VL, Jacobsen SJ, Pellikka PA. Prognostic value of treadmill exercise testing: A population-based study in Olmsted county, Minnesota. *Circulation.* 98:2836–2841.

120. Gulati M, Pandey DK, Arnsdorf MF, Lauderdale DS, Thisted RA, Wicklund RH, Al-Hani AJ, Black HR. Exercise capacity and the risk of death in women: The St. James women take heart project. *Circulation*. 2003;108:1554–1559.

121. Weinsier RL, Hunter GR, Heini AF, Goran MI, Sell SM. The etiology of obesity: Relative contribution of metabolic factors, diet & physical activity. *Am J Med*. 1998;105:145–150.

122. Prentice AM, Jebb SA. Obesity in Britain: Gluttony or sloth? *Br Med J*. 1995;311:437–439.

123. Mayer J, Marshall NB, Vitale JJ, Christensen JH, Mashayekhi MB, Stare FJ. Exercise, food intake and body weight in normal rats and genetically obese adult mice. *Am J Physiol*. 1954;177:544–548.

124. Mayer J, Purnima R, Mitra KP. Relation between caloric intake, body weight, and physical work: Studies in an industrial male population in West Bengal. *Am J Clin Nutr*. 1956;4:169–175.

125. Asikainen TM, et al. Randomized, controlled walking trials in post-menopausal women: The minimum dose to improve aerobic fitness. *Br J Sport Med*. 2002;36:189–194.

126. Mark DB, Lauer MS. Exercise capacity: The prognostic variable that doesn't get enough respect. *Circulation*. 2003;108:1534–1536.

5 Fat Distribution and Diabetes Mellitus

Danae A. Delivanis and Michael D. Jensen

CONTENTS

5.1 INTRODUCTION

The prevalence of diabetes in the United States is on the rise, with a projected increase of 54%, to more than 54.9 million Americans with diabetes by 2030.[1] Although there are many risk factors for type 2 diabetes (T2DM), including age, race, pregnancy, stress, medications, genetics, and family history, the single best predictor of T2DM is obesity. Almost 90% of people with T2DM are overweight or obese, and it is clear that the increase in the prevalence of diabetes has paralleled the increase in obesity prevalence—approximately 60% of US adults are now overweight or obese.[2]

Although obesity should be suspected in adults with a body mass index (BMI) greater than 30 kg/m², using BMI alone to define health risk is problematic. There is strong evidence that body-fat distribution is a better predictor of insulin resistance and cardiovascular consequences than obesity defined simply by BMI.[3] The preferential accumulation of upper-body fat is independently associated with insulin resistance,[4–6] and reductions of visceral fat via energy restriction reverses many metabolic abnormalities.[7–9] However, there are also associations between upper-body sub-cutaneous fat and insulin resistance in obese adults,[3,10,11] whereas lower-body fat is independently associated with a reduced risk of metabolic abnormalities.[12,13]

The relationship between regional fat distribution and the development of metabolic abnormalities is well recognized. Independent of total body fat, body-fat distribution is an important and established risk factor for cardiovascular disease.[14,15] Unfortunately, not enough is known about the mechanisms by which differences in regional fat storage exert protective or harmful roles in the development of insulin resistance and β-cell dysfunction. The mechanism(s) by which regional fat depots contribute to obesity-related metabolic abnormalities and insulin resistance remains an area of investigation.[16]

5.2 HUMAN BODY-FAT DISTRIBUTION

Adipose tissue is highly active as both a metabolic and endocrine tissue. Adipocytes are essential in buffering the daily influx of dietary fat and exert autocrine, paracrine, and endocrine effects via secretion of proteins such as leptin, adiponectin, tumor necrosis factor-α (TNF-α), interleukin-6 (IL-6) and interleukin-1β (IL-1β). The best-documented role of adipose tissue is managing lipid fuels. When the buffering capacity for lipid storage in adipose tissue is decreased, or adipose tissue becomes overloaded, other tissues are exposed to an excess influx of free fatty acids and triacylglycerols (TAGs). It is thought that this "lipotoxicity" results in insulin resistance in many tissues, but especially skeletal muscle and liver.[17]

Human body-fat depots can broadly be divided into lower- and upper-body subcutaneous fat, and visceral/intra-abdominal fat (omental and mesenteric).[18] In normal-weight adults, upper-body and lower-body subcutaneous fat comprise the majority of total body fat.[19] Upper-body subcutaneous fat includes deep and superficial (divided by Scarpa's fascia) truncal fat and arm and breast depots, whereas lower-body fat is anatomically defined as all subcutaneous fat below the inguinal ligament and the posterior superior iliac crest. Lower-body subcutaneous fat includes gluteal, thigh, and calf fat, but the adipose tissue between major muscle groups—so-called "marbling"[20]—is often considered a form of ectopic fat that has negative, rather than positive, health connotations. Although each of these smaller compartments has unique characteristics,[21] lower-body adiposity as a whole is independently associated with greater metabolic health in contrast to upper-body/visceral obesity.[22]

Upper-body abdominal adipose tissue is anatomically divided by the fascia superficialis (Scarpa's fascia) into superficial and deep subcutaneous abdominal fat.[23] Visceral intra-abdominal fat includes omental and mesenteric fat depots, which drain into the portal vein and thus can have a disproportionate impact on liver metabolism.[24] Visceral fat comprises the minor component of total body fat, and represents approximately 10% and 5% of total body fat in normal-weight men and women, respectively. Although perirenal fat is also anatomically located intra-abdominally, it is not typically characterized as visceral fat because its venous drainage is into the inferior vena cava. Deep subcutaneous fat and visceral abdominal fat are better correlated with the metabolic sequelae of obesity.[3]

There are numerous body composition assessment methods that can be classified as direct (total body water, body potassium counting, dual-energy x-ray absorptiometry [DXA], etc.), indirect (skinfold thickness, bioelectrical impedance spectroscopy, etc.), and criterion (computed tomography [CT], magnetic resonance imaging [MRI], etc).[25–28] In clinical practice, waist circumference and waist-to-hip ratio are commonly used to measure regional fat adiposity. For research purposes, imaging techniques such as CT or MRI scan, with or without DXA, are considered the gold standards for measurement of adipose tissue distribution.[25,26]

5.3 FACTORS INFLUENCING FAT DISTRIBUTION

There is strong evidence that human body-fat distribution is controlled by genetic/constitutional and environmental factors. In addition to the above, age, sex, race/ethnicity, and energy balance are additional correlates of body-fat distribution (Table 5.1).

With aging, there is often a loss of lower-body, and sometimes upper-body, subcutaneous fat,[29] resulting in a proportionately greater amount of abdominal, in particular visceral, fat.[29] This age-dependent increase in visceral fat seems to be more pronounced in men than in women.[30] Sex is

TABLE 5.1

Fat Distribution Independent of Fat Mass

	Upper Body Subcutaneous Fat	Lower Body Subcutaneous Fat	Visceral Fat (As % of Total Fat)
Old age	↓	↓	↑
Sex			
I. Male	↓	↓	↑
II. Female	↑	↑	↓
Race*			
I. Caucasian	–	–	↑
II. African American	–	–	↓
III. Mexican American	–	–	↑↑
IV. Asian	–	–	↑↑↑
Diet composition*			
I. Greater % protein	–	–	↓/↑
II. Greater % carbohydrate	–	–	↓/↑
III. Greater % fat	–	–	↓/↑
Increased physical activity	↓	↓	↓
Excess alcohol intake	↓/↑	↓/↑	↑
Tobacco	↓/↑	↓/↑	↑
Stress	–	–	↑
Childhood-onset obesity	–	–	↑
Medications			
I. *Thiazolidinedione*	↑	↑	No effect
II. Growth hormone	No effect	No effect	↓
Associated genes:			
FTO gene	↑	–	↑
NRXN3 gene			
NEGR1 gene			
LINGO2 gene			
LYPLAL1 gene			

"*" Data presented refers to % body fat rather than visceral fat.

another important contributor, as women tend to store more fat in the gluteal-femoral region ("pear"), and men store more fat in the visceral/abdominal region ("apple").[31,32] Indeed, men have twofold more visceral adipose tissue than premenopausal women.[33] In this context, sex hormones are the main mediators of some of the observed differences. During the postmenopausal state, the loss of estrogen and relative rise in androgens is associated with fat redistribution from the periphery to the intra-abdominal cavity.[34] On the other hand, men with low testosterone often have more visceral fat.[35] There are uncommon endocrine disorders that can be responsible for changes in fat distribution. Patients with Cushing's syndrome are characterized by fat redistribution from the periphery to the intra-abdominal region,[30] whereas untreated patients with acromegaly exhibit a reduction in central adiposity with an increase in intermuscular fat.[36]

There is also evidence that people with different racial backgrounds differ in body-fat distribution.[37,38] For a similar level of total adiposity, Asians have more visceral adipose tissue than Caucasians, who in turn have more visceral fat than those of African ancestry.[39] Similar results were reported from the National Health and Nutrition Examination Survey (NHANES) study[40] (Table 5.1). A woman's race is also an important determinant of body-fat distribution, with African-American women having less visceral adipose tissue for a given BMI than Caucasian women.[41,42]

A number of investigators have attempted to link nutritional factors with body-fat distribution, but variable results make it difficult to draw firm conclusions. Studies reporting both positive and negative associations between body fat and high-carbohydrate diets,[43,44] high-fat diets,[45–47] and high-protein diets[47–50] have appeared. Other investigators have failed to find any difference in body-fat distribution between participants with different macronutrient consumption patterns.[45,51] These conflicting results may result from unaccounted cofounders and measurement error in those studies that use self-reported dietary intake. Other studies have shown an association between dietary fatty acid composition and body-fat distribution patterns independent of overall adiposity.[52,53] As such, the Mediterranean diet that consists mostly of monounsaturated fatty acids reduces visceral fat gain and waist circumference values in both men and women, independent of BMI.[54,55]

In addition to diet composition, physical activity is also considered an important factor in body-fat distribution. Higher levels of physical activity are shown to be associated with lower levels of body fat in most studies, and a preferential loss of visceral fat over subcutaneous fat.[47,56–59] Exercise has been shown to reduce visceral fat virtually independent of total fat.[60–62] However, physical activity can vary in intensity, and different intensities have resulted in different results in body fat and distribution.[63] Time spent in television viewing has been used as a marker of sedentary behavior, and has been found to be associated with increased abdominal obesity and increased risk of T2DM.[64–66]

Additional environmental factors may contribute to differences in body-fat distribution. Alcohol,[67] cigarette smoking,[68] stress,[69] and the timing of onset of childhood obesity[70] are established risk factors known to be associated with increased central adiposity. There is only limited data on environmental associates of subcutaneous fat distribution,[71,72] as presented in Table 5.1.

There are also medications that influence body-fat distribution. Thiazolidinediones (TZDs) are agonists for the nuclear receptor PPAR-γ, a key transcription factor in the regulation of adipogenesis that is abundantly expressed in adipose tissue. TZDs preferentially increase subcutaneous fat and recruit new adipocytes that can better accommodate "excess" fatty acids; no significant effect on visceral fat is noted.[73,74] This is in contrast to the preferential visceral fat mobilization by diet and exercise. Growth hormone (GH) treatment of deficient adults has resulted in a preferential decrease in visceral fat, an increase in lean body mass, and improvements in serum lipids.[59,75] However, GH treatment of patients with low GH due solely to obesity can aggravate insulin resistance.

Body-fat distribution is also controlled by genetic factors independent of BMI and overall obesity.[76,77] This was nicely illustrated by studies of identical twins.[78] More recently, with the use of more advanced technology and new statistical approaches, well-powered genome-wide association studies (GWAS) have revealed novel genes/loci that are linked with body-fat distribution (Table 5.1.)[79–81]

5.4 FAT CELL SIZE AND NUMBER

While regional differences in body-fat distribution are better predictors of metabolic alterations than overall obesity,[39] adipocyte size, per se, is also associated with metabolic disease and adipose-tissue dysfunction. Multiple studies have linked enlarged abdominal subcutaneous adipocytes with an increased cardiometabolic risk.[82–84]

Obesity can be characterized based on the way adipose tissue expands in a given fat depot. Adipose-tissue expansion can occur either through adipocyte hyperplasia, hypertrophy, or a combination of both. The term *hypertrophic obesity* is used to describe fat gain that occurs preferentially with increased adipocyte size, and the term *hyperplastic obesity* to describe fat gain that is associated with a preferential increase in fat cell numbers.[21,85,86] Recruitment of new cells through differentiation of pre-adipocytes (hyperplasia) is considered a more benign way to gain weight because it is associated with fewer metabolic abnormalities. Adipocyte hyperplasia is the typical way of expansion of subcutaneous adipose tissue that occurs in the female or gynoid obesity phenotype.[87,88] In contrast, visceral fat depots expand mainly via adipocyte hypertrophy.[87,89]

As discussed, the majority of studies support that greater degrees of hypertrophic obesity are associated with insulin resistance,[90,91] and adipocyte hypertrophy has been proposed as being mechanistically linked to metabolic abnormalities.[92] While the majority of reports indicate a clear association between subcutaneous fat cell size and markers of insulin resistance,[83,85,91,93–95] a few have not.[96,97] For human obesity, the association between visceral fat cell size and markers of insulin resistance is not settled.[84,98,99] Several studies have reported an association between excess liver fat and subcutaneous adipocyte size,[84,100,101] whereas others have not.[102,103] Discrepancies between the studies can be explained by variation in the anthropometric adjustments in each study, as well as the existence of a non-linear relation between fat cell size and levels of obesity.

Another factor relating to the tendency to develop hypertrophic obesity is a family history of T2DM, with greater enlargement of abdominal adipocytes for equal increases in body fat in patients with a positive family history.[104] In a recent study, after adjusting for confounders, authors found that a family history of T2DM was a predictor of larger abdominal (but not femoral) adipocytes for females, but not for males.[105]

Mean adipocyte size increases as a function of obesity, up to a point.[91] The two main predictors of adipocyte size and number are sex and anatomical localization of the fat depots.[21,90,106] Lower-body subcutaneous adipocytes of women tend to be larger than those of men independent of adiposity level, whereas no significant sex variations are noted in abdominal subcutaneous adipocyte size.[19,21,106,107] Regarding visceral adipocytes, lean to moderately obese men have larger omental adipocytes than women.[106] Regarding adipocyte number, women have more adipocytes and more subcutaneous fat mass than men. Gene-expression studies have suggested that women's subcutaneous adipocytes expand mainly via adipocyte hyperplasia, whereas women's visceral adipocytes demonstrate mainly a hypertrophic expansion.[108] In normal-weight women, omental adipocytes are smaller than abdominal subcutaneous adipocytes that are, in turn, smaller than lower-body subcutaneous adipocytes.[106,109–111] In men, visceral and abdominal adipocytes are of similar size, implying that a similar expansion occurs.[112] In response to overfeeding, lower-body fat expands via hyperplasia in both women and men; sex differences in the increase in abdominal subcutaneous adipocyte size are not readily apparent.[88]

Fat cell size also affects lipolysis rate. Specifically, lipolysis correlates positively with fat cell size, so that larger adipocytes have greater basal lipolytic activity per cell.[113] Gluteal adipocytes from women that are larger than those from men have higher basal lipolytic rates.[114] In addition, the larger omental adipocytes in men than premenopausal women have a greater lipolytic capacity, but the reverse is true in postmenopausal women.[115] However, lipolytic activity per cell cannot be extrapolated easily into the in vivo situation. This information requires an understanding of the number of cells per gram of adipose tissue and the relationship between the conditions in the in vitro studies and the normal microenvironment of the adipocytes (e.g., insulin, growth hormone, sympathetic innervation).

In summary, women tend to store more fat in subcutaneous fat depots through adipocyte hyperplasia, whereas men typically store excess fat in visceral and upper-body subcutaneous adipose tissue through adipocyte hypertrophy.[39] These (largely hormone driven) adipose cell responses account for the sex differences in body fat and probably contribute to the accompanying differences in their metabolic profile.

5.5 BODY-FAT DISTRIBUTION AND ADIPOSE DYSFUNCTION: POTENTIAL MECHANISMS

Traditionally, adipose tissue has been viewed solely as a biological energy reservoir that expands in response to overnutrition, storing calories in as triglyceride lipid droplets formed largely from dietary fatty acids. In conditions of energy deficit, adipocytes hydrolyze more triglyceride than they store, and they release free fatty acids (FFAs) for oxidation in other organs. However, the delivery of *excess* FFA to the liver is shown to reduce the insulin-mediated suppression of glucose output, reduce insulin-mediated glucose uptake in the skeletal muscle, and mediate a direct toxic effect on pancreatic β-cells.[116]

Adipose tissue is also an endocrine organ that secretes numerous adipokines. Some, such as leptin, help control energy balance. Others, including the cytokines TNF-α, IL-6, and IL-1β, are thought to modulate systemic inflammation. Another adipose hormone, adiponectin, is thought to reduce insulin resistance, while adipose-derived complement and complement-related proteins (adipsin and complement factor B) are proposed to modulate immunity.[117,118]

Excess fat has been associated with metabolic syndrome; however, not all obese patients manifest features of the metabolic syndrome.[119] Furthermore, complete lack of adipose tissue, such as in patients with lipodystrophy, results in the paradoxical development of severe insulin resistance and diabetes.[120] These observations reveal that the role of adipose tissue in the development of metabolic syndrome is rather complex, and regional differences in adipocyte biology have provided new pathophysiological explanations of these noted differences.

5.5.1 THE PORTAL HYPOTHESIS

Many studies have found a strong correlation between the preferential gain of upper-body/visceral fat and insulin resistance.[121] This led investigators to suggest that visceral adipocytes, which have been found to be more lipolytically active in vitro,[122] were releasing large amounts of FFA into the portal vein and subsequently (via the hepatic vein) into the systemic circulation. This idea was termed the *portal hypothesis* and includes the effects of high portal venous FFA derived from visceral fat having adverse effects on the liver—increased lipid synthesis, gluconeogenesis, and ultimately insulin resistance.[123] This excess of FFA was thought to also inhibit skeletal muscle glucose uptake due to preferential use of FFA[124] and would result in peripheral insulin resistance. However, studies using hepatic vein catheterization techniques have shown that visceral fat contributes to only 15% of the systemic FFA, with the majority of FFA derived by non-splanchnic upper-body adipose tissue.[12] This observation raised important questions as to whether visceral adiposity was the culprit for insulin resistance and placed new emphasis on the theory of "ectopic fat" depots.

5.5.2 ECTOPIC FAT DEPOTS

Associations between the function of upper body subcutaneous fat and insulin resistance have emerged,[24,125] and given that subcutaneous fat doesn't drain to the portal vein, this made a pure version of the "portal theory" harder to support. The concept that visceral fat is another ectopic fat depot now seems to fit more of the observations.[126] Under ideal physiological conditions, humans primarily store fat in the upper- and lower-body subcutaneous fat depots. Although in lean adults, visceral adipose tissue avidly stores (and obviously releases) dietary fat,[127] with greater degrees of fatness, visceral adipose tissue stores dietary fat less well,[128] and direct FFA uptake is also impaired.[129] This argues against the concept that visceral fat is a pernicious depot that preferentially takes up fatty acids and then floods the body with inappropriate amounts of FFA. Instead, we interpret these data as indicating that visceral fat is expanding in the context of dysfunctional subcutaneous fat. This dysfunction may involve both excess FFA release[130] and less-efficient storage of circulating triglycerides.[128,131] Thus, with progressive hypertrophic obesity, subcutaneous fat functions abnormally, with excess FFA that can lead to excess lipid deposition into other non-adipose organs, including skeletal muscle (intramyocellular triglycerides), liver, pancreas, and perhaps the heart, thus forming the "ectopic fat depots." Lipid deposition in these ectopic sites leads to insulin resistance (impaired glucose uptake in muscle and increased glucose output in liver) and to impaired insulin secretion from the β-cells of the pancreas.

Patients with lipodystrophies are an example of "ectopic fat" theory. Lipodystrophy in humans is an acquired or hereditary syndrome in which patients are characterized by a decrease in adipose tissue mass but paradoxically develop marked insulin resistance.[132] The limited adipose storage capacity of these patients leads to excess triglycerides being diverted in the liver,[133] skeletal muscle, and pancreatic β-cells, leading to insulin resistance and diabetes.

5.5.3 SECRETION OF ADIPOKINES FROM THE ADIPOSE TISSUE

It is also possible that there are regional differences in adipocyte biology as it relates to secretion of adipokines that regulate multiple biological processes. Adipokines are secreted mainly by adipocytes and other inflammatory cells located in the adipose tissue.[39] Adipocytes located in the various fat depots respond differently to increased glycemic load, with an overexpression of cytokines, such as adiponectin, leptin, TNF-α, IL-6, and angiotensinogen.[134] Chronic, low-grade inflammation induced by these adipokines may alter glucose and lipid metabolism and contribute to insulin resistance.[123,135]

5.6 REGIONAL DIFFERENCES IN FREE FATTY ACID RELEASE

Independent of the exact underlying mechanism, high concentrations of FFA derived from the portal and systemic circulation have been strongly linked to obesity and insulin resistance.[136] FFAs originate almost entirely from hydrolysis of stored lipid droplets in the adipose tissue under postabsorptive conditions. During the postprandial time interval, some circulating FFAs are from the spillover of fatty acids from hydrolysis of triglyceride-rich lipoproteins.[137] Under fasting conditions, upper-body subcutaneous adipose tissue in both men and women is more lipolytically active than lower-body subcutaneous fat; approximately three-fourths of all circulating FFAs come from upper-body subcutaneous fat.[138] After a meal ingestion and in response to hyperinsulinemia, lower-body FFA release is much more readily suppressed than upper-body subcutaneous fat and the splanchnic bed (a marker of visceral adipose tissue lipolysis).[139]

Apart from its lipolytic function, adipose tissue is also a major site of meal fatty acid storage. Similar to its major role in systemic fatty acid release, upper-body subcutaneous fat is more efficient in storage of meal-derived fatty acids than lower-body subcutaneous and visceral fat stores more fat than either upper-body subcutaneous or lower-body subcutaneous fat in normal-weight men and women.[127,140,141]

Appropriate regulation of FFA availability is pivotal for optimal human health. Studies have shown that excess FFA can induce insulin resistance by inhibiting muscle glucose uptake,[142] induce resistance to insulin's ability to suppress endogenous glucose production,[143] attenuate hypertriglyceridemia,[144] reduce hepatic insulin clearance,[145] and impair β-cell insulin secretion.[146]

5.6.1 EFFECT OF INCREASED FREE FATTY ACIDS ON THE LIVER

Insulin acts directly on the liver to limit glucose output by inhibiting glycogen phosphorylation and indirectly by decreasing the flow of FFA and thus decreasing hepatic gluconeogenesis.[147] In those with upper-body/visceral obesity, the delivery of excess FFA to the liver from systemic and/or portal circulation[24] is likely to reduce the ability of insulin to inhibit hepatic glucose production and very low-density lipoprotein (VLDL)–triglyceride secretion, with the latter being more pronounced in patients with greater visceral adiposity.[148]

5.6.2 EFFECT OF INCREASED FREE FATTY ACIDS ON THE SKELETAL MUSCLE

Skeletal muscle is the predominant organ of glucose disposal in the human body,[149] thus muscle tissue dysfunction with respect to glucose uptake is central in the pathogenesis of insulin resistance. It is well documented that excess FFA results in reduced insulin sensitivity as measured by glucose uptake in skeletal muscle.[150] One theory is through the preferential oxidation of fatty acids in comparison to glucose, resulting in a decrease of glucose uptake and oxidation (the Randle cycle).[123] However, excess FFAs are also shown to interrupt muscle insulin receptor substrate-1 and its downstream signaling, resulting in impairment of insulin-mediated glucose uptake independent of muscle oxidative preferential substrate.[151] Elevation of plasma FFA is thought to drive production of long-chain acyl-CoAs, ceramides, and diacylglycerols, some of the culprit molecules thought to disrupt insulin-mediated signaling.[152] Considering that the majority of excess FFA is derived from upper-body subcutaneous adipose tissue, the upper-body subcutaneous fat depot is likely to be an important culprit for skeletal muscle–induced insulin resistance.[153]

5.6.3 EFFECT OF INCREASED FREE FATTY ACIDS ON β-CELL DYSFUNCTION

The presence of FFA is essential for glucose-mediated insulin secretion in pancreatic islet β-cells. However, persistent elevation of FFA augments glucose-mediated insulin secretion, which, when combined with elevated glucose concentrations, results in the eventual impairment of insulin synthesis and induction of β-cell apoptosis.[150,154] Several mechanisms have been proposed to mediate the toxic effect of excess FFA in the pancreatic β-cells; however, further research is being conducted in this field.[155]

5.7 REGIONAL DIFFERENCES IN INSULIN ACTION IN VISCERAL AND SUBCUTANEOUS FAT CELLS

We have come to understand that regional differences in the regulation of lipolysis exist, which has implications for the pathophysiology of obesity-related metabolic abnormalities. The primary modulators of lipolysis are insulin, catecholamines, cytokines, and possibly atrial natriuretic factor; growth hormone and cortisol have less-pronounced immediate effects but likely have important long-term regulatory actions. These hormones, catecholamines, and cytokines seem to have different potencies in different depots (visceral versus subcutaneous). The mechanism(s) through which this occurs is not entirely clear.

Insulin's role is to inhibit lipolysis, increase fat storage, and regulate fat cell glucose uptake.[156] Visceral adipocytes studied in vitro are more resistant to the antilipolytic effect of insulin and fat storage compared to subcutaneous adipose tissue. Functional differences in the insulin receptor and the post-receptor signaling between the two fat depots have been observed.[157] Nevertheless, visceral fat is not the source of excess systemic postprandial FFA in obesity, given that the greater postprandial FFA availability that is observed in upper-body obese women and type 2 diabetics is from upper body subcutaneous fat.[158]

5.8 REGIONAL DIFFERENCES IN THE CATECHOLAMINE-MEDIATED REGULATION OF LIPOLYSIS IN VISCERAL AND SUBCUTANEOUS FAT CELLS

The sympathetic nervous system also plays a pivotal role in the control of lipolysis in adipose tissue. Human adipocytes express both β- and α-adrenergic receptors; activation of β1- and β2-adrenoreceptors stimulates lipolysis, whereas activation of α2-adrenoreceptors inhibits lipolysis. Similar to insulin action, regional differences in catecholamine-induced lipolysis activity between subcutaneous and visceral adipose tissue have been reported.[104,159] In vitro studies in isolated fat cells have shown that the lipolytic response to catecholamines is less when the cells come from subcutaneous leg and abdominal fat than when visceral fat cells are studied.[160] These site-specific lipolytic defects can be explained by either a difference in the number or responsiveness of the adrenergic receptors or by an altered expression and/or function of the hormone-sensitive lipase and its associated proteins (i.e., adipocyte lipid-binding protein).[161,162]

Similarly, exercise-induced activation of the sympathetic system results in β-adrenoreceptor stimulation and enhancement of lipolysis equally from the two fat compartments (leg fat and splanchnic) in both men and women volunteers.[163,164] However, exercise-induced lipolysis is impaired in subcutaneous abdominal adipose tissue in obese men when compared with lean controls, and this is thought to occur due to activation of the antilipolytic effect of $\alpha 2$-adrenoceptors during exercise.[165]

5.9 EFFECT OF WEIGHT LOSS ON REGIONAL FAT DISTRIBUTION

There have been a number of studies documenting how the human body preferentially mobilizes fat from specific fat depots during conditions of energy deficits. Most studies suggest that, independent of the weight loss modality (diet, physical activity, or weight loss medications), the relative amount of visceral loss is the greatest.[166–168]

Specifically, in a study by Singh et al., normal-weight adults who lost weight through underfeeding after an experimentally induced weight gain showed that visceral and upper-body subcutaneous fat masses had returned to pre-overfeeding amounts, whereas lower-body fat had not.[169] This preferential mobilization of upper-body subcutaneous and visceral fat during weight loss may reflect the differences in storage capacity and lipolytic rates between the various fat compartments. In addition, this group found that decreases in both upper-body and lower-body subcutaneous fat mass during weight loss was due to decreases in fat cell size, but not in fat cell number. This observation has been supported by other studies.[170] Whether a similar caloric deficit induced by diet or by an exercise program will generate the same loss of visceral adipose tissue in a given individual is an area of debate,[168] with most studies supporting that caloric restriction leading to a moderate weight loss results in a greater relative change in visceral versus subcutaneous abdominal fat in comparison to exercise.[59] However, the advantage of vigorous regular exercise over caloric restriction is that it would preserve or, in some cases, increase lean muscle mass.[171,172]

In theory, surgical excision of upper-body fat should be effective in reducing metabolic abnormalities. In reality, however, liposuction (removal of subcutaneous fat) did not improve insulin sensitivity in skeletal muscle, liver, or adipose tissue, and had no significant effects on other cardiovascular risk factors.[8] Furthermore, although some studies on selective reduction of visceral fat have found improvement in metabolic parameters,[173,174] these were confounded by clinically important, if not statistically significant, differences in weight loss at follow-up. A number of other studies have not been able to document metabolic improvements from surgical removal of visceral fat.[7,175] These conflicting data may be a result of inconsistency in the outcomes measured, differences in baseline BMI between the groups studied (especially in studies that showed a significant beneficial effect), and the combination of omentectomy (visceral fat removal) with other surgical techniques, such as gastric bypass.

Weight loss after bariatric surgery is usually associated with an improvement in insulin resistance and other cardiovascular risk factors (i.e., hyperlipidemia, hypertension, and obstructive sleep apnea).[176] Limited data exist on the effect of bariatric surgery on subsequent effect on fat distribution. Olbers et al. documented preferential mobilization of visceral adipose tissue in women 1 year after Roux-en Y gastric bypass compared with vertical banded gastroplasty; however, in men, reduction in visceral adipose tissue was not significantly different.[177] In the study by Weiss et al., looking at early (6 months) changes in fat adiposity after bariatric surgery, a similar reduction was shown between visceral and subcutaneous fat adiposity.[178]

5.10 CONCLUSION

The prevalence of obesity worldwide has reached epidemic proportions, resulting in an exponential rise of obesity-related metabolic complications, such as insulin resistance. The fact that body fat distribution is an important predictor of the development of obesity-related metabolic complications strongly suggests that some fundamental properties of adipose tissue vary considerably, in concert with regional variation in fat gain. Factors such as age, sex, genetics, race, nutrition, and others regulate regional adipose tissue morphology.

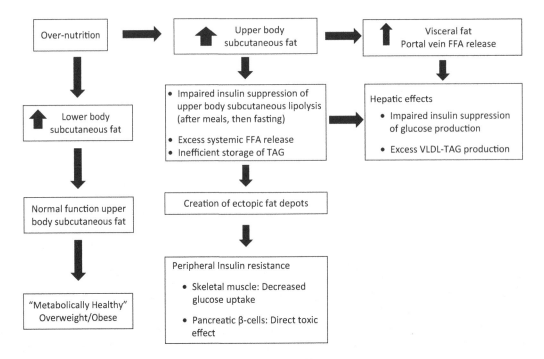

FIGURE 5.1   Schematic representation of how different fat depots contribute to insulin resistance via the fatty acid pathway. (FFA, free fatty acid; TAG, triaglycerol; VLDL, very low-density lipoprotein.)

Although visceral obesity is strongly linked with metabolic complications, evidence from studies that have measured regional FFA release, combined with studies that manipulate FFA, suggest that these metabolic derangements are at least partially a result of excess FFA derived from upper-body subcutaneous adipose tissue. The excess FFA from upper-body subcutaneous fat results in peripheral insulin resistance. Visceral fat is now being considered a marker of subcutaneous fat dysfunction, leading to undesired excess fat accumulation at the liver, skeletal muscle, pancreas, and heart (Figure 5.1). Understanding how regional adipose tissue handles excess caloric intake should provide clues on how to best identify patients at high risk for cardiometabolic complications and how to best counsel and manage these undesired metabolic consequences.

REFERENCES

1. Rowley WR, Bezold C, Arikan Y, Byrne E, Krohe S. Diabetes 2030: Insights from yesterday, today, and future trends. *Popul Health Manag* 2017; **20**(1): 6–12.
2. Hurt RT, Kulisek C, Buchanan LA, McClave SA. The obesity epidemic: Challenges, health initiatives, and implications for gastroenterologists. *Gastroenterol Hepatol* 2010; **6**(12): 780–92.
3. Smith SR, Lovejoy JC, Greenway F, et al. Contributions of total body fat, abdominal subcutaneous adipose tissue compartments, and visceral adipose tissue to the metabolic complications of obesity. *Metabolism* 2001; **50**(4): 425–35.
4. Carey VJ, Walters EE, Colditz GA, et al. Body fat distribution and risk of non-insulin-dependent diabetes mellitus in women. The Nurses' Health Study. *Am J Epidemiol* 1997; **145**(7): 614–9.
5. Chan JM, Rimm EB, Colditz GA, Stampfer MJ, Willett WC. Obesity, fat distribution, and weight gain as risk factors for clinical diabetes in men. *Diabetes Care* 1994; **17**(9): 961–9.
6. Welborn TA, Dhaliwal SS. Preferred clinical measures of central obesity for predicting mortality. *Eur J Clin Nutr* 2007; **61**(12): 1373–9.
7. Fabbrini E, Tamboli RA, Magkos F, et al. Surgical removal of omental fat does not improve insulin sensitivity and cardiovascular risk factors in obese adults. *Gastroenterology* 2010; **139**(2): 448–55.

8. Klein S, Fontana L, Young VL, et al. Absence of an effect of liposuction on insulin action and risk factors for coronary heart disease. *N Engl J Med* 2004; **350**(25): 2549–57.

9. Magkos F, Fraterrigo G, Yoshino J, et al. Effects of moderate and subsequent progressive weight loss on metabolic function and adipose tissue biology in humans with obesity. *Cell Metab* 2016; **23**(4): 591–601.

10. Abate N, Garg A, Peshock RM, Stray-Gundersen J, Adams-Huet B, Grundy SM. Relationship of generalized and regional adiposity to insulin sensitivity in men with NIDDM. *Diabetes* 1996; **45**(12): 1684–93.

11. Goodpaster BH, Thaete FL, Simoneau JA, Kelley DE. Subcutaneous abdominal fat and thigh muscle composition predict insulin sensitivity independently of visceral fat. *Diabetes* 1997; **46**(10): 1579–85.

12. Jensen MD, Johnson CM. Contribution of leg and splanchnic free fatty acid (FFA) kinetics to postabsorptive FFA flux in men and women. *Metabolism* 1996; **45**(5): 662–6.

13. Goodpaster BH, Krishnaswami S, Harris TB, et al. Obesity, regional body fat distribution, and the metabolic syndrome in older men and women. *Arch Intern Med* 2005; **165**(7): 777–83.

14. Lakka TA, Lakka HM, Salonen R, Kaplan GA, Salonen JT. Abdominal obesity is associated with accelerated progression of carotid atherosclerosis in men. *Atherosclerosis* 2001; **154**(2): 497–504.

15. Lakka HM, Lakka TA, Tuomilehto J, Salonen JT. Abdominal obesity is associated with increased risk of acute coronary events in men. *Eur Heart J* 2002; **23**(9): 706–13.

16. Ravussin E, Smith SR. Increased fat intake, impaired fat oxidation, and failure of fat cell proliferation result in ectopic fat storage, insulin resistance, and type 2 diabetes mellitus. *Ann N Y Acad Sci* 2002; **967**: 363–78.

17. Goossens GH. The role of adipose tissue dysfunction in the pathogenesis of obesity-related insulin resistance. *Physiol Behav* 2008; **94**(2): 206–18.

18. Ebbert JO, Jensen MD. Fat depots, free fatty acids, and dyslipidemia. *Nutrients* 2013; **5**(2): 498–508.

19. Tchoukalova YD, Koutsari C, Votruba SB, et al. Sex- and depot-dependent differences in adipogenesis in normal-weight humans. *Obesity (Silver Spring)* 2010; **18**(10): 1875–80.

20. Goodpaster BH, Thaete FL, Kelley DE. Thigh adipose tissue distribution is associated with insulin resistance in obesity and in type 2 diabetes mellitus. *Am J Clin Nutr* 2000; **71**(4): 885–92.

21. Tchoukalova YD, Koutsari C, Karpyak MV, Votruba SB, Wendland E, Jensen MD. Subcutaneous adipocyte size and body fat distribution. *Am J Clin Nutr* 2008; **87**(1): 56–63.

22. Snijder MB, Dekker JM, Visser M, et al. Trunk fat and leg fat have independent and opposite associations with fasting and postload glucose levels: The Hoorn study. *Diabetes Care* 2004; **27**(2): 372–7.

23. Kelley DE, Thaete FL, Troost F, Huwe T, Goodpaster BH. Subdivisions of subcutaneous abdominal adipose tissue and insulin resistance. *Am J Physiol Endocrinol Metab* 2000; **278**(5): E941–8.

24. Nielsen S, Guo Z, Johnson CM, Hensrud DD, Jensen MD. Splanchnic lipolysis in human obesity. *J Clin Invest* 2004; **113**(11): 1582–8.

25. Jensen MD, Kanaley JA, Reed JE, Sheedy PF. Measurement of abdominal and visceral fat with computed tomography and dual-energy x-ray absorptiometry. *Am J Clin Nutr* 1995; **61**(2): 274–8.

26. Poonawalla AH, Sjoberg BP, Rehm JL, et al. Adipose tissue MRI for quantitative measurement of central obesity. *J Magn Reson Imaging* 2013; **37**(3): 707–16.

27. Wagner DR, Heyward VH. Techniques of body composition assessment: A review of laboratory and field methods. *Res Q Exerc Sport* 1999; **70**(2): 135–49.

28. Duren DL, Sherwood RJ, Czerwinski SA, et al. Body composition methods: Comparisons and interpretation. *J Diabetes Sci Technol* 2008; **2**(6): 1139–46.

29. Kuk JL, Saunders TJ, Davidson LE, Ross R. Age-related changes in total and regional fat distribution. *Ageing Res Rev* 2009; **8**(4): 339–48.

30. Wajchenberg BL. Subcutaneous and visceral adipose tissue: Their relation to the metabolic syndrome. *Endocr Rev* 2000; **21**(6): 697–738.

31. Blaak E. Gender differences in fat metabolism. *Curr Opin Clin Nutr Metab Care* 2001; **4**(6): 499–502.

32. Krotkiewski M, Bjorntorp P, Sjostrom L, Smith U. Impact of obesity on metabolism in men and women. Importance of regional adipose tissue distribution. *J Clin Invest* 1983; **72**(3): 1150–62.

33. Kvist H, Chowdhury B, Grangard U, Tylen U, Sjostrom L. Total and visceral adipose-tissue volumes derived from measurements with computed tomography in adult men and women: Predictive equations. *Am J Clin Nutr* 1988; **48**(6): 1351–61.

34. Goss AM, Darnell BE, Brown MA, Oster RA, Gower BA. Longitudinal associations of the endocrine environment on fat partitioning in postmenopausal women. *Obesity (Silver Spring)* 2012; **20**(5): 939–44.

35. Seidell JC, Bjorntorp P, Sjostrom L, Kvist H, Sannerstedt R. Visceral fat accumulation in men is positively associated with insulin, glucose, and C-peptide levels, but negatively with testosterone levels. *Metabolism* 1990; **39**(9): 897–901.

36. Reyes-Vidal CM, Mojahed H, Shen W, et al. Adipose tissue redistribution and ectopic lipid deposition in active acromegaly and effects of surgical treatment. *J Clin Endocrinol Metab* 2015; **100**(8): 2946–55.

37. Lovejoy JC, de la Bretonne JA, Klemperer M, Tulley R. Abdominal fat distribution and metabolic risk factors: Effects of race. *Metabolism* 1996; **45**(9): 1119–24.

38. Kanaley JA, Giannopoulou I, Tillapaugh-Fay G, Nappi JS, Ploutz-Snyder LL. Racial differences in subcutaneous and visceral fat distribution in postmenopausal black and white women. *Metabolism* 2003; **52**(2): 186–91.

39. Tchernof A, Despres JP. Pathophysiology of human visceral obesity: An update. *Physiol Rev* 2013; **93**(1): 359–404.

40. Heymsfield SB, Peterson CM, Thomas DM, Heo M, Schuna JM, Jr. Why are there race/ethnic differences in adult body mass index-adiposity relationships? A quantitative critical review. *Obesity Rev* 2016; **17**(3): 262–75.

41. Albu JB, Murphy L, Frager DH, Johnson JA, Pi-Sunyer FX. Visceral fat and race-dependent health risks in obese nondiabetic premenopausal women. *Diabetes* 1997; **46**(3): 456–62.

42. Conway JM, Yanovski SZ, Avila NA, Hubbard VS. Visceral adipose tissue differences in black and white women. *Am J Clin Nutr* 1995; **61**(4): 765–71.

43. Miller WC, Lindeman AK, Wallace J, Niederpruem M. Diet composition, energy intake, and exercise in relation to body fat in men and women. *Am J Clin Nutr* 1990; **52**(3): 426–30.

44. Atlantis E, Martin SA, Haren MT, Taylor AW, Wittert GA. Lifestyle factors associated with age-related differences in body composition: The Florey Adelaide Male Aging Study. *Am J Clin Nutr* 2008; **88**(1): 95–104.

45. Larson DE, Hunter GR, Williams MJ, Kekes-Szabo T, Nyikos I, Goran MI. Dietary fat in relation to body fat and intraabdominal adipose tissue: A cross-sectional analysis. *Am J Clin Nutr* 1996; **64**(5): 677–84.

46. Tucker LA, Kano MJ. Dietary fat and body fat: A multivariate study of 205 adult females. *Am J Clin Nutr* 1992; **56**(4): 616–22.

47. Bowen L, Taylor AE, Sullivan R, et al. Associations between diet, physical activity and body fat distribution: A cross sectional study in an Indian population. *BMC Public Health* 2015; **15**: 281.

48. Koppes LL, Boon N, Nooyens AC, van Mechelen W, Saris WH. Macronutrient distribution over a period of 23 years in relation to energy intake and body fatness. *Br J Nutr* 2009; **101**(1): 108–15.

49. Soenen S, Westerterp-Plantenga MS. Changes in body fat percentage during body weight stable conditions of increased daily protein intake vs. control. *Physiol Behav* 2010; **101**(5): 635–8.

50. Vinknes KJ, de Vogel S, Elshorbagy AK, et al. Dietary intake of protein is positively associated with percent body fat in middle-aged and older adults. *J Nutr* 2011; **141**(3): 440–6.

51. de Souza RJ, Bray GA, Carey VJ, et al. Effects of 4 weight-loss diets differing in fat, protein, and carbohydrate on fat mass, lean mass, visceral adipose tissue, and hepatic fat: Results from the POUNDS LOST trial. *Am J Clin Nutr* 2012; **95**(3): 614–25.

52. Garaulet M, Hernandez-Morante JJ, Lujan J, Tebar FJ, Zamora S. Relationship between fat cell size and number and fatty acid composition in adipose tissue from different fat depots in overweight/obese humans. *Int J Obes (2005)* 2006; **30**(6): 899–905.

53. Garaulet M, Perez-Llamas F, Perez-Ayala M, et al. Site-specific differences in the fatty acid composition of abdominal adipose tissue in an obese population from a Mediterranean area: Relation with dietary fatty acids, plasma lipid profile, serum insulin, and central obesity. *Am J Clin Nutr* 2001; **74**(5): 585–91.

54. Paniagua JA, Gallego de la Sacristana A, Romero I, et al. Monounsaturated fat-rich diet prevents central body fat distribution and decreases postprandial adiponectin expression induced by a carbohydrate-rich diet in insulin-resistant subjects. *Diabetes Care* 2007; **30**(7): 1717–23.

55. Romaguera D, Norat T, Mouw T, et al. Adherence to the Mediterranean diet is associated with lower abdominal adiposity in European men and women. *J Nutr* 2009; **139**(9): 1728–37.

56. Moliner-Urdiales D, Ruiz JR, Ortega FB, et al. Association of objectively assessed physical activity with total and central body fat in Spanish adolescents; the HELENA Study. *Int J Obes (2005)* 2009; **33**(10): 1126–35.

57. Janssen I, Katzmarzyk PT, Boyce WF, et al. Comparison of overweight and obesity prevalence in school-aged youth from 34 countries and their relationships with physical activity and dietary patterns. *Obes Rev* 2005; **6**(2): 123–32.

58. Abe T, Sakurai T, Kurata J, Kawakami Y, Fukunaga T. Subcutaneous and visceral fat distribution and daily physical activity: Comparison between young and middle aged women. *Br J Sports Med* 1996; **30**(4): 297–300.

59. Chaston TB, Dixon JB. Factors associated with percent change in visceral versus subcutaneous abdominal fat during weight loss: Findings from a systematic review. *Int J Obes (2005)* 2008; **32**(4): 619–28.

60. Ross R, Rissanen J, Pedwell H, Clifford J, Shragge P. Influence of diet and exercise on skeletal muscle and visceral adipose tissue in men. *J Appl Physiol* 1996; **81**: 2445–55.

61. Ross R, Janssen I, Dawson J, et al. Exercise-induced reduction in obesity and insulin resistance in women: A randomized controlled trial. *Obes Res* 2004; **12**(5): 789–98.

62. Ross R, Dagnone D, Jones PJ, et al. Reduction in obesity and related comorbid conditions after diet-induced weight loss or exercise-induced weight loss in men. A randomized, controlled trial. *Ann Intern Med* 2000; **133**(2): 92–103.

63. Slentz CA, Houmard JA, Kraus WE. Exercise, abdominal obesity, skeletal muscle, and metabolic risk: Evidence for a dose response. *Obesity (Silver Spring)* 2009; **17 Suppl 3**: S27–33.

64. Cleland VJ, Schmidt MD, Dwyer T, Venn AJ. Television viewing and abdominal obesity in young adults: Is the association mediated by food and beverage consumption during viewing time or reduced leisure-time physical activity? *Am J Clin Nutr* 2008; **87**(5): 1148–55.

65. Chang PC, Li TC, Wu MT, et al. Association between television viewing and the risk of metabolic syndrome in a community-based population. *BMC Public Health* 2008; **8**: 193.

66. Hu FB. Sedentary lifestyle and risk of obesity and type 2 diabetes. *Lipids* 2003; **38**(2): 103–8.

67. Wannamethee SG, Shaper AG, Whincup PH. Alcohol and adiposity: Effects of quantity and type of drink and time relation with meals. *Int J Obes* 2005; **29**(12): 1436–44.

68. Canoy D, Wareham N, Luben R, et al. Cigarette smoking and fat distribution in 21,828 British men and women: A population-based study. *Obes Res* 2005; **13**(8): 1466–75.

69. Bjorntorp P. Do stress reactions cause abdominal obesity and comorbidities? *Obes Rev* 2001; **2**(2): 73–86.

70. Sachdev HS, Fall CH, Osmond C, et al. Anthropometric indicators of body composition in young adults: Relation to size at birth and serial measurements of body mass index in childhood in the New Delhi birth cohort. *Am J Clin Nutr* 2005; **82**(2): 456–66.

71. Komiya H, Mori Y, Yokose T, Tajima N. Smoking as a risk factor for visceral fat accumulation in Japanese men. *Tohoku J Exp Med* 2006; **208**(2): 123–32.

72. Molenaar EA, Massaro JM, Jacques PF, et al. Association of lifestyle factors with abdominal subcutaneous and visceral adiposity: The Framingham Heart Study. *Diabetes Care* 2009; **32**(3): 505–10.

73. Yang X, Smith U. Adipose tissue distribution and risk of metabolic disease: Does thiazolidinedione-induced adipose tissue redistribution provide a clue to the answer? *Diabetologia* 2007; **50**(6): 1127–39.

74. Shadid S, Jensen MD. Effects of pioglitazone versus diet and exercise on metabolic health and fat distribution in upper body obesity. *Diabetes Care* 2003; **26**(11): 3148–52.

75. Mekala KC, Tritos NA. Effects of recombinant human growth hormone therapy in obesity in adults: A meta analysis. *J Clin Endocrinol Metab* 2009; **94**(1): 130–7.

76. Bouchard C, Tremblay A, Despres JP, et al. The response to long-term overfeeding in identical twins. *N Engl J Med* 1990; **322**(21): 1477–82.

77. Bouchard C, Despres JP, Mauriege P. Genetic and nongenetic determinants of regional fat distribution. *Endocr Rev* 1993; **14**(1): 72–93.

78. Bouchard C, Tremblay A. Genetic influences on the response of body fat and fat distribution to positive and negative energy balances in human identical twins. *J Nutr* 1997; **127**(5 Suppl): 943s–7s.

79. Heard-Costa NL, Zillikens MC, Monda KL, et al. NRXN3 is a novel locus for waist circumference: A genome-wide association study from the CHARGE Consortium. *PLoS Genetics* 2009; **5**(6): e1000539.

80. Schleinitz D, Bottcher Y, Bluher M, Kovacs P. The genetics of fat distribution. *Diabetologia* 2014; **57**(7): 1276–86.

81. Fox CS, Liu Y, White CC, et al. Genome-wide association for abdominal subcutaneous and visceral adipose reveals a novel locus for visceral fat in women. *PLoS genetics* 2012; **8**(5): e1002695.

82. Bjorntorp P, Grimby G, Sanne H, Sjostrom L, Tibblin G, Wilhelmsen L. Adipose tissue fat cell size in relation to metabolism in weight-stabile, physically active men. *Horm Metab Res* 1972; **4**(3): 182–6.

83. Haller H, Leonhardt W, Hanefeld M, Julius U. Relationship between adipocyte hypertrophy and metabolic disturbances. *Endokrinologie* 1979; **74**(1): 63–72.

84. O'Connell J, Lynch L, Cawood TJ, et al. The relationship of omental and subcutaneous adipocyte size to metabolic disease in severe obesity. *PLoS One* 2010; **5**(4): e9997.

85. Bjorntorp P, Bengtsson C, Blohme G, et al. Adipose tissue fat cell size and number in relation to metabolism in randomly selected middle-aged men and women. *Metabolism* 1971; **20**(10): 927–35.

86. Salans LB, Cushman SW, Weismann RE. Studies of human adipose tissue. Adipose cell size and number in nonobese and obese patients. *J Clin Invest* 1973; **52**(4): 929–41.

87. Ryden M, Andersson DP, Bergstrom IB, Arner P. Adipose tissue and metabolic alterations: Regional differences in fat cell size and number matter, but differently: A cross-sectional study. *J Clin Endocrinol Metab* 2014; **99**(10): E1870–6.

88. Tchoukalova YD, Votruba SB, Tchkonia T, Giorgadze N, Kirkland JL, Jensen MD. Regional differences in cellular mechanisms of adipose tissue gain with overfeeding. *Proc Natl Acad Sci U S A* 2010; **107**(42): 18226–31.

89. Joe AW, Yi L, Even Y, Vogl AW, Rossi FM. Depot-specific differences in adipogenic progenitor abundance and proliferative response to high-fat diet. *Stem Cells (Dayton, Ohio)* 2009; **27**(10): 2563–70.

90. Bjorntorp P. Sjostrom L. Number and size of adipose tissue fat cells in relation to metabolism in human obesity. *Metabolism* 1971; **20**(7): 703–13.

91. Arner E, Westermark PO, Spalding KL, et al. Adipocyte turnover: Relevance to human adipose tissue morphology. *Diabetes* 2010; **59**(1): 105–9.

92. Laforest S, Labrecque J, Michaud A, Cianflone K, Tchernof A. Adipocyte size as a determinant of metabolic disease and adipose tissue dysfunction. *Critical reviews in clinical laboratory sciences* 2015; **52**(6): 301–13.

93. Kissebah AH, Vydelingum N, Murray R, et al. Relation of body fat distribution to metabolic complications of obesity. *J Clin Endocrinol Metab* 1982; **54**(2): 254–60.

94. Despres JP, Nadeau A, Tremblay A, et al. Role of deep abdominal fat in the association between regional adipose tissue distribution and glucose tolerance in obese women. *Diabetes* 1989; **38**(3): 304–9.

95. Weyer C, Foley JE, Bogardus C, Tataranni PA, Pratley RE. Enlarged subcutaneous abdominal adipocyte size, but not obesity itself, predicts type II diabetes independent of insulin resistance. *Diabetologia* 2000; **43**(12): 1498–506.

96. Joffe BI, Goldberg RB, Feinstein J, Kark A, Seftel HC. Adipose cell size in obese Africans: Evidence against the existence of insulin resistance in some patients. *J Clin Pathol* 1979; **32**(5): 471–4.

97. McLaughlin T, Sherman A, Tsao P, et al. Enhanced proportion of small adipose cells in insulin-resistant vs insulin-sensitive obese individuals implicates impaired adipogenesis. *Diabetologia* 2007; **50**(8): 1707–15.

98. Veilleux A, Caron-Jobin M, Noel S, Laberge PY, Tchernof A. Visceral adipocyte hypertrophy is associated with dyslipidemia independent of body composition and fat distribution in women. *Diabetes* 2011; **60**(5): 1504–11.

99. Hardy OT, Perugini RA, Nicoloro SM, et al. Body mass index-independent inflammation in omental adipose tissue associated with insulin resistance in morbid obesity. *Surg Obes Relat Dis* 2011; **7**(1): 60–7.

100. Anand SS, Tarnopolsky MA, Rashid S, et al. Adipocyte hypertrophy, fatty liver and metabolic risk factors in South Asians: The Molecular Study of Health and Risk in Ethnic Groups (mol-SHARE). *PLoS One* 2011; **6**(7): e22112.

101. Petaja EM, Sevastianova K, Hakkarainen A, Orho-Melander M, Lundbom N, Yki-Jarvinen H. Adipocyte size is associated with NAFLD independent of obesity, fat distribution, and PNPLA3 genotype. *Obesity (Silver Spring)* 2013; **21**(6): 1174–9.

102. Johannsen DL, Tchoukalova Y, Tam CS, et al. Effect of 8 weeks of overfeeding on ectopic fat deposition and insulin sensitivity: Testing the "adipose tissue expandability" hypothesis. *Diabetes Care* 2014; **37**(10): 2789–97.

103. Jansen HJ, Vervoort GM, van der Graaf M, Stienstra R, Tack CJ. Liver fat content is linked to inflammatory changes in subcutaneous adipose tissue in type 2 diabetes patients. *Clin Endocrinol (Oxf)* 2013; **79**(5): 661–6.

104. Arner P, Arner E, Hammarstedt A, Smith U. Genetic predisposition for Type 2 diabetes, but not for overweight/obesity, is associated with a restricted adipogenesis. *PLoS One* 2011; **6**(4): e18284.

105. Anthanont P, Ramos P, Jensen MD, Hames KC. Family history of type 2 diabetes, abdominal adipocyte size and markers of the metabolic syndrome. *Int J Obes* 2017; **41**(11): 1621–6.

106. Fried SK, Kral JG. Sex differences in regional distribution of fat cell size and lipoprotein lipase activity in morbidly obese patients. *Int J Obes* 1987; **11**(2): 129–40.

107. Mundi MS, Karpyak MV, Koutsari C, Votruba SB, O'Brien PC, Jensen MD. Body fat distribution, adipocyte size, and metabolic characteristics of nondiabetic adults. *J Clin Endocrinol Metab* 2010; **95**(1): 67–73.

108. Drolet R, Richard C, Sniderman AD, et al. Hypertrophy and hyperplasia of abdominal adipose tissues in women. *Int J Obes* 2008; **32**(2): 283–91.

109. Ostman J, Arner P, Engfeldt P, Kager L. Regional differences in the control of lipolysis in human adipose tissue. *Metabolism* 1979; **28**(12): 1198–205.

110. Rebuffe-Scrive M, Anderson B, Olbe L, Bjorntorp P. Metabolism of adipose tissue in intraabdominal depots in severely obese men and women. *Metabolism* 1990; **39**(10): 1021–5.

111. Tchernof A, Belanger C, Morisset AS, et al. Regional differences in adipose tissue metabolism in women: Minor effect of obesity and body fat distribution. *Diabetes* 2006; **55**(5): 1353–60.

112. Boivin A, Brochu G, Marceau S, Marceau P, Hould FS, Tchernof A. Regional differences in adipose tissue metabolism in obese men. *Metabolism* 2007; **56**(4): 533–40.

113. Jacobsson B, Smith U. Effect of cell size on lipolysis and antipolytic action of insulin in human fat cells. *J Lipid Res* 1972; **13**(5): 651–6.

114. Richelsen B. Increased alpha 2- but similar beta-adrenergic receptor activities in subcutaneous gluteal adipocytes from females compared with males. *Eur J Clin Invest* 1986; **16**(4): 302–9.

115. Rebuffe-Scrive M, Andersson B, Olbe L, Bjorntorp P. Metabolism of adipose tissue in intraabdominal depots of nonobese men and women. *Metabolism* 1989; **38**(5): 453–8.

116. Jensen MD. Role of body fat distribution and the metabolic complications of obesity. *J Clin Endocrinol Metab* 2008; **93**(11 Suppl 1): S57–63.

117. Trayhurn P, Beattie JH. Physiological role of adipose tissue: White adipose tissue as an endocrine and secretory organ. *Proc Nutr Soc* 2001; **60**(3): 329–39.

118. Fasshauer M, Bluher M. Adipokines in health and disease. *Trends Pharmacol Sci* 2015; **36**(7): 461–70.

119. Karelis AD, St-Pierre DH, Conus F, Rabasa-Lhoret R, Poehlman ET. Metabolic and body composition factors in subgroups of obesity: What do we know? *J Clin Endocrinol Metab* 2004; **89**(6): 2569–75.

120. Garg A, Misra A. Lipodystrophies: Rare disorders causing metabolic syndrome. *Endocrinol Metab Clin North Am* 2004; **33**(2): 305–31.

121. Dagenais GR, Yi Q, Mann JF, Bosch J, Pogue J, Yusuf S. Prognostic impact of body weight and abdominal obesity in women and men with cardiovascular disease. *Am Heart J* 2005; **149**(1): 54–60.

122. Bolinder J, Kager L, Ostman J, Arner P. Differences at the receptor and postreceptor levels between human omental and subcutaneous adipose tissue in the action of insulin on lipolysis. *Diabetes* 1983; **32**(2): 117–23.

123. Bjorntorp P. "Portal" adipose tissue as a generator of risk factors for cardiovascular disease and diabetes. *Arteriosclerosis (Dallas, Tex)* 1990; **10**(4): 493–6.

124. Randle PJ, Garland PB, Hales CN, Newsholme EA. The glucose fatty-acid cycle. Its role in insulin sensitivity and the metabolic disturbances of diabetes mellitus. *Lancet* 1963; **1**(7285): 785–9.

125. Guo ZK, Hensrud DD, Johnson CM, Jensen MD. Regional postprandial fatty acid metabolism in different obesity phenotypes. *Diabetes* 1999; **48**: 1586–92.

126. Rasouli N, Molavi B, Elbein SC, Kern PA. Ectopic fat accumulation and metabolic syndrome. *Diabetes Obes Metab* 2007; **9**(1): 1–10.

127. Jensen MD, Sarr MG, Dumesic DA, Southorn PA, Levine JA. Regional uptake of meal fatty acids in humans. *Am J Physiol Endocrinol Metab* 2003; **285**(6): E1282–8.

128. Votruba SB, Mattison RS, Dumesic DA, Koutsari C, Jensen MD. Meal fatty acid uptake in visceral fat in women. *Diabetes* 2007; **56**(10): 2589–97.

129. Ali AH, Koutsari C, Mundi M, et al. Free fatty acid storage in human visceral and subcutaneous adipose tissue: Role of adipocyte proteins. *Diabetes* 2011; **60**(9): 2300–7.

130. Guo Z, Hensrud DD, Johnson CM, Jensen MD. Regional postprandial fatty acid metabolism in different obesity phenotypes. *Diabetes* 1999; **48**(8): 1586–92.

131. Santosa S, Hensrud DD, Votruba SB, Jensen MD. The influence of sex and obesity phenotype on meal fatty acid metabolism before and after weight loss. *Am J Clin Nutr* 2008; **88**(4): 1134–41.

132. Tritos NA, Mantzoros CS. Clinical review 97: Syndromes of severe insulin resistance. *J Clin Endocrinol Metab* 1998; **83**(9): 3025–30.

133. Ludtke A, Genschel J, Brabant G, et al. Hepatic steatosis in Dunnigan-type familial partial lipodystrophy. *Am J Gastroenterol* 2005; **100**(10): 2218–24.

134. Einstein FH, Atzmon G, Yang XM, et al. Differential responses of visceral and subcutaneous fat depots to nutrients. *Diabetes* 2005; **54**(3): 672–8.

135. Fontana L, Eagon JC, Trujillo ME, Scherer PE, Klein S. Visceral fat adipokine secretion is associated with systemic inflammation in obese humans. *Diabetes* 2007; **56**(4): 1010–3.

136. Boden G. Interaction between free fatty acids and glucose metabolism. *Curr Opin Clin Nutr Metab Care* 2002; **5**(5): 545–9.

137. Roust LR, Jensen MD. Postprandial free fatty acid kinetics are abnormal in upper body obesity. *Diabetes* 1993; **42**: 1567–73.

138. Jensen MD. Gender differences in regional fatty acid metabolism before and after meal ingestion. *J Clin Invest* 1995; **96**(5): 2297–303.

139. Meek SE, Nair KS, Jensen MD. Insulin regulation of regional free fatty acid metabolism. *Diabetes* 1999; **48**(1): 10–4.

140. Marin P, Rebuffe-Scrive M, Bjorntorp P. Uptake of triglyceride fatty acids in adipose tissue in vivo in man. *Eur J Clin Invest* 1990; **20**(2): 158–65.

141. Romanski SA, Nelson RM, Jensen MD. Meal fatty acid uptake in adipose tissue: Gender effects in non-obese humans. *Am J Physiol Endocrinol Metab* 2000; **279**(2): E455–62.

142. Kelley DE, Mokan M, Simoneau JA, Mandarino LJ. Interaction between glucose and free fatty acid metabolism in human skeletal muscle. *J Clin Invest* 1993; **92**(1): 91–8.

143. Saloranta C, Franssila-Kallunki A, Ekstrand A, Taskinen MR, Groop L. Modulation of hepatic glucose production by non-esterified fatty acids in type 2 (non-insulin-dependent) diabetes mellitus. *Diabetologia* 1991; **34**(6): 409–15.

144. Kissebah AH, Alfarsi S, Adams PW, Wynn V. Role of insulin resistance in adipose tissue and liver in the pathogenesis of endogenous hypertriglyceridaemia in man. *Diabetologia* 1976; **12**(6): 563–71.

145. Hennes MM, Shrago E, Kissebah AH. Receptor and postreceptor effects of free fatty acids (FFA) on hepatocyte insulin dynamics. *Int J Obes* 1990; **14**(10): 831–41.

146. Zhou YP, Grill VE. Long-term exposure of rat pancreatic islets to fatty acids inhibits glucose-induced insulin secretion and biosynthesis through a glucose fatty acid cycle. *J Clin Invest* 1994; **93**(2): 870–6.

147. Ramnanan CJ, Edgerton DS, Rivera N, et al. Molecular characterization of insulin-mediated suppression of hepatic glucose production in vivo. *Diabetes* 2010; **59**(6): 1302–11.

148. Lewis GF, Uffelman KD, Szeto LW, Weller B, Steiner G. Interaction between free fatty acids and insulin in the acute control of very low density lipoprotein production in humans. *J Clin Invest* 1995; **95**(1): 158–66.

149. DeFronzo RA. Pathogenesis of type 2 diabetes mellitus. *Med Clin North Am* 2004; **88**(4): 787–835, ix.

150. McGarry JD. Banting lecture 2001: Dysregulation of fatty acid metabolism in the etiology of type 2 diabetes. *Diabetes* 2002; **51**(1): 7–18.

151. Dresner A, Laurent D, Marcucci M, et al. Effects of free fatty acids on glucose transport and IRS-1-associated phosphatidylinositol 3-kinase activity. *J Clin Invest* 1999; **103**(2): 253–9.

152. Kanaley JA, Shadid S, Sheehan MT, Guo Z, Jensen MD. Relationship between plasma free fatty acid, intramyocellular triglycerides and long-chain acylcarnitines in resting humans. *J Physiol* 2009; **587**(Pt 24): 5939–50.

153. Chung JO, Koutsari C, Blachnio-Zabielska AU, Hames KC, Jensen MD. Intramyocellular ceramides: Subcellular concentrations and fractional De Novo synthesis in postabsorptive humans. *Diabetes* 2017; **66**(8): 2082–91.

154. El-Assaad W, Buteau J, Peyot ML, et al. Saturated fatty acids synergize with elevated glucose to cause pancreatic beta-cell death. *Endocrinology* 2003; **144**(9): 4154–63.

155. Nolan CJ, Madiraju MS, Delghingaro-Augusto V, Peyot ML, Prentki M. Fatty acid signaling in the beta-cell and insulin secretion. *Diabetes* 2006; **55 Suppl 2**: S16–23.

156. Rutkowski JM, Stern JH, Scherer PE. The cell biology of fat expansion. *J Cell Biol* 2015; **208**(5): 501–12.

157. Zierath JR, Livingston JN, Thorne A, et al. Regional difference in insulin inhibition of non-esterified fatty acid release from human adipocytes: Relation to insulin receptor phosphorylation and intracellular signalling through the insulin receptor substrate-1 pathway. *Diabetologia* 1998; **41**(11): 1343–54.

158. Basu A, Basu R, Shah P, Vella A, Rizza RA, Jensen MD. Systemic and regional free fatty acid metabolism in type 2 diabetes. *Am J Physiol Endocrinol Metab* 2001; **280**(6): E1000–6.

159. Hellmer J, Marcus C, Sonnenfeld T, Arner P. Mechanisms for differences in lipolysis between human subcutaneous and omental fat cells. *J Clin Endocrinol Metab* 1992; **75**(1): 15–20.

160. Jansson PA, Smith U, Lonnroth P. Interstitial glycerol concentration measured by microdialysis in two subcutaneous regions in humans. *Am J Physiol* 1990; **258**(6 Pt 1): E918–22.

161. Jensen MD. Lipolysis: Contribution from regional fat. *Annu Rev Nutr* 1997; **17**: 127–39.

162. Arner P. Catecholamine-induced lipolysis in obesity. *Int J Obes Relat Metab Disord* 1999; **23 Suppl 1**: 10–3.

163. Ahlborg G, Felig P, Hagenfeldt L, Hendler R, Wahren J. Substrate turnover during prolonged exercise in man. Splanchnic and leg metabolism of glucose, free fatty acids, and amino acids. *J Clin Invest* 1974; **53**(4): 1080–90.

164. Burguera B, Proctor D, Dietz N, Guo Z, Joyner M, Jensen MD. Leg free fatty acid kinetics during exercise in men and women. *Am J Physiol Endocrinol Metab* 2000; **278**(1): E113–7.

165. Stich V, De Glisezinski I, Crampes F, et al. Activation of alpha(2)-adrenergic receptors impairs exercise-induced lipolysis in SCAT of obese subjects. *Am J Physiol Regul Integr Comp Physiol* 2000; **279**(2): R499–504.

166. Ross R, Rissanen J. Mobilization of visceral and subcutaneous adipose tissue in response to energy restriction and exercise. *Am J Clin Nutr* 1994; **60**(5): 695–703.

167. Kamel EG, McNeill G, Van Wijk MC. Change in intra-abdominal adipose tissue volume during weight loss in obese men and women: Correlation between magnetic resonance imaging and anthropometric measurements. *Int J Obes Relat Metab Disord* 2000; **24**(5): 607–13.

168. Strasser B, Spreitzer A, Haber P. Fat loss depends on energy deficit only, independently of the method for weight loss. *Ann Nutr Metab* 2007; **51**(5): 428–32.

169. Singh P, Somers VK, Romero-Corral A, et al. Effects of weight gain and weight loss on regional fat distribution. *Am J Clin Nutr* 2012; **96**(2): 229–33.

170. Gurr MI, Jung RT, Robinson MP, James WP. Adipose tissue cellularity in man: The relationship between fat cell size and number, the mass and distribution of body fat and the history of weight gain and loss. *Int J Obes* 1982; **6**(5): 419–36.

171. Stiegler P, Cunliffe A. The role of diet and exercise for the maintenance of fat-free mass and resting metabolic rate during weight loss. *Sports Med (Auckland, NZ)* 2006; **36**(3): 239–62.

172. Calbet JAL, Ponce-Gonzalez JG, Calle-Herrero J, et al. Exercise preserves lean mass and performance during severe energy deficit: The role of exercise volume and dietary protein content. *Front Physiol* 2017; **8**: 483.

173. Milleo FQ, Campos AC, Santoro S, et al. Metabolic effects of an entero-omentectomy in mildly obese type 2 diabetes mellitus patients after three years. *Clinics (Sao Paulo)* 2011; **66**(7): 1227–33.

174. Thorne A, Lonnqvist F, Apelman J, Hellers G, Arner P. A pilot study of long-term effects of a novel obesity treatment: Omentectomy in connection with adjustable gastric banding. *Int J Obes Relat Metab Disord* 2002; **26**(2): 193–9.

175. Herrera MF, Pantoja JP, Velazquez-Fernandez D, et al. Potential additional effect of omentectomy on metabolic syndrome, acute-phase reactants, and inflammatory mediators in grade III obese patients undergoing laparoscopic Roux-en-Y gastric bypass: A randomized trial. *Diabetes Care* 2010; **33**(7): 1413–8.

176. Buchwald H, Avidor Y, Braunwald E, et al. Bariatric surgery: A systematic review and meta-analysis. *JAMA* 2004; **292**(14): 1724–37.

177. Olbers T, Bjorkman S, Lindroos A, et al. Body composition, dietary intake, and energy expenditure after laparoscopic Roux-en-Y gastric bypass and laparoscopic vertical banded gastroplasty: A randomized clinical trial. *Ann Surg* 2006; **244**(5): 715–22.

178. Weiss R, Appelbaum L, Schweiger C, et al. Short-term dynamics and metabolic impact of abdominal fat depots after bariatric surgery. *Diabetes Care* 2009; **32**(10): 1910–5.

6 Combined Effect of Diet and Physical Activity in the Management of Obesity

Gary D. Miller

CONTENTS

6.1 INTRODUCTION

Obesity is widely defined as an excess accumulation of body fat. This is the result of a positive energy balance caused by a relative excess of energy intake as compared to energy expenditure. To assess and quantify obesity, accurate and reliable measurements of body fat are difficult to obtain, expensive, and rarely performed in usual-care clinical settings. However, body mass index (BMI) is highly correlated with body fat and simple to calculate based on weight (kg) divided by height (m^2). A BMI of 30 kg/m^2 or higher is the criteria for obesity, and it has a high, direct correlation with morbidity and mortality.

The initial line of treatment for obesity is lifestyle modifications that specifically target dietary behaviors and physical activity. This generally refers to an increase in physical activity to enhance energy expenditure and to lower energy intake through dietary modifications to restrict portion sizes, alter macronutrient content, or make lower-calorie selections. These modifications create a negative whole-body energy balance, leading to reductions in body weight and long-term body energy stores (i.e., adipose tissue).

Creating a negative energy balance is the cornerstone for treating obesity. Although it is a simple, thermodynamic process, our body protects ourselves from weight loss by altering our energy expenditure processes, as well as changing our drive for eating.[1] Even considering the physiological adaptations that occur, weight loss is apparent when energy expenditure exceeds energy intake. Traditionally, a deficit or excess of 7,700 kcals creates a loss or gain, respectively, of 1 kg (3,500 kcals for 1 lb) of body fat.[2] Although recent research demonstrates this overestimates weight loss,[1] this model is easily implemented and is understood by patients. However, Hall has challenged this traditional approach by proposing a newer model that accounts for metabolic adjustments, especially with a negative energy deficit.[1] This dynamic approach more closely models actual weight loss experiences in individuals compared to the static 7,700 kcals/kg of fat mass scenario.

An often-overlooked aspect of the negative energy balance is that altering one component, either energy intake or energy expenditure, leads to alterations with the other component through either physiological or behavioral changes (Figure 6.1). This is illustrated when hunger increases during weight loss, which is disproportionate to the decrease in energy expenditure caused by loss of total body and lean body mass. This is commonly referred to as the *energy gap*.[3] Recent observations have highlighted the challenge that the energy gap poses for continued weight loss and/or weight loss maintenance. A plausible explanation for the increase in hunger and reduction in satiety is the rise in circulating ghrelin, an orexigenic hormone, and/or the drop in leptin, glucagon-like peptide 1 (GLP-1), and other anorexigenic hormones. Similarly, the reduction in energy expenditure can be, at least in part, described by lower sympathetic nervous system activity, lower leptin, and an increase in energy efficiency. Although these actions help us defend against excessive weight loss, similar, but much less robust, mechanisms are in place to protect against excessive weight gain.

For adults, energy expenditure is comprised of resting energy expenditure, activity energy expenditure, and the thermic effect of food. While resting energy expenditure is generally

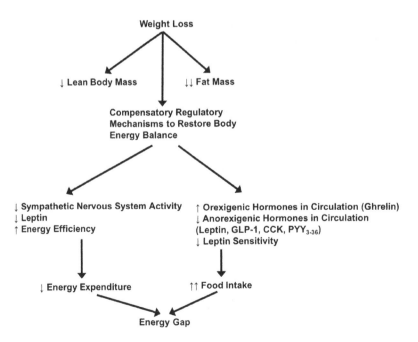

FIGURE 6.1 Compensatory regulatory mechanisms from weight loss for body energy balance. Magnitude of effect is based on number of *arrows* associated with it (either one or two upward-or downward-facing *arrows*). (CCK, cholecystokinin; GLP-1, glucagon-like peptide 1; PYY$_{3-36}$, pancreatic tyrosine tyrosine.)

the largest component of total daily energy expenditure (comprising approximately 60% of total expenditure), activity expenditure is the most variable. This latter category of energy expenditure includes energy used during structured exercise, but also in daily activities, such as house cleaning, shopping, and yard work. As discussed later in this chapter, increasing physical activity energy expenditure comprises a critical component of a lifestyle intervention for weight management.

Importantly, weight loss is not exclusively from fat mass. Approximately 80% of weight loss is anticipated from fat mass and 20% from lean mass,[4] although this ratio varies based on initial body fat levels, inclusion of strength and/or aerobic exercise, rate of weight loss, and dietary factors, such as protein intake.[5] A greater proportion of weight loss from lean mass further lowers resting energy expenditure, since lean mass largely determines resting energy expenditure.[6] Additionally, the loss in both fat and lean mass reduces activity energy expenditure when the activity is mass dependent, as it requires less energy to move. In practical terms, this decline in activity and resting energy expenditure with weight loss means an individual requires a greater restriction of energy intake to create a similar level of negative energy imbalance. If further dietary restriction is not employed, a plateau in weight loss occurs. This plateau frequently occurs at 6 months in research and clinic settings and is attributed to metabolic adaptations from the negative energy balance. Resting energy expenditure dropped by 11% in the first month of a program that utilized a very low-calorie diet (565–650 kcals/day) with exercise training,[4] which likely leads to weight loss that was only approximately two-thirds of predicted. It is also noteworthy that poor adherence to prescribed weight loss interventions are also common and may contribute significantly to the weight loss plateaus.[7]

This chapter explores variations and strategies for implementing both dietary and physical activity changes to achieve weight loss goals.

6.2 NUTRITIONAL CONSIDERATIONS FOR WEIGHT LOSS

6.2.1 MACRONUTRIENT ALTERATIONS

Because the energy content differs per unit of mass for carbohydrates, protein, and fats, manipulating the levels of these macronutrients has been a dietary strategy employed for weight management. In addition to altering total energy intake, these nutrients also have distinctive actions on other important aspects of weight loss programs, including energy metabolism, appetite, and satiety. Thus, frequent alterations include diets that are low fat and high carbohydrate; low carbohydrate and high fat; and high protein. In all cases, for weight loss, a restriction of total energy intake is the goal.

Research generally indicates that, during dietary energy restriction, weight loss occurs over a wide range of macronutrient composition.[8–10] Whether it is low carbohydrate, moderate carbohydrate, low fat, or high protein, clinical trials do not show one diet is better than others for long-term success. In a 2-year study comparing four diets that ranged in the proportion of kcals from fat (20%–40%), protein (15%–25%), and carbohydrates (35%–65%), all diets demonstrated similar weight loss.[9] For example, in a comparison of a low-carbohydrate versus a low-fat diet in healthy obese individuals, the low-carbohydrate diet had more than twice the weight loss at 6 months, but by 12 months, there were no differences between groups. It is noted that there was a high dropout rate (approximately 40%) in both groups.[11] Furthermore, ratings of hunger and satiety were similar for all diets. Weight loss success seems to hinge on adherence to the meal plan.[12] This further supports the importance of counseling to ensure that diets are personalized with consideration for taste and cultural preferences. However, with *ad libitum* intake—that is, no intentional food restrictions—lowering the proportion of intake from dietary fats reduced body weight.[11,13–16] This is attributed to a higher diet-induced thermogenesis and reduced energy intake with carbohydrates and protein than fat.

Historically, most dietary manipulations for weight loss have focused on altering either carbohydrates or fats, with protein remaining relatively constant in diets. However, manipulation of dietary protein has gained attention, and a couple of recent meta-analyses demonstrate that eating a protein-rich diet (> 1.05 g protein/kg body weight) during at least 4 weeks of dietary energy restriction leads to greater weight loss with maintenance of lean body mass compared to diets with lower protein content (≤ 1.05 g protein/kg body weight).[17,18] Theoretically, a higher-protein diet may provide additional benefits, as a higher-protein diet alters a number of physiological processes that affect energy balance, including increased metabolic rate during sleep, higher diet-induced thermogenesis, greater satiety, reduced sensations of hunger, and reduction of energy efficiency during positive energy balance.[19,20] In contrast, others have not supported the benefits of the high-protein diet for weight loss or weight maintenance, especially in longer-term (≥ 12 months) studies.[21–23] In a study that investigated the effect of animal and plant protein supplements on weight maintenance after an 8-week weight loss period, no differences were found over 24 weeks of follow-up in weight regain, fat mass regain, or changes in lean body mass. Mean daily intake of protein was 1.45 g/kg body weight for the protein-supplemented groups and 1.16 g/kg body weight for controls. However, the protein supplements, independent of source, lead to higher diet-induced thermogenesis and resting energy expenditure, as well as greater appetite suppression with a test meal challenge than a nonprotein-supplemented control.[24] Although hunger sensations were different, *ad libitum* energy intake was similar among groups.

6.2.2 CARBOHYDRATES: GLYCEMIC INDEX, GLYCEMIC LOAD, AND FIBER

Manipulation of the carbohydrate content and type of carbohydrates in the diet has been hypothesized to alter the meal's insulin response. The glycemic index is a measure of how the food or meal affects blood glucose levels, and the glycemic load considers the actual amount of carbohydrates in a food. However, it must be understood that classifying foods or a diet as being low or high glycemic index is difficult, as many factors influence it, including other foods consumed with the meal and the rate of gastric emptying.[25] Manipulation of the types of carbohydrates has been investigated as a potential strategy for weight loss diets. The South Beach Diet and the Zone Diet promote low-glycemic-index/load carbohydrates. A food with a high glycemic index or load increases blood glucose, which leads to a greater insulin secretion. This has the potential to inhibit fat oxidation and stimulate hunger through rebound hypoglycemia, leading to weight gain. Acute studies show that high-glycemic-index foods have reduced ability to induce satiety.[26,27] Currently, there is not overwhelming evidence to support consumption of a low-glycemic-load diet for weight management.[28–31] Fewer than 25% of controlled trials from a couple of recent reviews showed a significant weight loss benefit from a low-glycemic-index or -load diet as compared to a control diet.[30,31] Effects on body composition were also minimal with a low-glycemic-index or -load diet. Supporting the relatively minor impact of glycemic index on weight loss, an overall benefit of 1.1 kg more weight loss was seen in a meta-analysis examining low-glycemic-index or -load diets after up to 6 months of intervention.[29] Another study supported consumption of a low-glycemic-index or -load diet for weight loss, as more participants lost at least 5% weight after 12 weeks on this diet compared to diets that varied in levels of carbohydrates, protein, and glycemic index, but with similar fat and dietary fiber intake.[32] One large, multisite trial in Europe did show potential for altering one's dietary glycemic index for weight maintenance, as individuals on low-glycemic-index or high-protein *ad libitum* diets had less weight regain after an 11-kg weight loss as compared to other dietary manipulations.[28]

Although the glycemic index rating has received significant attention as a dietary weight loss strategy through the South Beach Diet and Zone Diet, a report from the World Health Organization stated that a high fiber intake was the only dietary factor that protected against weight gain.[33] In a systematic review of diet components that demonstrate successful weight maintenance and weight loss in research trials, increased dietary fiber was part of 21% of successful interventions, which was the second-most-frequent diet manipulation behind fat reduction.[34–40] These trials promoted up to 20 g of fiber per day,[35] with some emphasizing soluble fiber[36] in the form of increased intake of fruits, vegetables, and beans (pulses), often in conjunction with dietary energy restriction.[41] Risk for obesity was inversely correlated to fiber intake, such that men with the highest dietary fiber intake had the lowest risk for developing obesity.[42] Although the nutritional supplement polyglycoplex, which is a dietary fiber that is a combination of three soluble fibers, is sold and promoted as a weight loss supplement, randomized clinical trials do not support these claims.[43–46] One type of high-fiber food that has received considerable attention for weight loss is legumes, which are high in fiber and protein, and low in saturated fat, and have a low glycemic index. A pooled analysis of 21 studies suggest beans (pulses) have a modest impact on weight loss, with an additional 0.34 kg of lost weight over a median study duration of 6 weeks.[47] This effect is apparent in both intentional reduced-energy diets and in neutral-energy-balance diets. Part of the effect of the weight loss from legumes may be from their satiation-producing properties.[48]

Resistant starch is a broad category of dietary fiber and is defined as a starch that is not digested and absorbed in the small intestine. A number of studies have examined the effect of this particular type of dietary fiber on energy balance and body weight. To date, however, the findings from this research do not support the claims that resistant starch impacts body weight, energy intake, or energy expenditure.[49–56] However, resistant starch does appear to alter mechanisms that could potentially affect body weight and body composition, including the expression of mRNA of gut hormones (incretins), such as GLP-1 and PYY, and increased gut microbial community of butyrate-producing bacteria, both of which have been tied with improved weight management.[57] Thus, additional studies are warranted to further investigate the potential action of resistant starch as a dietary strategy for weight loss.

6.2.3 Dietary Energy Density

Research investigating regulatory factors for eating indicates that volume of food is an important factor in how much humans consume at a meal, independent of total energy content.[10,58,59] This concept has been applied through manipulation of the energy density of foods and meals. Increasing the water and fiber content of the diet, as well as reducing fat and sugar levels, can lower energy density. Practically, this is accomplished by adding fruits and vegetables to the diet. Thus, for the same volume of food, fewer kcals are consumed. Studies have shown that eating a broth-based soup or a salad, both which are low in energy density, at the start of a meal lowers the amount of energy eaten at that meal and over the next 1–2 days.[60–63] A number of trials lasting from 3 to 24 months demonstrate that consuming a lower-energy-density diet leads to greater weight loss and/or prevention of weight regain than a comparison diet in obese adults.[64–67] Specifically, a randomized, clinical trial showed greater weight loss at 12 months in participants who consumed a low energy dense soup twice a day as compared to an isocaloric, low vs. high energy dense snack.[64] Supporting the use of this dietary strategy is that increasing nutrient density and lowering energy density is a recommendation with the recent editions of the US Dietary Guidelines.

Following specific, healthy meal plans that are based on consuming specific food patterns is also a sound strategy for a weight loss program. The following sections describe modifications to eating patterns and the research that has investigated their effectiveness.

6.2.4 Adopting Different Eating Patterns

The most recent Dietary Guidelines[68–70] promote following healthy dietary patterns within an individual's own preferences. Included in these patterns are a vegetarian diet (and the many deviations of this pattern) and a Mediterranean diet. Other common eating patterns, especially for

TABLE 6.1

Dietary Patterns and Feeding Behaviors and Their Effects on Diet and Body Weight

Dietary Patterns	Actions Compared to Typical US Diets
Vegetarian diets—Vegans, Lacto, Lacto-Ovo	Low: Energy intake, energy density High: Nutrient density, water, fruits, vegetables, legumes, fiber ↓ Hunger, ↑ Satiety ↓ Body weight
Mediterranean diet	Low: Energy intake High: Nutrient density, plant oils, nuts, fruits, vegetables, whole grains, fiber, fish, poultry Low: Meat, animal fats ↓ Body weight
Paleolithic diet	Low: Energy intake High: Lean meats, fish, shellfish, fruits, vegetables, roots, eggs, nuts Low: Grains (wheat, rice, oats), dairy, salt, refined sugars and fats ↑ Satiety ± Body weight
Meal replacements	Low: Energy intake High: Nutrient density ↓ Body weight
Alternate-day fasting	Low: Energy intake ↓ Body weight

weight loss, are the Paleo diet, meal replacements, and alternate-day fasting. Each of these is briefly reviewed in the following sections and Table 6.1.

6.2.4.1 Vegetarian Dietary Pattern

Individuals following a variation of a vegetarian diet (vegans, lacto-, lacto-ovo-, pesco-, etc.) consume nearly 500 fewer kcals and are generally leaner and have a lower BMI than those adhering to an omnivorous-type diet. Thus, it may also be an option to promote weight loss in obese individuals.[68–70] These diets, although not without risk for nutrient deficiencies, especially for vegans, are considered to be low in energy density and high nutrient density due to the high fiber and water content of the high levels of fruits, vegetables, and legumes consumed. The high volume of food consumed increases satiety and lowers ratings of hunger.[71] Studies indicate that plant-based diets can be a viable dietary pattern for weight loss.[72–74] For example, in comparison to a National Cholesterol Education Program (NCEP) diet, a vegan diet produced a nearly 3-kg greater weight loss at both year 1 and year 2 of follow-up.[73] Another study demonstrated that, in overweight adults not intentionally trying to lose weight, a vegan diet as compared to other plant-based diets (allowing eggs, dairy, fish, or red meat and poultry occasionally) leads to greater weight loss after 6 months.[74] Importantly, all diets resulted in at least 3% weight loss, even though calorie restriction was not central to the intervention.

6.2.4.2 Mediterranean Dietary Pattern

Observational trials support weight loss, as well as reduce the risk for weight gain[75–81] in individuals who adhere to a Mediterranean diet. However, only a small number of randomized, controlled trials have examined the Mediterranean dietary pattern for weight loss in obese adults. A meta-analysis of these studies suggests almost a 2-kg greater weight loss with this type of diet compared to control diets. The Mediterranean diet pattern is higher in dietary fat than what has traditionally been prescribed for weight loss, owing to its higher contents of olive oil and nuts; however, the diet is also rich in fruits, vegetables, and dietary fiber from whole grains and legumes. This contributes to its low energy and high nutrient density.[82,83] High adherence to the dietary pattern is related to reduced weight gain and lower risk for obesity development.[81]

6.2.4.3 Paleo

The Paleolithic (or Paleo) diet contains staple foods such as lean meats, fish, shellfish, fruits, vegetables, roots, eggs, and nuts. Foods that likely are the result of agricultural farming and processing, such as grains, dairy products, salt, and refined fats and sugar, are to be avoided. Individuals in research studies express difficulty in adhering to this pattern, although there is a reduction in total energy intake and high ratings of satiety at meal times.[84] Improvements in many cardiometabolic variables (blood lipids, hemoglobin A1c, glucose tolerance, blood pressure, inflammation, blood clotting factors) are apparent with a Paleo diet.[33,85–93] Studies showing the effectiveness of the diet on weight loss are limited; however, a reduction in body weight has been seen in a few investigations.[84,90] The difficulty in adhering to the diet, and the relatively small weight loss, limits its use for sustained weight loss in the general obese population.

6.2.5 MEAL REPLACEMENTS

Meal replacements are already-proportioned food that limits consumption of total daily energy. When larger portions are provided at meals, research shows that individuals consume more food, beverages, and total energy intake.[94–96] Thus, food intake is reduced with use of meal replacements. These products are usually liquid products and may take the place of all foods in the diet (complete meal replacement) or may only replace one or two meals (partial meal replacement). In addition, conventional solid foods that are already proportioned can be an alternative approach. Typically, solid foods provide greater satiation versus liquid meals.[97,98] These products have a high acceptance rate, as they add structure to the program and minimize decisions on what and how much food to eat. These products are typically fortified with nutrients to provide daily recommendations of micronutrients, providing a more nutrient-dense diet than a weight-stable group.[99]

The acceptance of both complete and partial meal replacements in the research and clinical settings is evident from their use in several preeminent weight loss trials.[100–102] Recent reviews demonstrate their success, as greater weight loss and compliance are seen with meal replacements compared to lifestyle-change programs. Importantly, greater weight loss has been observed in individuals using the most number of meal replacements.[100] Use of meal replacements leads to a nearly 7-kg greater weight loss for up to 2 years of follow-up compared to a control group.[103,104] Although limited in number of studies, the results are consistent in that use of meal replacements (liquid and solid proportioned foods) produced greater weight loss compared to a self-selected diet that was targeted as similar in energy content.[105,106]

As presented, there is no magical diet for weight loss. Restricting energy intake across a variety of dietary patterns produces clinical meaningful weight loss. Long-term success of weight maintenance is dependent on adherence to healthy lifestyle behaviors. Particularly with dietary habits, recidivism is common, as it is difficult to maintain the reduced energy intake in light of the physiological drive to eat. Also, drastic changes from usual habits to a dietary pattern that may not be palatable or consistent with social habits is difficult to maintain over the long-term. In a meta-analysis, behavioral obesity treatment interventions, such as goal setting, motivational interviewing, and relapse prevention in randomized, clinical trials, demonstrates beneficial effects on adherence measures, such as session attendance and participation in physical activity.[107]

6.3   STRATEGIES FOR DIETARY MANIPULATIONS

By creating a negative energy balance, individuals can be successful in losing significant weight through a number of different types of diets that restrict energy intake and exercise programs that increase daily energy expenditure. The challenge is to maintain the weight loss and prevent weight regain, as only 15% keep the weight off over the long term.[108] The following section examines dietary different strategies to counter biological responses that are challenges for maintaining weight loss and preventing weight regain.

6.3.1 RATE OF WEIGHT LOSS

A gradual weight loss of 0.5–1.0 kg per week (1–2 lb) is the general guide for rate of weight loss,[109] based on the assumption that more rapid weight loss leads to a greater loss of lean body mass,[110] a reduction of resting energy expenditure more than predicted,[111] and ultimately greater potential for weight regain.[112] However, much of the clinical evidence suggests that an increased rate of weight loss using a greater energy restriction with a very low-calorie diet provides similar, if not better, long-term weight loss success[113–115] (Table 6.2). In a relatively short-term study, consuming 550 (women) to 660 (men) kcals per day for 4 weeks compared to 1,200 (women) to 1,500 (men) kcals per day for 8 weeks led to similar changes in weight and body composition. Furthermore, after 4 weeks of weight stability, there were no differences among groups in indices of metabolic adaptations, such as anorexigenic hormones, resting metabolic rate, and ratings of hunger and satiety.[115] In a larger and longer-term study, a rapid weight loss group had a target of 12.5% weight loss at 12 weeks, whereas a gradual group was to achieve this goal by 36 weeks.[113] Individuals were then followed during a 144-week weight maintenance phase. Approximately 50% of the gradual-weight-loss group and 81% of the rapid-weight-loss group reached the 12.5% weight loss goal. Furthermore, at

TABLE 6.2
Randomized Clinical Trials on Effect of Rate of Weight Loss on Weight Regain

References	Cohort	Design	Intervention	Findings
Coutinho et al. (2017)	16 W/M BMI > 30.0 kg/m² 18–65 yr	2 groups: • *Rapid* • *Gradual* Similar targeted WL for groups	**WL phase (≈ 10%)** *Rapid*: 550 (W) & 660 (M) kcal/d × 4 wk *Gradual*: 1,200 (W) & 1,500 (M) kcal/d × 8 wk **Maint phase** 1 mo each group	**WL & body composition** • No group differences after WL and maint
Purcell et al. (2014)	153 W/51 M BMI = 30–45 kg/m² 18–70 yr	2 groups: • *Rapid* • *Gradual* Similar targeted WL for groups	**WL phase (≈ 15%)** *Rapid*: 450–800 kcal/d × 12 wk *Gradual*: 400–500 kcal energy deficit diet × 36 wk **Maint phase** Subjects losing ≥12.5% (≈ 50% of *Gradual*; 81% of *Rapid*) during WL followed × 144 wk	**WL & body composition** • No group differences • After maint, both groups regained >70% of lost wt
Vink et al. (2016)	30 W/27 M BMI = 28–35 kg/m²	2 groups: • *Low-calorie diet (LCD)* • *Very low-calorie diet (VLCD)*	**WL phase (≈ 10%)** LCD: 1,250 kcal/d × 12 wk VLCD: 500 kcal/d × 5 wk **WS phase** 4 wk both groups **Follow-up** 9 mo both groups	**WL & body composition** • No group differences in WL • % FFM loss greater in VLCD vs LCD **Weight regain** • No group differences • % FFM loss associated with wt regain

BMI, body mass index; FFM, fat-free mass; M, men; Maint, maintenance; RMR, resting metabolic rate; WL, weight loss; W, women; wt, weight; WS, weight stable.

the end of the follow-up, both groups had regained nearly three-fourths of their lost weight, with no difference between rapid- and gradual-weight-loss groups. From these studies, rate of weight loss does not influence long-term weight loss success.

6.3.2 MODIFIED ALTERNATE-DAY FASTING

Generally, a weight loss diet includes reducing total caloric intake by 250–1,250 kcals every day. Alternate-day fasting is a model in which every other day, calories are restricted up to 75% of normal intake[116,117] or by 1,500–1,750 kcals. On alternate days, individuals consume their normal diet. Adherence over an 8-week study was 85% on this dietary pattern.[117] Enhancing adherence to this program is the recent demonstration that the time of day the food is consumed on the fasting days has little impact on weight loss, providing greater flexibility for the individual.[118] To date, only a limited number of trials have investigated weight loss with this type of eating strategy, and these are limited in their duration, and randomized versus nonrandomized. Weight loss was 3.2% more for individuals undergoing an alternate-day fasting program compared to a usual weight loss control group over a 12-week period.[119] In a single-arm study, those on an alternate-day fast lost 8% of body weight in 8 weeks.[120] Others showed a weight loss of 5–6 kg, or about 0.67 kg per week, which is comparable to a moderate calorie-restricted diet.[116,117] Importantly, this type of eating strategy may impart improvements in metabolic health, such as inflammatory biomarkers, glucose regulation, and blood lipids,[121] making it an attractive strategy for inducing weight loss.

In a most recent study, Byrne and colleagues examined the use of intermittent energy restriction in comparison with continuous energy restriction. The intermittent group completed 2 cycles of 8 weeks of energy restriction, followed by 7 weeks of energy balance, over a total of 30 weeks. The continuous-energy-restriction group completed 16 weeks of energy restriction at the same relative energy intake as the continuous group. Although both groups had similar energy restriction, the intermittent group showed greater weight loss and fat mass loss than the continuous group, demonstrating an improved weight loss efficiency.

6.3.3 TIME OF DAY FOR EATING

One approach for reducing energy intake is to restrict times eating is allowed to occur. This can be expressed as restricting nighttime eating. In a crossover study, normal-weight men having an 11-hour fasting period (from 19:00 to 06:00 hours) during the night over a 2-week period led to a difference of 2% in body weight as compared to a control group.[122] Whereas the nighttime fasting group showed no calorie intake during the night, the control group consumed approximately 700 kcals during this nighttime period. Thus, nighttime fasting, at least in the short term, reduces total daily energy intake.

The number of daily meals has been investigated, with the idea that fewer opportunities for eating will lead to weight reduction. Also, similar to intermittent fasting, metabolic benefits may be apparent from eating fewer meals per day. In a crossover trial, consuming one meal versus three meals per day of equal total daily energy intake for 8 weeks led to a reduction in body fat mass and body weight by 2.1 and 1.4 kg, respectively, for the one meal per day, but there were no changes for the three-meals-per-day diet.[123] Not surprisingly, consumption of only a single meal produced an increase in hunger. Metabolic effects, including a rise in blood pressure and blood cholesterol levels (total, low-density lipoprotein [LDL], and high-density lipoprotein [HDL]), were apparent when participants consumed one meal per day. Glucose regulation worsened and ghrelin increased when consuming one meal per day as compared to a three-meal-per-day eating regimen.[124]

A frequent strategy to reduce daily caloric intake for weight loss is to skip breakfast. The concern is that omitting this meal will result in overcompensation from the prolonged fast and lead to greater, or similar, daily caloric intake than experienced if breakfast is consumed. In an acute (1-day) study, when breakfast was skipped, individuals were hungrier at lunch, with higher ghrelin levels, than when they consumed breakfast, but they did not eat more calories at lunch.[125] They showed no difference in hunger or appetite later in the day between eating regimens. Over a 6-week, longitudinal study, there were no body weight differences between those who ate and those who did not eat breakfast.[126]

6.4   SEDENTARY AND PHYSICAL ACTIVITY BEHAVIORS IN WEIGHT MANAGEMENT

Health benefits incurred by being physically active are well documented, spanning conditions such as cardiovascular disease, diabetes, certain types of cancer, osteoporosis, and weight management. Similarly, reducing sedentary behaviors has positive effects on cardiometabolic risk, as well as body composition,[127] and, conversely, high levels of sedentary behaviors produce poor health consequences.[128,129] The additive effect of reducing sedentary behaviors and increasing physical activity potentially provide the best direction for weight management. Recommendations from prominent public health agencies (e.g., the U.S. Centers for Disease Control and Prevention, American College of Sports Medicine, and National Heart, Lung, and Blood Institute) promote physical activity behaviors as part of weight management.[109,130–133] Recent research evidence suggests that greater amounts of physical activity are needed for most individuals.[134] Expending energy equivalent to walking 4 miles every day of the week,[135] or exercising for 80 minutes per day of moderate-intensity exercise or 35 minutes per day of vigorous physical activity[136] have been demonstrated to prevent weight regain and obesity, respectively. Importantly, individuals vary in their response to physical activity with regards to health benefits, including weight management. Assuming alterations in energy intake do not occur with changes in physical activity and sedentary behaviors, increasing energy expenditure would lead to a negative energy balance and weight loss. Generally, a 1%–3% (up to 3 kg) loss in body weight is observed with a moderate increase in physical activity, which is dependent on the minutes of activity per week.[134] Participating in more than 225 minutes of activity per week lead to more than 5 kg of weight loss, whereas 150 minutes of activity produced 2–3 kg of weight loss.[134] Furthermore, in individuals followed for up to 16 years after bariatric surgery, those who had the most minutes of sitting time showed the lowest levels of weight loss.[127,137] Interrupting sitting time during an 8-hour work day with a 5-minute walk every hour computes to a nearly 10-lb weight loss (calculated using an additional energy expenditure of 130 kcals per work day).

Interestingly, clinical trials have shown that exercise duration and intensity have minimal impact on weight loss and weight maintenance.[138,139] In a study that compared four different combinations of moderate and vigorous intensity and moderate and vigorous duration in overweight and obese women,[138] there were no differences in weight loss at 12 or 24 months of follow-up. This was present even though the estimated activity energy expenditure was 1,000 kcals for moderate-duration groups and 2,000 kcals per week for vigorous-duration groups. However, confounding these results was the awareness of a low adherence to the exercise prescriptions. Thus, it is unknown if in reality there is no difference in weight loss with varying exercise intensities and duration, or whether the chosen exercise prescriptions were unachievable, and a more moderate approach needs to be tried. In a separate study that also compared varying exercise intensities and durations, no difference in weight loss occurred over 24 weeks between exercise groups that differed in exercise intensity and duration.[139] Importantly, individuals were instructed to maintain a similar energy intake throughout the study. Although weight loss was not a goal for the study, the exercising groups had greater reductions in waist circumference and weight than the nonexercising controls. In examining the effect of exercise energy expenditure over a short duration (11 weeks), similar differences in body fat change were observed in overweight young men and women who were randomized to either a moderate (300 kcals per day) or high (600 kcals per day) exercise training program.[140]

Physical activity is promoted and is a strong predictor for weight maintenance following loss of weight in obese and overweight individuals.[135,141] In observational studies, less weight is regained in individuals who participate in physical activity compared to those who are sedentary.[142] There also appears to be a dose-response effect, as greater amounts of exercise are more protective of weight regain than moderate levels of physical activity.[142] Unfortunately, randomized, controlled trials are few and show varying effects (negative, positive, and no effect) for engaging in physical activity after weight loss to prevent weight regain.[142,143] Recent work in this area shows that individuals engaging in at least 200 minutes per week of moderate-intensity physical activity show minimal weight regain after weight loss.[138,144,145] Interestingly, randomizing individuals into a targeted physical activity energy expenditure of 1,000 and 2,500 kcals per week showed no difference in weight loss at 6 months, but at 12 and 18 months, the group with the higher level of physical activity showed greater weight loss.[146] Caution must be applied in interpreting the results of this study, as adherence to the actual physical activity program showed great variation in individuals meeting the physical activity goals. Promoting "more is better" seems to hold in this case, but the absence of large randomized, clinical trials of sufficient duration give some hesitancy in wide-scale promotion of high levels of physical activity for weight loss maintenance. Based on available evidence, walking 4 miles per day (60 minutes) at a moderate intensity is associated with weight maintenance.[136,141,145,147]

Support for the impact physical activity energy expenditure has on weight management was demonstrated by Drenowatz and colleagues, who studied nearly 200 young men and women (21–35 years old) over a 2-year period.[148] Participants had no weight loss intentions during the study. Body weight, body composition, physical activity, total daily energy expenditure, and total daily energy intake were assessed serially throughout the study. After 2 years, approximately 15% of the cohort lost weight (mean = −6.9 kg), and nearly 30% gained weight (mean = 7.1 kg). Daily energy intake and daily energy expenditure did not change with either the weight loss or weight gain group. Importantly, moderate-to-vigorous physical activity increased by 35 minutes per day from baseline to 2 years in the weight loss group, whereas the weight gain group had a 35-minutes-per-day decrease.

6.4.1 Resistance versus Aerobic Exercise Training

Historically, aerobic training has been the cornerstone exercise modality for weight loss, since it increases energy expenditure. A recent position statement from the American College of Sports Medicine speaks of the benefits of resistance training as part of a weight loss program[134] and thus has brought attention to this mode of exercise. Use of resistance training during weight loss is purported to help dampen lean body mass from energy restriction. Since lean body mass is the primary determinant of resting energy expenditure, reducing or maintaining this component of body composition can aid in weight loss and maintenance. However, randomized, controlled trial evidence is limited comparing resistance and aerobic exercise training. Most evidence is derived from observational studies and secondary analyses. One important study addressing the different exercise modalities compared moderate aerobic training, moderate resistance training, and their combination on body weight and body composition changes.[149] Importantly, the study did not have specific diet restrictions or weight loss goals. The results bore out what would be expected, as the two aerobic training groups had similar weight and body fat loss, which were greater than the resistance training–only group. Also, lean body mass change was similar for both resistance training groups, which was greater than the aerobic training–only group. Combining both exercise forms leads to the greatest changes/benefits on body composition. However, because time is a barrier for participating in exercise, if only one type of training is possible, aerobic training is the optimal mode for weight and body fat loss.[150]

Behavioral approaches to enhance physical activity adherence and the impact of the timing of the physical activity intervention on weight loss were addressed by Jakicic and colleagues.[151] In this 18-month study, they compared three groups: a standard behavioral weight loss program, an arm with the standard program plus additional strategies during the first 9 months of the study, and an arm with the standard program plus additional strategies spread over the entire 18 months of the study. Greater weight loss was observed when the standard program was enhanced with further behavioral strategies that were spread over the 18-month study and not just the first 9 months. By providing support for enhancing physical activity behaviors throughout the duration of the study, greater weight loss is observed, which is an important strategy for implementing a weight loss program.

Based on research and clinical experiences, achieving significant weight loss using exercise alone is not to be expected. Goals for physical activity as part of a weight loss program should be to increase overall activity, with an emphasis on engaging in moderate- to vigorous-intensity activity. Similarly, a reduction in sedentary behaviors should be addressed.

6.5 SUMMARY

Unfortunately, the obesity epidemic continues to contribute to major health issues in the United States and globally. Implementing effective prevention and treatment strategies is critical. Dietary energy restriction and enhancing physical activity behaviors are the cornerstone for behavioral treatment of obesity. As reviewed here, many aspects of dietary alterations, including macronutrient manipulation, adherence to specific dietary patterns (Mediterranean diet, DASH diet), increasing dietary fiber levels, as well as alternate-day fasting, rate of weight loss, and time of day for meals, can provide benefits for weight loss efforts. However, one of the most important predictors remains adhering to a restricted-energy diet, independent of its content. Being physically active improves a number of health conditions, including weight management. More recent studies demonstrate that increasing levels of physical activity engagement provides greater weight loss and prevention of weight regain. Similar to diet approaches, enhancing physical activity adherence is a critical behavioral issue that needs future study.

REFERENCES

1. Hall, K. D. *et al.* Quantification of the effect of energy imbalance on bodyweight. *Lancet* **378,** 826–837 (2011).
2. Wishnofsky, M. Caloric equivalents of gained or lost weight. *Am. J. Clin. Nutr.* **6,** 542–546 (1958).
3. Melby, C. L., Paris, H. L., Foright, R. M. & Peth, J. Attenuating the biologic drive for weight regain following weight loss: Must what goes down always go back up? *Nutrients* **9,** (2017).
4. Byrne, N. M., Wood, R. E., Schutz, Y. & Hills, A. P. Does metabolic compensation explain the majority of less-than-expected weight loss in obese adults during a short-term severe diet and exercise intervention? *Int. J. Obes.* **36,** 1472–1478 (2012).
5. Hall, K. D. & Jordan, P. N. Modeling weight-loss maintenance to help prevent body weight regain. *Am. J. Clin. Nutr.* **88,** 1495–1503 (2008).
6. Javed, F. *et al.* Brain and high metabolic rate organ mass: Contributions to resting energy expenditure beyond fat-free mass. *Am. J. Clin. Nutr.* **91,** 907–912 (2010).
7. Thomas, D. M. *et al.* Effect of dietary adherence on the body weight plateau: A mathematical model incorporating intermittent compliance with energy intake prescription. *Am. J. Clin. Nutr.* **100,** 787–795 (2014).
8. Sacks, F. M. *et al.* Comparison of weight-loss diets with different compositions of fat, protein, and carbohydrates. *N. Engl. J. Med.* **360,** 859–873 (2009).
9. Johnston, B. C. *et al.* Comparison of weight loss among named diet programs in overweight and obese adults. *JAMA* **312,** 923–923 (2014).
10. Stubbs, R. J., Ritz, P., Coward, W. A. & Prentice, A. M. Covert manipulation of the ratio of dietary fat to carbohydrate and energy density: Effect on food intake and energy balance in free-living men eating ad libitum. *Am. J. Clin. Nutr.* **62,** 330–337 (1995).
11. Foster, G. D. *et al.* A randomized trial of a low-carbohydrate diet for obesity. *N. Engl. J. Med.* **348,** 2082–2090 (2003).
12. Dansinger, M. L., Gleason, J. A., Griffith, J. L., Selker, H. P. & Schaefer, E. J. Comparison of the Atkins, Ornish, Weight Watchers, and Zone diets for weight loss and heart disease risk reduction: A randomized trial. *JAMA* **293,** 43–53 (2005).
13. Samaha, F. F. *et al.* A low-carbohydrate as compared with a low-fat diet in severe obesity. *N. Engl. J. Med.* **348,** 2074–2081 (2003).

14. Stern, L. *et al.* The effects of low-carbohydrate versus conventional weight loss diets in severely obese adults: One-year follow-up of a randomized trial. *Ann. Intern. Med.* **140,** 778–785 (2004).

15. Astrup, A. *et al.* The role of dietary fat in body fatness: Evidence from a preliminary meta-analysis of ad libitum low-fat dietary intervention studies. *Br. J. Nutr.* **83 Suppl 1,** S25–32 (2000).

16. Thomas, C. D. *et al.* Nutrient balance and energy expenditure during ad libitum feeding of high-fat and high-carbohydrate diets in humans. *Am. J. Clin. Nutr.* **55,** 934–942 (1992).

17. Krieger, J. W., Sitren, H. S., Daniels, M. J. & Langkamp-Henken, B. Effects of variation in protein and carbohydrate intake on body mass and composition during energy restriction: A meta-regression 1. *Am. J.Clin. Nutr.* **83,** 260–274 (2006).

18. Wycherley, T. P., Moran, L. J., Clifton, P. M., Noakes, M. & Brinkworth, G. D. Effects of energy-restricted high-protein, low-fat compared with standard-protein, low-fat diets: A meta-analysis of randomized controlled trials. *Am. J. Clin. Nutr.* **96,** 1281–1298 (2012).

19. Lejeune, M. P. G. M., Westerterp, K. R., Adam, T. C. M., Luscombe-Marsh, N. D. & Westerterp-Plantenga, M. S. Ghrelin and glucagon-like peptide 1 concentrations, 24-h satiety, and energy and substrate metabolism during a high-protein diet and measured in a respiration chamber. *Am. J. Clin. Nutr.* **83,** 89–94 (2006).

20. Stock, M. J. Gluttony and thermogenesis revisited. *Int. J. Obes. Relat. Metab. Disord. J. Int. Assoc. Study Obes.* **23,** 1105–1117 (1999).

21. Schwingshackl, L. & Hoffmann, G. Long-term effects of low-fat diets either low or high in protein on cardiovascular and metabolic risk factors: A systematic review and meta-analysis. *Nutr. J.* **12,** 48 (2013).

22. Lepe, M., Bacardí Gascón, M. & Jiménez Cruz, A. Long-term efficacy of high-protein diets: A systematic review. *Nutr. Hosp.* **26,** 1256–1259 (2011).

23. Clifton, P. M., Condo, D. & Keogh, J. B. Long term weight maintenance after advice to consume low carbohydrate, higher protein diets—a systematic review and meta analysis. *Nutr. Metab. Cardiovasc. Dis. NMCD* **24,** 224–235 (2014).

24. Kjølbæk, L. *et al.* Protein supplements after weight loss do not improve weight maintenance compared with recommended dietary protein intake despite beneficial effects on appetite sensation and energy expenditure: A randomized, controlled, double-blinded trial. *Am. J. Clin. Nutr.* **106,** 684–697 (2017).

25. Pi-Sunyer, F. X. Glycemic index and disease. *Am. J. Clin. Nutr.* **76,** 290S–8S (2002).

26. Ludwig, D. S. Dietary glycemic index and obesity. *J. Nutr.* **130,** 280S–283S (2000).

27. Roberts, S. B. High-glycemic index foods, hunger, and obesity: Is there a connection? *Nutr. Rev.* **58,** 163–169 (2000).

28. Larsen, T. M. *et al.* Diets with high or low protein content and glycemic index for weight-loss maintenance. *N. Engl. J. Med.* **363,** 2102–2113 (2010).

29. Thomas, D. E., Elliott, E. J. & Baur, L. Low glycaemic index or low glycaemic load diets for overweight and obesity. *Cochrane Database Syst. Rev.* CD005105-CD005105 (2007). doi:10.1002/14651858. CD005105.pub2.

30. Esfahani, A., Wong, J. M. W., Mirrahimi, A., Villa, C. R. & Kendall, C. W. C. The application of the glycemic index and glycemic load in weight loss: A review of the clinical evidence. *IUBMB Life* **63,** 7–13 (2011).

31. Ajala, O., English, P. & Pinkney, J. Systematic review and meta-analysis of different dietary approaches to the management of type 2 diabetes. *Am. J. Clin. Nutr.* **97,** 505–516 (2013).

32. McMillan-Price, J. *et al.* Comparison of 4 diets of varying glycemic load on weight loss and cardiovascular risk reduction in overweight and obese young adults: A randomized controlled trial. *Arch. Intern. Med.* **166,** 1466–1475 (2006).

33. Jonsson, T. *et al.* A Paleolithic diet confers higher insulin sensitivity, lower C-reactive protein and lower blood pressure than a cereal-based diet in domestic pigs. *Nutr. Metab. Lond.* **3,** 39–39 (2006).

34. Cussler, E. C. *et al.* Maintenance of weight loss in overweight middle-aged women through the Internet. *Obes. Silver Spring Md* **16,** 1052–1060 (2008).

35. Itoh, K. *et al.* Association between blood pressure and insulin resistance in obese females during weight loss and weight rebound phenomenon. *Hypertens. Res. Off. J. Jpn. Soc. Hypertens.* **24,** 481–487 (2001).

36. Kuller, L. H. *et al.* The women on the move through activity and nutrition (WOMAN) study: Final 48-month results. *Obes. Silver Spring Md* **20,** 636–643 (2012).

37. Layman, D. K. *et al.* A moderate-protein diet produces sustained weight loss and long-term changes in body composition and blood lipids in obese adults. *J. Nutr.* 1–8 (2009). doi:10.3945/jn.108.099440. highly.

38. Thorpe, M. P. *et al.* A diet high in protein, dairy, and calcium attenuates bone loss over twelve months of weight loss and maintenance relative to a conventional high-carbohydrate diet in adults. *J. Nutr.* **138,** 1096–1100 (2008).

39. Yankura, D. J. *et al.* Weight regain and health-related quality of life in postmenopausal women. *Obes. Silver Spring Md* **16**, 2259–2265 (2008).

40. Ramage, S., Farmer, A., Eccles, K. A. & McCargar, L. Healthy strategies for successful weight loss and weight maintenance: A systematic review. *Appl. Physiol. Nutr. Metab. Physiol. Appl. Nutr. Metab.* **39**, 1–20 (2014).

41. Phelan, S., Wyatt, H. R., Hill, J. O. & Wing, R. R. Are the eating and exercise habits of successful weight losers changing? *Obes. Silver Spring Md* **14**, 710–716 (2006).

42. Langlois, K., Garriguet, D. & Findlay, L. Diet composition and obesity among Canadian adults. *Health Rep.* **20**, 11–20 (2009).

43. Onakpoya, I. J. & Heneghan, C. J. Effect of the novel functional fibre, polyglycoplex (PGX), on body weight and metabolic parameters: A systematic review of randomized clinical trials. *Clin. Nutr. Edinb. Scotl.* **34**, 1109–1114 (2015).

44. Kacinik, V. *et al.* Effect of PGX, a novel functional fibre supplement, on subjective ratings of appetite in overweight and obese women consuming a 3-day structured, low-calorie diet. *Nutr. Diabetes* **1**, e22 (2011).

45. Reimer, R. A. *et al.* Increased plasma PYY levels following supplementation with the functional fiber PolyGlycopleX in healthy adults. *Eur. J. Clin. Nutr.* **64**, 1186–1191 (2010).

46. Reimer, R. A. *et al.* Changes in visceral adiposity and serum cholesterol with a novel viscous polysaccharide in Japanese adults with abdominal obesity. *Obes. Silver Spring Md* **21**, E379–387 (2013).

47. Kim, S. J. *et al.* Effects of dietary pulse consumption on body weight: A systematic review and meta-analysis of randomized controlled trials. *Am. J. Clin. Nutr.* **103**, 1213–1223 (2016).

48. Li, S. S. *et al.* Dietary pulses, satiety and food intake: A systematic review and meta-analysis of acute feeding trials. *Obes. Silver Spring Md* **22**, 1773–1780 (2014).

49. Higgins, J. A. Resistant starch and energy balance: Impact on weight loss and maintenance. *Crit. Rev. Food Sci. Nutr.* **54**, 1158–1166 (2014).

50. Higgins, J. A. Resistant starch: Metabolic effects and potential health benefits. *J. AOAC Int.* **87**, 761–768 (2004).

51. de Roos, N., Heijnen, M. L., de Graaf, C., Woestenenk, G. & Hobbel, E. Resistant starch has little effect on appetite, food intake and insulin secretion of healthy young men. *Eur. J. Clin. Nutr.* **49**, 532–541 (1995).

52. Robertson, M. D., Bickerton, A. S., Dennis, A. L., Vidal, H. & Frayn, K. N. Insulin-sensitizing effects of dietary resistant starch and effects on skeletal muscle and adipose tissue metabolism. *Am. J. Clin. Nutr.* **82**, 559–567 (2005).

53. Johnston, K. L., Thomas, E. L., Bell, J. D., Frost, G. S. & Robertson, M. D. Resistant starch improves insulin sensitivity in metabolic syndrome. *Diabet. Med. J. Br. Diabet. Assoc.* **27**, 391–397 (2010).

54. Bodinham, C. L., Frost, G. S. & Robertson, M. D. Acute ingestion of resistant starch reduces food intake in healthy adults. *Br. J. Nutr.* **103**, 917–922 (2010).

55. Keogh, J. B., Lau, C. W. H., Noakes, M., Bowen, J. & Clifton, P. M. Effects of meals with high soluble fibre, high amylose barley variant on glucose, insulin, satiety and thermic effect of food in healthy lean women. *Eur. J. Clin. Nutr.* **61**, 597–604 (2007).

56. Sands, A. L., Leidy, H. J., Hamaker, B. R., Maguire, P. & Campbell, W. W. Consumption of the slow-digesting waxy maize starch leads to blunted plasma glucose and insulin response but does not influence energy expenditure or appetite in humans. *Nutr. Res. N. Y. N* **29**, 383–390 (2009).

57. Zhang, L. *et al.* Effect of dietary resistant starch on prevention and treatment of obesity-related diseases and its possible mechanisms. *Biomed. Environ. Sci. BES* **28**, 291–297 (2015).

58. Stubbs, R. J., Harbron, C. G., Murgatroyd, P. R. & Prentice, A. M. Covert manipulation of dietary fat and energy density: Effect on substrate flux and food intake in men eating ad libitum. *Am. J. Clin. Nutr.* **62**, 316–329 (1995).

59. Kral, T. V., Roe, L. S. & Rolls, B. J. Combined effects of energy density and portion size on energy intake in women. *Am. J. Clin. Nutr.* **79**, 962–968 (2004).

60. Rolls, B. J., Bell, E. A. & Thorwart, M. L. Water incorporated into a food but not served with a food decreases energy intake in lean women. *Am. J. Clin. Nutr.* **70**, 448–455 (1999).

61. Rolls, B. J., Roe, L. S. & Meengs, J. S. Salad and satiety: Energy density and portion size of a first-course salad affect energy intake at lunch. *J. Am. Diet. Assoc.* **104**, 1570–1576 (2004).

62. Bell, E. A. & Rolls, B. J. Energy density of foods affects energy intake across multiple levels of fat content in lean and obese women. *Am. J. Clin. Nutr.* **73**, 1010–1018 (2001).

63. Bell, E. A., Castellanos, V. H., Pelkman, C. L., Thorwart, M. L. & Rolls, B. J. Energy density of foods affects energy intake in normal-weight women. *Am. J. Clin. Nutr.* **67**, 412–420 (1998).

64. Rolls, B. J., Roe, L. S., Beach, A. M. & Kris-Etherton, P. M. Provision of foods differing in energy density affects long-term weight loss. *Obes. Res.* **13,** 1052–1060 (2005).

65. Ello-Martin, J. A., Roe, L. S., Ledikwe, J. H., Beach, A. M. & Rolls, B. J. Dietary energy density in the treatment of obesity: A year-long trial comparing 2 weight-loss diets. *Am. J. Clin. Nutr.* **85,** 1465–1477 (2007).

66. Raynor, H. A., Looney, S. M., Steeves, E. A., Spence, M. & Gorin, A. A. The effects of an energy density prescription on diet quality and weight loss: A pilot randomized controlled trial. *J. Acad. Nutr. Diet.* **112,** 1397–1402 (2012).

67. Lowe, M. R., Butryn, M. L., Thomas, J. G. & Coletta, M. Meal replacements, reduced energy density eating, and weight loss maintenance in primary care patients: A randomized controlled trial. *Obes. Silver Spring* **22,** 94–100 (2014).

68. Kennedy, E. T., Bowman, S. A., Spence, J. T., Freedman, M. & King, J. Popular diets: Correlation to health, nutrition, and obesity. *J. Am. Diet. Assoc.* **101,** 411–420 (2001).

69. Newby, P. K., Tucker, K. L. & Wolk, A. Risk of overweight and obesity among semivegetarian, lacto-vegetarian, and vegan women. *Am. J. Clin. Nutr.* **81,** 1267–1274 (2005).

70. Spencer, E. A., Appleby, P. N., Davey, G. K. & Key, T. J. Diet and body mass index in 38000 EPIC-Oxford meat-eaters, fish-eaters, vegetarians and vegans. *Int. J. Obes. Relat. Metab. Disord.* **27,** 728–734 (2003).

71. Howarth, N. C., Saltzman, E. & Roberts, S. B. Dietary fiber and weight regulation. *Nutr. Rev.* **59,** 129–139 (2001).

72. Burke, L. E. *et al.* A randomized clinical trial of a standard versus vegetarian diet for weight loss: The impact of treatment preference. *Int. J. Obes. 2005* **32,** 166–176 (2008).

73. Turner-McGrievy, G. M., Barnard, N. D. & Scialli, A. R. A two-year randomized weight loss trial comparing a vegan diet to a more moderate low-fat diet. *Obes. Silver Spring* **15,** 2276–2281 (2007).

74. Turner-McGrievy, G. M., Davidson, C. R., Wingard, E. E., Wilcox, S. & Frongillo, E. A. Comparative effectiveness of plant-based diets for weight loss: A randomized controlled trial of five different diets. *Nutrition* **31,** 350–358 (2015).

75. Goulet, J., Lamarche, B., Nadeau, G. & Lemieux, S. Effect of a nutritional intervention promoting the Mediterranean food pattern on plasma lipids, lipoproteins and body weight in healthy French-Canadian women. *Atherosclerosis* **170,** 115–124 (2003).

76. Andreoli, A. *et al.* Effect of a moderately hypoenergetic Mediterranean diet and exercise program on body cell mass and cardiovascular risk factors in obese women. *Eur. J. Clin. Nutr.* **62,** 892–897 (2008).

77. Beunza, J. J. *et al.* Adherence to the Mediterranean diet, long-term weight change, and incident overweight or obesity: The Seguimiento Universidad de Navarra (SUN) cohort. *Am. J. Clin. Nutr.* **92,** 1484–1493 (2010).

78. Martinez-Gonzalez, M. A. *et al.* A 14-item Mediterranean diet assessment tool and obesity indexes among high-risk subjects: The PREDIMED trial. *PLoS One* **7,** e43134–e43134 (2012).

79. Romaguera, D. *et al.* Mediterranean dietary patterns and prospective weight change in participants of the EPIC-PANACEA project. *Am. J. Clin. Nutr.* **92,** 912–921 (2010).

80. Mendez, M. A. *et al.* Adherence to a Mediterranean diet is associated with reduced 3-year incidence of obesity. *J. Nutr.* **136,** 2934–2938 (2006).

81. García-Fernández, E., Rico-Cabanas, L., Rosgaard, N., Estruch, R. & Bach-Faig, A. Mediterranean diet and cardiodiabesity: A review. *Nutrients* **6,** 3474–3500 (2014).

82. Mozaffarian, D., Hao, T., Rimm, E. B., Willett, W. C. & Hu, F. B. Changes in diet and lifestyle and long-term weight gain in women and men. *N. Engl. J. Med.* **364,** 2392–2404 (2011).

83. Good, C. K., Holschuh, N., Albertson, A. M. & Eldridge, A. L. Whole grain consumption and body mass index in adult women: An analysis of NHANES 1999-2000 and the USDA pyramid servings database. *J. Am. Coll. Nutr.* **27,** 80–87 (2008).

84. Jonsson, T. *et al.* Beneficial effects of a Paleolithic diet on cardiovascular risk factors in type 2 diabetes: A randomized cross-over pilot study. *Cardiovasc. Diabetol.* **8,** 35–35 (2009).

85. Lindeberg, S. *et al.* A Palaeolithic diet improves glucose tolerance more than a Mediterranean-like diet in individuals with ischaemic heart disease. *Diabetologia* **50,** 1795–1807 (2007).

86. Howlett, J. & Ashwell, M. Glycemic response and health: Summary of a workshop. *Am. J. Clin. Nutr.* **87,** 212S–216S (2008).

87. Livesey, G., Taylor, R., Hulshof, T. & Howlett, J. Glycemic response and health—a systematic review and meta-analysis: Relations between dietary glycemic properties and health outcomes. *Am. J. Clin. Nutr.* **87,** 258S–268S (2008).

88. Riccardi, G., Rivellese, A. A. & Giacco, R. Role of glycemic index and glycemic load in the healthy state, in prediabetes, and in diabetes. *Am. J. Clin. Nutr.* **87,** 269S–274S (2008).

89. Thomas, D. & Elliott, E. J. Low glycaemic index, or low glycaemic load, diets for diabetes mellitus. *Cochrane Database Syst. Rev.* CD006296-CD006296 (2009). doi:10.1002/14651858.CD006296.pub2.

90. Osterdahl, M., Kocturk, T., Koochek, A. & Wandell, P. E. Effects of a short-term intervention with a paleolithic diet in healthy volunteers. *Eur. J. Clin. Nutr.* **62,** 682–685 (2008).

91. Frassetto, L. A., Schloetter, M., Mietus-Synder, M., Morris Jr., R. C. & Sebastian, A. Metabolic and physiologic improvements from consuming a paleolithic, hunter-gatherer type diet. *Eur. J. Clin. Nutr.* **63,** 947–955 (2009).

92. Jonsson, T. *et al.* Subjective satiety and other experiences of a Paleolithic diet compared to a diabetes diet in patients with type 2 diabetes. *Nutr. J.* **12,** 105–105 (2013).

93. Boers, I. *et al.* Favourable effects of consuming a Palaeolithic-type diet on characteristics of the metabolic syndrome: A randomized controlled pilot-study. *Lipids Health Dis.* **13,** 160–160 (2014).

94. Rolls, B. J., Morris, E. L. & Roe, L. S. Portion size of food affects energy intake in normal-weight and overweight men and women. *Am. J. Clin. Nutr.* **76,** 1207–1213 (2002).

95. Rolls, B. J., Roe, L. S., Meengs, J. S. & Wall, D. E. Increasing the portion size of a sandwich increases energy intake. *J. Am. Diet. Assoc.* **104,** 367–372 (2004).

96. Rolls, B. J., Roe, L. S. & Meengs, J. S. Larger portion sizes lead to a sustained increase in energy intake over 2 days. *J. Am. Diet. Assoc.* **106,** 543–549 (2006).

97. Tieken, S. M. *et al.* Effects of solid versus liquid meal-replacement products of similar energy content on hunger, satiety, and appetite-regulating hormones in older adults. *Horm. Metab. Res.* **39,** 389–394 (2007).

98. Stull, A. J., Apolzan, J. W., Thalacker-Mercer, A. E., Iglay, H. B. & Campbell, W. W. Liquid and solid meal replacement products differentially affect postprandial appetite and food intake in older adults. *J. Am. Diet. Assoc.* **108,** 1226–1230 (2008).

99. Miller, G. D. Improved nutrient intake in older obese adults undergoing a structured diet and exercise intentional weight loss program. *J. Nutr. Health Aging* **14,** 461–466 (2010).

100. Wadden, T. A. *et al.* One-year weight losses in the Look AHEAD study: Factors associated with success. *Obes. Silver Spring* **17,** 713–722 (2009).

101. Ryan, D. H. *et al.* Look AHEAD (Action for Health in Diabetes): Design and methods for a clinical trial of weight loss for the prevention of cardiovascular disease in type 2 diabetes. *Control Clin. Trials* **24,** 610–628 (2003).

102. Messier, S. P. *et al.* The intensive diet and exercise for arthritis (IDEA) trial: Design and rationale. *BMC. Musculoskelet. Disord.* **10,** 93–93 (2009).

103. Hartmann-Boyce, J. *et al.* Behavioural weight management programmes for adults assessed by trials conducted in everyday contexts: Systematic review and meta-analysis. *Obes. Rev.* **15,** 920–932 (2014).

104. Rock, C. L. *et al.* Effect of a free prepared meal and incentivized weight loss program on weight loss and weight loss maintenance in obese and overweight women: A randomized controlled trial. *JAMA J. Am. Med. Assoc.* **304,** 1803–1810 (2010).

105. Foster, G. D. *et al.* A randomized comparison of a commercially available portion-controlled weight-loss intervention with a diabetes self-management education program. *Nutr. Diabetes* **3,** e63–e63 (2013).

106. Cheskin, L. J. *et al.* Efficacy of meal replacements versus a standard food-based diet for weight loss in type 2 diabetes: A controlled clinical trial. *Diabetes Educ.* **34,** 118–127 (2008).

107. Burgess, E., Hassmén, P., Welvaert, M. & Pumpa, K. L. Behavioural treatment strategies improve adherence to lifestyle intervention programmes in adults with obesity: A systematic review and meta-analysis. *Clin. Obes.* **7,** 105–114 (2017).

108. Ayyad, C. & Andersen, T. Long-term efficacy of dietary treatment of obesity: A systematic review of studies published between 1931 and 1999. *Obes. Rev. Off. J. Int. Assoc. Study Obes.* **1,** 113–119 (2000).

109. National Institute of Health, N. H. L. and B. I. Clinical guidelines on the identification, evaluation and treatment of overweight and obesity in adults - the evidence report. *Obes. Res.* **6,** 51S–209S (1998).

110. Chaston, T. B., Dixon, J. B. & O'Brien, P. E. Changes in fat-free mass during significant weight loss: A systematic review. *Int. J. Obes. 2005* **31,** 743–750 (2007).

111. Valtueña, S., Blanch, S., Barenys, M., Solà, R. & Salas-Salvadó, J. Changes in body composition and resting energy expenditure after rapid weight loss: Is there an energy-metabolism adaptation in obese patients? *Int. J. Obes. Relat. Metab. Disord. J. Int. Assoc. Study Obes.* **19,** 119–125 (1995).

112. Wadden, T. A., Foster, G. D. & Letizia, K. A. One-year behavioral treatment of obesity: Comparison of moderate and severe caloric restriction and the effects of weight maintenance therapy. *J. Consult. Clin. Psychol.* **62,** 165–171 (1994).

113. Purcell, K. *et al.* The effect of rate of weight loss on long-term weight management: A randomised controlled trial. *LANCET Diabetes Endocrinol.* **8587,** 1–9 (2014).

114. Vink, R. G., Roumans, N. J. T., Arkenbosch, L. A. J., Mariman, E. C. M. & van Baak, M. A. The effect of rate of weight loss on long-term weight regain in adults with overweight and obesity. *Obes. Silver Spring Md* **24,** 321–327 (2016).

115. Coutinho, S. R. *et al.* The impact of rate of weight loss on body composition and compensatory mechanisms during weight reduction: A randomized control trial. *Clin. Nutr. Edinb. Scotl.* (2017). doi:10.1016/j.clnu.2017.04.008.

116. Eshghinia, S. & Mohammadzadeh, F. The effects of modified alternate-day fasting diet on weight loss and CAD risk factors in overweight and obese women. *J. Diabetes Metab. Disord.* **12,** 4–4 (2013).

117. Varady, K. A., Bhutani, S., Church, E. C. & Klempel, M. C. Short-term modified alternate-day fasting: A novel dietary strategy for weight loss and cardioprotection in obese adults. *Am. J. Clin. Nutr.* **90,** 1138–1143 (2009).

118. Hoddy, K. K. *et al.* Meal timing during alternate day fasting: Impact on body weight and cardiovascular disease risk in obese adults. *Obes. Silver Spring* **22,** 2524–2531 (2014).

119. Bhutani, S., Klempel, M. C., Kroeger, C. M., Trepanowski, J. F. & Varady, K. A. Alternate day fasting and endurance exercise combine to reduce body weight and favorably alter plasma lipids in obese humans. *Obes. Silver Spring Md* **21,** 1370–1379 (2013).

120. Johnson, J. B. *et al.* Alternate day calorie restriction improves clinical findings and reduces markers of oxidative stress and inflammation in overweight adults with moderate asthma. *Free Radic. Biol. Med.* **42,** 665–674 (2007).

121. Patterson, R. E. & Sears, D. D. Metabolic effects of intermittent fasting. *Annu. Rev. Nutr.* **37,** 371–393 (2017).

122. LeCheminant, J. D., Christenson, E., Bailey, B. W. & Tucker, L. A. Restricting night-time eating reduces daily energy intake in healthy young men: A short-term cross-over study. *Br. J. Nutr.* **110,** 2108–2113 (2013).

123. Stote, K. S. *et al.* A controlled trial of reduced meal frequency without caloric restriction in healthy, normal-weight, middle-aged adults. *Am. J. Clin. Nutr.* **85,** 981–988 (2007).

124. Carlson, O. *et al.* Impact of reduced meal frequency without caloric restriction on glucose regulation in healthy, normal-weight middle-aged men and women. *Metabolism.* **56,** 1729–1734 (2007).

125. Chowdhury, E. A. *et al.* The causal role of breakfast in energy balance and health: A randomized controlled trial in obese adults. *Am. J. Clin. Nutr.* **103,** 747–756 (2016).

126. Chowdhury, E. A., Richardson, J. D., Tsintzas, K., Thompson, D. & Betts, J. A. Effect of extended morning fasting upon ad libitum lunch intake and associated metabolic and hormonal responses in obese adults. *Int. J. Obes. 2005* **40,** 305–311 (2016).

127. Healy, G. N. *et al.* Breaks in sedentary time: Beneficial associations with metabolic risk. *Diabetes Care* **31,** 661–666 (2008).

128. Booth, F. W., Gordon, S. E., Carlson, C. J. & Hamilton, M. T. Waging war on modern chronic diseases: Primary prevention through exercise biology. *J. Appl. Physiol. 1985* **88,** 774–787 (2000).

129. Hamilton, M. T., Hamilton, D. G. & Zderic, T. W. Role of low energy expenditure and sitting in obesity, metabolic syndrome, type 2 diabetes, and cardiovascular disease. *Diabetes* **56,** 2655–2667 (2007).

130. Saris, W. H. *et al.* How much physical activity is enough to prevent unhealthy weight gain? Outcome of the IASO 1st Stock Conference and consensus statement. *Obes. Rev.* **4,** 101–114 (2003).

131. Haskell, W. L. *et al.* Physical activity and public health: Updated recommendation for adults from the American College of Sports Medicine and the American Heart Association. *Med. Sci. Sports Exerc. JID - 8005433* **39,** 1423–1434 (2007).

132. Report of the Dietary Guidelines Advisory Committee on the Dietary Guidelines for Americans, 2010. (2010).

133. Pate, R. R. *et al.* Physical activity and public health. A recommendation from the Centers for Disease Control and Prevention and the American College of Sports Medicine. *JAMA* **273,** 402–407 (1995).

134. Donnelly, J. E. *et al.* Appropriate physical activity intervention strategies for weight loss and prevention of weight regain for adults. *Med. Sci. Sports Exerc.* **41,** 459–471 (2009).

135. Klem, M. L., Wing, R. R., McGuire, M. T., Seagle, H. M. & Hill, J. O. A descriptive study of individuals successful at long-term maintenance of substantial weight loss. *Am. J. Clin. Nutr.* **66,** 239–246 (1997).

136. Schoeller, D. A., Shay, K. & Kushner, R. F. How much physical activity is needed to minimize weight gain in previously obese women? *Am. J. Clin. Nutr.* **66,** 551–556 (1997).

137. Herman, K. M., Carver, T. E., Christou, N. V. & Andersen, R. E. Physical activity and sitting time in bariatric surgery patients 1-16 years post-surgery. *Clin. Obes.* **4,** 267–276 (2014).

138. Jakicic, J. M., Marcus, B. H., Lang, W. & Janney, C. Effect of exercise on 24-month weight loss maintenance in overweight women. *Arch. Intern. Med.* **168,** 1550–1559; discussion 1559–1560 (2008).

139. Ross, R., Hudson, R., Stotz, P. J. & Lam, M. Effects of exercise amount and intensity on abdominal obesity and glucose tolerance in obese adults. *Ann. Intern. Med.* **162,** 325–325 (2015).

140. Reichkendler, M. H. *et al.* Only minor additional metabolic health benefits of high as opposed to moderate dose physical exercise in young, moderately overweight men. *Obesity* **22,** 1220–1232 (2014).

141. Tate, D. F., Jeffery, R. W., Sherwood, N. E. & Wing, R. R. Long-term weight losses associated with prescription of higher physical activity goals. Are higher levels of physical activity protective against weight regain? *Am. J. Clin. Nutr.* **85,** 954–959 (2007).

142. Fogelholm, M., Kujala, U., Kaprio, J. & Sarna, S. Predictors of weight change in middle-aged and old men. *Obes. Res.* **8,** 367–373 (2000).

143. Perri, M. G. *et al.* Effects of four maintenance programs on the long-term management of obesity. *J. Consult. Clin. Psychol.* **56,** 529–534 (1988).

144. Jakicic, J. M., Marcus, B. H., Gallagher, K. I., Napolitano, M. & Lang, W. Effect of exercise duration and intensity on weight loss in overweight, sedentary women: A randomized trial. *JAMA* **290,** 1323–1330 (2003).

145. Jakicic, J. M., Winters, C. & Wing, R. R. Effects of intermittent exercise and on adherence, weight loss, and fitness in overweight women. *October* **02906,** 1554–1560 (1999).

146. Jeffery, R. W., Wing, R. R., Sherwood, N. E. & Tate, D. F. Physical activity and weight loss: Does prescribing higher physical activity goals improve outcome? *Am. J. Clin. Nutr.* **78,** 684–689 (2003).

147. Ewbank, P. P., Darga, L. L. & Lucas, C. P. Physical activity as a predictor of weight maintenance in previously obese subjects. *Obes. Res.* **3,** 257–263 (1995).

148. Drenowatz, C., Hill, J. O., Peters, J. C., Soriano-Maldonado, A. & Blair, S. N. The association of change in physical activity and body weight in the regulation of total energy expenditure. *Eur. J. Clin. Nutr.* **71,** 377–382 (2017).

149. Willis, L. H. *et al.* Effects of aerobic and/or resistance training on body mass and fat mass in overweight or obese adults. *J. Appl. Physiol. 1985* **113,** 1831–1837 (2012).

150. Davidson, L. E. *et al.* Effects of exercise modality on insulin resistance and functional limitation in older adults: A randomized controlled trial. *Arch. Intern. Med.* **169,** 122–131 (2009).

151. Jakicic, J. M. *et al.* Time-based physical activity interventions for weight loss: A randomized trial. *Med. Sci. Sports Exerc.* **47,** 1061–1069 (2015).

7 Pharmacological Treatment of Obesity

Amie A. Ogunsakin and Ayotunde O. Dokun

CONTENTS

7.1 INTRODUCTION

The prevalence of obesity and overweight has risen substantially in the past few decades. It is a public health problem that is associated with significant increase in morbidity and mortality, and a reduction in health-related quality of life [1,2]. *Obesity* is defined by the World Health Organization (WHO) based on body mass index (BMI). *BMI* is defined as an individual's weight in kilograms divided by height in meters squared. A BMI between 18.5 and 25 is considered to be a normal weight, a BMI between 25 and 30 is classified as overweight, and a BMI of more than 30 is considered obese [3,4]. Among Asians, a BMI of 23 or higher is overweight, and a BMI of 27 or higher is obese, due to increased incidence of obesity-related complications at lower BMI.

Obesity raises the risk of morbidity from hypertension, dyslipidemia, type 2 diabetes mellitus, coronary heart disease (CHD), stroke, nonalcoholic fatty liver disease (NAFLD), polycystic ovarian syndrome (PCOS), osteoarthritis, decreased lung function, obstructive sleep apnea (OSA), urinary incontinence, disability, and some cancers [5–10]. Obesity has also been implicated in chronic kidney disease and cognitive decline [11,12].

Comprehensive lifestyle modification is recommended for all individuals who are overweight or obese. A structured lifestyle intervention program designed for weight loss should include caloric restriction, an increase in physical activity, and behavioral interventions. Physical activity should be individualized to include activities and exercise regimens within the physical and health-related capabilities of the individual. Exercise can be initiated with gradual increments, with a goal of a total of at least 150 minutes per week of moderate exercise performed during three to five daily sessions per week and should include resistance training two to three times per week. It recommended that lifestyle intervention and support should be intensified if individuals do not achieve a 2.5% weight loss in the first month of treatment, as early weight reduction is a key predictor of long-term weight loss success. Addressing underlying mental health issues, such as depression, anxiety, psychosis, eating disorders, and other psychological problems that can undermine the effectiveness of lifestyle intervention, is critical to increase likelihood of success. Nevertheless, even when lifestyle intervention is implemented with the above approach in mind, maintaining weight loss through lifestyle interventions alone is often difficult due to obesity-related hormonal, metabolic, and neuronal adaptations that favor weight gain. These include changes in leptin, ghrelin, and other gut hormones that augment appetite, reduced physical activity, and decreased resting energy expenditure [13–16]. Typically, comprehensive lifestyle modification produces average weight losses of 5%–10% of initial weight in a 6-month period. Thereafter, most patients will equilibrate (caloric intake balancing energy expenditure) and require adjustment of energy balance if they are to lose additional weight [16]. There is currently strong evidence from clinical trials that the addition of pharmacotherapy produces greater weight loss and weight loss maintenance compared with lifestyle modification alone [17–22].

Decades prior, the only pharmacologic agents available to treat obesity were approved only for short-term use ($\leq$ 12 weeks) by the US Food and Drug Administration (FDA) and include diethylpropion, phendimetrazine, benzphetamine, and phentermine [23]. However, short-term of use of these weight loss medications did not demonstrate long-term health benefits [14,15]. More recently, the FDA approved a number of medications for longer-term treatment of obesity [17–22]. Given this understanding, recent guidelines now advocate a more comprehensive approach to achieving long-term weight loss [24,25]. Recommendations of the US Preventive Service Task Force, American Association of Clinical Endocrinologists (AACE)/American College of Endocrinology(ACE) and Endocrine Society now incorporate the use of pharmacotherapy as key components of a long-term weight loss strategy [24,25]. The guidelines also include consideration for concurrent initiation of lifestyle modification and pharmacotherapy in individuals with weight-related complications that can be improved by weight loss. Additionally, they recommend that pharmacotherapy should be considered and offered to patients with obesity, when potential benefits outweigh the risks, for the chronic treatment of the disease. Hence, pharmacologic agents are now indicated for chronic weight management in obese adults (a BMI of 30 kg/m^2 or greater) or in overweight patients (BMI of 27 kg/m^2 or greater) with at least one weight-related comorbid condition (e.g., hypertension, type 2 diabetes, or dyslipidemia) [26] as an adjunct to lifestyle modification.

7.2 PHARMACOLOGIC AGENTS

Currently, there are five medications that have been approved for management of obesity for long-term weight loss. They are orlistat, lorcaserin, naltrexone-bupropion, phentermine-topiramate, and liraglutide. A systematic review and meta-analysis of 28 randomized, clinical trials conducted among overweight and obese adults treated with these agents for long-term weight loss showed that, compared to placebo, these agents were each associated with achieving at least 5% weight loss at 52 weeks of treatment [27]. Available data across various randomized, controlled trials leading to the approval of the currently available weight loss medications, however, showed differences in efficacy in terms of mean percentage weight loss and proportion of individuals who attained 5% and 10% weight loss. Phentermine topiramate showed the greatest placebo subtracted weight loss at 8%, followed by naltrexone/bupropion and liraglutide at 6%, and orlistat and lorcaserin at 4.0%–4.5% [28–32] (Tables 7.1 and 7.2).

7.2.1 PHENTERMINE/TOPIRAMATE (QYSMIA)

Phentermine is a noradrenergic and possibly dopaminergic sympathomimetic amine that was originally approved for obesity in 1959; the drug was used on-label until 1977, when an amendment to the Food Drug and Cosmetic Act required that the FDA approve new drugs based on efficacy as well as safety. There was concern for addiction potential; hence it was approved for short-term use. Topiramate is a neuro-stabilizer and anti-seizure medication that suppresses appetite by unknown mechanism. Topiramate was FDA approved for treatment of refractory epilepsy in 1996, with weight loss noted as a side effect. The FDA approved fixed-dose phentermine/topiramate for long-term management of obesity in 2012. Phentermine/topiramate is a once-daily, extended-release capsule combining two separate drugs with different pharmacokinetics. Combining the two drugs into one formulation provides an immediate release of phentermine and delayed release of topiramate, which

TABLE 7.1
Pharmacologic Agents for Long-Term Therapy in Obesity Management

Name	Dose	Mode of Action	Typical Weight Loss, kg (%); Study Duration	FDA Approval Status
Phentermine (P)/ topiramate (T)	3.75 mg P/23 mg T ER QD (starting dose) 7.5 mg P/46 mg T ER daily (recommended dose) 15 mg P/92 mg P/T ER daily (high dose)	GABA receptor modulation (T) plus norepinephrine-releasing agent (P)	Recommended dose 8.1 kg (7.8) High dose 10.2 kg (9.8) placebo 1.4 kg (1.2); 56 weeks	FDA approved in 2012 for chronic weight management
Naltrexone/ bupropion	32 mg/360 mg 2 tablets QID (high dose)	Reuptake inhibitor of dopamine and norepinephrine (bupropion) and opioid antagonist (naltrexone)	6.2 kg (6.4) placebo 1.3 kg (1.2); 56 weeks	FDA approved in 2014 for chronic weight management
Lorcaserin (10 mg)	10 mg BID	5HT2c receptor agonist	5.8 kg (5.8) placebo 2.2 kg (2.2); 52 weeks	FDA approved in 2012 for chronic weight management
Orlistat, prescription (120 mg)	120 mg TID	Pancreatic and gastric lipase inhibitor	8.8 kg (8.8) placebo 5.8 kg (5.8); 52 weeks	FDA approved in 1999 for chronic weight management
Liraglutide	3 mg daily subcutaneous	Slows gastric emptying and increases satiety by central pathways	8.4 kg (8.0) placebo 2.8 kg (2.6); 56 weeks	FDA approved in 2014 for chronic weight management

5HT2c, selective serotonin 2c receptor agonist; BID, twice daily; ER, extended release; FDA, US Food and Drug Administration; GABA, gamma-aminobutyric acid; QID, four times daily; TID, three times daily.

TABLE 7.2

Common Side Effects of Available Pharmacologic Agents for the Treatment of Obesity

Name	Common Side Effects	Consider for Use in Patients with
Phentermine (P)/ topiramate (T)	Dry mouth, constipation, insomnia, dizziness, dysgeusia, tingling of the hands and feet	Hypertension
Naltrexone/ bupropion	Headache, nausea, vomiting, diarrhea, constipation, dry mouth, insomnia, hypoglycemia in patients with diabetes	Active smokers motivated to quit
Lorcaserin	Headache, dizziness, fatigue, nausea, dry mouth; do not take with SSRI or MAO inhibitors	Hypertension, cardiovascular disease
Orlistat	Fecal incontinence, bloating, diarrhea, abdominal pain	Hypertension, cardiovascular disease, adolescents, patients with anxiety and\or depression
Liraglutide	Nausea, vomiting, abdominal pain, hypoglycemia	Diabetes, cardiovascular disease, patients with anxiety and depression

MAO, monoamine oxidase; SSRI, selective serotonin reuptake inhibitors.

theoretically provides better appetite suppression throughout the day. Phentermine/topiramate has been associated with cleft lip and palate and should not be used in individuals who are pregnant or planning to become pregnant while being treated with phentermine-topiramate. Other contraindications include glaucoma, hyperthyroidism and recent monoamine inhibitor use during or within 14 days as well as allergies to either topiramate or symptanomimetic amines [33,34].

A typical starting dose is 3.75 mg/23 mg, one tablet daily for 14 days, and then it can be increased to 7.5 mg/46 mg daily. Dose titration should be made after being on the current dose for at least 2 weeks. The maximum dose is 15 mg/92 mg. This medication should be discontinued if, after 12 weeks of treatment with phentermine/topiramate, a patient has not achieved at least a 5% weight loss since its initiation. When a decision to stop phentermine/topiramate is made, it has to be gradually tapered off to prevent the risk of seizures. There is currently no data available to guide the use of the medication in nursing mothers [39–41].

Metabolic acidosis, increased heart rate, anxiety, insomnia, and elevated creatinine levels have been associated with the use of phentermine/topiramate. Dysgeusia and paresthesia, as well as cognitive impairment, can occur with phentermine/topiramate. This drug has abuse potential, due to the phentermine component; therefore, it is a Schedule IV controlled substance [39–41].

7.2.2 NALTREXONE/BUPROPION (CONTRAVE)

This is a fixed-dose combination of naltrexone and bupropion. It was FDA approved in September of 2014 for management of obesity. Naltrexone is an opioid antagonist, and bupropion is an aminoketone antidepressant that inhibits dopamine and norepinephrine re-uptake inhibitors, which stimulates pro-opiomelanocortin (POMC) neurons. The exact mechanism of the naltrexone/bupropion combination leading to weight loss is not fully understood [35]. The combination is theorized to work synergistically in the hypothalamus and the mesolimbic dopamine circuit to promote satiety, reduce food intake, and enhance energy expenditure. POMC cells located in the arcuate nucleus of the hypothalamus produce melanocyte-stimulating hormone (alpha-MSH) and beta-endorphin, an endogenous opioid [36,37]. The alpha-MSH activates the melanocortin-4 receptor (MC4R), leading to decreased food intake, increased energy expenditure, and weight loss [38,39]. Beta-endorphin reduces activity of POMC cells by binding

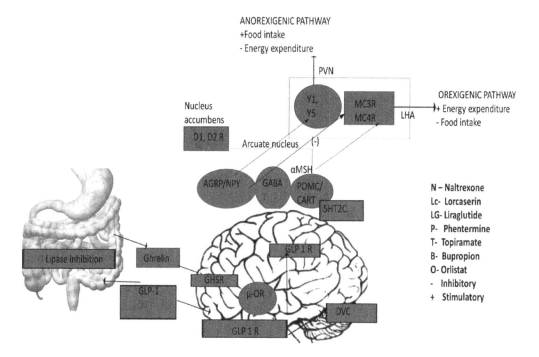

FIGURE 7.1   Major target sites of obesity drugs. (5HT2c, serotonin 2C; AGRP, agouti-related peptide; CART, cocaine amphetamine-related transcript; D1, dopamine 1 receptor; D2, dopamine 2 receptor; DVC, dorsal vagal complex; GABA, gamma-aminobutyric acid; GHSR, GH secretagogue receptor; GLP1R, glucagon-like receptor; LHA, lateral hypothalamus; MC3R, melanocortin 3 receptor; MC4R, melanocortin 4 receptor; αMSH, α-melanocyte-stimulating; NPY, neuropeptide Y; μ-OR, μ-opioid receptor; POMC, proopiomelanocortin; PVN, paraventricular nucleus; Y1/Y5R, Y1/Y5 receptor.)

to the inhibitory mu-opioid receptor (MOP-R) [40]. Bupropion, a weak dopamine and norepinephrine reuptake inhibitor, enhances POMC cell production and release of alpha-MSH and beta-endorphin [41]. Naltrexone, an opioid antagonist, blocks the MOP-R; therefore, it disrupts beta-endorphin inhibitory feedback on POMC cells [41] (Figure 7.1).

The naltrexone/bupropion combination enhances the effect of POMC signaling more than either drug alone [35].

Each tablet contains 8 mg of naltrexone and 90 mg of bupropion. A typical starting dose is one tablet taken by mouth in the morning for 1 week. At the start of week 2, another tablet should be added to the regimen in the evening. This titration should continue weekly until the optimal dosing of two tablets, twice daily, is reached at week 4, for a total daily dose of 32 mg of naltrexone and 360 mg of bupropion.

If patients do not achieve a 5% reduction in weight by week 12, it should be discontinued as it is unlikely to result in weight loss. The drug has not been evaluated in patients with renal or hepatic impairment [42]. The naltrexone component of naltrexone/bupropion may prevent patients from achieving maximal effect from concomitant opioid use, due to its intrinsic opioid antagonist effect. Naltrexone/bupropion should be discontinued, and standard doses of the opioid should not be exceeded, if intermittent treatment with opioid is required. In situations of chronic opioid use, the opioid should be discontinued for 7–10 days before naltrexone/bupropion is initiated to prevent precipitation of opioid withdrawal [42]. The concomitant use of bupropion with a monoamine oxidase inhibitor (MAOI) is contraindicated due to risk of hypertensive reactions. A 14-day washout period is recommended before the initiation of naltrexone/bupropion or an MAOI after the discontinuation of the prior medication [43,44]. Bupropion has a dose-related propensity to cause seizures, and caution should be used when prescribed in individuals with an increased risk of seizure. Bupropion is a strong inhibitor of cytochrome P450 (CYP 450) 2D6 isozyme. The use of concomitant drugs that are metabolized through the CYP 450 system may require a reduction in the dose of the drug. Naltrexone/bupropion should not exceed one tablet in the morning and evening when used concomitantly with CYP2B6 inhibitors. Naltrexone/bupropion may be used in patients with mild to moderate renal impairment but is not recommended for use in individuals with end-stage renal disease. No dose adjustments are required for mild renal disease. In moderate to severe renal failure, the recommended dose is one tablet twice per day. It can also be used in individuals with mild to severe hepatic impairment at a recommended dose of one tablet daily [42].

The effect of naltrexone/bupropion in pediatric patients younger than 18 years is unknown due to the lack of clinical trials, and use in this age group is not recommended. For individuals older than 65 years, caution is advised. Elderly patients are more likely to have polypharmacy, impaired cognition, and abnormalities in renal and hepatic function; hence they may be more likely to suffer side effects from the individual subcomponents of this drug [42].

The most common adverse drug effects (ADEs) reported in randomized, clinical trials with naltrexone/bupropion use were nausea (32.5%), constipation (19.2%), headache (17.6%), vomiting (10.7%), dizziness (9.9%), insomnia (9.2%), dry mouth (8.1%), and diarrhea (7.1%).

Naltrexone/bupropion carries the antidepressant-class boxed warnings for suicidality and neuropsychiatric reactions. Naltrexone/bupropion has been associated with increases in resting heart rate and average blood pressure [42].

Naltrexone/bupropion has not been shown to have abuse potential and therefore is not a Schedule IV controlled substance like phentermine/topiramate and lorcaserin.

7.2.3 Liraglutide (Saxenda)

Liraglutide is an analogue of the incretin hormone glucagon-like peptide 1 (GLP-1), and it has a 97% amino acid sequence homology to native GLP-1. Liraglutide at a maximum daily dose of 1.8 mg subcutaneous injection was initially approved by the FDA in 2010 as an adjunct therapy to diet and exercise for management of type 2 diabetes. Results from clinical trials consistently demonstrated the ability of GLP-1 analogues to induce weight loss [45,46]. As a result, liraglutide was also developed as a weight loss agent, and its 3-mg daily subcutaneous dose was approved by the FDA in December 2014. Weight loss is primarily mediated by reducing appetite and caloric intake [47]. GLP-1 is released predominantly from the small intestine in response to food intake. It reduces fasting and postprandial glycemia and enhances glucose-dependent insulin secretion [48–50]. It also inhibits glucagon secretion, slows gastric emptying, and increases satiety by central pathways that affect food intake and metabolism via hindbrain and hypothalamic activation, as well as those brain areas associated with motivation and reward processes [51] (Figure 7.1). The most common reported adverse effects (AEs) from liraglutide use are gastrointestinal side effects such as nausea, diarrhea, constipation, vomiting, dyspepsia, abdominal pain, and increased lipase. Other AEs include hypoglycemia, headache, fatigue, and dizziness.

Liraglutide should be used with caution in individuals with impaired kidney or liver function [52] but has been shown to be safe and did not affect kidney function in patients with moderate renal impairment [53]. Patients starting liraglutide should be cautioned about the risks of acute pancreatitis, acute gallbladder disease, serious hypoglycemia, heart rate increase, hypersensitivity reactions, and suicidal behavior. Liraglutide is contraindicated in patients with a personal or family history of medullary thyroid cancers (MTCs) or multiple endocrine neoplasia, as it has been shown to cause thyroid C-cell tumors in rats and mice; however, no increased risk for MTC has been observed in humans [52]. Liraglutide is also contraindicated in pregnancy. It is not recommended in nursing mothers, children, or individuals taking other GLP-1 agonists [46,52]. Finally, although liraglutide (as well as other GLP-1 agonists) increases heart rate to a small degree, the clinical significance is unclear [46,54]. Liraglutide may be a particularly effective choice among obese patients with type 2 diabetes and can be considered for those at high risk for cardiovascular disease, given a beneficial effect in cardiovascular outcomes seen in the 1.8-mg formulation in a diabetes population. However, the effects of the 3-mg formulation on cardiovascular morbidity and mortality have not been established.

A typical starting dose is 0.6 mg per day and should be titrated up on a weekly basis to achieve a maintenance dose of 3 mg daily. If a dose is missed for more than 72 hours, it is recommended that patients be instructed to resume dosing at 0.6 mg daily and restart the titration schedule (in order to reduce gastrointestinal side effects).

7.2.4 LORCASERIN (BELVIQ)

Lorcaserin is a selective serotonin 2c receptor agonist (5HT-2C). It was FDA approved in June 2012. Lorcaserin acts at $5\text{-}HT_{2C}$ receptors in the central nervous system (CNS), particularly the hypothalamus, to reduce appetite [55,56]. It stimulates $5\text{-}HT_{2C}$ receptors on the POMC neurons in the arcuate nucleus; this causes the release of alpha-melanocortin-stimulating hormone (alpha-MSH), which acts on melanocortin-4 receptors in the paraventricular nucleus to suppress appetite (Figure 7.1). Potential drug interactions may occur with medications that affect serotonergic pathways. There is a risk of serotonin syndrome and neuroleptic malignant syndrome if used in combination with other serotonergic agents.

The recommended dose is 10 mg orally twice daily. Lorcaserin may be used in patients with mild to moderate hepatic impairment and mild renal impairment. Caution is recommended for moderate renal impairment and severe hepatic impairment. The use of lorcaserin in patients with severe renal impairment or end-stage renal failure is not recommended [55].

The effect of lorcaserin in pediatric patients younger than 18 years old and individuals older than 65 years has not been established. Lorcaserin is contraindicated in pregnant women, and it is listed as a pregnancy Category X medication. There are no data supporting the use of the medication in nursing mothers.

Common ADEs reported in randomized, clinical trials with lorcaserin use were hypoglycemia associated with weight loss in individuals who had diabetes (29.3%), headache (14.5%–16.8%), and nasopharyngitis (11.3%–13.1%). Other ADEs include upper respiratory infections (13.7%), dizziness (7.0%–8.5%), fatigue (7.2%–7.4%), nausea (8.3%–9.4%), and dry mouth (5.3%) [20,31,56,57].

In clinical trials, no significant increase in valvular disease was observed for lorcaserin when compared with placebo. Priapism was noted in rodent studies, and caution is advised in individuals at risk for priapism or who are on medications for erectile dysfunction. Leukopenia, hyperprolactinemia, and cognitive impairment have been reported with lorcaserin. At doses higher than 20 mg per day, psychotic tendencies and behavior have been described [58,59].

7.2.5 ORLISTAT (XENICAL)

Orlistat is a lipase inhibitor that reduces fat absorption from intestines. It was FDA approved in 1999. Orlistat, a semisynthetic derivative of lipstatin, is a potent and selective inhibitor of these enzymes, with little or no activity against amylase, trypsin, chymotrypsin, and phospholipases. Orlistat acts by binding covalently to the serine residue of the active site of gastric and pancreatic lipases (Figure 7.1). When administered with fat-containing foods, orlistat partially inhibits hydrolysis of triglycerides, thus reducing the subsequent absorption of monoacylglycerides and free fatty acids [60–62]. Orlistat blocks absorption of 25%–30% of fat calories and is not appreciably absorbed systemically. The drug is available over the counter at a dosage of 60 mg TID. The recommended prescription dosage is 120 mg TID, and this dose should not be exceeded, as there is no evidence from clinical trials that efficacy is greater at higher dosages. Orlistat 120 mg TID has been studied and approved for treatment of adolescents with obesity [23,31,33].

7.3 PREFERRED DRUGS IN SELECT DISORDERS

7.3.1 CORONARY ARTERY DISEASE, CARDIAC ARRYTHMIAS

The preferred weight loss agents for use in individuals with coronary artery disease or arrhythmias are orlistat, lorcaserin, and liraglutide. Phentermine/topiramate and naloxone/bupropion can be used with caution, with careful monitoring of heart rate and blood pressure.

7.3.2 TYPE 2 DIABETES

All weight-loss medications can be used in the individual with type 2 diabetes. However, there is the added benefit of glycemic control with the use of liraglutide, and this should be strongly considered if there are no other contraindications to liraglutide use.

7.3.3 PREDIABETES/METABOLIC SYNDROME

In the individual with prediabetes or metabolic syndrome, all the currently available agents can be used; however, there is insufficient data for lorcaserin and naltrexone/bupropion for the prevention of diabetes mellitus type 2 prevention, and caution is advised with the use of either of these agents in this population.

7.3.4 ANXIETY AND DEPRESSION

In individuals with anxiety and depression, orlistat and liraglutide can be safely used. Phentermine/topiramate can be used in doses smaller than the maximal dose of 15–92 mg.

7.3.5 ALCOHOL ABUSE OR DRUG ADDICTION

When a history of alcohol abuse or drug addiction exists, liraglutide or orlistat is the preferred weight loss medication.

7.3.6 CHRONIC OPIOID USE

In individuals requiring chronic administration of opioid or opiate medications, phentermine/topiramate extended release (ER), lorcaserin, liraglutide 3 mg, and orlistat are the preferred weight loss medications. Naltrexone/bupropion is not recommended for use in individuals with opioid use.

7.3.7 BARIATRIC SURGERY

Individuals who have undergone bariatric surgery and have regained excess weight ($\geq$ 25% of the lost weight), who have not responded to intensive lifestyle intervention and are not candidates for reoperation, may be considered for treatment with liraglutide 1.8–3.0 mg. There is limited data to support the use of phentermine/topiramate ER. The safety and efficacy of other weight loss medications have not been assessed in these patients.

7.3.8 SMOKING

In the individual with a history of smoking, with no pre-existing contraindications, the use of naltrexone/bupropion can be considered to aid smoking cessation.

7.3.9 CONGESTIVE HEART FAILURE

There is insufficient data to guide the use of any of the currently approved agents in congestive heart failure.

7.3.10 PSYCHOTIC DISORDERS

There is insufficient data to guide the use of any of the currently approved agents in psychotic disorders.

7.3.11 PREGNANCY AND LACTATION

None of these agents is recommended in pregnancy or breast-feeding females. Furthermore, contraception is recommended with the use of all of these agents in any woman within the reproductive age group.

7.3.12 HEPATIC IMPAIRMENT

All weight loss medications should be used with caution in patients with hepatic impairment. No dose adjustments are needed in mild hepatic impairment. In moderate hepatic impairment, the maximum recommended dose of naltrexone ER/bupropion ER is one tablet (8 mg/90 mg) in the morning, and the maximum recommended dose of phentermine/topiramate is 7.5 mg/46 mg. All of these agents are contraindicated in severe hepatic impairment.

7.3.13 HYPERTENSION

In patients with existing hypertension, orlistat, lorcaserin, phentermine/topiramate ER, and liraglutide 3 mg are preferred weight-loss medications. Heart rate should be carefully monitored in patients receiving liraglutide 3 mg and phentermine/topiramate ER. Naltrexone/bupropion ER should be avoided if other weight loss medications can be used, since weight loss assisted by naltrexone ER/bupropion ER cannot be expected to produce blood pressure lowering, and the drug is contraindicated in uncontrolled hypertension.

7.3.14 ELDERLY (>65 YEARS)

Weight loss medications should be used with extra caution in elderly patients. Additional studies are needed to assess efficacy and safety of weight loss medications in the elderly.

7.3.15 SEIZURE DISORDER/HIGH RISK FOR SEIZURES

Phentermine/topiramate, lorcaserin, liraglutide, and orlistat are the preferred weight loss medications in individuals with a history of seizure disorder, or at risk for seizures, such as withdrawal seizures in chronic alcohol use. The use of naltrexone ER/bupropion ER should be avoided in these patients.

7.3.16 Chronic Kidney Disease

Weight loss medications should not be used in the setting of end-stage renal disease, with the exception that orlistat and liraglutide 3 mg can be considered in selected patients with a high level of caution.

All weight-loss medications can be used with caution in patients with mild (50–79 mL/min) and moderate (30–49 mL/min) renal impairment, except that in moderate renal impairment, the dose of naltrexone/bupropion should not exceed 8 mg/90 mg twice a day, and the daily dose of phentermine/topiramate ER should not exceed 7.5 mg/46 mg.

7.3.17 Nephrolithiasis

Naltrexone ER/bupropion ER, lorcaserin, and liraglutide 3.0 mg are the preferred weight loss medications in patients with a history, or at risk, of nephrolithiasis. Caution should be exercised in treating patients with phentermine/topiramate ER and orlistat who have a history of nephrolithiasis.

7.4 CONCLUSIONS

The availability of these FDA-approved medication for use as an adjunct to lifestyle intervention in the management of obesity ushers in a new era in the management of obesity as a chronic disease. However, a number of challenges and obstacles remain to widespread use of these therapies. These include (1) recognizing and understanding that obesity is a preventable, treatable, and chronic disease that requires long-term treatment to maintain weight loss; (2) the limited education of the public on the availability of pharmacotherapy as a viable and recommended treatment option for obesity; (3) the prohibitive costs of weight loss medications; (4) many physicians' discomfort prescribing medications for obesity management due to lack of expertise in obesity management; (5) safety concerns regarding long-term use (i.e., > 5 years) of these agents.

Current guidelines provide a general guide for physicians in the use of pharmacotherapy in obesity management, but treatment must be individualized, with careful consideration paid to the side effect profile and efficacy of the medications, along with the unique clinical characteristics of each patient. Specific head-to-head trials of currently available agents may help further guide the choice of agents. Additionally, studies assessing the safety and effectiveness of combinations of these agents would likely increase treatment options. Finally, education of the public, policy makers, and medical professionals, and specialty training in obesity are pivotal to ensuring that pharmacotherapy for treatment of obesity is widely available, affordable, and readily deployed as part of a comprehensive strategy for the management of obesity.

REFERENCES

1. Ng M, Fleming T, Robinson M, et al. Global, regional, and national prevalence of overweight and obesity in children and adults during 1980–2013: A systematic analysis for the Global Burden of Disease Study 2013. *Lancet.* 2014;384(9945):766–781.
2. Jia H, Lubetkin EI. The impact of obesity on health-related quality-of-life in the general adult US population. *J Public Health (Oxf).* 2005;27(2):156–164.
3. Flegal KM, Kruszon-Moran D, Carroll MD, Fryar CD, Ogden CL. Trends in obesity among adults in the United States, 2005 to 2014. *JAMA.* 2016;315:2284–2291.
4. Centers for Disease Control and Prevention (CDC) Defining Overweight and Obesity. Updated April 27, 2012 Available at: www.cdc.gov/obesity/adult/defining.html
5. Flegal KM, Graubard BI, Williamson DF, Gail MH. Excess deaths associated with underweight, overweight, and obesity. *JAMA.* 2005;293:1861–1867.
6. Campos P, Saguy A, Ernsberger P, Oliver E, Gaesser G. The epidemiology of overweight and obesity: Public health crisis or moral panic? *Int J Epidemiol.* 2006;35:55–60.
7. Sims EAH. Are there persons who are obese, but metabolically healthy? *Metabolism.* 2001;50:1499–1504.

8. Willett WC, Hu FB, Thun M. Overweight, obesity, and all-cause mortality. *JAMA*. 2013;309:1681–1682.
9. Flegal KM, Kit BK, Orpana H, Graubard BI. Association of all-cause mortality with overweight and obesity using standard body mass index categories: A systematic review and meta-analysis. *JAMA*. 2013;309:71–82.
10. Spiegelman BM, Flier JS. Obesity and the regulation of energy balance. *Cell*. 2001;104:531–543.
11. Kovesdy CP, Furth SL, Zoccali C; World Kidney Day Steering Committee. Obesity and kidney disease: Hidden consequences of the epidemic. *Future Sci OA*. 2017;3(3):FSO159. doi:10.415.
12. Chao Hse-Huang, Liao Yin-To, Chen Vincent Chin-Hung, Li Cheng-Jui, McIntyre Roger S, Lee Yena, Weng Jun-Cheng. Correlation between brain circuit segregation and obesity. *Behav Brain Res*. 2018;337:218–227. doi:10.1016/j.bbr.2017.09.017.
13. MacLean PS, Wing RR, Davidson T, et al. NIH working group report: Innovative research to improve maintenance of weight loss. *Obesity*. 2015;23(1):7–15.
14. Parsons WB. Controlled-release diethylpropion hydrochloride used in a program for weight reduction. *Clin Ther*. 1981;3(5):329–335.
15. Carney DE, Tweddell ED. Double blind evaluation of long acting diethylpropion hydrochloride in obese patients from a general practice. *Med J Aust*. 1975;1(1):13–15.
16. Sumithran P, Prendergast LA, Delbridge E, et al. Long-term persistence of hormonal adaptations to weight loss. *N Engl J Med*. 2011;365(17):1597–1604.
17. Kelley DE, Bray GA, Pi-Sunyer FX, et al. Clinical efficacy of orlistat therapy in overweight and obese patients with insulin-treated type 2 diabetes: A 1-year randomized controlled trial. *Diabetes Care*. 2002;25(6):1033–1041.
18. Miles JM, Leiter L, Hollander P, et al. Effect of orlistat in overweight and obese patients with type 2 diabetes treated with metformin. *Diabetes Care*. 2002;25(7):1123–1128.
19. Garvey WT, Ryan DH, Bohannon NJ, et al. Weight loss therapy in type 2 diabetes: Effects of phentermine and topiramate extended release. *Diabetes Care*. 2014;37(12):3309–3316.
20. O'Neil PM, Smith SR, Weissman NJ, et al. Randomized placebo-controlled clinical trial of lorcaserin for weight loss in type 2 diabetes mellitus: The BLOOM-DM study. *Obesity (Silver Spring)*. 2012;20(7):1426–1436.
21. Hollander P, Gupta AK, Plodkowski R, et al. CORDiabetes Study Group. Effects of naltrexone sustained release/bupropion sustained-release combination therapy on body weight and glycemic parameters in overweight and obese patients with type 2 diabetes. *Diabetes Care*. 2013;36(12):4022–4029.
22. Davies MJ, Bergenstal R, Bode B, et al. NN8022-1922 Study Group. Efficacy of liraglutide for weight loss among patients with type 2 diabetes: The SCALE diabetes randomized clinical trial. *JAMA*. 2015;314(7):687–699.
23. Velazquez A, Apovian CM. Pharmacological management of obesity. *Minerva Endocrinol*. 2017. doi:10.23736/S0391-1977.17.02654-2.
24. US Preventive Services Task Force. Screening for obesity in adults: Recommendations and rationale. *Ann Intern Med*. 2003;139(11):930–932.
25. Apovian CM, Aronne LJ, Bessesen DH, et al.; Endocrine Society. Pharmacological management of obesity: An endocrine Society clinical practice guideline. *J Clin Endocrinol Metab*. 2015;100(2):342–362.
26. Wadden TA, Berkowitz RI, Sarwer DB, Prus- Wisniewski R, Steinberg C. Benefits of lifestyle modification in the pharmacologic treatment of obesity: A randomized trial. *Arch Intern Med*. 2001;161(2):218–227.
27. Khera R, Murad MH, Chandar AK, Dulai PS, Wang Z, Prokop LJ, Loomba R, Camilleri M, Singh S. Association of pharmacological treatments for obesity with weight loss and adverse events. A systematic review and meta-analysis. *JAMA*. 2016;315(22):2424–2434. doi:10.1001/jama.2016.7602.
28. Greenway FL, Fujioka K, Plodkowski RA, et al.; COR-I Study Group. Effect of naltrexone plus bupropion on weight loss in overweight and obese adults (COR-I): A multicentre, randomised, double-blind, placebo-controlled, phase 3 trial. *Lancet*. 2010;376(9741):595–605.
29. Pi-Sunyer X, Astrup A, Fujioka K, et al.; SCALE Obesity and Prediabetes NN8022-1839 Study Group. A randomized, controlled trial of 3.0 mg of liraglutide in weight management. *N Engl J Med*. 2015;373(1):11–22.
30. Gadde KM, Allison DB, Ryan DH, et al. Effects of low-dose, controlled-release, phentermine plus topiramate combination on weight and associated comorbidities in overweight and obese adults (CONQUER): A randomised, placebo-controlled, phase 3 trial. *Lancet*. 2011;377(9774):1341–1352.
31. Fidler MC, Sanchez M, Raether B, et al. A one-year randomized trial of lorcaserin for weight loss in obese and overweight adults: The BLOSSOM trial. *J Clin Endocrinol Metab*. 2011;96(10):3067–3077.
32. Hauptman J, Lucas C, Boldrin MN, Collins H, Segal KR. Orlistat in the long-term treatment of obesity in primary care settings. *Arch Fam Med*. 2000;9(2):160–167.

33. McGovern L, Johnson JN, Paulo R, Hettinger A, Singhal V, Kamath C, Erwin PJ, Montori VM. Treatment of pediatric obesity: A systematic review and meta-analysis of randomized trials. *J Clin Endocrinol Metab.* 2008;93(12):4600–4605.

34. Hendricks EJ, Rothman RB. RE: Pulmonary hypertension associated with use of phentermine? *Yonsei Med J.* 2011;52(5):869–870.

35. Billes SK, Sinnayah P, Cowley MA. Naltrexone/bupropion for obesity: An investigational combination pharmacotherapy for weight loss. *Pharmacol Res.* 2014;84:1–11.

36. Cone RD. Studies on the physiological functions of the melanocortin system. *Endocr Rev.* 2006;27(7):736–749.

37. Liotta AS, Advis JP, Krause JE, et al. Demonstration of *in vivo* synthesis of pro-opiomelanocortin-, beta-endorphin-, and alpha-melanotropin-like species in the adult rat brain. *J Neurosci.* 1984;4(4):956–965.

38. Brady LS, Smith MA, Gold PW, Herkenham M. Altered expression of hypothalamic neuropeptide mRNAs in food-restricted and food-deprived rats. *Neuroendocrinology.* 1990;52(5):441–447.

39. Fan W, Voss-Andreae A, Cao W-H, Morrison SF. Regulation of thermogenesis by the central melano-cortin system. *Peptides.* 2005;26(10):1800–1813.

40. Pennock RL, Hentges ST. Differential expression and sensitivity of presynaptic and postsynaptic opioid receptors regulating hypothalamic proopiomelanocortin neurons. *J Neurosci.* 2011;31(1):281–288.

41. Greenway FL, Whitehouse MJ, Guttadauria M, et al. Rational design of a combination medication for the treatment of obesity. *Obesity (Silver Spring).* 2009;17(1):30–39.

42. Contrave (naltrexone HCl/bupropion HCl) prescribing information. Deerfield, IL: Takeda Pharmaceuticals America; 2014.

43. Billes SK, Greenway FL. Combination therapy with naltrexone and bupropion for obesity. *Expert Opin Pharmacother.* 2011;12(11):1813–1826.

44. Sherman MM, Ungureanu S, Rey JA. Naltrexone/Bupropion ER (Contrave): Newly approved treatment option for chronic weight management in obese adults. *Pharm Ther.* 2016;41(3):164–172.

45. Monami M, Dicembrini I, Marchionni N, Rotella CM, Mannucci E. Effects of glucagon-like peptide-1 receptor agonists on body weight: A meta-analysis. *Exp Diabetes Res.* 2012;2012:672658.

46. Mehta A, Marso SP, Neeland IJ. Liraglutide for weight management: A critical review of the evidence. *Obes Sci Pract.* 2017;3(1):3–14.

47. Van Can J, Sloth B, Jensen CB, Flint A, Blaak EE, Saris WHM. Effects of the once-daily GLP-1 analog liraglutide on gastric emptying, glycemic parameters, appetite and energy metabolism in obese, non-diabetic adults. *Int J Obes (2005).* 2014;38(6):784–793.

48. Holst JJ, Deacon CF. Glucagon-like peptide-1 mediates the therapeutic actions of DPP-IV inhibitors. *Diabetologia.* 2005;48(4):612–615.

49. Orskov C, Wettergren A, Holst JJ. Secretion of the incretin hormones glucagon-like peptide-1 and gastric inhibitory polypeptide correlates with insulin secretion in normal man throughout the day. *Scand J Gastroenterol.* 1996;31(7):665–670.

50. Wettergren A, Schjoldager B, Mortensen PE, Myhre J, Christiansen J, Holst JJ. Truncated GLP-1 (proglucagon 78–107-amide) inhibits gastric and pancreatic functions in man. *Dig Dis Sci.* 1993;38(4):665–673.

51. Ladenheim EE. Liraglutide and obesity: A review of the data so far. *Drug Des Devel Ther.* 2015;9:1867–1875.

52. Saxenda [package insert]. Novo Nordisk: Plainsboro, NJ, 2015.

53. Davies MJ, Bain SC, Atkin SL, et al. Efficacy and safety of liraglutide versus placebo as add-on to glucose-lowering therapy in patients with type 2 diabetes and moderate renal impairment (LIRA-RENAL): A randomized clinical trial. *Diabetes Care.* 2016;39:222–230.

54. Robinson LE, Holt TA, Rees K, Randeva HS, O'Hare JP. Effects of exenatide and liraglutide on heart rate, blood pressure and body weight: Systematic review and meta-analysis. *BMJ Open.* 2013;3. doi:10.1136/bmjopen-2012-001986.

55. FDA Center for Drug Evaluation and Research Belviq NDA 022529 drug label, June 27, 2012.

56. Gustafson A, King C, Rey JA. Lorcaserin (Belviq): A selective serotonin 5-HT$_{2C}$ agonist in the treatment of obesity. *Pharm Ther.* 2013;38(9):525–534.

57. Smith SR, Weisserman NJ, Anderson CM, et al. Multicenter, placebo-controlled trial of lorcaserin for weight management. *N Engl J Med.* 2010;363:245–256.

58. Smith BM, Smith JM, Tsai JH, et al. Discovery and structure–activity relationship of (1*r*)-8-chloro-2,3,4,5-tetrahydro-1-methyl-1*h*-3-benzazepine (lorcaserin), a selective serotonin 5-HT$_{2C}$ receptor agonist for the treatment of obesity. *J Med Chem.* 2008;51:305–313.

59. Geyer MA, Vollenweider FX. Serotonin research: Contributions to understanding psychosis. *Trends Pharmacol Sci.* 2008;29:445–453.

60. Bakris G, Calhoun D, Egan B, Hellmann C, Dolker M, Kingma I. Orlistat improves blood pressure control in obese subjects with treated but inadequately controlled hypertension. *J Hypertens.* 2002;20(11):2257–2267.
61. Zavoral JH. Treatment with orlistat reduces cardiovascular risk in obese patients. *J Hypertens.* 1998;16(12 pt 2):2013–2017.
62. Derosa G, Maffioli P, Salvadeo SA, et al. Comparison of orlistat treatment and placebo in obese type 2 diabetic patients. *Expert Opin Pharmacother.* 2010;11(12):1971–1982.

8 The Role of Gut Microbiota in the Pathogenesis and Treatment of Obesity

Stephen J. Walker and Puja B. Patel

CONTENTS

8.1 INTRODUCTION

Obesity is a condition, influenced by a number of factors, that results in an excessive accumulation of adipose tissue [1]. It has become more prevalent both in developing and industrialized countries, currently thought to impact more than 500 million people worldwide [2]. Obesity occurs when caloric intake exceeds expenditure, resulting in a net gain in body fat [2,3]. It can emerge from interactions among genes and environmental elements, such as diet, food components, and/or lifestyle [2]. Obesity is associated with the onset of a number of other diseases, including cancer, diabetes, nonalcoholic fatty liver disease, cardiovascular disease, and some immune-related disorders [2].

Research has begun to focus on the association between gut microbiota and obesity. The gut flora of humans is comprised of trillions of bacterial microbes that inhabit the gastrointestinal tract [2,3]. Researchers have found that, by controlling the gut microbiota and its metabolic pathways, they may be able to impact the metabolism and adiposity of the host [1]. Research also suggests that, along with the gut microbiota, the bacterial genome is responsible for the regulation of energy, storage of fat, and attainment of nutrients [2]. A growing body of evidence suggests that even from the beginning phases of life, modifying the gut flora can influence the microbiota's ability to manage host energy metabolism, as well as the host's capability to gain and lose weight; this, in turn, can lead to the development of obesity and other associated metabolic conditions [2,3]. The microbiota begins to colonize during pregnancy as it is transmitted from the mother to the fetus. This transmission is regulated by multiple factors, including diet, length of pregnancy, antibiotic exposure, and method of delivery (natural birth versus cesarean section). During the first 3 years of life, one's diet and surroundings play a crucial role in microbiota colonization; this time allows for proper development of the immune system and neurological systems [4].

The human body has a symbiotic relationship with the gut microbiota, which is able to complete vital functions that the human body cannot (Figure 8.1). This makes the gut microbiota crucial in its role of preserving routine immune and gastrointestinal function, as well as allowing effective nutrient digestion [2]. Gut microbiota interacts with host physiology for many beneficial roles, including synthesis of vitamins and nutrients, defense against pathogens (enteric), metabolism of carcinogens, conversion of cholesterol and bile acids, immune system modulation, intestinal function regulation, host metabolism, blood vessel formation (intestinal angiogenesis), development of enterocytes, and improvement of nutrient digestibility via fermentation of indigestible nutrients [2,4–6].

The natural gut microbiota of humans is composed of multiple microbes, including viruses, fungi, archaea, protozoans, and bacteria, which make up the dominant portion [4]. The most plentiful phyla members in the gut microbiota are Firmicutes and Bacteroidetes, which comprise approximately 90% of bacterial species found in the gut; the least plentiful are Actinobacteria, Verrucomicrobia, and Proteobacteria [1,4]. Research has shown that in both animal and human models, the diversity

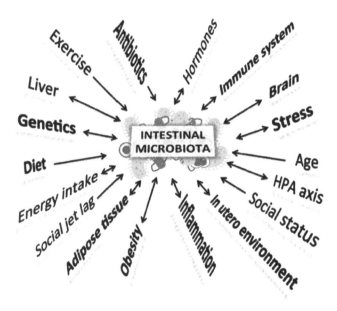

FIGURE 8.1 Environmental factors and the bidirectional interaction with host organ systems shape the intestinal microbiome. Studies over the past decade have revealed that many environmental factors, including diet, antibiotic exposure, energy intake (EI), and exercise, can dramatically influence the intestinal microbiome (both membership and functional capacity). In addition to environment, further research has revealed a bidirectional interaction between host organ systems and the intestinal microbiome in shaping host metabolic outcomes. HPA, hypothalamic-pituitary-adrenal. (Reprinted from *Cell Host Microbe*, 22, Maruvada, P. et al., The human microbiome and obesity: Moving beyond associations, 589–599, Copyright 2010, with permission from Elsevier.)

in the arrangement of gut microbiota can be correlated to obesity. For example, a common finding in most studies is that an increase in Firmicutes, paired with a decrease in Bacteroidetes, leads to an "obesogenic microbiota" [1]. Additional factors that contribute to the development of obesity include genetics and epigenetics, as these factors have also been shown to alter an individual's gut microbiota. These confounding variables can be investigated in twin studies. For example, in a twin study in which participants were discordant for body mass index (BMI), researchers found higher levels of Actinobacteria and lower levels of Bacteroidetes in obese participants versus lean [1].

8.2 MECHANISMS UNDERLYING GUT MICROBIOTA INDUCED OBESITY

Figure 8.1 is an illustration of the various factors, including diet, energy intake, exercise, and antibiotic use that interact with an individual's intestinal microbiome to control body weight.

8.2.1 INFLUENCE OF ANTIBIOTICS ON OBESITY

Antibiotic overuse and overexposure, as contributing factors to the development of obesity, are an important area of study right now. Farmers are using low doses of antibiotics to increase the weight of their livestock, and researchers believe that passive or active vulnerability to these antibiotics may be a key factor in the recent increase in the rate of obesity. Research in human infants and mice has indicated that premature antibiotic use may lead to eventual progression of obesity and adiposity [1]. Medically, antibiotics are used to treat infections by preventing unwanted bacterial colonization in the body. However, as most do not target specific species of bacteria and instead have broad-spectrum activity, even a brief exposure to antibiotics can affect the gut microbiota for years to come [7,8].

Gut microbiota is believed to play an important role in obesity, and research has suggested that controlling the gut bacterial environment may impact the trajectory towards obesity. Evidence has shown that gut microbiota can be altered through antibiotic exposure, and while one can quickly recuperate following a brief period of antibiotic exposure, frequent use can lead to adverse and long-lasting outcomes. For the past 60 years, antibiotics have been administered to encourage growth and weight gain in farm animals and livestock, after it was shown that antibiotics given in low dosages to chicks led to growth. Research in germ-free chickens found that antibiotics were not responsible for growth; instead, it is the alteration of the microbiota that causes the promotion of growth effect. However, recent research in mice has shown that the weight gain due to antibiotics is only seen when subjects are exposed to antibiotics early in life. Mice that, at birth, were given small-dose penicillin had greater body mass than those mice that were given antibiotics at weaning. Studying the mice a few weeks after antibiotic exposure showed that the effects were still seen, demonstrating that even temporary disturbances at the beginning of life may lead to lasting effects. Germ-free mice were transplanted with microbiota from mice with penicillin exposure, and these mice gained more weight than mice that were transplanted with the microbiota of the control mice. This evidence demonstrates that the transferred microbiota is itself capable of promoting obesity [2].

The ability of antibiotics to influence the development of obesity is dependent on the amount of antibiotic administered. Higher dosages of antibiotics given to mice have been shown to lead to a decrease in body fat, weight, and resistance to insulin, which is most likely due to the fact that higher dosages decrease the presence of bacteria and the ability of gut microbiota to extract calories from diet [2]. Until recently, there were very few published human studies that looked specifically at the long-term effects of antibiotic exposure, so the significance of these studies was not fully appreciated until a clearer association between obesity and gut microbiota had been demonstrated. Because of the paucity of available data, researchers in many countries initiated studies to assess the effect of antibiotic exposure in infancy on the development of obesity, and they have found evidence to suggest that antibiotic treatment in early stages of life correlates to a larger BMI. This implies that extensive antibiotic exposure/use within the past few decades may be an important contributing factor to the increase obesity rates seen in Western countries [2].

Antibiotics can alter the structure and, in turn, the role of the gut microbiota. For example, in a study in which vancomycin was intravenously administered for 6 weeks as treatment for infective endocarditis, patients experienced weight gain; the authors concluded that this was most likely due to a shift of the microbiota towards *Lactobacillus* species, as *Lactobacilli* have an intrinsic resistance to vancomycin [7,8]. In another study, in which obese males were given a 7-day oral treatment of vancomycin, there was a decrease in the quantity of gram-positive bacteria (especially the Firmicutes), accompanied by a worsened peripheral insulin resistance. However, amoxicillin (a β-lactam antibiotic) administration, typically used to target gram-negative bacteria, had no impact on Firmicutes or insulin sensitivity. This evidence shows the importance of the role of Firmicutes in the gut and how it arbitrates insulin resistance caused by obesity [9,10].

A study by Cho et al. showed a significant increase in adiposity in 10-week-old mice that had been given multiple antibiotics at "subtherapeutic doses" starting at 4 weeks of age. There was also an elevated ratio of Firmicutes to Bacteroidetes, with enhanced presence of genes that are responsible for converting carbohydrates into short-chain fatty acids (SCFAs). There was also an increase in gut hormone levels that may control "energy metabolism and growth" [11]. Similarly, in human studies, when infants (up to 6 months old) were exposed to antibiotics, by 38 months they also showed extreme adiposity, which was measured by increasing BMI scores. This suggests that antibiotics may put children at an increased risk for obesity. The particular impact of antibiotic exposure in and after early infancy may be associated with changes in gut microbiota related to the weaning process, which occurs at around 6 months in humans [10]. Antibiotics can negatively impact the infant gut microbiota by lowering levels of obligate anaerobes. By diminishing the bacterial variety in an infant's intestinal flora, the infant is at more risk for asthma, allergic sensitization, allergic rhinitis, and peripheral blood eosinophilia [7]. Fouhy and colleagues conducted a study of infant gut flora after exposure to gentamicin and ampicillin, and found that the gut microbiota changed, with an increase in Proteobacteria and a decrease in Actinobacteria and *Lactobacillus*, when compared to untreated infants. They noted that, after 8 weeks, a return to pre-antibiotic levels of the bacteria was still not complete, indicating that the development of the infant gut microbiota can be significantly influenced by even the early periods of antibiotic exposure [12].

8.2.2 INCREASED ENERGY HARVESTING BY GUT MICROBIOTA

Obesity can be defined as the excessive storage of energy as adipose tissue, due to disparity between energy intake and expenditure [1]. It has been suggested that obese individuals, when compared to lean individuals, have a gut microbiota that is more effective at extricating energy from their food consumption. This suggestion has been supported by multiple studies that show that germ-free mice gained body fat and mass after receiving gut microbiota from obese mice. This observed weight gain can be explained by several gut bacteria–related mechanisms, including the microbial fermentation of indigestible dietary polysaccharides into absorbable monosaccharides and the generation of SCFAs that are converted to more complex lipids in the liver [1].

Multiple studies have shown that, when compared to their lean littermates, diet-induced obese mice and genetically obese mice have a decrease of Bacteroidetes, accompanied by an elevation in Firmicutes levels. The phyla Firmicutes is responsible for the production of the SCFA butyrate. When dietary carbohydrates, proteins, and peptides undergo bacterial fermentation in the colon, they create SCFAs. Along with production of SCFAs like acetate, butyrate, and propionate, there are also products of heat and gases such as CO_2, CH_4, and H_2 as a result of the fermentation reaction. Saccharolytic bacteria located mostly in the proximal colon are responsible for fermenting carbohydrates and creating SCFAs, H_2, and CO_2. Proteolytic bacteria are responsible for fermenting amino acids and proteins and creating SCFAS, H_2, CO_2, CH_4, amines, and phenols, all of which affect the rate of cholesterol creation [1]. Butyrate is used primarily as an energy source for colonic epithelial cells, propionate is used for gluconeogenesis, and acetate is used for hepatic lipogenesis [1–3,8,13]. SCFAs also modulate gene expression and commonly bind to G-protein–coupled receptors (GPRs), such as GPR41 (FFAR3) and GPR43 (FFAR2) [2–4,8,10,13]. These receptors are present in adipocytes, endocrine cells, and epithelial cells. GPR43 is commonly stimulated by acetate and GPR41 by butyrate, and both are activated by propionate [2].

Activation of GPR41 in enteroendocrine cells causes the release of the gut hormone peptide YY (PYY), which stimulates satiety and decreases food consumption [10]. When GPR41 was not activated, researchers observed diminished levels of PYY, reduced hepatic lipogenesis, and decreased uptake of energy via diet. Mice who were GPR43-deficient had a lower body mass and diminished insulin resistance; GPR43 inhibition correlated with higher food consumption, increased body temperature, and more energy utilization [13]. Binding to GPR43 suppresses adipogenesis and also causes higher expression of GLP-1, which enhances insulin secretion [3,10]. GLP-1 also impacts L-cells, adipose tissue, and leptin [2,3]. When GPR41 is expressed in adipose tissue, it stimulates leptin release [10].

A recent study used mice to investigate the association between energy metabolism and microbiota that may cause obesity. The study concluded that gut microbiota in animals with obesity were more likely to harvest energy and that this was due to a leptin deficiency. Leptin, produced by adipocytes, is a hormone responsible for inhibiting hunger. Mice with altered leptin genes consumed greater amounts of food, and when the microbiota from these mice were transplanted into germ-free mice, the recipient mice experienced an increase in body mass [3].

In a human study investigating the impact of gut microbial metabolites, obese patients were given propionate, which increased PYY levels and stimulated GLP-1 release, and were found to have a decreased weight gain and adiposity [10]. GPR43 may stimulate fat storage, as researchers discovered GPR43$^{-/-}$ mice were able to resist obesity caused by diet. In another study, germ-free GPR41$^{-/-}$ mice that were transplanted with a microbiota gained less body mass than wild-type littermates. The researchers believe that, due to the lack of GPR41 signaling, PYY levels in the blood were low, causing greater gut motility and reduced energy harvest via diet. GPR41 and GPR43 may regulate host energy expenditure via gut flora–dependent effects [2].

Jumpertz and colleagues conducted a study to investigate the association between energy harvest and gut flora in humans. For 3 days, 12 obese and nine lean males were randomly placed on 2,400 or 3,400 kcal per day diets. Each individual then had a 3-day washout period in which he consumed weight maintenance diets. Using pyrosequencing, the researchers determined the bacterial composition of participants' feces and, using bomb calorimetry, calculated the consumed and stool calories. Due to the differences in calorie intake, researchers saw a quick association to modifications in the bacterial species of the gut flora. With either the 2,400 or 3,400 kcal per day diet, evidence showed an increase in quantities of Firmicutes and a decrease in Bacteroidetes. In the lean participants, researchers saw a negative correlation with proportional alterations in Firmicutes and positive correlation for proportional alterations in Bacteroidetes. At the end of the study, researchers concluded there was a likely effect of gut microbiota on energy harvest, as they observed a 20% decrease in Bacteroidetes and 20% increase in Firmicutes with a 150-kcal host energy harvest [14].

8.2.3 Changes in Metabolic Pathways

8.2.3.1 Changes in Carbohydrate, Lipid, and Amino Metabolism

The gut microbiome has been associated with changes in both carbohydrate and lipid metabolism. In a study in which germ-free mice received the microbiota from normal mice, the recipient mice showed a 60% increase in body fat and also insulin resistance. The study authors attributed these results to an increase in bioavailability of monosaccharides and the subsequent induction of de novo hepatic lipogenesis [1]. The livers of conventionalized (i.e., those that receive a microbiota transplant from normal mice) animals display elevated levels of triglyceride due to de novo fatty acid synthesis. Hypertrophy and triglyceride accumulation in the adipocytes were linked to suppression of fasting-induced adipocyte factor (Fiaf), a circulating lipoprotein lipase inhibitor (LPL), by the conventionalized microbiota resulting in fat storage in white adipose tissue [1].

Choline, obtained from food such as eggs and red meat, is important for lipid metabolism and is considered a crucial part of cell membranes. Research in both animals and humans has shown that the microbial activity of dietary choline can modify the arrangement of gut microbiota, which can then influence the occurrence of obesity. The metabolism of dietary choline into trimethylamine-N-oxide (TMAO) is linked to cardiovascular disease and atherosclerosis, which suggests a possible correlation between consumption of dietary choline and gut microbiota and a heightened possibility of obesity and metabolic disease [1].

Likewise, essential amino acid metabolic pathways are also linked with insulin resistance and obesity. The genes that function in these specific metabolic pathways were elevated in germ-free mice that received the gut microbiome from their obese twin, versus germ-free mice who received the microbiome of their lean twin. Essential amino acid pathways including lysine, phenylalanine, leucine, isoleucine, and valine, as well as nonessential amino acid pathways including tyrosine, arginine, and cysteine were impacted. However, when compared to the microbiome of obese-twin donors, the transferred lean-twin gut microbiomes were abundant in genes associated with decomposition and fermentation of diet polysaccharides [1].

8.2.3.2   Influence of Gut Microbiota on Plasma Lipids

Dyslipidemia refers to the presence of abnormal amounts of lipids in the blood and is known to correlate with obesity and metabolic syndrome. Dyslipidemia affects weight gain and metabolic disorders, and abundant research has shown that the gut microbiota exerts influence on lipid metabolism in the host. As early as the 1960s, Wostmann and colleagues suggested that, although germ-free animals more readily absorb dietary cholesterol than conventional control animals, they still present with lower levels of plasma cholesterol [15]. This topic was studied again recently, and researchers discovered that in a comparison of germ-free and conventional mice fed a high-fat diet (HFD), the germ-free mice displayed increased fecal lipid excretion and reduced plasma free fatty acid and liver triglyceride levels [2,16]. A disrupted cholesterol metabolism may be associated with the loss of cholesterol transformation by intestinal bacteria.

In the 1930s, researchers discovered the transformation of cholesterol to saturated product coprostanol via microorganisms in the intestine. Coprostanol is not easily absorbed by the human intestine; a converse association has been seen between serum cholesterol levels and the coprostanol-to-cholesterol ratio in human feces [2]. The transformation of cholesterol to coprostanol by the gut microbiota may cause a decline in cholesterol uptake, which causes cholesterolemia. In addition to cholesterol, when conventional and germ-free mice were compared, it was shown that the gut microbiota altered many lipid species in the liver, adipose tissue, and serum, with the highest impact on the phosphatidylcholine and triglyceride species. Phosphatidylcholine is significant when considering the function of gut microbiota in cardiovascular diseases; gut microbiota are responsible for the conversion of phosphatidylcholine and dietary choline to trimethylamine (TMA); then the absorbed TMA is metabolized to TMAO, a proatherosclerotic metabolite, by hepatic flavin monooxygenases [2]. Gut microbiota may also participate in bile acid metabolism that may help control serum lipids. Bile acids are considered exceptionally efficient detergents that stimulate solubilization and uptake of dietary lipids in the intestine [2]. Bile acids are able to forego enterohepatic circulation and instead go through bacterial metabolism in the large intestine, a process that accounts for the presence of more than 20 varying secondary bile acids in human feces [2]. When the enzyme bile salt hydrolase (BSH) decouples bile acids, it causes a modification to cholesterol levels in the blood. The deconjugation of bile acids allows glycine and taurine to separate from the steroid moiety of the molecule, which is responsible for the creation of free bile acids that are not readily absorbed like conjugated bile acids [2]. This leads to the excretion of these deconjugated acids in the feces. Cholesterol is then fragmented to compensate for processed bile acids, which leads to diminishing levels of serum cholesterol [2].

8.2.4 INDUCTION OF LOW-GRADE INFLAMMATION

Obesity is correlated to low-grade inflammation, which has been shown to be involved in the progression of insulin resistance and metabolic syndrome. Although the reason for this inflammation is unclear, many researchers propose that the abundance of lipopolysaccharide (LPS) in the blood, which comes from the cell membrane of gram-negative bacteria, may be responsible [2,7,13,17]. This hypothesis is supported by the following evidence: (1) LPS attaches to the CD14–toll-like receptor 4 (TLR4) complex on the immune cell surface and stimulates the release of proinflammatory cytokines [1,2,13,18]; (2) lysis of gram-negative bacteria causes the continual creation of LPS, which is transported to intestinal capillaries via a TLR4 mechanism [2]; and (3) LPS travels from the intestine via a chylomicron mechanism, which is created from epithelial cells due to high fat consumption [2,18].

In a study in which mice were fed a high-fat diet (HFD) for 2–4 weeks, Cani et al. observed elevated levels of LPS and coined the term *metabolic endotoxemia*, which they described as an increase in circulating LPS levels [2,7,18,19]. They also conducted a study in which they constantly infused mice with LPS and discovered that the mice exhibited symptoms similar to a HFD phenotype, such as steatosis, hyperglycemia, weight gain, insulin resistance, and adipose tissue macrophage invasion. When they took CD-14 (an LPS receptor) knockout mice and gave them either an LPS infusion or HFD, the mice were protected from any metabolic disease that could be caused by LPS infusion or high fat consumption [19]. These results were supported by other animal studies that found TLR4-deficient mice were protected from diet-induced obesity. Consequently, researchers proposed that germ-free mice could also be protected from diet-induced obesity because they have no LPS present in their gut. As a follow-up on their research to examine how much gut microbiota influences metabolic disorders, they conducted a study in which they administered antibiotics to the intestines of genetically obese mice or HFD mice. They found that the gut flora composition changed due to the antibiotics; however, the metabolic endotoxemia was crippled. They also found that gut permeability was elevated due to HFD consumption, as well as decreased levels of *Bifidobacteria*, *Clostridium coccoides*, and *Bacteroides* [2].

Bifidobacteria has been shown to improve gut functionality and diminish LPS levels in mice. The researchers wished to determine whether metabolic conditions seen as a result of HFDs are associated with a reduction in *Bifidobacteria*. To do this, they utilized prebiotic dietary fibers, in high-fat-fed mice, which elevated the levels of *Bifidobacteria* in the gut. As previous research had indicated, mice that consumed an HFD exhibited greater endotoxemia, but the administration of prebiotics eradicated the endotoxemia completely. Additionally, in mice that received the prebiotics, *Bifidobacteria* was negatively associated with body mass gain and endotoxemia, but was positively associated with an improved glucose tolerance [2,18]. Prebiotic administration also improved (i.e., decreased) the gut permeability of the mice, likely due to heightened expression of tight junction mRNA and a better circulation of proteins. The improved functionality of the gut barrier was associated with a decrease in blood LPS levels and low-grade inflammatory tone (i.e., decreases in hepatic and circulating cytokines) [18]. They also found that utilizing prebiotics to decrease systemic inflammation was coincident with reduction of inflammation and oxidative stresses in liver tissue [18].

8.2.4.1 Role of Dietary Fat and Microbiota

Inflammation in an individual that is presumed to be caused by bacteria and related to obesity and type 2 diabetes is speculated to arise from two factors related to high-protein diets: increased LPS concentration and increased permeability of the intestinal barrier [5]. LPS, large molecules consisting of a lipid and a polysaccharide, are located in the outer membrane of gram-negative bacteria and are capable of causing inflammatory responses such that researchers believe they may be responsible for the inflammation correlated with obesity and type 2 diabetes. In humans and mice, higher LPS levels are related to a greater intake of HFDs. HFDs are also responsible for directly stimulating an inflammatory feedback by saturated fat, which then decreases the integrity of the intestinal barrier; this heightened intestinal permeability brought on by HFDs may be due to reduced stability of gut epithelial tight-junction proteins. In mice, researchers saw decreased expression of genes encoding zona-occludens-1 and -occluding, which are tight junction proteins, in animals that were subjected to HFDs [5]. Everard and colleagues discovered that a plethora of *Akkermansia muciniphila*, a mucus-deteriorating bacteria, is directly associated with the density of the mucus layer; when obese mice were given these bacteria, metabolic conditions caused by HFDs were reversed [20].

8.3   DIETARY FAT AND HIGH-FAT DIETS

Diet is a critically important factor capable of shaping and defining the gut microbiota. The gut microbiota of healthy adults is considerably balanced; however, research has shown that short-term adjustments in diet can quickly impact microbiota composition and can manifest within 1–4 days of a diet change, and while these short-term changes can usually be reversed, longer dietary changes may cause a lasting effect [5,8]. HFDs correlate with elevated levels of Erysipelotrichia, within the phyla Firmicutes, especially *Clostridium ramosum*. Research has shown that the presence of *Clostridium ramosum* can cause diet-induced obesity in germ-free mice; it is also responsible for heightened expression of glucose transporter 2 (Glut2) and fatty acid translocase (CD36); both are responsible for an increased absorption of carbohydrates and fat [1]. In animal models of research, when there is a diet change, there is a modification to levels of intestinal bacteria, namely Bacteroidetes and Firmicutes. When mice were fed HFDs, there was an increase in the amount of Firmicutes and decrease in the amount of Bacteroidetes [8].

8.3.1   EFFECTS OF HIGH-FAT DIET ON MICROBIOTA COMPOSITION

Research in animal studies has shown that HFDs result in significant modifications in specific taxonomic groups of the gut microbiota compared to control diets. However, there have not been many controlled human interventional studies that explore how gut microbiota composition is impacted by HFDs [5]. Wu et al. investigated changes in gut microbiota in 10 individuals who were given either a low-fiber/HFD or high-fiber/low-fat diet. They discovered that differences between individuals in microbiota layout possibly disguised differences due to short-term diet alterations. For the duration of the 10-day study, each participant was designated with an enterotype identity, distinguished by levels of specific bacterial genera, such as *Bacteroides* and *Prevotella*. These enterotype identities stayed constant, regardless of quick changes in gut microbiota, in 1 day of dietary interference [21]. Duncan et al. conducted a human study in which they observed how gut microbiota was affected when going from a weight maintenance diet to a high-fat/protein, low-carbohydrate diet (HPLC diet). The researchers observed a decrease in bacteria that ferment fiber, such as *Eubacterium rectale*, *Roseburia* spp., and *Bifidobacterium* [22]. The type of fat (saturated, monosaturated, or polyunsaturated fatty acid) also seems to affect how each will influence gut microbiota. In one animal study, researchers discovered that gut microbiota diversity was diminished in mice that received a diet with high amounts of saturated fat; however, there was no microbial effect due to diets with high amounts of polyunsaturated fatty acids (PUFAs) [5]. De Filippo et al. conducted a study in which they compared gut flora of children from Burkina Faso who ate a high-fiber diet, to European children who ate a Western high-fat/high-sugar diet. The West African children had diminished levels of Firmicutes and elevated levels of Bacteroidetes, together with bacterial species such as *Prevotella* and *Xylanibacter* (which specialize in fiber breakdown). These last two species were not present in European children. European children had elevated levels of Firmicutes and Proteobacteria. When a similar study was conducted in animals given a high-fat, high-sugar, Western diet, researchers observed modifications to the gut flora. They saw a rise in Mollicutes, of the phyla Firmicutes, and restrained Bacteroidetes. When the flora of these Mollicutes-rich mice was transplanted into germ-free mice, researchers observed an increase in

TABLE 8.1

Summary of High-Fat Diet Effects on Gut Microbiota Studies

Dietary Intervention	Subjects	Effect on Microbiota	References
Habitual long-term diet	Healthy human	Protein and animal fat: ↑ *Bacteroides* Carbohydrates: ↑ *Prevotella*	[21]
Controlled HF/low-fiber and LF/high-fiber diets	Healthy human	Stable enterotype identity	[21]
HFD Normal chow diet	Male C57BL/6J mice	HFD: ↑ Firmicutes and Proteobacteria, ↓ Bacteroidetes Chow: addition of normal chow diet caused HFD-induced microbiota taxonomic shifts to revert back to similar compositions found in control normal chow diet	[24]
High-saturated-fat diet	Female C57BL/6J mice	↑ Firmicutes and ↓ Bacteroidetes. At species level, ↓ *Lactobacillus* and ↑ *Oscillibacter*	[25]
HFD not supplemented HFD with oleic acid–derived compound HFD with n-3 fatty acids (EPA and DHA)	Female outbred mice	↑ Firmicutes and order Enterobacteriales ↓ *Clostridium* cluster XIVa and Enterobacteriales ↑ *Bifidobacterium* and Bacteroidetes ↑ Firmicutes and the group *Lactobacillus*	[26]

Source: Adapted from Portune, K.J., et al., *Mol Nutr Food Res*, 61, 2017.

EPA, aicosapentaneoic acid; DHA, docosahexaenoic acid; HF, high fat; LF, low fat; HFD, high-fat diet.

adiposity compared to transplantation with microbiota of lean mice [23]. Other studies examining the effect of HFDs on gut microbiota are summarized in Table 8.1 [5].

8.3.2 MEDIATION BY BACTERIAL METABOLITES

High dietary fat consumption is associated with increased adiposity, chronic low-grade inflammation, insulin resistance, and increased bile acid production. This may lead to diseases such as obesity, metabolic syndrome, type 2 diabetes, and colon cancer [5]. There is little information on possible bioactive metabolites that are created via an indirect or direct impact of dietary fat on gut bacteria and how this may relate to obesity or other metabolic changes [5]. Haghikia and colleagues observed that long-chain fatty acids, commonly present in Western diets, are responsible for enhancing differentiation and proliferation of T helper 1 (Th1) and/or Th17 cells; they are also able to decrease gut SCFAs, a finding that suggests this pro-inflammatory environment could have an adverse outcome for obesity [27]. It was also found that, to see this effect of Th cells, gut microbiota must be present, which suggests that this impact on the immune cells may come from a bacterial-type compound [27].

Gut microbiota is involved in enhancing absorption of fatty acids and also promoting the arrangement of lipid droplets in the liver and intestinal epithelium of zebrafish, providing a possible mechanistic role of gut microbiota in host adiposity in animal models [5]. In this study, it was also shown that bacteria of the Firmicutes phyla, along with related metabolic outputs, were responsible for increasing the number of lipid droplets; however, another type of bacteria was responsible for change in size of lipid droplets. These findings suggest that fatty acid absorption is controlled by the mediation of multiple different microbial species [5]. Mice with HFD-induced obesity were given *Bacteroides uniformis* CECT 7771 bacterium and exhibited a decrease of fat absorption by enterocytes, which supports the idea that specific components of the human microbiota could interfere with dietary lipid absorption, although the mechanism or bacterial components mediating this effect were not investigated [5].

8.3.3 DIETARY FAT, MICROBIOTA, AND BILE ACIDS

High dietary fat intake has been shown to stimulate the discharge of primary bile acids in the small intestine. Primary bile acids are formed by combining with glycine or taurine in the liver; this enhances the process of bile acid uptake in the distal ileum, as well as their transfer back to the liver [5]. Bacteria can deconjugate and dehydroxylate primary bile acids in the distal ileum, which restricts uptake, allowing the bile acids to enter the colon, where the gut microbiota can metabolize them into secondary bile acids [28]. The bacterial processes could possibly alter the solubilization and uptake of dietary lipids within the small intestine, as well as raise the amount of bile excreted in feces. This activity then boosts the formation of extra bile acids from liver cholesterol, which adjusts cholesterol quantity by cooperation with enterohepatic farnesoid X receptors [5]. Bile acid bacterial activity could possibly impact the bile acid–induced activation of the G-protein–coupled membrane bile acid receptor (M-BAR) on enteroendocrine L cells, which leads to secretion of glucagon-like peptide 1 (GLP-1) secretion, an enteroendocrine peptide that regulates appetite, insulin sensitivity, and glucose metabolism [5].

Recent studies have shown that Firmicutes phyla bacteria participate in the metabolism of bile acids in humans. In rats, secondary bile acids have been shown to be responsible for cecal microbiota modifications, causing alterations that are almost identical to alterations caused by HFD to gut microbiota. Secondary bile acids, together with fatty acids, are believed to be involved in gastrointestinal cancers due to genotoxic and cytotoxic damage of cells [29].

8.4 EFFECT OF DIETARY FIBER ON MICROBIOTA

Digestion of carbohydrate is a complex process that utilizes multiple enzymes and is dependent on the particular carbohydrate being consumed. While most of the dietary carbohydrates that are digestible are absorbed by the small intestine, the nondigestible carbohydrates travel to the colon, where anaerobic bacteria are responsible for fermenting them. Most research examining the impact of particular nutrients on the gut microbiota target fiber because it is the favored source of carbon for the large intestine microbiota. Although many primary studies have looked at the impact of fiber on restricted bacterial groups, such as *Bifidobacterium* and *Lactobacillus*, newer studies have shown that some groups of Firmicutes, Bacteroidetes, and Actinobacteria are elevated when there is a larger intake of fiber, although effects differ according to the type of fiber being studied and the specific microbiota makeup [5].

Whole-grain (WG) cereals go through minimum processing after they are harvested; this is done to conserve the naturally occurring amount of germ, endosperm, and bran (which has the largest amount of fiber). Research involving human dietary interventions shows that consuming WG cereals causes a bifidogenic effect, coincident with elevated abundance of Firmicutes and Actinobacteria (see Table 8.2) [5]. Inulin is a combination of approximately 60 fructose monomers with a terminal glucosyl moiety that can be broken down to produce shorter-chain fructooligosaccharides (FOS) [5]. Galactooligosaccharides (GOS) are made of galactose chain units with variations in chain length and link types between the monomers. The architectural variety between FOS and GOS is responsible for their impact on gut microbiota composition. Inulin, FOS, and GOS are responsible for elevated quantities of *Faecalibacterium prausnitzii* in human feces (Table 8.2), whereas inulin and FOS have also been shown to increase the presences of *Bifidobacterium* and *Lactobacillus* (Table 8.2). In contrast, it has been observed that consumption of fructans and galactans may lead to a decrease in *Bacteroides*, *Prevotella*, and *F. prausnitzii*. Nondigestible starch or resistant starch (RS) avoids degradation at the proximal parts of the gastrointestinal tract and is able to continue to the distal regions of the large intestine, which is why it is believed to affect the gut microbiota.

TABLE 8.2

Summary of High-Fiber-Diet Effects on Gut Microbiota Studies

	Dietary Intervention	Subjects	Effect on Microbiota	References
WG	WG wheat	Healthy human	↑ *Bifidobacterium*, lactobacillus	[31]
	Maize-based WG	Healthy human	↑ *Bifidobacterium*	[32]
	WG barley	Healthy human	↑ *Blautia*; slight ↑ in *Roseburia*, *Bifidobacterium*, *Dialister*	[33]
FOS, inulin, and GOS	Inulin	Women with low iron levels	↑ *Bifidobacteria*	[34]
	Inulin + FOS	Women receiving radiotherapy	↑ *Lactobacillus* and *Bifidobacterium*	[35]
	Inulin + oligofructose	Obese women	↑ *Bifidobacterium* and *F. prausnitzii* ↓ *Bacteroides intestinalis*, *Bacteroides vulgatus* and *Propionibacterium*	[36]
	Jerusalem artichoke inulin	Healthy human	↑ *Bifidobacteria* ↓ *Bacteroides/Prevotella*, *C. histolyticum/C. lituseburense* and *C. coccoides/Eubacterium rectale*	[37]
	Chicory inulin		↑ *Bifidobacteria* ↓ *Bacteroides/Prevotella*, *C. histolyticum/C. lituseburense* and *C. coccoides/E.* rectale ↑ Enterobacteriaceae	
	GOS	Healthy human	↑ *Bifidobacteria*, ↑ Firmicutes (some individuals) ↓ *Bacteroides*	[38]
RS	RS (RS2) RS (RS4)	Healthy human	↑ *Ruminococcus bromii* and *E. rectale* ↑ Actinobacteria and Bacteroidetes ↓ Firmicutes	[39]
	RS (RS3)	Obese men	↑ *Ruminococcus bromii*, *E. rectale*, *Roseburia*, *Oscillibacter*	[30]

Source: Portune, K.J. et al., *Mol. Nutr. Food Res*, 61, 2017.
WG, whole grain; FOS, fructooligosaccharides; GOS, galactooligosaccharides; RS, resistant starch.

When humans are given an RS diet, *Ruminococcus bromii* comprises 17% of the fecal microbiota, and it is responsible for the degradation of type RS3 in the large intestine (Table 8.2) [30].

8.4.1 Effects of Dietary Fiber on Microbiota Metabolites and Host Physiology

Diets high in fiber have a favorable impact on health, indirectly by producing SCFAs through fermentation, and directly by controlling nutrient uptake, which impacts lipid and glucose metabolism. The most common SCFAs formed by gut microbiota after fiber consumption are butyrate, acetate, and propionate. They are commonly found in the large intestine, where 95% is taken in by colonocytes and utilized for energy with the following order of preference: butyrate > propionate > acetate. Most of the butyrate is used for energy by colonocytes, allowing propionate and acetate to move through the portal vein and to the liver; from there, acetate enters systemic circulation and travels to peripheral tissues. Acetate and propionate are often utilized as substrates for lipogenesis and gluconeogenesis;

acetate has also been utilized for the biosynthesis of cholesterol [5]. Propionate can also be used to inhibit the synthesis of cholesterol, diminish the quantity of hepatic triglycerides, and decrease food consumption by stimulating intracellular signaling molecules, which then discharge anorexigenic peptides [40]. Many studies have investigated the association between a decrease in the availability of SCFAs to colonocytes and a variety of gut immune disorders. There has been some indirect support for this in a study examining the feces of inflammatory bowel disease patients, in which a reduction in the abundance of gut microbiota butyrate producers was found [41]. Research has also shown that butyrate can elevate internal creation of glucagon-like peptide 2 (GLP-2). The presence of GLP-2 may improve the functionality of the mucosal barrier by stimulating villus elongation and crypt cell generation, and reducing apoptosis. Butyrate has also been shown to be crucial in regulating anti-inflammatory processes through the following mechanisms: stimulating regulatory T cells to suppress inflammatory responses in the large intestine, regulating the action of macrophages of the intestine to downregulate the generation of TLR4 receptor and proinflammatory cytokines, intervening in the differentiation and maturation of monocyte-derived dendritic cells, and promoting the creation of anti-inflammatory cytokine IL-10 via binding to GPR109A receptors on intestinal macrophages and dendritic cells [5]. In mice, propionate and butyrate have shown protective effects against obesity caused by diet, as well as insulin resistance. In mice, free fatty receptors such as FFAR3 (GPR41) and FFAR2 (GPR43) are known to control how cells respond to SCFAs; however, when SCFAs stimulate GLP-1, the effect seems to be independent of FFAR3 [40]. Thus, depending on cell type, SCFA signaling through these receptors will result in a variety of functions.

8.5 TREATMENT

8.5.1 PROBIOTICS

Probiotics are live microorganisms that, when administered in adequate amounts to allow colonization of the colon, confer a health benefit on the host [2,7,18,42]. The more prevalent groups are of the genera *Bifidobacterium* and *Lactobacillus* [7,8,42]. Administering probiotics to humans and mice results in variations in expression of microbiome-encoded enzymes associated with plant polysaccharide metabolism. Probiotic administration has also been shown to maintain the normal microbial community structure, inhibit the invasion of pathogens in the human gut by increasing the amount of mucus secretion, improve the mucosal integrity, and reduce gut permeability [7]. Probiotics comprised of *Bifidobacterium* were found to be beneficial in mice and rats that were on HFDs. This was due to a boost in gut barrier action, which leads to reduced bacterial translocation and endotoxemia, and improvement of inflammation, insulin sensitivity, fat accumulation, as well as cholesterol and triglyceride serum levels [2].

In animal models, probiotics comprised of *Lactobacillus* were shown to be efficient in decreasing body fat mass, as well as improving lipid panels and glucose homeostasis. The prospective systems for these results are conjugated linoleic acid production, bile salt hydrolase (BSH) activity, stimulation of fatty acid oxidation, or inhibition of lipoprotein lipase activity [2]. Multiple studies have shown that *Bifidobacteria* are capable of decreasing endotoxin levels in the intestine, as well as amending the gut barrier. Probiotics can affect the immune system of the gut and impact the gut epithelium and immune cells sensitivity to microbes in the gut lumen [7]. Another benefit of probiotics is their ability to decrease necrotizing enterocolitis in premature infants. They also help to inhibit infections in patients who have exposed immune systems.

Newer studies have proposed that, in obese human individuals, *Lactobacillus gasseri* may reduce body mass and stomach adiposity, which in turn would improve postprandial serum lipid responses [2]. A meta-analysis, which included 51 reports on farm animals, 17 randomized human clinical trials, and 14 experimental models, concluded that the effect probiotics comprised of *Lactobacillus* have on weight control is strain-dependent [2]. *L. acidophilus* use caused noteworthy body mass increase in both humans and animals, whereas *L. fermentum* and *L. ingluviei* had the same effect but only in animals. Conversely, *L. plantarum* was correlated with body mass decrease in animals, whereas *L. gasseri* produced the same effect in both obese humans and animals [43]. *L. casei* was given to diet-induced obese mice, and researchers saw both antidiabetic and anti-inflammatory effects [8].

A study conducted using diet-induced obese mice investigated the influence of human-originated bacterium, *L. rhamnosus* PL60. Diet-induced obese mice underwent 8 weeks of *L. rhamnosus* PL60 feeding and experienced a reduction in body mass and epididymal and perirenal white adipose tissue, all without decreased energy intake [7,44]. Another study on germ-free mice found that *L. paracasei* was responsible for a reduction in fat storage, as well as higher levels of Angptl4, a lipoprotein lipase inhibitor that regulates triglyceride accumulation in adipocytes [7].

In an in vivo study by Griffiths and colleagues, *Bifidobacteria* were shown to be capable of improving the function of the gut barrier. For 28 days, newborn Balb/c mice received *B. infantis* and *B. bifidum*, and the mice that were given probiotics had significantly decreased intestinal endotoxin levels compared to the mice that were given only the vehicle [44]. Yin and colleagues examined the impact that four different strains of *Bifidobacterium* extracted from healthy human feces had on rats with HFD-induced obesity. In contrast to HFD mice, one strain reduced body mass, one strain increased body mass, and the other two strains produced no noteworthy change on body mass. This provides additional support for the notion that the putative anti-obesity impact of *Bifidobacterium* is strain-specific [45]. However, interestingly, all four strains were able to lower serum and liver triglyceride levels and alleviate lipid deposition in the liver [8]. An et al. blended three strains of *Bifidobacterium* (*B. pseudocatenulatum* SPM 1204, *B. longum* SPM 1205, and *B. longum* SPM 1207), all extracted from the guts of healthy Korean participants, to evaluate the effects of the blended strains on obese, HFD rats. The rats were given an HFD augmented with the strain mixture for 7 weeks, which resulted in a decrease in body mass and fat build-up, and improvements in lipid profiles and glucose-insulin homeostasis [44].

Although there are not many human studies on this subject, the few available reports do advocate for the possibility of probiotic use to manage weight. Kadooka et al. conducted a randomized, double-blind, placebo-controlled intervention study with 43 obese human participants (BMI, 24.2–30.7 kg/m^2). For 12 weeks, participants drank 200 g per day of fermented milk with probiotic strain *L. gasseri* SBT2055 (LG2055) or fermented milk alone. Participants who got the probiotic experienced a significantly reduced abdominal visceral and subcutaneous fat area, body mass, and waist circumference [46]. In another study, for 4 weeks before their scheduled delivery date until 6 months postnatal, mothers continuously consumed the probiotic strain *L. rhamnosus* GG. In a 10-year follow-up, it was concluded that the continuous probiotic intake correlated with an aversion of extreme weight gain [44].

Ironically, probiotics can also improve growth and have been put to use in the animal farming industry because they have proven to encourage fattening of mice, poultry, and livestock. Due to this evidence, many researchers have proposed that by modifying the intestinal flora, probiotics could have a similar impact on humans. Researchers have shown that increased amounts of intestinal lactobacilli can heighten the risk of hyperglycemia and obesity in adults [7]. However, the impact of probiotics on body mass and obesity is said to be strain-specific. Experiments have shown that *L. ingluviei* and *L. acidophilus* correlate with a weight-gain effect, but *L. casei/paracasei*, *L. plantarum*, and *L. gasseri* correlate with an anti-obesity effect [7].

8.5.2 PREBIOTICS

Prebiotics are indigestible but fermentable polysaccharides that selectively stimulate the growth or activity of one or multiple gut microbes that are beneficial to their human hosts [2,7,8,42,44]. Prebiotics also stimulate the production of SCFAs and promote growth of good gut bacteria, such as *Lactobacillus* and *Bifidobacterium* [7,8,44]. The prebiotics that have been researched most are inulin and different forms of FOS and GOS, which, in animal models, are shown to alter the gut microbiota to encourage the growth of favorable bacteria such as *Bifidobacteria* and *Lactobacillus* [2,7]. By controlling the gut microbiota, one can see a decrease in body fat, mass, and adipocyte size. These decreases are moderated via dietary intervention (mostly decreasing food consumption and appetite) and decreasing storage of fatty acids. By mending the stability of the gut barrier, one can improve glucose tolerance and insulin sensitivity.

Prebiotics mediate a reduction of a diet-induced inflammatory state. HFDs are known to increase the levels of LPS in gut microbiota, as well as downregulate levels of *Bifidobacteria*. Because of this, the body enters an inflammatory state also known as *metabolic endotoxemia*, which is followed by weight gain and insulin resistance. However, prebiotics, which consist of oligofructose (OFS), promote the growth of *Bifidobacteria*, which can decrease the amount of circulating LPS. In studies with human participants who were given OFS *Bifidobacteria*, participants returned to normal levels and regulated blood endotoxin levels, which led to improved glucose tolerance, increased satiety, and weight reduction [8]. Cani and colleagues showed that the impact of OFS was regulated by the GLP1-dependent pathway. Diabetic mice who were fed an HFD received OFS therapy and showed an improved glucose tolerance, reduction in weight, and diminished gluconeogenesis. However, when using GLP-1 knockout mice or GLP-1 receptor antagonist exendin 9–39, researchers saw none of the aforementioned favorable effects of OFS, thus suggesting a role of the GLP-1 dependent pathway [8,42,44,47]. Translating these findings to human subjects is inconclusive; however, depending on the dose, OFS may diminish energy intake and increase levels of PYY in plasma. There are still conflicting views on the effects it may have on satiety in humans. OFS fermentation also impacts how extracellular acetate and lactate produce butyrate, which suggests the possibility for use as a prebiotic therapy [8].

The use of prebiotics therapeutically to manage obesity in humans is supported by a few studies. In a study by Genta et al., obese and premenopausal women, characterized by a BMI greater than 30 kg/m^2, were given either a placebo or OFS-rich syrup from an Andean tuber named *yacon*. Participants who consumed the syrup saw a significant reduction in body mass, BMI, and waist circumference, as well as heightened satiety. Over the 120-day test period, these participants experienced a loss of an average of 15 kg, together with a 50% decrease in levels of fasting insulin and 30% decrease in levels of low-density lipoprotein (LDL) cholesterol [48]. In a double-blind study by Parnell and Reimer, 48 overweight adults, characterized by a BMI greater than 25 kg/m^2, were randomly given 21 g of a placebo (maltodextrin) or a prebiotic (OFS) daily for 12 weeks. When compared to the placebo group, the prebiotic group decreased body mass by 1.0 ± 0.4 kg, together with "Please provide closing quotes.decreased secretion of ghrelin, increased circulating PYY levels, reduced calorie intake, and lowered plasma glucose and insulin [44,49].

8.5.3 FECAL MICROBIOTA TRANSPLANT

Fecal microbiota transplant (FMT) has been used to improve gut health through the transfer of fecal-derived microbiota from a healthy donor into the gastrointestinal tract of an unhealthy participant [2,8,18]. FMT was originally used to treat enteric infections such as *Clostridium difficile*, usually caused by antibiotic use [8,18,42]. Because of this, recently there has been an interest in how FMT may regulate metabolism and metabolic disorders. It has been hypothesized that FMT may be efficient in the improvement of glucose and lipid homeostasis [2]. Studies have shown that, when lean donors donate their microbiota, recipients experience an increase in peripheral insulin sensitivity in just 6 weeks post-FMT when compared to their peripheral insulin sensitivity pre-FMT [2]. In a pilot study, the intestinal microbiota from lean human participants was transplanted via a postpyloric enteral feeding tube to participants with metabolic syndrome. Recipients of lean donor microbiota saw a raise in their peripheral insulin sensitivity 6 weeks post-FMT when contrasted with pre-FMT peripheral insulin sensitivity. However, there was no significant change in the recipients' adiposity or body weight. These changes are most likely due to diversification of gut microbiota, in addition to an increase in the quantity of *Eubacterium hallii*, a butyrate producer [2].

Many animal studies have shown that when germ-free mice receive feces from conventional mice, they experience elevated levels of insulin resistance, as well as an increase in body mass [8,18].

Mice, when conventionalized with human feces, show conservation of variety and structure of the donor gut microbiota; there was also a conservation of adiposity and cholesterol metabolism of the donor [8]. To see if these findings could be translated to humans, researchers conducted a study in which obese men with metabolic syndrome were transplanted with either allogenic or autologous fecal microbiota from healthy and lean donors. These transplants were carried out via a duodenal tube and into the small intestine. Six weeks post-FMT, the allogenic group saw an improvement in median insulin sensitivity, as measured by glucose disappearance rate during euglycemic hyper-insulinemic clamps [18]. This observed effect was variable, as some individuals responded, but others did not. The microbiota diversity in the obese group was initially low; however, upon allogenic transplantation, the diversity increased. Participants' fecal and small intestine microbial samples also saw elevated levels of bacteria that produce butyrate. Researchers continued to follow participants for 3 months after the FMT to assess gut microbiota resilience [8,18]. They found new species along with pre-existing species, most of which were phylogenetically linked. For most participants, the degree of engraftment, when blood-forming cells received on transplant day begin to grow and make healthy blood cells, varied, as did resistance to colonization of donor microbiota. Further study of healthy donor microbiota revealed that the microbiota of one particular donor was able to occupy several receivers [8,18].

8.5.4 Bariatric Surgery

Roux-en-Y gastric bypass (RYGB) is a surgical remedy usually reserved for morbidly obese patients. This therapy allows patients to undergo considerable and continuous weight loss, accompanied by improvement in inflammatory and metabolic conditions [8]. Research suggests that RYGB is successful because it causes constant reorganization of innate gut microbiota, which, when paired with restriction of calories and malabsorption, allows for increased host glucose tolerance and insulin sensitivity [10]. Many studies have been able to associate the preoperative metabolic state with changes seen in gut microbiota postoperatively. Preoperatively, researchers saw increased levels of H_2-generating Prevotellacea (subgroup of Bacteroidetes), along with increased levels of H_2-utilizing methanogens (Archaea). The transmission of H_2 between these two bacteria is responsible for a rise in energy absorption by the intestine; methanogens have the ability to extract fermentation intermediates from polysaccharides [8]. This allows for larger quantities of SCFAs to be taken in by the intestinal epithelium. A pilot study demonstrated that post-surgery, quantities of Prevotellacea and methanogens had reduced, and the primary control of Firmicutes diminished. These human results were supported by an animal study. Non-obese rats that underwent RYGB saw a reduced level of Firmicutes and Bacteroidetes, but a much higher concentration of Proteobacteria, versus sham-operated rats [8]. Liou and colleagues also conducted an animal study in which they relocated the cecal matter of RYGB donors to germ-free, lean mice. The mice that received the contents saw a significant reduction in body mass; however, control germ-free mice and mice that had received the cecal matter of those who had sham surgery did not show weight loss. The researchers believed this change was associated with SCFAs [50].

Zhang and colleagues showed Firmicutes levels in patients who went through the RYGB procedure were reduced versus obese and normal-weight patients [51]. Furet and colleagues supported these findings by showing that pre-RYGB, there was a higher ratio of Firmicutes to Bacteroidetes in obese patients, then at 3 months and 6 months post-RYGB surgery, along with body mass reduction, patients saw a reduction in this ratio. After the RYGB procedure, the stomach is much less acidic, which allows for probiotics to be used to regulate gut microbiota. In a randomized trial, post-RYGB participants were given either a placebo or *Lactobacillus* probiotic, and those that received the probiotic saw 9% more body mass reduction after 3 months versus those who received the placebo [52].

8.6 CONCLUSIONS

Obesity is a disease affecting more than 500 million people worldwide. The main cause is an excessive accumulation of adipose tissue due to a higher energy intake than expenditure, which leads to a gain in body mass. Recent research has focused on how the gut microbiota may influence the pathogenesis and treatment of obesity. Our gut flora, composed of trillions of bacterial microbes, is responsible for regulating energy, nutrient attainment, and storage of fat. The gut flora can be manipulated by many factors, including antibiotics, diet, hormones, and genetics. Most research finds an association of gut microbiota composition with obesity, indicating that a decrease in Bacteriodetes and an increase in Firmicutes lead to an obesogenic microbiome. Gut microbiota can also influence the immune system, causing low-grade inflammation as obesity causes an abundance of lipopolysaccharide in the blood. Current research is now focused on how to target the gut microbiota for therapeutic treatment for obese patients. There has been a rise in the use of products such as probiotics and prebiotics, as they colonize the colon and influence the gut flora to improve the health of patients with metabolic disorders. Although many animal studies have shown promising results, the effectiveness of prebiotics and probiotics in humans is still uncertain. Future research aims to target this uncertainty so affected individuals may receive the beneficial effects of probiotics and prebiotics.

REFERENCES

1. Sanmiguel C, Gupta A, Mayer EA. Gut microbiome and obesity: A plausible explanation for obesity. *Curr Obes Rep.* 2015 Jun; 4(2): 250–261.
2. Gérard P. Gut microbiota and obesity. *Cell Mol Life Sci.* 2016 Jan; 73(1): 147–162.
3. Omer E, Atassi H. The microbiome that shapes us: Can it cause obesity? *Curr Gastroenterol Rep.* 2017 Oct 27; 19(12): 59.
4. Murugesan S, Nirmalkar K, Hoyo-Vadillo C, García-Espitia M, Ramírez-Sánchez D, García-Mena J. Gut microbiome production of short-chain fatty acids and obesity in children. *Eur J Clin Microbiol Infect Dis.* 2017 Dec 2.
5. Portune KJ, Benítez-Páez A, Del Pulgar EM, Cerrudo V, Sanz Y. Gut microbiota, diet, and obesity-related disorders- The good, the bad, and the future challenges. *Mol Nutr Food Res.* 2017 Jan; 61(1).
6. Maruvada P, Leone V, Kaplan LM, Chang EB. The human microbiome and obesity: Moving beyond associations. *Cell Host Microbe.* 2017 Nov 8; 22(5): 589–599.
7. Chen J, He X, Huang J. Diet effects in gut microbiome and obesity. *J Food Sci.* 2014 Apr; 79(4): R442–451.
8. Kootte RS, Vrieze A, Holleman F, Dallinga-Thie GM, Zoetendal EG, de Vos WM, Groen AK, Hoekstra JB, Stroes ES, Nieuwdorp M. The therapeutic potential of manipulating gut microbiota in obesity and type 2 diabetes mellitus. *Diabetes Obes Metab.* 2012 Feb; 14(2): 112–120.
9. Caricilli AM, Saad MJ. Gut microbiota composition and its effects on obesity and insulin resistance. *Curr Opin Clin Nutr Metab Care.* 2014 Jul; 17(4): 312–318.
10. Li X, Shimizu Y, Kimura I. Gut microbial metabolite short-chain fatty acids and obesity. *Biosci Microbiota Food Health.* 2017 Aug 25; 36(4): 135–140.
11. Cho I, Yamanishi S, Cox L, Methé BA, Zavadil J, Li K, Gao Z, Mahana D, Raju K, Teitler I, Li H, Alekseyanko AV, Blaser MJ. Antibiotics in early life alter the murine colonic microbiome and adiposity. *Nature.* 2012 Aug 30; 488(7413): 621–626.
12. Fouhy F, Guinane CM, Hussey S, Wall R, Ryan CA, Dempsey EM, Murphy B, Ross RP, Fitzgerald GF, Stanton C, Cotter PD. High-throughput sequencing reveals the incomplete, short-term recovery of infant gut microbiota following parenteral antibiotic treatment with ampicillin and gentamicin. *Antimicrob Agents Chemother.* 2012 Nov; 56(11): 5811–5820.
13. Esteve E, Ricart W, Fernández-Real JM. Gut microbiota interactions with obesity, insulin resistance and type 2 diabetes: Did gut microbiote co-evolve with insulin resistance? *Curr Opin Clin Nutr Metab Care.* 2011 Sep; 14(5): 483–490.
14. Jumpertz R, Le DS, Turnbaugh PJ, Trinidad C, Bogardus C, Gordon JI, Karkoff J. Energy-balance studies reveal associations between gut microbes, caloric load, and nutrient absorption in humans. *Am J Clin Nutr.* 2011 Jul; 94(1): 58–65.

15. Wostmann BS. Intestinal bile acids and cholesterol absorption in the germfree rat. *J Nutr.* 1973 Jul; 103(7): 982–990.
16. Rabot S, Membrez M, Bruneau A, Gérard P, Harach T, Moser M, Raymond E, Mansourian R, Chou CJ. Germ-free C57BL/6J mice are resistant to high-fat-diet-induced insulin resistance and have altered cholesterol metabolism. *FASEB J.* 2010 Dec; 24(12): 4948–4959.
17. Cani PD, Delzenne NM. The gut microbiome as therapeutic target. *Pharmacol Ther.* 2011 May; 130(2): 202–212.
18. Dao MC, Clément K. Gut microbiota and obesity: Concepts relevant to clinical care. *Eur J Intern Med.* 2018 Feb; 48: 18–24.
19. Cani PD, Amar J, Iglesias MA, Poggi M, Knauf C, Bastelica D, Neyrinck AM, et al. Metabolic endotoxemia initiates obesity and insulin resistance. *Diabetes.* 2007 Jul; 56(7): 1761–1772.
20. Everard A, Belzer C, Geurts L, Ouwerkerk JP, Druart C, Bindels LB, Guiot Y, et al. Cross-talk between Akkermansia muciniphila and intestinal epithelium controls diet-induced obesity. *Proc Natl Acad Sci U S A.* 2013 May 28; 110(22): 9066–9071.
21. Wu GD, Chen J, Hoffmann C, Bittinger K, Chen YY, Keilbaugh SA, Bewtra M, et al. Linking long-term dietary patterns with gut microbial enterotypes. *Science.* 2011 Oct 7; 334(6052): 105–108.
22. Duncan SH, Belenguer A, Holtrop G, Johnstone AM, Flint HJ, Lobley GE. Reduced dietary intake of carbohydrates by obese subjects results in decreased concentrations of butyrate and butyrate-producing bacteria in feces. *Appl Environ Microbiol.* 2007 Feb; 73(4): 1073–1078.
23. De Filippo C, Cavalieri D, Di Paola M, Ramazzotti M, Massart S, Collini S, Pieraccini G, Lionetti P. Impact of diet in shaping gut microbiota revealed by a comparative study in children from Europe and rural Africa. *Proc Natl Acad Sci U S A.* 2010 Aug 17; 107(33): 14691–14696.
24. Zhang C, Zhang M, Pang X, Zhao Y, Wang L, Zhao L. Structural resilience of the gut microbiota in adult mice under high- fat dietary perturbations. *ISME J.* 2012 Oct; 6(10): 1848–1857.
25. Lam YY, Ha CW, Campbell CR, Mitchell AJ Dinudom A, Oscarsson J, Cook DI, Hunt NH, Caterson ID, Holmes AJ, Storlien LH. Increased gut permeability and microbiota change associate with mesenteric fat inflammation and metabolic dysfunction in diet-induced obese mice. *PLoS One.* 2012; 7(3): e34233.
26. Mujico JR, Baccan GC, Gheorghe A, Díaz LE, Marcos A. Changes in gut microbiota due to supplemented fatty acids in diet-induced obese mice. *Br J Nutr.* 2013 Aug; 110(4): 711–720.
27. Haghikia A, Jörg S, Duscha A, Berg J, Manzel A, Waschbisch A, Hammer A, et al. Dietary fatty acids directly impact central nervous system autoimmunity via the small intestine. *Immunity.* 2016 Apr 19; 44(4): 951–953.
28. Tremaroli V, Bäckhed F. Functional interactions between the gut microbiota and host metabolism. *Nature.* 2012 Sep 13; 489(7415): 242–249.
29. Bernstein H, Bernstein C, Payne CM, Dvorakova K, Garewal H. Bile acids as carcinogens in human gastrointestinal cancers. *Mutat Res.* 2005 Jan; 589(1): 47–65.
30. Walker AW, Ince J, Duncan SH, Webster LM, Holtrop G, Ze X, Brown D, et al. Dominant and diet-responsive groups of bacteria within the human colonic microbiota. *ISME J.* 2011 Feb; 5(2): 220–230.
31. Costabile A, Klinder A, Fava F, Napolitano A, Fogliano V, Leonard C, Gibson GR, Tuohy KM. Whole-grain wheat breakfast cereal has a prebiotic effect on the human gut microbiota: A double-blind, placebo-controlled, crossover study. *Br J Nutr.* 2008 Jan; 99(1): 110–120.
32. Carvalho-Wells AL, Helmolz K, Nodet C, Molzer C, Leonard C, McKevith B, Thielecke F, Jackson KG, Tuohy KM. Determination of the in vivo prebiotic potential of a maize-based whole grain breakfast cereal: A human feeding study. *Br J Nutr.* 2010 Nov; 104(9): 1353–1356.
33. Martínez I, Lattimer JM, Hubach KL, Case JA, Yang J, Weber CG, Louk JA, et al. Gut microbiome composition is linked to whole grain-induced immunological improvements. *ISME J.* 2013 Feb; 7(2): 269–280.
34. Petry N, Egli I, Chassard C, Lacroix C, Hurrell R. Inulin modifies the bifidobacteria population, fecal lactate concentration, and fecal pH but does not influence iron absorption in women with low iron status. *Am J Clin Nutr.* 2012 Aug; 96(2), 325–331.
35. García-Peris P, Velasco C, Lozano MA, Moreno Y, Paron L, de la Cuerda C, Bretón I, Camblor M, García-Hernández J, Guarner F, Hernández M. Effect of a mixture of inulin and fructo-oligosaccharide on Lactobacillus and Bifidobacterium intestinal microbiota of patients receiving radiotherapy: A randomised, double- blind, placebo-controlled trial. *Nutr Hosp.* 2012 Nov-Dec; 27(6): 1908–1915.

36. Dewulf EM, Cani PD, Claus SP, Fuentes S, Puylaert PG, Neyrinck AM, Bindels LB, de Vos WM, Gibson GR, Thissen JP, Delzenne NM. Insight into the prebiotic concept: Lessons from an exploratory, double blind intervention study with inulin-type fructans in obese women. *Gut.* 2013 Aug; 62(8): 1112–1121.

37. Kleessen B, Schwarz S, Boehm A, Fuhrmann H, Richter A, Henle T, Krugger M. Jerusalem artichoke and chicory inulin in bakery products affect faecal microbiota of healthy volunteers. *Br J Nutr.* 2007 Sep; 98(3): 540–549.

38. Davis LM, Martinez I, Walter J, Goin C, Hutkins RW. Barcoded pyrosequencing reveals that consumption of galactooligosaccharides results in a highly specific bifidogenic response in humans. *PLoS One.* 2011; 6(9): e25200.

39. Martínez I, Kim J, Duffy PR, Schlegel VL, Walter J. Resistant starches types 2 and 4 have differential effects on the composition of the fecal microbiota in human subjects. *PLoS One.* 2010 Nov 29; 5(11): e15046.

40. Lin HV, Frassetto K, Kowalik EJ Jr, Nawrocki AR, Lu MM, Kosinski JR, Hubert JA, Szeto D, Yao X, Forrest G, Marsh DJ. Butyrate and propionate protect against diet-induced obesity and regulate gut hormones via free fatty acid receptor 3-independent mechanisms. *PLoS One.* 2012; 7(4): e35240.

41. Takahashi K, Nishida A, Fujimoto T, Fujii M, Shioya M, Imaeda H, Inatomi O, Bamba S, Sugimoto M, Andoh A. Reduced abundance of butyrate-producing bacteria species in the fecal microbial community in Crohn's disease. *Digestion.* 2016; 93(1): 59–65

42. John GK, Mullin GE. The gut microbiome and obesity. *Curr Oncol Rep.* 2016 Jul; 18(7): 45.

43. Million M, Angelakis E, Paul M, Armougom F, Leibovici L, Raoult D. Comparative meta-analysis of the effect of Lactobacillus species on weight gain in humans and animals. *Microb Pathog.* 2012 Aug; 53(2): 100–108.

44. Shen J, Obin MS, Zhao L. The gut microbiota, obesity and insulin resistance. *Mol Aspects Med.* 2013 Feb; 34(1): 39–58

45. Yin YN, Yu QF, Fu N, Liu XW, Lu FG. Effects of four Bifidobacteria on obesity in high-fat diet induced rats. *World J Gastroenterol.* 2010 Jul 21; 16(27): 3394–3401.

46. Kadooka Y, Sato M, Imaizumi K, Ogawa A, Ikuyama K, Akai Y, Okano M, Kagoshima M, Tsuchida T. Regulation of abdominal adiposity by probiotics (Lactobacillus gasseri SBT2055) in adults with obese tendencies in a randomized controlled trial. *Eur J Clin Nutr.* 2010 Jun; 64(6), 636–643.

47. Cani PD, Neyrinck AM, Fava F, Knauf C, Burcelin RG, Tuohy KM, Gibson GR., Delzenne NM. Selective increases of bifidobacteria in gut microflora improve high-fat-diet-induced diabetes in mice through a mechanism associated with endotoxaemia. *Diabetologia.* 2007 Nov; 50(11): 2374–2383.

48. Genta S, Cabrera W, Habib N, Pons J, Carillo IM, Grau A, Sanchez S. Yacon syrup: Beneficial effects on obesity and insulin resistance in humans. *Clin Nutr.* 2009 Apr; 28(2): 182–187.

49. Parnell JA, Reimer RA. Weight loss during oligofructose supplementation is associated with decreased ghrelin and increased peptide YY in overweight and obese adults. *Am J Clin Nutr.* 2009 Jun; 89(6): 1751–1759.

50. Liou AP, Paziuk M, Luevano JM Jr, Machineni S, Turnbaugh PJ, Kaplan LM. Conserved shifts in the gut microbiota due to gastric bypass reduce host weight and adiposity. *Sci Transl Med.* 2013 Mar 27; 5(178): 178ra41.

51. Zhang H, DiBaise JK, Zuccolo A, Kudma D, Braidotti M, Yu Y, Parameswaran P, Crowell MD, Wing R, Rittmann BE, Krajmalnik-Brown R. Human gut microbiota in obesity and after gastric bypass. *Proc Natl Acad Sci U S A.* 2009 Feb 17; 106(7): 2365–2370.

52. Furet JP, Kong LC, Tap J, Poitou C, Bouillot JL, Mariat D, Corthier G, Doré J, Henegar C, Rizkalla S, Clément K. Differential adaptation of human gut microbiota to bariatric surgery-induced weight loss: Links with metabolic and low-grade inflammation markers. *Diabetes.* 2010 Dec; 59(12): 3049–3057.

9 Bariatric Surgery

Adolfo Z. Fernandez, Jr.

CONTENTS

9.1 INTRODUCTION

The obesity epidemic continues without slowing in the United States. In the last report from the National Health and Nutrition Examination Survey (NHANES), the obesity trends across all groups were either unchanged or growing [1]. Despite the focus on obesity prevention and treatment, there has been little impact on this epidemic. *Obesity* is defined as a body mass index (BMI) greater than 30 kg/m^2 (Table 9.1). The group with the worst form of the disease, Class III obesity, is the most difficult to treat. The options for treatment in this group include pharmacotherapy, behavior modification, and surgery. Surgery has been shown to have the greatest impact and success in this group compared to any other form of treatment [2].

The qualifications for surgery have, for the most part, remained unchanged over the last 40 years [3]. The weight criteria is that a candidate's BMI be higher than 40 kg/m^2, or if certain health conditions exist, it can be between 35 and 40 kg/m^2. The health conditions that typically qualify patients for the lower BMI criteria are diabetes mellitus (DM), hypertension (HTN), obstructive sleep apnea (OSA), and disabling degenerative joint disease (DJD). Candidates will also need to undergo nutritional and psychological evaluation and counseling prior to being deemed appropriate surgical candidates. After completing the evaluation process, a patient can move forward with weight loss surgery.

Bariatric surgery has evolved and changed tremendously since its beginning with the jejunal-ileal bypass (JIB) in 1954 [4]. Bariatric procedures have been classically categorized into either restrictive, malabsorptive, or combination procedures. Restrictive procedures are those that reduce the capacity of the stomach, thereby inducing weight loss by limiting the amount of calories consumed. The category of purely restrictive procedures includes the horizontal gastroplasty (HG),

TABLE 9.1
Weight Classification by BMI

Body Mass Index (BMI)	Classification
< 18.5 kg/m^2	Underweight
18.5–24.9 kg/m^2	Normal
25.0–29.9 kg/m^2	Overweight
30.0–34.9 kg/m^2	Class I obesity
35.0–39.9 kg/m^2	Class II obesity
> 40.0 kg/m^2	Class III obesity

vertical banded gastroplasty (VBG), adjustable gastric band (AGB), and vertical sleeve gastrectomy (VSG). Malabsorptive procedures are those that limit the absorptive capacity of the gastrointestinal (GI) tract, inducing weight loss by reducing the absorption of the calories consumed. The JIB is an example of a purely malabsorptive procedure. The combination procedures are those that use both a restrictive and malabsorptive mechanism for weight loss. These include the Roux-en-Y gastric bypass (RYGB), bilio-pancreatic diversion (BPD), bilio-pancreatic diversion—duodenal switch (DS), mini-gastric bypass (MGB), and single anastomosis duodenal-ileal bypass with sleeve gastrectomy (SADI). This mechanistic approach to categorizing the different types of surgeries is quite simplistic. Many hormonal mechanisms have been postulated and identified for these procedures, far beyond what is explained by simple restriction or malabsorption alone. These mechanisms are yet to be wholly defined and are beyond the scope of this review.

The bariatric surgeon has quite an armamentarium of choices for patients. The four most common procedures performed today include the VSG, RYGB, AGB, and DS. Each of these procedures is different in its effectiveness as it relates to weight loss and improvement or resolution of obesity-related diseases. Like all surgeries, these procedures carry both short- and long-term morbidity related to the procedures themselves and the changes they induce. This discussion will be limited to these four procedures, as the others mentioned are of historical significance only or are considered investigational.

9.2 PROCEDURES

9.2.1 Adjustable Gastric Banding

The first "banding" of the stomach was performed by Drs. Peloso and Wilkinson in 1976 [5]. This band was not adjustable and resulted in poor weight loss and significant morbidity. Over the next decade, multiple modifications of the gastric band were attempted. In 1985 and 1986, two AGBs were developed and placed in humans [6,7]. These bands went on to be known as the *Swedish adjustable gastric band* (SAGB) and the laparoscopic adjustable gastric band (*Lap Band*). These were the two commercially available bands in the United States. The lap band system gained approval from the US Food and Drug Administration (FDA) in 2001; the SAGB gained approval in 2007. The AGB gained popularity in the United States in the early 2000s, until its peak in 2011. Multiple reports came out then that called into question the long-term safety and effectiveness of the AGB [8]. The popularity of the AGB began to decline sharply among both patients and bariatric surgeons. The company providing the SAGB in the United States stopped production in 2016.

The AGB is constructed from silicone, with an inner inflatable bladder that is connected to a reservoir located under the skin (Figure 9.1). The AGB is placed laparoscopically around the superior portion of the stomach, partitioning the stomach into an upper pouch with a volume between

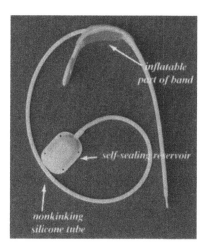

FIGURE 9.1 Band developed by Dr Kuzmak. (From Kuzmak, L.I. et al., *AORN J.*, 51, 1307–1324, 1990.)

15 and 30 cc. The food must traverse through the AGB in order to pass into the remainder of the stomach and GI tract are made by accessing the subcutaneous reservoir with a needle depending on the individual's symptoms. The goal of the adjustments is to help patients achieve a sense of satiety with small portions, while avoiding any obstructive symptoms. This will result in a lower caloric intake and weight loss when the appropriate amount of restriction is achieved. The weight loss induced by the AGB has been shown to positively impact the person's overall health and quality of life.

The AGB proved to be an effective weight loss device. In early published series, the AGB was found to produce 40%–60% excess weight loss (%EWL) in patients 4–6 years out from surgery [10–13]. The AGB-induced weight loss resulted in significant improvement or even resolution of the co-morbid conditions associated with their obesity. One recent systematic review looking for studies that described outcomes in bariatric surgery patients with more than 2-year outcomes and follow-up of at least 80% in the initial cohort identified nine prospective and five retrospective cohorts meeting criteria in AGB patients [14]. The goal of the review was to assess the quality of the evidence and assess the effectiveness of bariatric surgery in severely obese adults. Thirty-one percent of the AGB studies showed a %EWL of greater than 50%. The mean sample-size-weighted %EWL for AGB was 45% ($n = 4,109$), compared to 65.7% for RYGB studies ($n = 3,544$). This same systematic review looked at remission rates for type 2 diabetes (DM), HTN, and hyperlipidemia (HL). Diabetes remission was defined as glycated hemoglobin less than 6.5% without medication. HTN remission was defined as a blood pressure less than 140/90 without medication, and hyperlipidemia remission was defined as a total cholesterol less than 200 mg/dl, high-density lipoprotein greater than 40 mg/dl, low-density lipoprotein less than 160 mg/dl, and triglycerides less than 200 mg/dl. The remission rates for diabetes, HTN, and HL for the AGB studies were 28.6% ($n = 96$), 17.4% ($n = 247$), and 22.7% ($n = 97$), respectively. The AGB produced less weight loss and remission than the RYGB but was significantly better than intensive lifestyle modification.

The AGB had many advantages over other weight loss surgeries being performed when it was first introduced. These included reversibility, laparoscopic placement, very low peri-operative morbidity, and adjustability [13]. These advantages helped the AGB gain popularity and opened weight loss surgery to a group of individuals that would not have considered it prior to the introduction of the AGB. The Achilles heel of the AGB was the need for continuous, frequent follow-up and surveillance to ensure successful weight loss. The required follow-up and adjustments proved to be expensive and time-consuming for both patients and providers. Furthermore, problems with increasing gastro-esophageal reflux disease (GERD), "slips," erosions, and poor weight loss led to a nearly 50% rate of explantation and 60% re-operation rates long term in one center's experience [8]. This paper was reported in 2011 and shortly thereafter, there was a sharp decline in the demand and popularity for the AGB in the United States.

9.2.2 VERTICAL SLEEVE GASTRECTOMY

The VSG is the restrictive portion of the DS. The DS is recommended for patients with a BMI higher than 50 kg/m^2. When the DS was transitioning to a laparoscopic approach, the morbidity was high, particularly in patients with BMIs higher than 60 kg/m^2 [15]. In cases in which the intestinal portion of the procedure could not be performed, it was found that patients did well with the VSG alone. It then developed into a staging strategy for high-risk and high-BMI patients. Some patients did very well with the VSG alone, which led to the development of the VSG as a primary bariatric procedure from 2003 to 2009. After 2010, it gained acceptance as a validated primary procedure for weight loss, was given its own procedure code, and gained coverage by government and private payers. The VSG skyrocketed in popularity at this time, just as the AGB's popularity was declining. The VSG had numerous benefits that made it attractive to both patients and surgeons. The procedure was simple and low risk, and there was no foreign body.

The VSG is performed laparoscopically, which benefits patients with less post-operative pain, less risk for incisional complications like infections or hernias, quicker recovery, and shorter hospital stay. The VSG does not require any anastomosis, which reduces the risk of the surgery, and has low risk for malabsorption, which reduces long-term risk for vitamin or mineral deficiencies. The procedure itself is performed by placing a sizing bougie between 32 and 40 French into the stomach (Figure 9.2 [16]). The greater curve of the stomach is mobilized from the left crus distally to 3–6 cm from the pyloric channel. The stomach is then transected with a surgical stapler, using the bougie as a guide to reduce the stomach. The majority of the stomach (roughly 66%–75%) is removed. The procedure is not reversible.

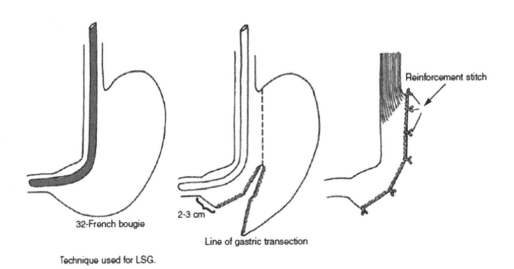

FIGURE 9.2 Technique for the vertical sleeve gastrectomy (VSG), as described by Braghetto et al. [16]. *Left*: stomach with the sizing device to guide the stapler cutter. *Middle*: stomach as the transection has begun. *Right*: remaining stomach after the resection has been completed.

The operative risk of the procedure is low. The mortality rate for the procedure is roughly 1 in 1,000. The most significant morbidities are staple line leaks or bleeding, but the risk of these is less than 1%. Leaks most commonly occur at the angle of His and can be associated with stenosis at the incisura. Early identification is important, as a delay in diagnosis can lead to poor outcomes. Treatment usually requires re-operation and management of the stenosis and leak. Another rare complication of the procedure is mesenteric vein thrombosis. This has been reported to occur in 0.4% of patients [17,18]. The majority of patients identified present with abdominal pain and require a hypercoagulable work-up. If identified early and anti-coagulation therapy is initiated quickly, major complications like bowel or liver ischemia can be avoided. Long term, the most prominent risks of the VSG include weight gain and GERD. Management of these two conditions in some patients may require operative conversion to either the RYGB or DS.

A review of the early experience of the VSG from 2003 to 2009 revealed 36 studies that described the weight loss and its risks [19]. Within this review, there was data from more than 2,400 patients with follow-up that ranged from 3 months to 5 years. In the studies that looked at the VSG as a primary procedure, the average BMI was 46.6 kg/m². This was reduced to 32.2 kg/m². The average %EWL was 60.7% with a follow-up that ranged between 3 months and 3 years. The mean complication rate was low at 6.2%, and overall mortality was 0.17%. The VSG was shown to produce significant weight loss with low morbidity and mortality. This led to its rapid rise in popularity and its adoption as a procedure for weight loss in the United States around 2010–2011. Unfortunately, there are still little long-term published results for the VSG.

The impact of the VSG on obesity-related co-morbid conditions is significant. Multiple series have demonstrated early resolution and improvements in DM, HTN, and HL. The rates of resolution varied widely between the reports, as differing definitions of *resolution* were used [20–22]. The improvement and resolution rates for DM in these reports ranged from 11% to 86% and 14% to 81%, respectively. There were similar ranges for HTN and HL. A systematic review published by Switzer focused on 5-year outcomes of the VSG and DM [23]. They found 11 studies that met their inclusion criteria, encompassing 1,134 patients, of which 29.7% (402 patients) had DM pre-operatively. The mean age and BMI for the group were 45.3 ± 6.9 years and 48.4 ± 10.8 kg/m², compared to 51.1 ± 5.9 years and 44.6 ± 11.8 kg/m² for the patients with diabetes. The whole group lost an average of 15.5 kg/m², for a mean BMI of 33.2 ± 4.7 kg/m² at 5 years. The average resolution of DM was 60.8%. Unfortunately, there were limitations to this review. Only one-half of the patients had follow-up at 5 years. Furthermore, the definition of *DM resolution* was mixed between the studies that were identified.

The VSG is a good option for patients. It is a simpler procedure than the RYGB and DS, with less operative risk and long-term risk. The mortality risk is one-half of the RYGB and the DS. Since the VSG has no malabsorption, the risk for vitamin and mineral deficiencies is much less than the DS and RYGB. Compared to the AGB, it produces more weight loss and impact on co-morbid conditions without the complications related to the Band device. It does have limitations, including weight recidivism and GERD. Weight recidivism may occur in up to 20% of patients and may require a second revisional procedure in up to 5%–10% of patients [24].

9.2.3 ROUX-EN-Y GASTRIC BYPASS

The RYGB is the second-most-common procedure performed today in the United States. It was developed in 1966 by Drs. Ito and Mason and is one of the oldest procedures for weight loss [25]. Despite all of its successes, many other procedures have come and gone during its existence. The RYGB transitioned to laparoscopy in the mid-1990s, which, along with the introduction of the AGB, led to a dramatic rise of bariatric surgery in the United States. The RYGB has

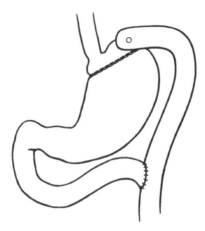

FIGURE 9.3 From Pories et al. Depiction of a typical RYGB performed through an open approach, in which the stomach is stapled but not divided. In the laparaoscopic approach, the stomach is usually stapled and divided into two separate compartments. In the Greenville modification of the gastric bypass, the stomach is partitioned to form at 20 to 30 mL proximal pouch that is connected to a 40 to 60 cm Roux-en-Y loop with an 8 to 10 mm double-layered gastroenterostomy. The biliopancreatic limb also measures 40 to 60 cm, depending on the mobility of gut.

maintained a steady demand due to its success in producing long-term weight loss and amelioration of obesity-related conditions like DM.

The procedure in the majority of cases is performed laparoscopically. A small pouch is created from the top portion of the stomach (Figure 9.3 [26]). The pouch will hold a volume of approximately 30 cc. The small intestine is then divided approximately 30–50 cm distal to the ligament of Treitz. The distal end of the small intestine is connected to the gastric pouch, and the proximal end is connected back to the small intestine, no more than 100 cm from the pouch. This creates a Roux limb length of approximately 100 cm. This is considered a standard RYGB; other versions of the RYGB include the long limb and distal. The long-limb RYGB has a Roux limb length of 150 cm and has been shown to cause slightly more weight loss than the standard RYGB in the short term but no difference in weight loss long term [27]. The distal RYGB has a Roux limb length of 100 cm but a common channel length of only 150 cm. This procedure did produce significantly more weight loss than the standard RYGB but had a 25% incidence of malnutrition, requiring lengthening of the common channel [28]. The standard RYGB is by far the most common version performed.

This risk of the surgery has dramatically improved with the advent of laparoscopy [29]. The largest impact was seen in the wound complications. The open RYGB had a wound complication rate of nearly 25%, including wound infection, seroma, or hernia. This rate is less than 5% with the laparoscopic approach. The risk of mortality is roughly 1 in 500. The most common perioperative complications include nausea and dehydration. GI leak for an anastomosis or staple line is low and, in some large series, non-existent [30,31]. Like the VSG, early detection and aggressive treatment help to improve outcomes after this devastating complication. Long-term issues include anastomotic complications like marginal ulceration and stenosis, hyperoxaluria and kidney stone formation, chronic anemia, and weight gain. The anastomotic complications are exacerbated by tobacco or Non-steroidal anti-inflammatory drugs (NSAIDs) use, which may lead to hemorrhage or GI perforation. These anastomotic complications usually require surgical revision and remediation, up to and including reversal of the procedure.

Many reports and series have been written about the benefits of the RYGB in effecting weight loss and treating medical co-morbid conditions of obesity, like DM, HTN, and hyperlipidemia. A landmark paper was published in 1995 by Dr. Pories and his group from East Carolina

University [26]. It was titled "Who would have thought it? An operation proves to be the most effective therapy for adult onset diabetes mellitus." Their series reported on more than 600 patients with follow-up to 14 years after surgery. In their report, there were 608 patients with an average initial BMI of 49.7 kg/m². Twenty-seven percent of the patients had DM, and an additional 27% had impaired glucose tolerance (IGT). The average %EWL was 70%, 58%, 55%, and 49% at 2 years, 5 years, 10 years, and 14 years, respectively. The follow-up was 96% for the entire group, but only 10 patients were 14 years out from the procedure at the time of the report. The most remarkable finding in the report was that 82.9% of the DM and 98.7% of the IGT patients reverted to euglycemia after surgery. Though the long-term follow-up was limited, the series demonstrated that the RYGB achieved sustained weight loss and had a dramatic impact on DM in the severely obese patient.

A prospective observational study from Utah has produced similar long-term results [32]. The study from Utah included 1,156 patients with a follow-up rate at 12 years of more than 90%. The patients were divided into three groups: those who sought and underwent the RYGB ($n = 418$), those who sought but did not undergo the RYGB (non-surgery group 1; $n = 417$), and those who did not seek out surgery (non-surgery group 2; $n = 321$). At 12 years, the RYGB group lost an average of 35 kg or 26.9% body weight loss. Seventy percent of the surgery group maintained at least a 20% body weight loss at 12 years. The other groups lost 2.9 and 0 kg, respectively, for an average body weight loss of 2% and 0.9%. The study defined *diabetes remission* as an HgbA1c of less than 6.5% or a fasting blood glucose level less than 126 mg per dl without any antidiabetic medications. Among the patients with type 2 DM in the surgery group, 51% (43 of 84) had complete remission at 12 years. Conversely, the incidence of DM in the surgery group was 3% (8 of 303 patients) at 12 years, compared to 26% (42 out of 164) in non-surgery group 1 and 26% (47 out of 184) in non-surgery group 2. The remission rate of HTN was statistically higher in the surgery group compared with non-surgery group 1. The remission rate of dyslipidemia was also statistically higher in the surgery group compared to both of the non-surgery groups. This observational study demonstrated that the RYGB had long-term, durable weight loss and was effective in the treatment and prevention of DM, HTN, and dyslipidemia.

These two reports demonstrate the long-term effect and success of the RYGB in the treatment of severe obesity. The RYGB is an effective procedure for weight loss and treatment of obesity-related conditions, especially DM. The risk profile of this surgery has dramatically improved since its inception in the 1960s. In patients with the combination of severe obesity and DM, it is one of the more effective treatment options available and should be considered early in the course of their care. Numerous studies have shown that RYGB is more effective in remitting DM if it is performed soon after the diagnosis is made and treatment begun. The RYGB is less effective in remitting the disease if the DM has been in place for longer duration or if patients require insulin for its treatment. Even though its risk profile is slightly more than the VSG, it is a more metabolically beneficial procedure for severely obese patients with metabolic derangement such as DM.

9.2.4 Bilio-Pancreatic Diversion—Duodenal Switch

The DS is a modification of the bilio-pancreatic diversion initially developed by Dr. Nicola Scopinaro in Italy. Dr. Scopinaro first described it in 1979 [33]. The BPD was very successful in producing significant weight loss and amelioration of obesity-related conditions. The BPD produced long-term, sustained weight loss and near-total remission of DM, OSA, and dyslipidemia. The downside to BPD was complications with ulcers, dumping syndrome, diarrhea, and malnutrition. The DS was a modification of the BPD to help reduce these issues by Drs. Marceau and Hess in 1988 [34,35].

The procedure can be performed laparoscopically. The stomach is reduced by performing a resection of the greater curve, preserving the antral pump and pylorus as in the VSG. The volume is reduced and calibrated with a 60-French bougie. The duodenum is then divided just past the

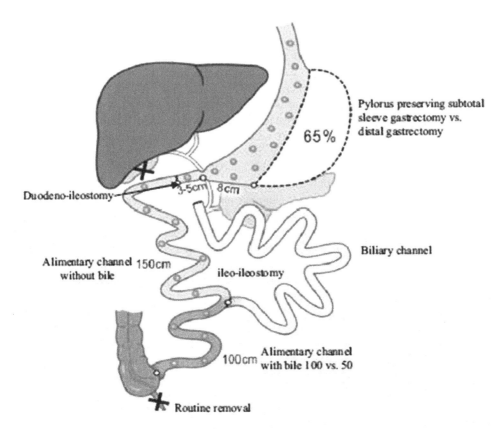

FIGURE 9.4 Bilio-pancreatic diversion with duodenal switch, BPD-DS. Modification of Scopinaro's BPD. Procedure described by Marceau et al. in their outcomes report from 2015. (From Marceau, P. et al., *Obes. Surg.*, 25, 1584–1593, 2015; Himpens, J. et al., *Arch. Surg.*, 146, 802–807, 2011.)

pylorus. The alimentary channel is measured 250 cm from the ileo-cecal valve in Dr. Marceau's version (Figure 9.4 [36]). The small intestine is transected here. The distal end of the transection is connected to the duodenum. The proximal end is connected back to the alimentary limb 100 cm from the ileocecal valve. In Dr Hess's version, he measured the entire length of the small bowel (Figure 9.5 [35]). He then would create an alimentary limb in 25-cm increments that was 40% of the small bowel length and a common channel that was 10% of the small bowel length. In his experience, the alimentary limb was most commonly between 250 and 325 cm long, and the common channel was between 50 and 100 cm long.

The DS is the most complex of the four bariatric procedures described here. In the best reports, the procedure can be performed with a mortality of 1 in 500 [36]. In the reports from Drs. Hess and Marceau, early complications occurred in approximately 8%–10% of patients [35,36]. The most common serious complications included GI leak, intra-abdominal abscess, sepsis, pancreatitis, and entero-cutaneous fistula. Readmission rates vary between 6% and 8%, and re-operation rates from 4% to 13%. Fortunately, with experience and laparoscopy, these rates continue to improve to even lower levels. The most common complications for the DS are related to the malabsorption of this procedure. These complications include anemia, vitamin or mineral deficiencies, osteoporosis, and protein-calorie malnutrition. With appropriate follow-up and supplementation, these issues occur less than 2% of the time [36]. Unfortunately, with poor follow-up and supplementation, these problems can be significant and require a re-operation [35]. That aside, the DS is still very safe and one of the most effective weight loss surgeries.

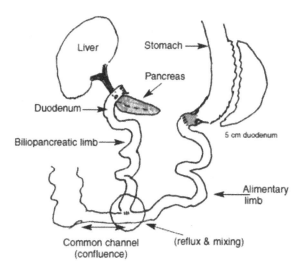

FIGURE 9.5 Original drawing from Hess et al. describing their configuration of the bilio-pancreatic diversion—duodenal switch (DS). BPD/DS as performed by the authors. 40% of total small bowel length is the alimentary (*including* common) limb. Common channel measures 10% of entire small bowel length.

With more than 10 years of experience and follow-up, Drs. Hess and Marceau have published their groups' results with the DS. Dr Hess's cohort consisted of 1,150 patients, of whom 182 were more than 10 years out from the DS, and had a 92% follow-up rate [35]. The mean follow-up in Dr. Marceau's series was almost 10 years in a group comprised of more than 2,000 patients—more than 800 of whom had follow-up of at least 10 years [36]. The mean weight loss expressed in %EWL was 75% and 71%, respectively. In more concrete terms, the Marceau group lost an average of 20 BMI units and more than 70% of the patients achieved a BMI less than 35 kg/m^2. The only series that can claim similar long-term follow-up and consistent weight loss are those from the Swedish Obesity Subjects (SOS) and Dr Pories' group. The long-term weight loss in these two series is less by comparison. The only other series with similar weight loss and follow-up is the series from Dr. Scopinaro and the BPD [37]. The common string between these groups is the significant malabsorption that is caused by the DS and BPD compared to the VSG and RYGB. With the significant impact on weight, the DS also impacts the co-morbid conditions like DM, HTN, and hyperlipidemia more than the other procedures.

The DS's biggest impact is on diabetes. It is generally accepted that the remission rate with the DS is better than 90% and is a rate that seems to be maintained long term. This is best seen in the data published from Dr. Marceau's group [36]. In the initial group, nearly 40% were diabetic—more than 900 patients, including patients on insulin, oral medications, and diet controlled. At 10 years, 92.7% had stopped all medications or treatments and maintained an HgbA1c of less than 6.5%. This was despite recurrence in 10.8% of the insulin-dependent group and 2.5% in both of the oral medication and diet-controlled groups. The impact on HTN and dyslipidemia was similarly significant; 68% of the group had HTN, and 64% remitted and 31% saw improvement. Dyslipidemia was present in 633 (24.2%) patients pre-operatively and resolved in 80%. The greatest impact was seen in the reductions of total cholesterol, LDL, and triglycerides. HDL levels did not significantly change. Multiple other series have shown equivalent results with the DS.

The DS is a durable weight loss surgery that has the best weight loss and metabolic impact of all the surgeries offered. It also offers the least weight recidivism—approximately 5%. It is probably the best procedure for patients with a BMI higher than 50 kg/m^2 and multiple medical co-morbid conditions, including insulin-dependent DM. The downside is that it carries the most peri-operative and long-term risk. Fortunately, the peri-operative risks have improved significantly with the development of the laparoscopic technique. The long-term risks for the most part can be mitigated with good follow-up and diligence with vitamin and mineral supplementation. Despite its benefits, this procedure is rarely performed in the United States, although its popularity is growing.

9.3   SWEDISH OBESITY SUBJECTS

The SOS is a prospective, non-randomized, controlled study. Two thousand and ten patients were recruited between 1987 and 2001 and were matched with 2,037 obese controls [38]. The study was conducted through 25 public surgical departments and 480 primary health centers throughout Sweden. The surgery group was divided between nonadjustable or adjustable gastric banding (376 patients or 18.7%), VBG (1,369 patients or 68.1%), and RYGB (265 patients or 13.2%). The control group received usual care. This trial was unique in that it allowed comparisons to be made between the different surgical types and between surgery and usual care over a very long period of time with excellent follow-up. One of the weaknesses of other surgical series is the high attrition of patients lost to follow-up.

The primary end point of the study was mortality. Mortality data were published in 2007, with a mean follow-up of 10.9 years [39]. The surgery group had significantly fewer deaths than the control group, 101 versus 129, unadjusted hazard ratio 0.76 ($P = .04$). When adjusted for sex, age, and risk factors, the hazard ratio was 0.71 ($P = .01$) (Figure 9.6). The most common causes of death were myocardial infarction (25 control deaths versus 13 surgery deaths) and cancer (47 controls versus 29 surgery patients). The surgery group had sustained and significant weight loss compared to the control group (Figure 9.7 [40]). The mean changes in body weight after 10, 15, and 20 years was −17%, −16%, and −18% in the surgery group, compared to 1%, −1%, and −1% in the control group. In the surgery group, the weight loss was further broken down by procedure. At 10 years, the mean change in body weight was −25%, −16.5%, and −13.2% for the RYGB, VBG, and banding subgroups.

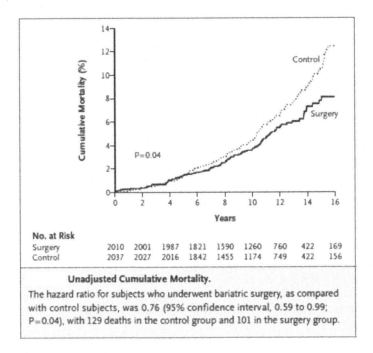

FIGURE 9.6   From the 2007 Swedish Obesity Subjects (SOS) report, showing a survival benefit in the bariatric surgery group compared to the control group. The surgery group had less cancer and myocardial infarction–related deaths.

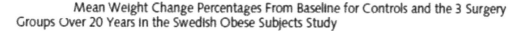

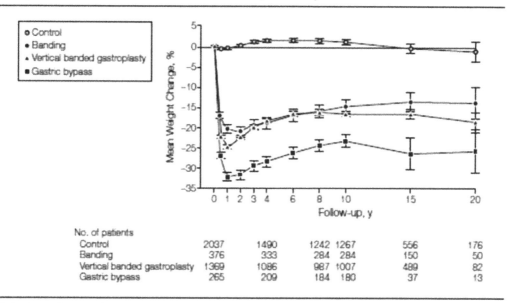

Data shown for controls obtaining usual care and for surgery patients obtaining banding, vertical banded gastroplasty, or gastric bypass at baseline. Percentage weight changes from the baseline examination and onward are based on data available on July 1, 2011. Error bars represent 95% CIs.

FIGURE 9.7 The 2012 Swedish Obesity Subjects (SOS) study report showed continued weight loss maintenance in the surgery group compared to controls.

The SOS series also looked at the long-term impact of bariatric surgery on DM and cardiovascular events [40,41]. *DM remission* was defined as fasting blood glucose levels less than 110 mg/dl without diabetes medication. The remission was highest at 2 years, 16.4% for the control group and 72.3% for the surgery group. At 15 years, the remission rates decreased to 6.5% and 30.4%, respectively. The surgery group benefited from the higher DM remission in that it also experienced less microvascular and macrovascular complications of DM long term than the control group. Higher DM remission was associated with shorter diabetes duration at baseline. This is very valuable in evaluating and treating patients with diabetes, as those who have a surgical intervention earlier are more likely to gain the most benefit from the surgical intervention. Similarly, with cardiovascular events (myocardial infarction or stroke), the surgery group experienced fewer cardiovascular deaths (28 versus 49, $P = .002$) and fewer first-time cardiovascular events, fatal and non-fatal (199 versus 234, $P < .001$), compared to the control group. The benefit of the sustained weight loss from bariatric surgery is clear from these results. Of course, the authors point out that one of the weaknesses of this study is that it is not randomized to procedure or treatment. Ideally, long-term, randomized, controlled trials would be needed to validate these findings. It is hard to dismiss the results of the SOS study because of the strength of the numbers and length of follow-up.

9.4 RANDOMIZED, CONTROLLED TRIALS

Multiple randomized, controlled trials have been initiated since the mid-2000s. The purpose of the trials was to further support bariatric surgery in its effectiveness as treatment not only for obesity but also for type 2 DM. Unfortunately, few studies have presented follow-up to 5 years. Two trials that compared surgery to medical treatment for obese patients with DM have reported their 5-year outcomes [42,43]. One other group has reported the 5-year outcomes of their trial comparing the RYGB and DS in patients with a BMI higher than 50 kg/m² [44].

The group from Sweden randomized 60 patients whose BMI was between 50 and 60 kg/m² to either a laparoscopic RYGB or DS. The main outcome measured was weight loss. Secondary outcomes included cardiometabolic risk factors and quality of life. Of the 60 patients who were initially recruited, 55 completed the study (27 RYGB and 28 DS). There was a statistically greater total body weight loss for the DS patients (40.3% versus 26.4%; $P < .001$) after 5 years. The RYGB patients lost a mean 13.6 BMI units compared to 22.1 BMI units for the DS group ($P < .001$). The reductions in total cholesterol, LDL cholesterol, triglycerides, and fasting glucose were significantly greater in the DS patients. As expected, the DS group had more GI adverse effects and more vitamin deficiencies. Although the DS patients in this study had more re-operations and re-admissions, the authors attributed this to their relative inexperience with the procedure. Overall, this study established that the DS provided better weight loss and impact on cardiometabolic risk factors than the RYGB. As a result of the greater malabsorption, the DS had more risk, adverse GI effects, and vitamin deficiencies than the RYGB. The authors were able to confirm in a randomized fashion what was commonly known in the bariatric surgery literature.

Two other groups performed randomized, controlled trials involving bariatric surgery and intensive medical management of obesity and type 2 DM [42,43]. The trials randomized patients to either medical treatment, RYGB, or another surgical procedure. The other surgical group in the US trial was the VSG and, in the Italian trial, was the BPD. The primary end point for both studies was slightly different. The Italian end point was to identify DM remission, defined as a HgbA1c level below 6.5% without the use of diabetes medications. The American end point was to achieve a HgbA1c less than 6%, with or without the use of diabetic medications. Other end points for both studies included weight loss, quality of life, and other cardiometabolic risk factors.

The American trial was called *Surgical Treatment and Medications Potentially Eradicate Diabetes Efficiently* (STAMPEDE) [43]. It randomized 150 individuals with DM to intensive medical therapy alone or in combination with ether the RYGB or VSG in a 1:1:1 fashion. Eligible patients were between 20 and 60 years old and diabetic, with an HgbA1c higher than 7% and a BMI between 27 and 43 kg/m². Of about 134 patients completed the 5-year trial, 38 in the medical group, 49 in the RYGB group, and 47 in the VSG group. Two in the medical group, 14 in the RYGB group, and 11 in the VSG group achieved an HgbA1c less than 6% with or without medications at 5 years. The only significant predictors of this outcome were a diabetes duration of less than 8 years or random assignment to the RYGB group. The surgical groups required less medication than the medical group. At 5 years, 89% of the patients in the surgical groups were not taking insulin and maintained an average HgbA1c of 7%, compared to 61% of the medical group with an average HgbA1c of 8.5%. Furthermore, 45% of the RYGB group was off all DM medication, compared to 25% in the VSG group ($P < .05$). As expected, the surgical groups lost significantly more weight than the medical groups and had significant improvements in the triglyceride levels, HDL levels, and quality of life scores compared to the medical group. Overall, the benefits of the surgical interventions far outweighed the risk. In fact, the only significant adverse outcome was four operative interventions in year 1 and mild anemia in the surgical group. The other adverse outcome measures were comparable between the groups. The results of this study further confirm that earlier intervention in obesity and DM with the RYGB and VSG is superior to medical therapy alone.

The Italian study randomized 60 individuals to either medical therapy or RYGB or BPD [42]. Eligible individuals were between 30 and 60 years old, had a BMI higher than 35 kg/m², and a history of type 2 DM for more than 5 years. They were randomly assigned to each group (1:1:1). Fifty-three of the patients completed the 5-year trial—15 in medical group, 19 in the RYGB group, and 19 in the BPD group. Fifty percent of the surgical patients achieved remission at 5 years (7 of 19 [37%] in the RYGB group and 12 of 19 [63%] in the BPD group) compared to none in the medical group. Furthermore, the surgical groups had significantly more weight loss, and there was no significant difference in weight loss between the RYGB and BPD groups. The surgery groups resulted in greater reduction of cardiovascular risk and medication use—antihypertensive medication, lipid-lowering agents, antidiabetic medications, and insulin—and diabetes-related complications. The quality of life measures were also better for the surgery group. The medical group had fewer intervention-related complications than the surgery group and, compared to the BPD group, fewer nutritional side effects. Similar to STAMPEDE, the surgical complications were rather benign, and no deaths related to the surgical groups occurred. The main limitation of this study, like the other two, has been the small sample size.

Despite the small sample sizes and relatively short follow-up (5 years), all three of these randomized trials have confirmed that surgical intervention is superior to medical management in treating obesity and type 2 DM. Furthermore, the complications from surgery have not been significant, as demonstrated in the significantly better quality-of-life scores. The one common conclusion from the two diabetes trials is that earlier surgical intervention results in even better diabetic outcomes. The more malabsorptive procedures have more GI and nutritional adverse outcomes, but they do have greater diabetic and cardiometabolic impact.

9.5 CONCLUSIONS

Bariatric surgery continues to accumulate more support for its role in the management of not only obesity, but the obesity-related diseases like diabetes, HTN, and dyslipidemia. The literature support is vast and improving, as randomized, controlled trials in the last 10 years have further confirmed the role of bariatric surgery in the management of obesity and its associated diseases. Fortunately, the complications related to the surgical procedures continue to decline. This will, one hopes, help change the perceptions of individuals and referring providers so that surgery will be considered earlier in the disease process and treatment. Multiple series and trials have shown that earlier intervention, particularly with DM, is more beneficial for the patient.

The surgeons' armamentarium of procedures continues to grow so that they can tailor the procedure to each particular patient. The VSG is the simplest and least "invasive." Yet it carries significant benefit for weight loss, with less GI adverse effects and metabolic impact than other surgeries. Individuals who may need more metabolic impact to help remedy or control problems such as DM or dyslipidemia will benefit more from the RYGB or DS. The RYGB will have more metabolic impact and weight loss than the VSG but with more negative GI and nutritional impact. The DS will have the greatest metabolic and weight loss impact compared to the VSG and RYGB, but at the cost of more significant negative operative and nutritional effects. Ultimately, bariatric surgery continues to play an important role in the treatment of obesity and the medical conditions that are made worse or exacerbated by it.

REFERENCES

1. Flegal KM, Kruszon-Moran D, Carroll MD, Fryar CD, Ogden CL. Trends in obesity among adults in the United States, 2005 to 2014. *JAMA* 2016; 315:2284–2291.
2. Buchwald H, Avidor Y, Braunwald E, Jensen MD, Pories W, Fahrbach K, Schoelles K. Bariatric surgery: A systematic review and meta-analysis. *JAMA* 2004; 292:1724–1737.
3. National Institutes of Health Consensus Development Panel. Gastrointestinal surgery for severe obesity. *Ann Intern Med* 1991; 115:956–961.
4. Kremen AJ, Linner JH, Nelson CH. An experimental evaluation of the nutritional importance of proximal and distal small intestine. *Ann Surg* 1954; 140:439–448.
5. Wilkinson LH, Peloso OA. Gastric (reservoir) reduction for morbid obesity. *Arch Surg* 1981; 116:602–605.
6. Hallberg D, Forsell O. Ballongband vid behandling av massiv överwikt. *Svinsk Kirurgi* 1985; 344:106–108.
7. Kuzmak LI. Silicone gastric banding: A simple and effective operation for morbid obesity. *Contemp Surg* 1986; 28:13–18.

8. Himpens J, Cadiere GB, Bazi M, Vouche M, Cadiere B, Dapri G. Long-term outcomes of laparoscopic adjustable gastric banding. *Arch Surg* 2011; 146:802–807.

9. Kuzmak LI, Yap IS, McGuire L, Dixon JS, Young MP. Surgery for morbid obesity: Using an inflatable gastric band. *AORN J* 1990; 51:1307–1324.

10. Dargent J. Surgical treatment of morbid obesity by adjustable gastric band: The case for a conservative strategy in the case of failure – a 9-year series. *Obes Surg* 2004; 14:986–990.

11. Parikh MS, Fielding GA, Ren CJ. U.S. experience with 749 laparoscopic adjustable gastric bands. *Surg Endosc* 2005; 19:1631–1635.

12. Belachew M, Belva P, Desaive C. Long-term results of laparoscopic adjustable gastric banding for the treatment of morbid obesity. *Obes Surg* 2002; 12:567–568.

13. OBrien P, Dixon J. Laparoscopic adjustable gastric banding in the treatment of morbid obesity. *Arch Surg* 2003; 138:377–382.

14. Puzziferri NP, Roshek TB, Mayo HB, Gallagher R, Belle SH, Livingston EH. Long-term follow-up after bariatric surgery: A systematic review. *JAMA* 2014; 312:934–942.

15. Regan JP, Inabnet WB, Gagner M, et al. Early experience with two-stage laparoscopic Roux-en-Y gastric bypass as an alternative in the super-super obese patient. *Obes Surg* 2003; 13:861–864.

16. Braghetto I, Korn O, Valladares H, et al. Laparoscopic sleeve gastrectomy: Surgical technique, indications and clinical results. *Obes Surg* 2007; 17:1442–1450.

17. Villagrán R, Smith G, Rodriguez W, et al. Portomesenteric vein thrombosis after laparoscopic sleeve gastrectomy: Incidence, analysis and follow-up in 1236 consecutive cases. *Obes Surg* 2016; 26:2555–2561.

18. Parikh M, Adelsheimer A, Somoza E, et al. Factor VIII elevation may contribute to portomesenteric vein thrombosis after laparoscopic sleeve gastrectomy: A multicenter review of 40 patients. *Surg Obes Relat Dis* 2017; 13:1835–1839.

19. Brethauer SA, Hammel JP, Schauer PR. Systematic review of sleeve gastrectomy as staging and primary bariatric procedure. *Surg Obes Relat Dis* 2009; 5:469–475.

20. Hamoui N, Anthone GJ, Kaufman HS, Crookes PF. Sleeve gastrectomy in the high-risk patient. *Obes Surg* 2006; 16:1445–1449.

21. Weiner RA, Weiner S, Pomhoff I, et al. Laparoscopic sleeve gastrectomy – influence of sleeve size and resected gastric volume. *Obes Surg* 2007; 17:1297–1305.

22. Cottam D, Qureshi FG, Mattar SG, et al. Laparoscopic sleeve gastrectomy as an initial weight-loss procedure for high-risk patients with morbid obesity. *Surg Endosc* 2006; 20:859–863.

23. Switzer NJ, Prasad S, Debru E, Church N, Mitchell P, Gill RS. Sleeve gastrectomy and type 2 diabetes mellitus: A systematic review of long-term outcomes. *Obes Surg* 2016; 26:1616–1621.

24. Switzer NJ, Karmali S. The sleeve gastrectomy and how and why it can fail? *Surgery Curr Res* 2014; 4: 180–183.

25. Mason EE. Gastric bypass. *Ann Surg* 1969; 170:329–339.

26. Pories WJ, Swanson MS, MacDonald KG, et al. Who would have thought it? An operation proves to be the most effective therapy for adult-onset diabetes mellitus. *Ann Surg* 1995; 222: 339–352.

27. Christou NV, Look D, MacLean LD. Weight gain after short- and long-limb gastric bypass in patients followed for longer than 10 years. *Ann Surg* 2006; 244:734–740.

28. Sugerman HJ, Kellum JM, DeMaria EJ. Conversion of proximal to distal gastric bypass for failed gastric bypass for superobesity. *J Gastrointest Surg* 1997; 1:517–525.

29. Wittgrove AC, Clark GW, Tremblay LJ. Laparoscopic gastric bypass, Roux-en-Y: Preliminary report of five cases. *Obesity Surg*.1994; 4:353–357.

30. Carrasquilla C, English WJ, Esposito P, Gianos J. Total stapled, total intra-abdominal (TSTI) laparoscopic Roux-en-Y gastric bypass: One leak in 1,000 cases. *Obes Surg* 2004; 14:613–617.

31. McCarty TM, Arnold DT, Lamont JP, Fisher TL, Kuhn JA. Optimizing outcomes in bariatric surgery: Outpatient laparoscopic gastric bypass. *Ann Surg* 2005; 242: 494–501.

32. Adams TD, Davidson LE, Litwin SE, et al. Weight and metabolic outcomes 12 years after gastric bypass. *N Engl J Med* 2017; 377:1143–1155.

33. Scopinaro N, Gianetta E, Civalleri D, Bonalumi U, Bachi V. Bilio-pancreatic by-pass for obesity. II. Initial experience in man. *Br J Surg* 1979; 66:618–620.

34. Marceau P, Hould FS, Simard S, Lebel S, Bourque RA, Potvin M, Biron S. Biliopancreatic diversion with duodenal switch. *World J Surg* 1998; 22:947–954.

35. Hess DS, Hess DW, Oalkley RS. The biliopancreatic diversion with duodenal switch: Results beyond 10 years. *Obes Surg* 2005; 15:408–416.

36. Marceau P, Biron S, Marceau S, et al. Long-term metabolic outcomes 5 to 20 years after biliopancreatic diversion. *Obes Surg* 2015; 25:1584–1593.

37. Scopinaro N, Adami GF, Marinari GM, et al. Biliopancreatice diversion. *World J Surg* 1998; 22:936–946.
38. Sjöström L, Lindroos A-K, Peltonen M, et al. Lifestyle, diabetes, and cardiovascular risk factors 10 years after bariatric surgery. *N Engl J Med* 2004; 351:2683–2693.
39. Sjöström L, Narbro K, Sjöström CD, et al. Effects of bariatric surgery on mortality in Swedish obese subjects. *N Engl J Med* 2007; 357:741–752.
40. Sjostrom L, Peltonen M, Jacobson P, et al. Bariatric surgery and long-term cardiovascular events. *JAMA* 2012; 307(1):56–65.
41. Sjöström L, Peltonen M, Jacobson P, et al. Association of bariatric surgery with long-term remission of type 2 diabetes and with microvascular and macrovascular complications. *JAMA* 2014; 311:2297–2304.
42. Mingrone G, Panunzi S, De Gaetano A, et al. Bariatric–metabolic surgery versus conventional medical treatment in obese patients with type 2 diabetes: 5 year follow-up of an open-label, single-centre, randomised controlled trial. *Lancet* 2015; 386:964–973.
43. Schauer PR, Bhatt DL, Kirwan JP, et al. Bariatric surgery versus intensive medical therapy for diabetes—5-year outcomes. *N Engl J Med* 2017; 376:641–651.
44. Risstad H, Søvik TT, Engström M, et al. Five-year outcomes after laparoscopic gastric bypass and laparoscopic duodenal switch in patients with body mass index of 50 to 60: A randomized clinical trial. *JAMA Surg* 2015; 150:352–361.

10 Postoperative Nutritional Management of the Bariatric-Surgery Patient

Gary D. Miller

CONTENTS

10.1 INTRODUCTION

It is well-recognized that the obesity epidemic is a critical global health issue. Currently, more than 36% of adults and 17% of youth in the United States[1] have a body mass index (BMI) higher than 30.0 kg/m²; globally, 650 million individuals are affected worldwide.[2] Pointedly, addressing the health implications of this condition needs to be a high priority.

A number of treatment options are available to combat obesity. Typically, behavior modification of dietary and physical activity habits is the first line of therapy. Unfortunately, behavioral weight loss therapy, even during well-controlled clinical research and in clinic settings, is modest at best, achieving around 5%–10% weight loss around 6 months. There is also tremendous variability in the weight loss outcome, but this approach can be categorized as having limited success. Additionally, recidivism is high. Alternatively, bariatric surgery has proven long-term weight loss success and is considered the most effective treatment of severe obesity.[3–10] Importantly, bariatric weight loss surgeries demonstrate success in the treatment and prevention of obesity-related comorbidities.[4,11–14]

Other chapters detail the various weight loss surgeries; briefly, these are categorized into restriction, malabsorptive, or a combination of these. Laparoscopic sleeve gastrectomy (SG) is a restrictive procedure, and laparoscopic Roux-en-Y gastric bypass (RYGB) combines both restriction and malabsorption; they are globally the two most frequently performed operations, with approximately 500,000 procedures performed annually.[15–17] Nearly 50% of operations are SG, and 43% are RYGB. Another procedure is the biliopancreatic diversion with duodenal switch (BPD+DS). This has both malabsorptive and restrictive properties, as the stomach revision is similar to sleeve gastrectomy, and the stomach empties its contents into the ileum.

The success of bariatric surgery is demonstrated, with 31.5%–39.0% weight loss at 3 years (62% excess weight loss) for RYGB.[18–20] Maximum weight loss is observed around 18-months after surgery.[21] More than 90% of patients lost more than 50% of their excess weight.[22] Although not as frequent or extensive as with behavioral therapy treatments, weight regain remains an issue in patients, as weight regain of 10%–20% of minimum weight achieved (i.e., maximum weight loss) has been observed[23] in 30%–50% of patients by 18–24 months post-surgery.[19,21] However, even after 7–10 years of follow-up post-surgery, weight regain is only 23%–25% of maximum weight loss for RYGB.[19,24] When examining weight regain based on level of initial weight loss, those who had the most success in absolute weight loss were more successful in long-term weight outcomes.[19]

Because of the anatomical changes that accompany bariatric procedures (both restrictive and malabsorptive procedures), nutrition-related complications can arise. These include symptoms such as nausea and vomiting, dumping syndrome, acid reflux, and nutrient deficiencies.[25,26] Development of food intolerances and dietary adjustments recommended post-surgery, such as reduced calorie intake, can also lead to nutrition concerns. These issues are more prominent in patients who do not comply with the post-surgical dietary and supplement recommendations.

10.2 OBESITY (PRE-SURGERY) NUTRIENT DEFICIENCIES

Demonstrating the presence of nutritional inadequacies in the face of energy excess, a number of studies show that a significant proportion of bariatric surgery patients are at risk for nutrient deficiencies prior to surgery.[27,28] Their medical history of chronic diseases, medication use, poor diet quality, and the required pre-surgery weight loss compromises nutritional status.[29] Having nutrient deficiencies in the presence of overconsumption of calories with positive energy balance is counter-intuitive and often overlooked. The pre-surgery deficiencies should be addressed and targeted in treatment for an extensive period post-surgery. As part of pre-surgery care, patients should be evaluated by the surgeon and registered dietitian to identify nutrient deficiencies and to develop a treatment plan for these, which may include dietary changes or use of supplements, or a combination of these. Poor nutritional outcomes, which ultimately can progress to poor surgical and health outcomes, are common in post-surgical patients, with reports that more than 80% of patients have deficiency in one or more nutrients.[30–33] Correction of pre-surgery deficiencies is important, as this is a strong predictor of postoperative deficiency.[27] Pre-surgery recommendations to assess nutrient status are shown in Table 10.1.

Caron et al. reported the prevalence of nutrient deficiencies pre-surgery as assessed by biochemical markers at 62% for vitamin D, 30% for vitamin B12, 20% for iron, and 8% for vitamin A.[28] They also show that hyperparathyroidism, anemia, and hypoalbuminemia were present in 23%, 14%, and 1% of patients, respectively, prior to surgery. Although others found a low prevalence of hypoalbuminemia in pre-surgery patients, measuring serum levels of prealbumin instead of albumin was more sensitive to low-protein status, as nearly four times more patients had lower levels of prealbumin versus albumin.[34] De Luis also showed that moderate vitamin D deficiency was 71.3% and severe vitamin deficiency was 26.1%.[34] Consistent with others and as further evidence of the vitamin D deficiency, hyperparathyroidism was reported in 22.6% of the patients prior to surgery. Besides vitamin D, other fat-soluble vitamins were adequate in all patients.[34] Deficiencies in folic acid (25.2%), vitamin B12 (9.5%), and trace minerals copper (67.8%) and zinc (73.9%) have also been reported.[34] Taken together, these and other studies illustrate the nutritional problems in this population.

In addition to use of biomarkers to indicate nutrient inadequacy, dietary intake can be used to assess nutritional health. Not surprisingly, there is an extreme variability, as intake ranged from less than 1,000 to more than 7,000 kcals per day in obese individuals.[35,36] The range for relative distribution of calories from fat, carbohydrate, and protein ranged from 33% to 40%, 45% to 55%, and 14% to 17%, respectively.[35,36] At least 40% of obese participants scheduled to undergo bariatric weight loss surgery were below recommended dietary intake values for dietary fiber (94.1%), vitamin D (100%),

TABLE 10.1
Recommended Nutrient Assessments for Pre-Bariatric Surgery Patients

Nutrient	Laboratory Tests
Protein	Serum albumin/prealbumin
	Serum protein
Vitamin A	Serum vitamin A
	Plasma retinol
	Retinol-binding protein
Vitamin D	25-OH cholecalciferol (vitamin D)
	Parathyroid hormone
Vitamin E	Plasma alpha-tocopherol
	Serum vitamin E
Vitamin K	Prothrombin time/INR
	Clotting factor
	Plasma phylloquinone
Vitamin B1	Urinary thiamin
	Red blood cell transketolase
	Serum thiamin
Vitamin B6	Plasma pyridoxal phosphate
	Homocysteine
Vitamin B12	Complete blood count
	Serum vitamin B12
	Homocysteine
	Methylmalonic acid
Folate	Complete blood count
	Serum folate
	Red blood cell folate
	Homocysteine
	Methylmalonic acid
Iron	Complete blood count
	Total iron binding capacity
	Transferrin
	Ferritin
	Serum iron
Zinc	Plasma zinc
	Red and white blood cell zinc
	Alkaline phosphatase
Copper	Serum copper
Selenium	
Calcium	Parathyroid hormone
	25-OH cholecalciferol (vitamin D)
	Serum calcium
	Dual-energy X-ray absorptiometry
Magnesium	Serum magnesium

INR, international normalized ratio.

vitamin E (52.9%), vitamin C (41.2%), folate (47.1%), calcium (52.9%), magnesium (58.8%), and potassium (94.1%).[36] Biomarkers were not measured in the study by Miller et al. to confirm adequacy or deficiency in nutrients. However, others have found that a large proportion of patients were deficient in at least one micronutrient as assessed by biomarkers, despite more than adequate total energy intake.[35,37–39] The most common micronutrient deficiencies were folate, iron, vitamin D, and vitamin B12.

10.3   PRE-SURGERY NUTRITION RECOMMENDATIONS

Patients who adapt from their current pre-surgery diet to established bariatric surgical guidelines have higher compliance with dietary restrictions after surgery, which translates into greater success with weight loss (i.e., reduction of slow weight loss, weight regain, weight plateaus) and reducing nutritional complications (dehydration, abdominal pain and discomfort, heartburn, and dumping syndrome).[26,40] This pre-surgery phase starts as early as from 6 months to 2 weeks prior to surgery.

During the pre-surgery period (6 months to 2 weeks prior to the procedure), patients are encouraged to begin a diet that will lead to weight loss and reduce liver size (in patients with nonalcoholic steatohepatitis). The typical diet for this period is a low-fat program that contains a high-protein meal replacement that is used 2–3 times a day, a serving of fruit, consumption of nonstarchy raw vegetables (leafy greens, tomatoes, carrots, broccoli, etc.), and a 400-kcal meal.[40]

Patients may have clear liquids up to 2 hours and solid foods up to 6 hours prior to delivering anesthesia for the surgery. Furthermore, use of carbohydrate loading prior to surgery has metabolic and clinical benefits in patients undergoing major abdominal elective surgery. The ingestion of an iso-osmolar carbohydrate drink 2–3 hours before anaesthesia reduced hospital stay and enhanced recovery.[42–44]

Additionally, during the period beginning 2 weeks prior to their procedure, patients are encouraged to try and become familiar with the post-surgical diet progression (see description below). This aids health professionals following the patient to identify patient attitudes towards food, willingness to follow the diets, and potential plan for further nutrition education and psychological follow-up.[40,41]

10.4   POST-SURGERY RECOMMENDED DIETARY PROGRESSION

Recommendations for post-surgical dietary and lifestyle guidelines have been previously reported.[37] Briefly, these include life-long use of vitamin and mineral supplements that include iron, folic acid, zinc, copper, thiamine, calcium, and vitamin D, and other micronutrients are recommended post-surgery, dependent on biochemical markers of nutrient adequacy for individual vitamins and minerals. Adequate protein intake (> 60 g protein/day) is encouraged through consumption of supplements or protein-rich foods. Meal patterns include eating up to 6 meals a day that are balanced in nutrients. It is also important to ensure sufficient water intake and consume fluids separate from foods.

Post-surgery diet progression goals are to reduce the risk for gastrointestinal issues, maximize weight loss, and preserve lean body mass. Because dehydration is an immediate concern after surgery, slow, repetitive fluid intake is recommended. This includes drinking clear liquids initially in 15-mL doses every 10–15 minutes and increasing gradually to 100 mL every 30 minutes on the first postoperative day. Hydration status remains a concern throughout the post-surgical follow-up, with fluids consumed slowly and achieving a daily intake of more than 1.5 L.[45] Clear liquids are then continued for 2 full days after leaving the hospital. To reduce consuming excess air, straws and gulping drinks are avoided. Use of low-sugar drinks that contain electrolytes and limited kcals helps heal surgical wounds and restore function of the intestinal tract.[26] By day 3 post-surgery, patients are transitioned to a full-liquid, low fat diet for up to 10 days. This diet delivers protein and some energy, and helps maintain hydration. Besides using protein supplement drinks 1–2 times a day, other foods in this diet may include milk, yogurt, pureed soup and broths, applesauce, and fruit juices (without pulp).

Patients are transitioned to a soft-foods diet around 10–14 days post-surgery at a medical assessment follow-up. These are soft, moist, chopped, ground, or mashed low-fiber foods and may include pureed fruit, canned fish and poultry, fruit and vegetable juices, white rice, noodles, and cottage cheese. Typically, patients tolerate this diet well and remain on it for 2–3 weeks. At the 1-month medical follow-up, patients are assessed for food tolerance/intolerance, hydration, and micronutrient status. If well-tolerated at this point, the soft diet can be progressed to a low-sugar, low-fat, high-protein, solid-food diet. Throughout the diet progression, patients should chew solid foods thoroughly and not drink beverages at the same time as eating. Interestingly, food intolerances remain fairly high, even more than 1 year post-surgery. In a sample of more than 100 post-surgery patients, 30% of the sample reported food intolerances, with the most frequent being red meat, rice, and sausage.[46]

Supplements begin as soon as the patient tolerates the full-liquid diet. The recommended dosages for vitamin and mineral supplements are described below. Specific nutrient dosages for the supplements are described in a section below. For the first 3-months, supplements are used in the chewable or liquid form. After this time, patient will progress to gel-encapsulated supplements. Every 3-months for the first-year post-surgery, patients should be evaluated for tolerance and micronutrient status. Long-term supplementation of micronutrients is warranted post-surgery, as there is continued risk for nutrient deficiencies even 5 or more years after surgery.[28]

10.5   POST-SURGERY DIETARY INTAKE

Measurement of dietary intake post-surgery provides an overview of nutrient intake and helps guide potential alterations to diets to improve nutritional health. Four-day food records were obtained from patients undergoing RYGB, and nutrient and food group intake were measured at baseline and then 3 weeks, 3 months, 6 months, and 12 months post-surgery.[36] As expected, mean energy intake decreased from baseline (2,150 kcals) to 649 kcals at 3-weeks, 877 kcals at 3 months, 1,076 kcals at 6 months, and 1,307 kcals at 12 months. Macronutrients followed a similar pattern, with drastic reduction at 3 weeks followed by gradually increased intake through 12 months, although 12-month intake was lower than baseline for all macronutrients. Dietary micronutrients (not including supplement intake) remained below baseline, even at 12 months, for the following: magnesium, zinc, copper, sodium, potassium, vitamin A, vitamin K, vitamin B1, and vitamin B3. Interestingly, intake of vegetables, grains, and dairy were all lower still at 12 months compared to baseline. This observation for meat intake returning to baseline is consistent with others.[47] Inherent with this low energy intake is a decrease of essential nutrients from critical foods. A high proportion of patients (> 50%) in this study were below the estimated average requirement or adequate intake at 6 or 12 months post-surgery for protein, dietary fiber, vitamin D, vitamin E, vitamin C, vitamin B1, folate, calcium, magnesium, iron, copper, and potassium. These results substantiate the need for dietary counseling in post-surgery patients and that this should still be emphasized even up to 12 months after surgery.

10.6   RECOMMENDATIONS FOR POST-SURGERY NUTRITION MANAGEMENT

Screening of patients for nutritional deficiency begins before surgery (see Table 10.1) with supplements recommended for at-risk nutrients; these screenings are continued post-surgery (see Table 10.2). During post-surgical follow-up, patients should visit a bariatric nutritionist for at least six meetings during the first year, and then have one to three appointments annually.[48] Maintaining support with a multidisciplinary team including nutritionist, psychologist, and medical professionals is recommended, as these communications provide the greatest success in maintaining surgical weight loss, as well as to monitor nutrient status, as nutrient insufficiencies and deficiencies may arise several years after surgery.[49] Furthermore, utilizing a registered dietitian along with the surgeon to deliver care in post-surgery patients provided better long-term outcomes, such as fewer readmissions from diet-related problems, lower cardiometabolic risk factors (blood lipids), and improved nutrient biomarkers as compared to the surgeon alone.[50]

Despite the documented nutrient deficiencies in pre-surgery patients and the benefits for recovery and surgery success when nutrient deficiencies are corrected, claims data from 21,000 patients in a health insurance database showed only a fraction of pre-surgery patients were tested for micronutrient deficiencies.[51] Similarly, monitoring deficiencies post-surgery occurred in fewer than 50% of patients for vitamin D, folate, and iron and in more than 50% of patients only for vitamin B12

TABLE 10.2

Recommended Micronutrient Status Evaluation—Schedule of Selected Biomarkers Based on Surgery Type

Laboratory Test	4 Wk	3 Mo	6 Mo	Year 1	Years 2–5
Hemoglobin	All	All	All	All	All
Ferritin	—	All	All	RYGB/BPD+DS	RYGB/BPD+DS
Iron	—	All	All	RYGB/BPD+DS	RYGB/BPD+DS
Zinc	—	All	All	RYGB/BPD+DS	RYGB/BPD+DS
Potassium	All	All	All	All	All
Calcium	All	All	All	All	All
Magnesium	—	All	RYGB/BPD+DS	RYGB/BPD+DS	RYGB/BPD+DS
Vitamin A	—	BPD+DS	BPD+DS	BPD+DS	BPD+DS
Vitamin E	—	—	—	All	—
Vitamin D3 (25-OH D3)	—	All	All	All	All
Vitamin B1	All	All	All	All	—
Vitamin B2	—	—	All	All	All
Vitamin B6	—	—	—	All	All
Vitamin B12	—	—	All	All	All
Folic acid in RBC	—	—	All	All	All
Parathyroid hormone	—	—	All	All	All

Source: Flegal, K.M. et al. *JAMA*, 315, 2284–2284, 2016; NCD Risk Factor Collaboration (NCD-RisC). *Lancet Lond Engl* 2017. doi:10.1016/S0140-6736(17)32129-3; Colquitt JL, Pickett K, Loveman E, Frampton GK. *Cochrane Database Syst Rev* 2014;8:CD003641–CD003641.

RBC, red blood cell; RYGB, Roux-en-Y gastric bypass surgery; BPD+DS, biliopancreatic diversion plus duodenal switch.

(60% of patients). Although micronutrient deficiencies are relatively common, many patients did not receive pre- or post-surgery monitoring.

Starting on day 1 after discharge from the hospital, a high-potency multivitamin and mineral supplement is recommended that contains at least 200% of the daily value for more than two-thirds of the micronutrients in RYGB and BPD+DS patients.[26] Use of specialized bariatric formulations is desired, as they do not have the enteric coating or are time-released. Because of the competitive interaction with absorption, avoid taking supplements that contain iron and calcium within a 2-hour window.

Adherence to dietary recommendations was examined in SG patients during the first 12 months post-surgery.[48] Data were collected at baseline and 3, 6, and 12 months post-surgery. Most patients (approximately 80%) reported eating 4–6 meals a day; however, patients who reported meeting the minimum recommended protein intake of 60 g per day were in the minority at each time point (3 months = 15%; 6 months = 33%; 12 months = 40%). Furthermore, only 40% of patients attended at least six meetings with a dietitian by month 12. Sixty percent of patients reported adherence to the guidelines for supplements at each of the follow-up periods, with the highest adherence observed at 3 months (80% of patients) and decreases at 6 and 12 months. Supporting the efficacy of supplement use, adherence to supplement guidelines was positively associated with measures of serum levels of folic acid, iron, hemoglobin, vitamin D, and vitamin B12.[48] The low-protein intake in this cohort supports an emphasis to use protein supplements to increase protein intake. The importance of dietary protein lies in its role in preserving lean body mass, enhancing satiety, improving overall nutrient status, and weight management.[37,49]

In a medical chart review of SG patients followed for a mean of nearly 3 years, 90% of patients reported taking a multivitamin and mineral supplement.[28] Individual micronutrient supplements used included iron (24.4% of patients), calcium (38.5%), vitamin D (58.2%), and vitamin A (7.5%).

Clements et al. also presented a high self-reported compliance of 96% in supplement use at 2 years post-surgery.[30] Others, however, found fewer than 60% of patients reported taking their supplement on the prescribed dosage at 12 months post-surgery.[52] In post-RYGB patients followed for 2 years, nutrient deficiencies were common, even with standard multivitamin and mineral supplements.[32] When assessed, additional supplements were routinely prescribed when reference values were below the lower point of the reference range. More than 95% of patients at 2 years were prescribed at least one additional supplement besides the multivitamin and mineral supplement. A mean of nearly three additional supplements were recommended, with the most common being vitamin B12 (80%), iron (60%), calcium and vitamin D (60%), and folic acid (45%).

The development of a nutrition pyramid for post-bariatric surgery patients provides a practical approach for patients to follow.[53] The primary points are energy restriction, adequate protein, low fat, restricted carbohydrate intake, reduction of sugar and concentrated sweets, micronutrients, and hydration. A recent study compared diet behaviors in patients at least 6 months post-surgery to the recommendations of a bariatric food pyramid.[54] Overall, individuals were below recommendations on the intake of protein, fruits, vegetables, vegetable oils, water, and use of vitamin and mineral supplements. The intake of carbohydrates, sugars, and fats was higher, and water intake was lower, than the pyramid.

10.7 POST-SURGERY NUTRIENT CONCERNS AND SUPPLEMENT GUIDELINES

The shortcoming of research in this area is that most studies are retrospective medical chart reviews with a limited number of randomized, controlled trials that have examined the effectiveness of supplements or dietary manipulation on deficiency outcomes. The impact of the surgery on nutrient status and recommendations for treatment options must be considered in this context.

Mechanisms for nutrient deficiencies in post-bariatric surgery patients are multifactorial, depending on the surgery type. In the RYGB procedure, the reduction in stomach volume to 30 mL and bypass of duodenum and proximal jejunum causes not only restriction and malabsorption, but also, importantly, alterations in incretin secretion, gut hormone release, and microbiome.[55–57] In addition to low food intake and dietary restrictions, the exclusion of the inferior stomach decreases acid production needed for vitamin B12 and cation absorption (e.g., calcium, iron, copper, zinc), and malabsorption from exclusion of portions of the small intestine, particularly the duodenum, as it is the primary location for the absorption of a number of macro- and micronutrients.[33,58] Furthermore, the degree of malabsorption of nutrients is affected by different points of anastomosis (proximal, distal, and intermediate) in RYGB procedures. Presence of anemia was higher postoperatively in individuals with a more distal connection.[59] Other biochemical indicators of metabolic deficiency were observed for vitamin A, vitamin D, calcium, and protein in distal versus proximal limb anastomosis.[59] Support for this was also observed in a swine model that compared nutrient digestion between SG and RYGB procedures.[60] The investigators showed that protein, calcium, fat, and ash digestibility was lower for RYGB than SG.

Furthermore, the impact of the surgical procedure on compromised nutritional status is time dependent. Because of adequate tissue stores in well-nourished individuals, biomarkers for nutrient deficiencies are not always affected in the acute post-surgery period. However, with extended follow-up, nutrient depletion often ensues, owing in part to poor compliance with supplement intake.[28] Additionally, with compromised nutrient bioavailability secondary to the surgical procedure, marginal intake over a lengthy period can lead to nutrient depletion in tissue stores that manifest deficiencies up to several years after surgery. Because of supplement use that begins in the pre-surgery period, nutrient status may improve from pre-surgery to the first year postoperatively.[27,61,62]

This section of the chapter details selected nutrients of concern in the post-bariatric surgery patient. These are discussed in relation to biomarkers and symptoms of deficiencies. Protein and several micronutrients (calcium, iron, vitamin B12, and vitamin D) are routinely monitored in post-surgery patients for deficiencies, especially in malabsorptive procedures. However, as some of the research indicates, the duration of monitoring may fall short. Patients are frequently counseled on use of supplements for these nutrients. However, a number of other nutrients, including vitamin B1, vitamin B6, folate, vitamin K, vitamin A, zinc, and copper, are not sufficiently monitored and pose substantial risks in post-surgery patients. Lastly, recommendations for vitamin and mineral supplements in post-surgery patients are presented in Table 10.3.

Monitoring protein status receives significant attention in the post-bariatric surgery patient. The consequence of protein malnutrition is significant, as it leads to postoperative complications, such as poor wound healing and increased risk for infections. Furthermore, lean body mass loss may promote insulin resistance and reduced resting metabolic rate, thereby hindering weight loss maintenance. In a 5-year follow-up of SG patients, hypoalbuminemia was most prominent at 1 year post-surgery, increasing sixfold from pre-surgery measures (1.1% of patients at postoperative to 6.6% at 1 year postoperative).[28] The altered protein metabolism from this restrictive surgical procedure may be the result of reduced stomach size, reduced hydrochloric acid and pepsinogen secretion, selected food intolerance, lower dietary intake, and higher gastric emptying rate.[28,63] Instead of using serum albumin levels as an indicator for protein status, pre-albuminemia levels may be a more sensitive indicator of acute protein status based on its shorter half-life. This shows a much higher prevalence of protein malnutrition, as 14%–52% of surgery patients have low prealbumin levels at 1 year post-operative, even with protein supplementation.[64,65] Similarly, adjustable gastric banding, an alternate restrictive procedure, also demonstrated protein deficiency at 3 months post-surgery, with nearly

TABLE 10.3
Daily Dose Recommendations of Supplements for Prevention of Micronutrients Deficiency Differentiated by Surgery Type

Micronutrient	Dietary Reference Intake	SG and RYGB	BPD+DS
High-potency multivitamin/ mineral supplement		200% of RDA for most nutrients	200% of RDA for most nutrients
Vitamin A	900 µg	3000 µg	3000 µg
Vitamin D	5 µg	10–20 µg	50 µg
Vitamin E	15 mg	15 mg	15 mg
Vitamin K	150 µg	90–120 µg	300 µg
Vitamin B1	1.2 mg	12–50 mg	12–50 mg
Vitamin B12	2.4 µg	Up to 500 µg orally or 1,000 µg monthly injections	Up to 500 µg orally or 1,000 µg monthly injections
Folic acid	400 µg	400–800 µg and 800–1,000 µg for women of child-bearing age	400–800 µg and 800–1,000 µg for women of child-bearing age
Vitamin C	75–90 mg	200	400
Calcium (mg)	1,000 mg	1,500–2,000 mg in divided daily doses	1,800–2,400 mg in divided daily doses
Copper	900 µg	2 mg and 1 mg per 15 mg zinc	2 mg and 1 mg per 15 mg zinc
Iron	8–18 mg	At least 18–27 mg and 45–60 mg in menstruating females	At least 18–27 mg and 45–60 mg in menstruating females
Selenium	55 µg	33	66
Zinc	8–11 mg	8–22 mg	16–22 mg
Magnesium (mg)	—	300 mg	300 mg

Source: Flegal KM, et al. *JAMA* 2016;315:2284–2284; NCD Risk Factor Collaboration (NCD-RisC), *Lancet Lond Engl*, 2017; Colquitt, J.L. et al., *Cochrane Database Syst. Rev.*, 8, CD003641–CD003641, 2014.

63% of patients having low pre-albuminemia.[66] Increased intake of protein post-surgery has beneficial effects with weight management as it leads to increased satiety, enhanced weight loss, and improved body composition, and may be important for preventing weight regain.[67–69] Because of the low total energy intake, protein consumption is compromised. Focus during the post-surgery period is on a protein-rich diet, including supplements, from high-quality sources. These provide the 10 g of leucine per day that aids in stimulating protein synthesis.[70,71] A carbohydrate-to-protein ratio of less than 1.0–1.5 helps with blood lipids and insulin sensitivity.[72–75] The consensus for recommended protein intake is 1.5–2.1 g/kg of ideal body weight (0.95 g/kg current weight) with consumption of a minimum of 30 g for at least one meal per day, and to emphasize protein consumption at breakfast to alter the catabolic state from overnight fasting.[76–78] It must also be recognized that consuming the recommended protein intake may be hard in restrictive procedures, as 30%–50% do not meet these requirements.[77]

The high prevalence of iron deficiency and anemia in obese individuals and in bariatric pre-surgery patients is affected by the chronic pro-inflammatory state on iron absorption. This is evident in that, in obese patients prior to bariatric surgery, anemia was present in 5%–22% and iron deficiency was found in up to 50% of patients.[27,79–85] The increased activity of the immune system disturbs iron homeostasis. Hepcidin, an adipose tissue cytokine that is increased during inflammation, blocks intestinal iron absorption.[86–88] Normally, iron deficiency leads to a decrease in hepcidin and a subsequent increase in iron bioavailability. However, the chronic inflammatory condition and raised hepcidin present in obesity reduces iron absorption. Importantly, perioperative anemia is linked with increased postoperative morbidity and mortality.[85]

The impact of bariatric surgery on iron deficiency is inconsistent, as some research indicates that weight loss reduces inflammation and thus improves iron homeostasis through its effect on hepcidin.[88,89] However, more frequently, prevalence of iron deficiency and anemia does not improve and likely worsens[85,86] based on a number of factors, including the prolonged inflammatory state of the surgical procedure, intestinal anatomical changes that diminish gastric acid secretion and absorptive area of the duodenum, and food intolerances, including avoidance of high-iron source foods, such as red meat.[85] Complicating the issue is that a frequent biomarker measured for iron deficiency, serum ferritin, is an acute phase protein and is elevated with systemic inflammation, and thus may mask the presence of iron deficiency.[90,91] In a recent report, biomarkers of iron status (iron binding capacity, serum ferritin, and hemoglobin) were worse post-surgery than pre-surgery, and these had not returned to pre-surgery levels even after 4 years of follow-up.[23] Others showed that, over a short post-surgery follow-up period, serum ferritin remained normal, but more than one-third of patients had low ferritin at 5 years post-surgery.[92] Over an extended follow-up, new-onset anemia at 3 months was present in 34.6% of patients, and this increased to 80.6% of patients at 4 years.[28] Additionally, from one-third to two-thirds of cases of anemia post-surgery are in individuals who are non-compliant with diet recommendations or use of iron supplements.[93]

Unfortunately, once anemia develops post-surgery, it is frequently refractory to oral treatment,[86,94] and parenteral treatment is required.[95,96] Marin et al. recently reported that an intensive iron treatment, starting with oral supplementation of iron at a dose of the patient's recommended daily allowance (RDA) for 1 month and then adjusting the dose to twice the RDA for 6 months post-surgery, improved iron metabolism better than a standard RDA oral supplement of iron provided for a 6-month period post-surgery.[89] Specifically, the intensive therapy had lower transferrin concentrations and higher transferrin saturation index than the conventional therapy.

Because anemia has a multifactorial etiology, its treatment may be difficult. It is caused not only by iron deficiency, but also by low levels of copper, folate, and vitamin B12. Folate and vitamin B12 deficiency cause macrocytic anemia, differentiating it from microcytic anemia apparent with iron deficiency. Both folate and vitamin B12 deficiencies are frequently present in bariatric surgery patients prior to the procedure, and they persist post-surgery. In pre-surgery patients, folate and vitamin B12 deficiency may be as high as 32% and 13% of patients, respectively.[27,34] Although prevalence of folate deficiency improved, more patients were vitamin B12 deficient at 1-year follow-up. Reduced intrinsic factor from stomach resections, lower acid production, and decreased food intake in post-surgical patients leads to vitamin B12 deficiencies.[28] Use of supplements appears to be sufficient to maintain normal, circulating levels of vitamin B12. However, continued monitoring of vitamin B12 levels is important, as it may take 3–4 years to deplete stores and reduce blood levels. Low levels of folic acid may increase up to a prevalence of 40% of patients after surgery,[97–99] with the primary risk factors being low intake from diet and poor adherence to taking folic acid supplements and not malabsorption.[100] Dosage of folic acid supplements should be no more than 1,000 µg to prevent masking vitamin B12 deficiency.

Although copper deficiency is rare in the general population, anatomic changes from bariatric surgery can lead to copper deficiency in bariatric surgery patients. The reduction in gastric acid from stomach resection and bypassing the duodenum reduces copper bioavailability. Signs of copper deficiency are anemia, leukopenia, neutropenia, thrombocytopenia, and neuropathies affecting muscle weakness, peripheral numbness, and paresthesias. Approximately 20% of RYGB patients were copper deficient at 24 months post-surgery.[101] Interestingly, no difference in copper intake was seen between copper-deficient and copper-sufficient patients, suggesting that the reduced bioavailability is the mechanism for compromised copper. Complicating assessment of copper status is that serum copper and ceruloplasmin, both biomarkers for copper status, are elevated with inflammation,[102] which may hinder the detection of copper deficiency.

Similar to copper, zinc bioavailability is reduced post-bariatric surgery from low stomach acid and reduced absorption area.[103] This is supported by the increased prevalence of zinc deficiency from 4% to 9% in pre-surgery patients to 20%–24% at 18 months post-surgery.[103] Adding to the zinc deficiency are the dietary changes observed in these post-surgery patients, including avoidance of meat and low compliance to supplements.[104,105] Symptoms of zinc deficiency including hair loss, poor wound healing, and loss of taste acuity are nonspecific and observed in post-bariatric surgery patients, making it difficult to detect. One must use caution in treating zinc deficiency with high-dose supplements, as this upregulates expression of metallothionein and may lead to copper deficiency, as it reduces copper absorption through its binding to enterocytes.[106]

There is a decrease in circulating vitamin D levels in obesity. Possible mechanisms for this includes reduced synthesis in the kidney, less sun exposure, inability to use sunlight to initiate vitamin D synthesis, reduced intestinal absorption, and sequestration of vitamin D in adipose tissue.[107,108] Up to 90% of these individuals have vitamin D insufficiency.[27,28,76] Globally, there is a 2.4 times greater odds of vitamin D insufficiency in individuals who are obese versus non-obese.[109] Although vitamin D is well recognized for its actions in calcium metabolism, its role in regulating insulin action, immune function, and cell proliferation is less appreciated.[110] As fat mass decreases with weight loss, this mobilizes vitamin D from adipose tissue and subsequently temporarily increases circulating vitamin D.[33] However, long-term studies still demonstrate vitamin D deficiency in post-surgery patients.[28,111,112] The prevalence of low vitamin D levels decreased from 63.2% in pre-surgery patients to 24.3% at 5 years of follow-up.[28] Generally, the main concern with vitamin D deficiency is increased risk of osteoporosis. Whereas total bone loss was observed in a cohort following bariatric surgery, bone mineral density was maintained, thereby keeping risk of osteoporosis low.[113] Supplementation with both calcium and vitamin D at daily dosages of 1,200–1,500 mg of calcium and above 3,000 IU vitamin D may attenuate bone loss following bariatric surgery.[25]

The interrelationship between calcium, vitamin D, and hyperparathyroidism is well-established. Vitamin D levels higher than 80 nmol/L are needed for optimal calcium absorption and to ameliorate hyperparathyroid hormone secretion.[114] Hyperparathyroidism was present in 23% of presurgery patients, and after SG, prevalence decreased to 12.5% at 18 months, but rose again to 20.8% at 5 years.[28] Others found an incidence of hyperparathyroidism in 41% of pre-surgery patients[27] and in 50% of patients with vitamin D deficiency.[24,115,116]

Fat-soluble vitamins have compromised status prior to surgery based on low levels of biochemical markers. After both restrictive and malabsorptive procedures, vitamin A insufficiency worsened compared to pre-surgery values, but this may be dependent upon duration of follow-up. Prevalence of insufficient vitamin A levels (< 1.4 µM/L) was 7.9% pre-surgery, and by 3 months post-SG, nearly 30% of patients had insufficient levels.[28] However, at 2 years post-surgery, prevalence of insufficient vitamin A levels returned to pre-surgery values. More severe vitamin A status (*deficiency* defined as < 0.7 µM/L) was not apparent throughout a 5-year follow-up in these patients.

Current guidelines also suggest that, in patients with BPD+DS, lifelong supplementation with fat and selected water-soluble vitamins is necessary due to malabsorption of these nutrients.[40] Slater et al. showed in a 4-year follow-up that after BPD+DS, low serum vitamin A was observed in 52% of patients at year 1, 58% in year 2, and 69%–70% in years 3 and 4.[117] In this same study, low vitamin K was seen in 13%–21% of patients during years 1–3, but by year 4, 68% of patients had low levels of vitamin K. Low levels of vitamin D were also seen in 46%–63% of the patients during this 4-year follow-up. In a study that compared RYGB with BPD+DS, individuals were followed for 12 months post-surgery. BPD+DS patients had lower biomarkers for vitamin A and vitamin D and a faster rate of decline in vitamin B1 than RYGB.[118] Vitamin K is at risk for deficiency in post-surgery patients due to abnormally low bile and pancreatic secretions, especially in BPD+DS procedures, and alteration of gut microflora, which provides a significant amount of the body's vitamin K.[119] An oral supplement of 5–20 mg per day or parental administration is recommended.[119] Lower hemoglobin, as well as total cholesterol, were also seen in the BPD+DS as compared to RYGB patients. No differences were observed among groups for other nutrients, including vitamins B2, B6, C, and E; these all remained stable or increased post-surgery. Confounding these findings from this observational study is that adherence to taking supplements was higher for BPD+DS (55%) than RYGB (26%) patients.

Potential for thiamine deficiency is noteworthy, as it is a major nutritional complication following RYGB surgery.[120] This appears to be the result of bacterial overgrowth as oral antibiotic therapy corrected low thiamine levels in post-RYGB surgery patients.[120] The clinical presentations of thiamine deficiency include cardiovascular, neuromuscular, and neuropsychiatric symptoms. The dosage for thiamine in patients is 100 mg twice a day, up to 250 mg given parenterally in those experiencing deficiency symptoms.[119]

In selected special populations, such as pregnant women, there are additional concerns with nutrient deficiencies. For example, offspring from women following bariatric surgery have shorter gestational age, higher risk of being small for gestational age, and lower birth weight than from women matched for BMI, age, and parity without undergoing bariatric surgery, with RYGB showing potentially worse outcomes.[121–124] Interestingly, bariatric surgery helps conception, but there are higher risks for developmental problems from the pregnancy. It is thought that the adverse outcomes reflect poor nutritional status, such as deficiencies in vitamin B12, folic acid, iron, and calcium, and higher anemia rates.[121,125] Importantly, special consideration must be made for folic acid before conception and prophylactic supplementation of folate and vitamin B12, due to its importance for preventing neural tube defects in infants.[126]

10.8 SUMMARY

Even during positive energy balance, nutrient deficiencies are apparent, as evident in the obese pre-bariatric surgery patient. Assessing and then addressing these nutrient deficiencies with dietary modifications and supplements improves surgical outcomes. Based on the anatomical and physiological changes associated with the various bariatric surgery procedures, nutrient deficiencies post-surgery are apparent. Additionally, restricted intake and food intolerances and avoidances can lead to concerns with specific nutrients, both with protein and micronutrients. Life-long monitoring of nutritional health and vitamin and mineral supplementation are recommended. This review details selected nutrients of concern in this cohort and guidelines for preventing nutrient concerns.

REFERENCES

1. Flegal, K. M. et al. Trends in obesity among adults in the United States, 2005 to 2014. *JAMA* **315**, 2284–2284 (2016).
2. NCD Risk Factor Collaboration (NCD-RisC). Worldwide trends in body-mass index, underweight, overweight, and obesity from 1975 to 2016: A pooled analysis of 2416 population-based measurement studies in 128·9 million children, adolescents, and adults. *Lancet Lond. Engl.* (2017). doi:10.1016/S0140-6736(17)32129-3
3. Colquitt, J. L., Pickett, K., Loveman, E. & Frampton, G. K. Surgery for weight loss in adults. *Cochrane Database Syst. Rev.* **8**, CD003641–CD003641 (2014).
4. Mingrone, G. et al. Bariatric surgery versus conventional medical therapy for type 2 diabetes. *N. Engl. J. Med.* **366**, 1577–1585 (2012).
5. Schauer, D. P. Gastric bypass has better long-term outcomes than gastric banding. *Evid. Based Med.* **20**, 18 (2014).
6. Dixon, J. B. et al. Adjustable gastric banding and conventional therapy for type 2 diabetes: A randomized controlled trial. *JAMA* **299**, 316–323 (2008).
7. O'Brien, P. E. et al. Laparoscopic adjustable gastric banding in severely obese adolescents: A randomized trial. *JAMA* **303**, 519–526 (2010).
8. Benoit, S. C., Hunter, T. D., Francis, D. M. & De La Cruz-Munoz, N. Use of bariatric outcomes longitudinal database (BOLD) to study variability in patient success after bariatric surgery. *Obes. Surg.* **24**, 936–943 (2014).
9. Buchwald, H. & Buchwald, J. N. Evolution of operative procedures for the management of morbid obesity 1950-2000. *Obes. Surg.* **12**, 705–717 (2002).
10. Saber, A. A., Elgamal, M. H. & McLeod, M. K. Bariatric surgery: The past, present, and future. *Obes. Surg.* **18**, 121–128 (2008).
11. Douglas, I. J., Bhaskaran, K., Batterham, R. L. & Smeeth, L. Bariatric surgery in the United Kingdom: A cohort study of weight loss and clinical outcomes in routine clinical care. *PLoS Med.* **12**, e1001925 (2015).
12. Hao, Z. et al. Does gastric bypass surgery change body weight set point? *Int. J. Obes. Suppl.* **6**, S37–S43 (2016).
13. Schauer, P. R., Nor Hanipah, Z. & Rubino, F. Metabolic surgery for treating type 2 diabetes mellitus: Now supported by the world's leading diabetes organizations. *Cleve. Clin. J. Med.* **84**, S47–S56 (2017).
14. Adams, T. D. et al. Long-term mortality after gastric bypass surgery. *N. Engl. J. Med.* **357**, 753–761 (2007).
15. Angrisani, L. et al. Bariatric surgery worldwide 2013. *Obes. Surg.* **25**, 1822–1832 (2015).
16. Schauer, P. R., Mingrone, G., Ikramuddin, S. & Wolfe, B. Clinical outcomes of metabolic surgery: Efficacy of glycemic control, weight loss, and remission of diabetes. *Diabetes Care* **39**, 902–911 (2016).
17. Khorgami, Z. et al. Trends in utilization of bariatric surgery, 2010-2014: Sleeve gastrectomy dominates. *Surg. Obes. Relat. Dis. Off. J. Am. Soc. Bariatr. Surg.* **13**, 774–778 (2017).
18. Courcoulas, A. P. et al. Weight change and health outcomes at 3 years after bariatric surgery among individuals with severe obesity. *JAMA* **15213**, 2416–2425 (2013).
19. Cooper, T. C., Simmons, E. B., Webb, K., Burns, J. L. & Kushner, R. F. Trends in weight regain following Roux-en-Y gastric bypass (RYGB) bariatric surgery. *Obes. Surg.* **25**, 1474–1481 (2015).
20. Buchwald, H. et al. Bariatric surgery: A systematic review and meta-analysis. *JAMA* **292**, 1724–1737 (2004).
21. Magro, D. O. et al. Long-term weight regain after gastric bypass: A 5-year prospective study. *Obes. Surg.* **18**, 648–651 (2008).
22. Capella, J. F., York, N., York, N. & Capella, R. F. The weight reduction operation of choice: Vertical banded gastroplasty or gastric bypass. *Am. J. Surg.* **171**, 74–79 (1996).
23. Nicoletti, C. F. et al. Influence of excess weight loss and weight regain on biochemical indicators during a 4-year follow-up after Roux-en-Y gastric bypass. *Obes. Surg.* **25**, 279–284 (2015).
24. Sjostrom, L. et al. Lifestyle, diabetes, and cardiovascular risk factors 10 years after bariatric surgery. *N. Engl. J. Med.* **351**, 2683–2693 (2004).
25. Mechanick, J. I. et al. American Association of Clinical Endocrinologists, the Obesity Society, and American Society for Metabolic & Bariatric Surgery medical guidelines for clinical practice for the perioperative nutritional, metabolic, and nonsurgical support of the bariat. *Obesity* **17**, S3–S72 (2009).

26. Aills, L., Blankenship, J., Buffington, C., Furtado, M. & Parrott, J. ASMBS allied health nutritional guidelines for the surgical weight loss patient. *Surg. Obes. Relat. Dis.* **4**, S73–108 (2008).

27. Ben-Porat, T. et al. Nutritional deficiencies after sleeve gastrectomy: Can they be predicted preoperatively? *Surg. Obes. Relat. Dis. Off. J. Am. Soc. Bariatr. Surg.* **11**, 1029–1036 (2015).

28. Caron, M. et al. Long-term nutritional impact of sleeve gastrectomy. *Surg. Obes. Relat. Dis. Off. J. Am. Soc. Bariatr. Surg.* **13**, 1664–1673 (2017).

29. Frame-Peterson, L. A., Megill, R. D., Carobrese, S. & Schweitzer, M. Nutrient deficiencies are common prior to bariatric surgery. *Nutr. Clin. Pract. Off. Publ. Am. Soc. Parenter. Enter. Nutr.* **32**, 463–469 (2017).

30. Clements, R. H. et al. Incidence of vitamin deficiency after laparoscopic Roux-en-Y gastric bypass in a university hospital setting. *Am. Surg.* **72**, 1196–1202; discussion 1203–1204 (2006).

31. Higa, K., Ho, T., Tercero, F., Yunus, T. & Boone, K. B. Laparoscopic Roux-en-Y gastric bypass: 10-year follow-up. *Surg. Obes. Relat. Dis. Off. J. Am. Soc. Bariatr. Surg.* **7**, 516–525 (2011).

32. Gasteyger, C., Suter, M., Gaillard, R. C. & Giusti, V. Nutritional deficiencies after Roux-en-Y gastric bypass for morbid obesity often cannot be prevented by standard multivitamin supplementation. *Am J Clin Nutr* **87**, 1128–1133 (2008).

33. Gletsu-Miller, N. & Wright, B. N. Mineral malnutrition following bariatric surgery. *Adv. Nutr.* **4**, 506–517 (2013).

34. De Luis, D. A. et al. Micronutrient status in morbidly obese women before bariatric surgery. *Surg. Obes. Relat. Dis.* **9**, 323–327 (2013).

35. Sánchez, A. et al. Micronutrient deficiencies in morbidly obese women prior to bariatric surgery. *Obes. Surg.* **26**, 361–368 (2016).

36. Miller, G. D., Norris, A. & Fernandez, A. Changes in nutrients and food groups intake following laparoscopic Roux-en-Y gastric bypass (RYGB). *Obes. Surg.* **24**, 1926–1932 (2014).

37. Dagan, S. S. et al. Nutritional status prior to laparoscopic sleeve gastrectomy surgery. *Obes. Surg.* **26**, 2119–2126 (2016).

38. Lefebvre, P. et al. Nutrient deficiencies in patients with obesity considering bariatric surgery: A cross-sectional study. *Surg. Obes. Relat. Dis.* **10**, 540–546 (2014).

39. Peterson, L. A. et al. Malnutrition in bariatric surgery candidates: Multiple micronutrient deficiencies prior to surgery. *Obes. Surg.* **26**, 833–838 (2016).

40. Leahy, C. R. & Luning, A. Review of nutritional guidelines for patients undergoing bariatric surgery. *AORN J.* **102**, 153–160 (2015).

41. Thorell, A. et al. Guidelines for perioperative care in bariatric surgery: Enhanced Recovery After Surgery (ERAS) Society recommendations. *World J. Surg.* **40**, 2065–2083 (2016).

42. Awad, S., Varadhan, K. K., Ljungqvist, O. & Lobo, D. N. A meta-analysis of randomised controlled trials on preoperative oral carbohydrate treatment in elective surgery. *Clin. Nutr. Edinb. Scotl.* **32**, 34–44 (2013).

43. Lemanu, D. P. et al. Randomized clinical trial of enhanced recovery versus standard care after laparoscopic sleeve gastrectomy. *Br. J. Surg.* **100**, 482–489 (2013).

44. Ronellenfitsch, U. et al. The effect of clinical pathways for bariatric surgery on perioperative quality of care. *Obes. Surg.* **22**, 732–739 (2012).

45. Stocker, D. J. Management of the bariatric surgery patient. *Endocrinol. Metab. Clin. North Am.* **32**, 437–457 (2003).

46. Ortega, J., Ortega-Evangelio, G., Cassinello, N. & Sebastia, V. What are obese patients able to eat after Roux-en-Y gastric bypass? *Obes. Facts* **5**, 339–348 (2012).

47. Giusti, V. et al. Energy and macronutrient intake after gastric bypass for morbid obesity: A 3-y observational study focused on protein consumption. *Am. J. Clin. Nutr.* **103**, 18–24 (2016).

48. Dagan, S. S. et al. Do bariatric patients follow dietary and lifestyle recommendations during the first postoperative year? *Obes. Surg.* **27**, 2258–2271 (2017).

49. McGrice, M. & Don Paul, K. Interventions to improve long-term weight loss in patients following bariatric surgery: Challenges and solutions. *Diabetes Metab. Syndr. Obes. Targets Ther.* **8**, 263–274 (2015).

50. Garg, T. et al. A postoperative nutritional consult improves bariatric surgery outcomes. *Surg. Obes. Relat. Dis. Off. J. Am. Soc. Bariatr. Surg.* **12**, 1052–1056 (2016).

51. Gudzune, K. A. et al. Screening and diagnosis of micronutrient deficiencies before and after bariatric surgery. *Obes. Surg.* **23**, 1581–1589 (2013).

52. Boyce, S. G., Goriparthi, R., Clark, J., Cameron, K. & Roslin, M. S. Can Composite nutritional supplement based on the current guidelines prevent vitamin and mineral deficiency after weight loss surgery? *Obes. Surg.* **26**, 966–971 (2016).

53. Moizé, V. L., Pi-Sunyer, X., Mochari, H. & Vidal, J. Nutritional pyramid for post-gastric bypass patients. *Obes. Surg.* **20**, 1133–1141 (2010).

54. Soares, F. L. et al. Food quality in the late postoperative period of bariatric surgery: An evaluation using the bariatric food pyramid. *Obes. Surg.* **24**, 1481–1486 (2014). doi:10.1007/s11695-014-1198-x.

55. Nannipieri, M. et al. The role of beta-cell function and insulin sensitivity in the remission of type 2 diabetes after gastric bypass surgery. *J. Clin. Endocrinol. Metab.* **96**, E1372–1379 (2011).

56. Bradley, D. et al. Gastric bypass and banding equally improve insulin sensitivity and β cell function. *J. Clin. Invest.* **122**, 4667–4674 (2012).

57. Laferrere, B. et al. Effect of weight loss by gastric bypass surgery versus hypocaloric diet on glucose and incretin levels in patients with type 2 diabetes. *J. Clin. Endocrinol. Metab.* **93**, 2479–2485 (2008).

58. Poitou Bernert, C. et al. Nutritional deficiency after gastric bypass: Diagnosis, prevention and treatment. *Diabetes Metab.* **33**, 13–24 (2007).

59. Brolin, R. E. et al. Malabsorptive gastric bypass in patients with superobesity. *J. Gastrointest. Surg.* **6**, 195–205 (2002).

60. Gandarillas, M., Hodgkinson, S. M., Riveros, J. L. & Bas, F. Effect of three different bariatric obesity surgery procedures on nutrient and energy digestibility using a swine experimental model. *Exp. Biol. Med. Maywood NJ* **240**, 1158–1164 (2015).

61. Damms-Machado, A. et al. Pre- and postoperative nutritional deficiencies in obese patients undergoing laparoscopic sleeve gastrectomy. *Obes. Surg.* **22**, 881–889 (2012).

62. van Rutte, P. W. J., Aarts, E. O., Smulders, J. F. & Nienhuijs, S. W. Nutrient deficiencies before and after sleeve gastrectomy. *Obes. Surg.* **24**, 1639–1646 (2014).

63. Behrns, K. E., Smith, C. D. & Sarr, M. G. Prospective evaluation of gastric acid secretion and cobalamin absorption following gastric bypass for clinically severe obesity. *Dig. Dis. Sci.* **39**, 315–320 (1994).

64. Verger, E. O. et al. Micronutrient and protein deficiencies after gastric bypass and sleeve gastrectomy: A 1-year Follow-up. *Obes. Surg.* **26**, 785–796 (2016).

65. Moizé, V. et al. Long-term dietary intake and nutritional deficiencies following sleeve gastrectomy or Roux-En-Y gastric bypass in a Mediterranean population. *J. Acad. Nutr. Diet.* **113**, 400–410 (2013).

66. Aron-Wisnewsky, J. et al. Nutritional and protein deficiencies in the short term following both gastric bypass and gastric banding. *PLoS One* **11**, e0149588 (2016).

67. Faria, S. L., De Oliveira Kelly, E., Lins, R. D. & Faria, O. P. Nutritional management of weight regain after bariatric surgery. *Obes. Surg.* **20**, 135–139 (2010).

68. Faria, S. L., Faria, O. P., Buffington, C., de Almeida Cardeal, M. & Ito, M. K. Dietary protein intake and bariatric surgery patients: A review. *Obes. Surg.* **21**, 1798–1805 (2011).

69. Schollenberger, A. E. et al. Impact of protein supplementation after bariatric surgery: A randomized controlled double-blind pilot study. *Nutr. Burbank Los Angel. Cty. Calif* **32**, 186–192 (2016).

70. Layman, D. K. The role of leucine in weight loss diets and glucose homeostasis. *J. Nutr.* **133**, 261S–267S (2003).

71. Layman, D. K. Protein quantity and quality at levels above the RDA improves adult weight loss. *J. Am. Coll. Nutr.* **23**, 631S–636S (2004).

72. Layman, D. K., Shiue, H., Sather, C., Erickson, D. J. & Baum, J. Increased dietary protein modifies glucose and insulin homeostasis in adult women during weight loss. *J. Nutr.* **133**, 405–410 (2003).

73. Volek, J. S. & Sharman, M. J. Cardiovascular and hormonal aspects of very-low-carbohydrate ketogenic diets. *Obes. Res.* **12 Suppl 2**, 115S–23S (2004).

74. Farnsworth, E. et al. Effect of a high-protein, energy-restricted diet on body composition, glycemic control, and lipid concentrations in overweight and obese hyperinsulinemic men and women. *Am. J.Clin. Nutr.* **78**, 31–39 (2003).

75. Shai, I. et al. Weight loss with a low-carbohydrate, Mediterranean, or low-fat diet. *N. Engl. J. Med.* **359**, 229–41 (2008).

76. Heber, D. et al. Endocrine and nutritional management of the post-bariatric surgery patient: An Endocrine Society Clinical Practice Guideline. *J. Clin. Endocrinol. Metab.* **95**, 4823–4843 (2010).

77. Moize, V. et al. Related to protein intolerance up to 1 year following Roux-en-Y gastric bypass. 23–28 (2003).

78. Schinkel, E. R. et al. Impact of varying levels of protein intake on protein status indicators after gastric bypass in patients with multiple complications requiring nutritional support. *Obes. Surg.* **16**, 24–30 (2006).

79. Skroubis, G. et al. Comparison of nutritional deficiencies after Roux-en-Y gastric bypass and after biliopancreatic diversion with Roux-en-Y gastric bypass. *Obes. Surg.* **12**, 551–558 (2002).

80. Coupaye, M. et al. Nutritional consequences of adjustable gastric banding and gastric bypass: A 1-year prospective study. *Obes. Surg.* **19**, 56–65 (2009).

81. Flancbaum, L., Belsley, S., Drake, V., Colarusso, T. & Tayler, E. Preoperative nutritional status of patients undergoing Roux-en-Y gastric bypass for morbid obesity. *J. Gastrointest. Surg. Off. J. Soc. Surg. Aliment. Tract* **10**, 1033–1037 (2006).

82. Yanoff, L. B. et al. Inflammation and iron deficiency in the hypoferremia of obesity. *Int. J. Obes. 2005* **31**, 1412–1419 (2007).

83. Menzie, C. M. et al. Obesity-related hypoferremia is not explained by differences in reported intake of heme and nonheme iron or intake of dietary factors that can affect iron absorption. *J. Am. Diet. Assoc.* **108**, 145–148 (2008).

84. Guralnik, J. M., Eisenstaedt, R. S., Ferrucci, L., Klein, H. G. & Woodman, R. C. Prevalence of anemia in persons 65 years and older in the United States: Evidence for a high rate of unexplained anemia. *Blood* **104**, 2263–2268 (2004).

85. Jáuregui-Lobera, I. Iron deficiency and bariatric surgery. *Nutrients* **5**, 1595–1608 (2013).

86. Muñoz, M., Botella-Romero, F., Gómez-Ramírez, S., Campos, A. & García-Erce, J. A. Iron deficiency and anaemia in bariatric surgical patients: Causes, diagnosis and proper management. *Nutr. Hosp.* **24**, 640–654 (2009).

87. Cheng, H. L. et al. The relationship between obesity and hypoferraemia in adults: A systematic review. *Obes. Rev. Off. J. Int. Assoc. Study Obes.* **13**, 150–161 (2012).

88. Cepeda-Lopez, A. C. et al. The effects of fat loss after bariatric surgery on inflammation, serum hepcidin, and iron absorption: A prospective 6-mo iron stable isotope study. *Am. J. Clin. Nutr.* **104**, 1030–1038 (2016).

89. Marin, F. A. et al. Micronutrient supplementation in gastric bypass surgery: Prospective study on inflammation and iron metabolism in premenopausal women. *Nutr. Hosp.* **34**, 369–375 (2017).

90. Vanarsa, K. et al. Inflammation associated anemia and ferritin as disease markers in SLE. *Arthritis Res. Ther.* **14**, R182 (2012).

91. Weiss, G. & Goodnough, L. T. Anemia of chronic disease. *N. Engl. J. Med.* **352**, 1011–1023 (2005).

92. Gillon, S., Jeanes, Y. M., Andersen, J. R. & Våge, V. Micronutrient status in morbidly obese patients prior to laparoscopic sleeve gastrectomy and micronutrient changes 5 years post-surgery. *Obes. Surg.* **27**, 606–612 (2017).

93. Song, A. & Fernstrom, M. H. Nutritional and psychological considerations after bariatric surgery. *Aesthet. Surg. J.* **28**, 195–199 (2008).

94. Brolin, R. E. et al. Are vitamin B12 and folate deficiency clinically important after roux-en-Y gastric bypass? *J. Gastrointest. Surg. Off. J. Soc. Surg. Aliment. Tract* **2**, 436–442 (1998).

95. Schröder, O. et al. Intravenous iron sucrose versus oral iron supplementation for the treatment of iron deficiency anemia in patients with inflammatory bowel disease—a randomized, controlled, open-label, multicenter study. *Am. J. Gastroenterol.* **100**, 2503–2509 (2005).

96. Kulnigg, S. et al. A novel intravenous iron formulation for treatment of anemia in inflammatory bowel disease: The ferric carboxymaltose (FERINJECT) randomized controlled trial. *Am. J. Gastroenterol.* **103**, 1182–1192 (2008).

97. Shankar, P., Boylan, M. & Sriram, K. Micronutrient deficiencies after bariatric surgery. *Nutr. Burbank Los Angel. Cty. Calif* **26**, 1031–1037 (2010).

98. von Drygalski, A. & Andris, D. A. Anemia after bariatric surgery: More than just iron deficiency. *Nutr. Clin. Pract. Off. Publ. Am. Soc. Parenter. Enter. Nutr.* **24**, 217–226 (2009).

99. Madan, A. K., Orth, W. S., Tichansky, D. S. & Ternovits, C. A. Vitamin and trace mineral levels after laparoscopic gastric bypass. *Obes. Surg.* **16**, 603–606 (2006).

100. Stein, J., Stier, C., Raab, H. & Weiner, R. Review article: The nutritional and pharmacological consequences of obesity surgery. *Aliment. Pharmacol. Ther.* **40**, 582–609 (2014).

101. Gletsu-Miller, N. et al. Incidence and prevalence of copper deficiency following roux-en-y gastric bypass surgery. *Int. J. Obes. 2005* **36**, 328–335 (2012).

102. Prohaska, J. R., Wittmers, L. E. & Haller, E. W. Influence of genetic obesity, food intake and adrenalectomy in mice on selected trace element-dependent protective enzymes. *J. Nutr.* **118**, 739–746 (1988).

103. Ruz, M. et al. Zinc absorption and zinc status are reduced after Roux-en-Y gastric bypass: A randomized study using 2 supplements. *Am. J. Clin. Nutr.* **94**, 1004–1011 (2011).

104. Di Martino, G. et al. Relationship between zinc and obesity. *J. Med.* **24**, 177–183 (1993).

105. Sallé, A. et al. Zinc deficiency: A frequent and underestimated complication after bariatric surgery. *Obes. Surg.* **20**, 1660–1670 (2010).

106. Whittaker, P. Iron and zinc interactions in humans. *Am. J. Clin. Nutr.* **68**, 442S–446S (1998).

107. Himbert, C., Ose, J., Delphan, M. & Ulrich, C. M. A systematic review of the interrelation between diet- and surgery-induced weight loss and vitamin D status. *Nutr. Res. N. Y. N* **38**, 13–26 (2017).

108. Wortsman, J., Matsuoka, L. Y., Chen, T. C., Lu, Z. & Holick, M. F. Decreased bioavailability of vitamin D in obesity. *Am. J. Clin. Nutr.* **72**, 690–693 (2000).

109. Marceau, P. et al. Duodenal switch: Long-term results. *Obes. Surg.* **17**, 1421–1430 (2007).

110. Holick, M. F. Vitamin D deficiency. *N. Engl. J. Med.* **357**, 266–281 (2007).

111. Sánchez-Hernández, J. et al. Effects of bariatric surgery on vitamin D status and secondary hyperparathyroidism: A prospective study. *Obes. Surg.* **15**, 1389–1395 (2005).

112. Yu, E. W. et al. Two-year changes in bone density after Roux-en-Y gastric bypass surgery. *J. Clin. Endocrinol. Metab.* **100**, 1452–1459 (2015).

113. Vilarrasa, N. et al. Evaluation of bone mineral density loss in morbidly obese women after gastric bypass: 3-year follow-up. *Obes. Surg.* **21**, 465–472 (2011).

114. Compher, C. W., Badellino, K. O. & Boullata, J. I. Vitamin D and the bariatric surgical patient: A review. *Obes. Surg.* **18**, 220–224 (2008).

115. Stroh, C. et al. A nationwide survey on bariatric surgery in Germany—results 2005–2007. *Obes. Surg.* **19**, 105–112 (2009).

116. Goldner, W. S. et al. Prevalence of vitamin D insufficiency and deficiency in morbidly obese patients: A comparison with non-obese controls. *Obes. Surg.* **18**, 145–150 (2008).

117. Slater, G. H. et al. Serum fat-soluble vitamin deficiency and abnormal calcium metabolism after malabsorptive bariatric surgery. *J. Gastrointest. Surg. Off. J. Soc. Surg. Aliment. Tract* **8**, 48–55; discussion 54–55 (2004).

118. Aasheim, E. T. et al. Vitamin status after bariatric surgery: A randomized study of gastric bypass and duodenal switch. *Am J Clin Nutr* **90**, 15–22 (2009).

119. Koch, T. R. & Finelli, F. C. Postoperative metabolic and nutritional complications of bariatric surgery. *Gastroenterol. Clin. North Am.* **39**, 109–124 (2010).

120. Lakhani, S. V. et al. Small intestinal bacterial overgrowth and thiamine deficiency after Roux-en-Y gastric bypass surgery in obese patients. *Nutr. Res. N. Y. N* **28**, 293–298 (2008).

121. Belogolovkin, V. et al. Impact of prior bariatric surgery on maternal and fetal outcomes among obese and non-obese mothers. *Arch. Gynecol. Obstet.* **285**, 1211–1218 (2012).

122. Lesko, J. & Peaceman, A. Pregnancy outcomes in women after bariatric surgery compared with obese and morbidly obese controls. *Obstet. Gynecol.* **119**, 547–554 (2012).

123. Santulli, P. et al. Obstetrical and neonatal outcomes of pregnancies following gastric bypass surgery: A retrospective cohort study in a French referral centre. *Obes. Surg.* **20**, 1501–1508 (2010).

124. Kjær, M. M., Lauenborg, J., Breum, B. M. & Nilas, L. The risk of adverse pregnancy outcome after bariatric surgery: A nationwide register-based matched cohort study. *Am. J. Obstet. Gynecol.* **208**, 464.e1–5 (2013).

125. Bebber, F. E. et al. Pregnancy after bariatric surgery: 39 pregnancies follow-up in a multidisciplinary team. *Obes. Surg.* **21**, 1546–1551 (2011).

126. American College of Obstetricians and Gynecologists. ACOG Committee opinion no. 549: Obesity in pregnancy. *Obstet. Gynecol.* **121**, 213–217 (2013).

Section II

Pathophysiology and Treatment of Diabetes

11 Health and Economic Burdens of Diabetes and Its Complications

William F. Kendall, Jr.

CONTENTS

11.1 INTRODUCTION

Diabetes is a prevalent disorder that affects a large segment of the population worldwide. In a conversation with Dr. Joshua M. Pogorelec, describing the economic burden of diabetes and its complications, he summed it up in one phrase: "bad disease; very expensive" (personal communication, 2018). While this chapter will go into more detail, that thought captures the essence of the matter. This chapter will not provide an exhaustive dialogue on the voluminous amount of information that has been published but will address the major associated issues.

11.1.1   What Is Diabetes?

Many diabetes definitions and categories have been developed and published throughout the years. In 1965, the World Health Organization (WHO) proposed the first widely accepted laboratory standard for diabetes mellitus, utilizing 2-hour venous plasma glucose levels after oral glucose loading, with clinical variables considered depending on the patient's age.[1] In 1979, the National Diabetes Data Group proposed new diagnostic criteria, based on observations made on venous plasma glucose distribution in studies performed on Pima Indians and Narouan people.[1] The WHO made new technical recommendations in 1980 and again in 1985.[1] The American Diabetes Association (ADA) released criteria in 1995 that were adopted by the WHO in 1999.[1] The ADA refined and modified its criteria in 2003 and again in 2010, and they were adopted by the WHO in 2011.[1]

Although several other categorizations exist, diabetes is typically divided into four main groups: type 1 diabetes, type 2 diabetes, gestational diabetes, and "other types of diabetes."[2]

Type 1 diabetes occurs due to auto-immune destruction of pancreatic beta-cells. Approximately 90% of patients will have markers of auto-immune destruction at the time of diagnosis, including antibodies to islet cells, tyrosine phosphatases IA-2 and IA-2b, insulin, and glutamic acid decarboxylase.[2] Type 1 diabetes may occur at any age.[2] In younger individuals, there tends to be a rapid rate of beta-cell destruction and development of ketoacidosis.[2] Older individuals tend to have a more indolent course and later development of ketoacidosis, leading to that group often being labeled as having *latent autoimmune diabetes*.[2]

Type 2 diabetes involves insulin resistance.[2] In the majority of patients, initially plasma insulin concentration tends to be increased, although inadequately to obtain glucose homeostasis due to insulin receptor resistance.[2] Over time, due to progressive beta-cell failure, absolute insulin deficiency tends to develop. A small number of patients diagnosed with type 2 diabetes will have severe insulinopenia with normal or near-normal insulin sensitivity at the time of diagnosis.[2] Gestational diabetes occurs when glucose intolerance is identified during pregnancy.

Diabetes is thought to also be caused by various other etiologies, including genetic defects, diseases of the exocrine pancreas, endocrinopathies, infections, and drugs.[2] The genetic defects include mature-onset diabetes of the young (MODY), which exhibits impaired insulin secretion with little or no insulin resistance.[2] It can occur within the first 6 months of life (neonatal) and can be transient or permanent.[2] It can also occur at later age, although most exhibit mild hyperglycemia at an early age. It has an autosomal-dominant inheritance, with the natural history varying depending on the underlying genetic defect.[2] There are various genetic disorders that can involve mutations of the insulin receptor and lead to insulin resistance.[2] Additionally, there are several genetic disorders that lead to diabetes due to unclear mechanisms.[2] Fibrotic changes to the pancreatic parenchyma, due to diseases such as cystic fibrosis or chronic pancreatitis, can lead to diabetes. In addition, diseases such as pancreatic cancer or pancreatic trauma can also lead to diabetes. In the presence of pre-existing beta-cell failure, other endocrinopathies, such as cortisol, growth hormone, glucagon, and epinephrine, can exacerbate insulin resistance. Infectious disease, such as congenital rubella, can predispose to development of diabetes. Other infectious agents are thought to predispose to diabetes.[3] Additionally, various drugs can induce insulin resistance and impair beta-cell function.[2]

11.1.2   Prediabetes

Prior to developing type 2 diabetes, individuals tend to have a variable period during which they have impaired fasting glucose or impaired glucose tolerance.[4] This state has been defined as *prediabetes*.[4] This diagnosis is significant, as the International Diabetes Federation estimated in 2015 that there were approximately 318 million adults with impaired glucose tolerance worldwide, with a projected increase to 482 million by 2040.[5] In addition, the annual progression rate from prediabetes to diabetes mellitus is estimated to be approximately 5%–10%.[5] Older individuals and individuals with severe insulin resistance, low insulin secretion, and other diabetes risk factors are at even higher risk of progression to diabetes.[5] Laboratory confirmation of the diagnosis includes 75-g oral glucose tolerance test with a fasting plasma glucose of 100–125 mg/dL, a 2-hour post-load plasma glucose from 140 to 199 mg/dL, or a hemoglobin A1c from 5.7% to 6.4%.[4] Several other markers have been proposed to aid with the diagnosis of prediabetes. These include glycated hemoglobin; 1,5-anhydroglucitol; adiponectin; fetuin-A; certain amino acids, such as isoleucine, leucine, valine, and tyrosine; α-hydroxybutyrate; linoleoyl glycerophosphocholine; lipoprotein A; triglycerides and high-density lipoprotein; ceramide; ferritin and transferrin; mannose-binding lectin serine peptidase; thrombospondin-1; glycosylphosphatidyl-inositol specific phospholipase D1; acyl-carnitine; micro-RNAs; and certain inflammatory markers (i.e., c-reactive protein [CRP] and interleukin [IL]-6, plasminogen activator-inhibitor 1, IL-18, IL-1 receptor antagonist); and even white blood cell, fibrinogen, and hematologic indices.[5]

The dysglycemia that is associated with the prediabetic states has been linked to an increased risk of cardiovascular events such as myocardial infarction, stroke, and cardiovascular death.[4] In addition, microvascular complications that are associated with diabetes, such as retinopathy, peripheral neuropathy, and nephropathy, have been documented in individuals with prediabetes.[4] The mechanism whereby these complications occur within this subgroup remains incompletely understood.[4] However, it is thought that differing genotypes and phenotypes that affect various insulin receptors and receptor types in different individuals, including brain insulin receptors, subphenotypes of obesity, fatty liver, fatty pancreas, and variations in perivascular fat, collectively and individually impact the varying responses that are seen in different individuals.[6]

11.2 PREVALENCE OF DIABETES

In 2016, the worldwide prevalence of diabetes was estimated to be more than 422 million adults, with a projected increase to 600 million adults by the year 2040.[7] Based on data available at that time, indications are that the top 10 nations with highest diabetes burden include China (109.6 million), India (99.2 million), the United States (29.3 million), Brazil (14.3 million), Russian Federation (12.1 million), Mexico (11.5 million), Indonesia (10 million), Egypt (7.8 million), Japan (7.2 million), and Bangladesh (7.1 million).[7] According to 2017 reports from the US Centers for Disease Control and Prevention (CDC), there were estimated to be approximately 30.3 million people (9.4% of the US population) with diabetes in 2015.[8,9] Of that total amount, approximately 1.25 million have type 1 diabetes.[8] Also of that total, approximately 7.2 million were undiagnosed.[8,9] It is estimated that approximately 1.5 million new cases of diabetes are diagnosed in the United States annually.[8,9]

A meta-analysis looking at 751 studies from 1980 to 2014 that included 4,372,000 adults from 146 countries (Table 11.1) showed increased prevalence of diabetes over that period of time, in all countries with highest incidence of diabetes.[10]

Table 11.2 shows the ethnic distribution of diabetes prevalence in the United States. Interestingly, it was estimated that approximately 33.9% of individuals ages 18 and older (approximately 84.1 million people) were diagnosed with prediabetes in 2015.[8,9]

Although the data for individuals under the age of 18 years is thought not to be very accurate, in 2015, it was estimated that approximately 193,000 individuals under the age of 20 years (approximately 0.24% of that population) had diagnosed diabetes.[9] Also in 2011–2012, the annual incidence of diagnosed diabetes in individuals younger than 18 years was estimated to be approximately 17,900 with diagnosed type 1 diabetes, and 5,300 with diagnosed type 2 diabetes.[9]

TABLE 11.1

Change in Prevalence from 1980 to 2014 in Top 10 Countries with Diabetes

Country	1980 Millions of Adults with Diabetes	1980 % of Global Diabetes	2014 Millions of Adults with Diabetes	2014 % of Global Diabetes
China	20.4	18.9	102.9	24.4
India	11.9	11.0	64.5	15.3
USA	8.1	7.5	22.4	5.3
Russia	7.1	6.6	10.7	2.5
Japan	4.7	4.4	10.8	2.6
Germany	3.4	3.2	5.1	1.2
Brazil	2.7	2.5	11.7	2.8
Ukraine	2.4	2.2	3.4	0.8
Italy	2.4	2.2	4.3	1.0
UK	2.3	2.1	3.8	0.9
Indonesia	2.1	1.9	11.7	2.8
Pakistan	1.7	1.6	11.0	2.6
Mexico	1.7	1.6	8.6	2.0
Egypt	1.5	1.4	8.6	2.0

TABLE 11.2

Ethnic Diabetes Incidence in the United States

Ethnicity	Ethnic Subgroup	Percentage with Diagnosed Diabetes	Subgroup Percentages
American Indians/ Alaskan natives		15.1%	
Non-Hispanic blacks		12.7%	
Hispanics		12.1%	
	Mexicans		13.8%
	Puerto Ricans		12%
	Cubans		9%
	Central and South Americans		8.5%
Asian Americans		8%	
	Asian Indians		11.2%
	Filipinos		8.9%
	Asian Americans		8.5%
	Chinese		4.3%

Source: National Diabetes Statistics Report, 2017. Estimates of diabetes and its burden in the United States, 1–19, American Diabetes Association. Statistics about Diabetes, Overall numbers, diabetes, and prediabetes, http://www.diabetes.org/diabetes-basics/statistics/, Accessed 10/14/2017.

11.3   COMPLICATIONS OF DIABETES

Diabetes tends to be an "end-organ disease" that is associated with various complications. These complications involve deleterious impact on various organs, including the eyes, stomach, kidneys, heart, pudenda, and peripheral nerves. The hyperglycemia caused by diabetes and its sequelae is thought to be the primary causative factor behind many, if not all, of its complications.

11.3.1   Diabetic Retinopathy

The Diabetes Control and Complications Trial clearly showed that, although there was an initial worsening of symptoms observed in individuals that underwent intensive insulin management of their blood glucose, there was ultimately a delay in onset and slowed progression of clinically relevant retinopathy.[11] It is well established that diabetes mellitus is a known cause of multiple ophthalmic issues in adults. These issues include diabetic retinopathy, macular edema, microvascular paralytic strabismus, refractive change, and cataracts.[12] Diabetes has been shown to be the leading cause of blindness in the United States, with 12,000–24,000 individuals with diabetic retinopathy and macular edema, progressing to blindness.[12] Fortunately, although some studies have reported the prevalence of diabetic retinopathy in children to range from 9% to 28%, with the youngest being 5.5 years and the youngest documented case of severe diabetic retinopathy occurring at 15 years old, several others have found no cases of diabetic retinopathy in large cohorts of children ranging from age 0 to 16 years of age.[12] Current guidelines from the American Academy of Ophthalmology recommend commencing annual screenings for diabetic retinopathy 5 years after the diagnosis of diabetes mellitus; the American Academy of Pediatrics recommends either commencing annual exams 3–5 years after the diagnosis of diabetes mellitus or after the child reaches 9 years old, whichever comes later.[12]

11.3.2   Periodontal Disease

Although there is a paucity of "hard data," there is some evidence that the resultant hyperglycemia from periodontal disease may worsen the control and adversely impact the complications of diabetes by serving as a source of chronic infection and inflammatory mediators.[13,14] In addition, there is some concern that diabetes may increase the incidence of periodontal disease, with increased issues such as loss of bone growth and gingivitis.[13,14] The increased periodontal disease is thought to be due to increased formation of advanced glycation end products (AGEs), owing to prolonged high blood sugar levels that occur, especially in patients with poorly controlled diabetes mellitus.[15] The increased hyperglycemia also upregulates the AGE receptors (RAGE), which then causes increased production of pro-inflammatory cytokines and increased tissue degradation, including increased bone resorption and decreased bone formation.[15] This phenomenon, coupled with the adverse effect of prolonged hyperglycemia on neutrophil function (suppressed responsiveness), is thought to contribute to the increased incidence of periodontal disease in patients with diabetes.[15,16]

11.3.3   Cerebrovascular Disease

Diabetes has been linked to cerebrovascular disease, with an increased link in cognitive decline noted in patients with diabetes mellitus, with a prevalence as high as 40% noted in patients with severe, longstanding diabetes.[17] There seems to be a stronger association between dementia and type 2 diabetes than there is with type 1 diabetes, with at least a 50% increase in dementia noted in individuals with type 2 diabetes compared to individuals without diabetes.[18] The associated vascular disease and its impact on cerebrovascular flow and autoregulation is thought to play a role in this process.[17] Although the process remains incompletely understood, it is thought to at least in part be due to interactions between insulin and insulin growth factor (IGF) polypeptides and their receptors in the brain.[19] This interplay affects and regulates a broad variety of neuronal and glial activities, including growth, survival, gene expression, metabolism, protein synthesis, cytoskeletal assembly, synapse formation, neurotransmitter functions, and plasticity.[19]

Studies such as the Rotterdam Study and the Honolulu Aging Study have shown a significantly increased risk of development of dementia in patients with diabetes mellitus.[19] Alzheimer disease (AD) is the most common cause of dementia in North America.[19] Sporadic AD, which makes up approximately 90% of the incidence of AD (5%–10% of the incidence of AD is inheritable), is thought to be related to the effects of brain insulin and IGF resistance.[19] The brain insulin resistance and its adverse impact on IGF-1 and IGF-2 networks is thought to lead to the reduced activation of the receptors and the resultant decreased downstream neuronal survival and plasticity mechanisms.[19] As a result of this and other related findings, some researchers have proposed that AD be reclassified as type 3 diabetes.[19] There is also thought to be an association between diabetes mellitus and vascular dementia, with several studies suggesting that type 2 diabetes contributes to both AD and vascular dementia.[20] The physiologic milieu and the vascular changes associated with diabetes may contribute to some of the changes that are commonly associated with vascular dementia in some individuals. These changes include white matter hyperintensities, cerebral microbleeds, silent infarcts, and cerebral atrophy.[21] Also, the Atherosclerosis Risk in Communities Study showed a fourfold increase in "strokes" in patients with diabetes mellitus when compared to non-diabetic controls, with a correlation noted with their degree of hyperglycemia, based on HgbA1c levels.[17]

11.3.4 DEPRESSION

Diabetes and depression tend to occur frequently.[22] Depression and anxiety are the fourth cause of disability-adjusted life years, and diabetes is the eighth cause of disability-adjusted life years in developed countries.[23] Approximately 25% of individuals with diabetes have depressive symptoms, and approximately 10%–15% of patients with diabetes have formal depressive diagnoses.[22] There is evidence that the presence of elevated depressive symptoms in patients with comorbid diabetes is associated with poorer cognitive outcomes than in patients who have fewer symptoms.[24]

It is not uncommon for depression to be unrecognized and underdiagnosed in older patients with diabetes, in part because some of the symptoms associated with diabetes, as well as symptoms associated with other health conditions, such as thyroid disorders, sleep apnea, polypharmacy, alcohol and drug abuse, and other disorders, may overlap with the symptoms of depression.[25] In addition, some older individuals may present with atypical symptoms of depression.[25] Patient and provider barriers, such as stigma attached to mental health issues, reluctance to report symptoms, prioritization of other health issues, or lack of a good support system, may also contribute to difficulty in diagnosing depression in older individuals.[25] It is estimated that less than 25% of cases are successfully identified and treated in clinical practice.[25] It is also estimated that approximately 75% of people who suffer a depressive episode will have a relapse within 5 years.[25]

Studies in children and adolescents are sparse, but the few studies that have been done suggest that the incidence of depression range from 9% to 26% in that age group.[22] General population risk factors for depression, such as female sex, marital status, childhood adversity, and social deprivation also play a role in the development of depression in individuals with diabetes.[22] Interestingly, one study showed that there was an increased prevalence of depression in individuals with both undiagnosed, as well as diagnosed, diabetes.[23] In addition, there are certain risk factors that are specific to individuals with diabetes.[22] Although the cause is unclear, the rates of depression are higher among insulin users than individuals who are being treated with noninsulin medications, dietary, or lifestyle interventions.[22]

Development of complications of diabetes, such as sexual dysfunction, painful peripheral neuropathy, nephropathy, recurrent hypoglycemia, and poor glycemic control tend to predispose to development of depression.[22] In one study, the presence of two or more complications was associated with a more than twofold increase in the risk of depression.[22] There are some biological changes that occur in both diabetes and depression that are thought to contribute to each one's predisposing to formation of the other.[22] For example, hyperglycemia and hypoglycemia can affect brain function in areas of mood and cognition.[22] It has been noted that prefrontal glutamate-glutamine-gamma-aminobutyric acid levels are higher in patients with type 1 diabetes than in non-diabetic controls, with levels that correlate with mild depressive symptoms.[22] It has also been shown that diabetes affects hippocampal integrity and neurogenesis, which may affect neuroplasticity and contribute to mood symptoms.[22] Both depression and diabetes can affect the hypothalamic-pituitary-adrenal axis and cause subclinical hypercortisolism, blunted diurnal cortisol rhythm, or hypocortisolism with their related effects.[22] Depression can disrupt sleep patterns; and oppositely, poor sleep quality and disrupted circadian rhythms can increase insulin resistance and risk of diabetes development.[23] There is some data that suggests that the use of antidepressant medications may lead to the development of diabetes in some individuals. In addition, HbA1c levels may increase in individuals with diabetes who use these medications.[23]

Chronic inflammation caused by diabetes can predispose to development of depression.[22] Multiple environmental factors including childhood adversity, poverty, and poor physical (i.e., physical disorder, traffic, noise, decreased walkability) and social environments (i.e., lower social cohesion and social capital, increased violence, and decreased residential stability) are associated with worse diet and lower physical activity patterns that can predispose to comorbidities such as diabetes and depression.[22]

A separate but related entity, called *diabetes distress* has been noted to occur among older individuals who are living with diabetes.[25] It includes symptoms such as frustration with self-care, concerns about diabetes complications and the future, concerns about the quality of medical care and the cost of the care, and perceived lack of support from family and friends.[25] The prevalence of diabetic distress is thought to be higher than that of depression, with a prevalence of 18%–35%.[25] Similar to depression, it is associated with poor adherence to treatment and worsening glycemic control, with associated higher rates of diabetic complications, reduced self-care, and increased morbidity.[25,26] A few tools, such as the Diabetes Distress Scale or the Problem Areas in Diabetes, can help to identify this entity.[25] Unfortunately, only a few validated treatments are available.[25]

11.3.5 Cardiac Disease

Diabetes is associated with development of coronary artery disease, with small, diffuse, calcified, multi-vessel disease along with autonomic neuropathy.[27] Cardiac autonomic neuropathy has been estimated to occur in 17%–66% of patients with type 1 diabetes and 31%–73% of patients with type 2 diabetes.[27] Although there is some controversy, several risk factors, such as duration of diabetes, glycemic control, presence of cardiovascular risk factors, gender, and presence of other microvascular complications, are thought to predict or play a role in the development of cardiac autonomic neuropathy.[27] The resultant parasympathetic denervation and sympathetic predominance is thought to lead to progressive issues including reduced heart rate variability, resting tachycardia or bradycardia, reduced exercise tolerance, orthostatic hypotension, QT prolongation, loss of nocturnal decline in blood pressure, and silent ischemia.[27,28]

Cardiac autonomic neuropathy can lead to cardiomyopathy and contribute to lower-limb complications; chronic kidney disease; increased risk of anesthetic-related complications, due to inability to vasoconstrict correctly; and increased risk of perioperative morbidity and mortality due to propensity to intraoperative hypothermia.[27] Interestingly, in patients with diabetes without known cardiovascular complications, although nonspecific, some characteristic electrocardiogram (EKG) changes have been noted to occur, which include tachycardia, shortening of the QRS and QT intervals, increased dispersion of the QT interval, and decrease in T-wave amplitude.[29] Although controversial, the anatomic and physiologic changes that occur in individuals with diabetes are thought to increase the occurrence of arrhythmias, such as atrial fibrillation and ventricular arrhythmias, and contribute to the associated morbidity and mortality.[30]

The ACCORD trial has shown cardiac autonomic neuropathy to be an independent predictor of all-cause mortality.[27] In addition, the EURODIAB IDDM Complication Trial has shown cardiac autonomic neuropathy to have the strongest association with mortality, when compared to other factors.[27] Also, some studies have shown a 5-year mortality rate of 16%–50% in both type 1 and type 2 diabetes once cardiac autonomic neuropathy had been diagnosed, with most mortality attributed to sudden cardiac death.[27]

11.3.6 DIABETIC GASTROPARESIS

Gastroparesis is defined as delayed gastric emptying without mechanical obstruction.[31] Although other causes can lead to gastroparesis, diabetes is the most common causative etiology.[31] Incidence is estimated to be approximately 4.8%–5.0% in individuals with type 1 diabetes, 1% in those with type 2 diabetes, and 0.1%–1.0% in individuals without diabetes.[31,32] Diabetic gastroparesis is thought to be due to development of autonomic and enteric nervous system dysfunction.[31] Although the natural history of diabetic gastroparesis is not well understood, there does seem to be a negative impact on quality of life (increased complaints of upper abdominal pain or discomfort) and a mortality rate of 4%–38%, although it is not clear that the mortality is related directly to gastroparesis.[32] Interestingly, up to 40% of individuals with gastroparesis are asymptomatic.[32] In addition to diabetic gastroparesis, up to 75% of individuals with diabetic neuropathy can also present with various symptoms that include nausea, bloating, abdominal pain, diarrhea, constipation, delayed gastric emptying, impaired oral drug absorption, and malnutrition.[33] These and other related symptoms can lead to poor quality of life and high rates of hospitalization.[32]

11.3.7 DIABETIC NEPHROPATHY

Diabetic renal disease occurs in 20%–40% of patients with diabetes.[34] Elevated albumin excretion and reduced glomerular filtration rate are utilized in the definition of diabetic renal nephropathy.[34] Although other classification schemes, such as the Banff classification, exist for renal allograft pathology, one of the recent classification schemes designed specifically for diabetic nephropathy, the Tervaert classification, describes four different types of lesions that can be identified in diabetic nephropathy.[35–37] These include: class 1 (mild or nonspecific changes on light microscopy and confirmed glomerular basement membrane (GBM) thickening proven by electron microscopy); class 2a (mild mesangial expansion in > 25% of observed mesangium; area of mesangial proliferation < area of capillary activity); class 2b (severe mesangial expansion in > 25% of observed mesangium; area of mesangial proliferation < area of capillary activity); class 3 (at least one convincing nodular sclerosis [Kimmelstein-Wilson lesion]); class 4 (advanced diabetic glomerulosclerosis in > 50% of glomeruli).[35] Approximately one-third of patients with diabetes show microalbuminuria after 15 years of disease duration, with fewer than one-half developing real clinical nephropathy.[34] When diabetic nephropathy occurs, it tends to occur in stages: stage 1 (glomerular filtration rate [GFR] is either normal or decreased; tends to last around 5 years from the onset of diabetes; size of kidneys tends to increase by 20% and renal plasma flow tends to increase by 10%–15%, but no albuminuria or hypertension tends to be present); stage 2 (may begin as soon as 2 years after the onset of disease; thickening of basement membrane and mesangial proliferation, but GFR remains normal with no clinical signs of the disease; many patients remain in this stage for life); stage 3 (first clinical detectable sign of glomerular damage and microalbuminuria [albumin 30–300 mg/day]; tends to occur 5–10 years after the onset of the disease, with or without hypertension); stage 4 (irreversible proteinuria [> 300 mg/day]; GFR < 60 mL/min per 1/73 m^2 and sustained hypertension; and stage 5 (GFR < 15 mL/min/1.73m^2).[34] Nearly one-half of patients who progress to stage 5 renal disease will require some form of replacement therapy (peritoneal dialysis, hemodialysis, or renal transplantation).[34]

11.3.8 Lower-Extremity Complications

Diabetic complications in the lower extremities are multifactorial and result from complex interplay between diabetic vasculopathy, neuropathy, structural deformity, and decreased immunity.[38] Lower-limb atherosclerosis tends to occur more distally in diabetic subjects and preferentially affects the arteries below the knees.[38] Ten percent to 18% of people have peripheral neuropathy at the time of their diagnosis; after 5 years of disease duration, approximately 26% have peripheral neuropathy, and at 10 years, approximately 41% have peripheral neuropathy, with at least 50% of people with diabetes eventually developing peripheral neuropathy.[39] Charcot osteopathic neuropathy is a chronic condition affecting the bones, joints, and soft tissues, most commonly of the foot and ankle. It is estimated to occur in 0.4%–13% of patients with diabetes. As a result of multiple factors, including the ones mentioned above, there is also a related propensity to development of fat atrophy, callus formation, ulceration sinus tracts, and avascular necrosis of pedal bones, which can lead to cellulitis and abscess formation, and can also lead to development of worsening sequelae such as osteomyelitis and necrotizing fasciitis.[38,40]

11.3.9 Urologic Complications

Approximately 50% of males and females with diabetes develop some degree of bladder cystopathy.[40] The resultant diminished bladder filling sensation and decreased contractility, with its resultant increased post-void residual, predisposes these individuals to increased risk of infections, lithiasis, and renal damage.[41] Sexual dysfunction (decreased libido, orgasmic abnormalities, and erectile dysfunction) affects both male and female individuals with diabetes.[41] The pathophysiology of diabetic sexual dysfunction is multifactorial and is due to vascular, neurologic, and hormonal causes.[42] It is estimated that 46% of males with type 2 diabetes have sexual dysfunction, in comparison to 32% of males without diabetes.[41] Seventy-one percent of women with type 1 diabetes and 42% of women with type 2 diabetes have sexual dysfunction, in comparison to a 25%–63% sexual dysfunction occurrence in women without diabetes.[41]

11.4 OTHER COMPLICATIONS

11.4.1 Benign Tumor and Cancer Associations

Diabetic mastopathy, also known as sclerosing lymphocytic lobulitis and lymphocytic mastopathy, is an uncommon, non-malignant, mass-forming lesion that has been noted in patients with diabetes.[43] It is more commonly in those with longstanding type 1 diabetes, although it has been seen in patients with type 2 diabetes.[43] It has been seen in patients with autoimmune disorders such as Hashimoto's thyroiditis.[43] Additionally, it has been seen in patients without diabetes or autoimmune disorders.[42] It occurs most commonly in premenopausal women, although it has been seen in postmenopausal women and men.[43–45] Although the cause is not fully understood, several possible causative theories exist: (1) It is postulated that hyperglycemia causes stromal matrix expansion and accumulation of advanced glycosylation end products, which then ultimately lead to an inflammatory B-cell response[43,44]; (2) it may be caused by extracellular expansion secondary to stimulated transcription of fibroblast mRNA due to a prolonged hyperglycemic state[45]; (3) it may be caused by extracellular matrix expansion secondary to stimulated transcription of fibroblast mRNA related to the hyperglycemic state; (4) it may develop due to an immunologic response to exogenous insulin.[42]

Evidence suggests that diabetes may contribute to breast cancer risk.[46] Up to 16% of patients with breast cancer have type 2 diabetes.[46] Conversely, type 2 diabetes has been associated with a 10%–20% excessive risk of breast cancer.[46] Several studies have implicated the role of sustained hyperglycemia, hyperinsulinemia, insulin resistance, hyperinsulinemia-related increase of insulin-like growth-factor, and the long-term pro-inflammatory condition associated with the dysregulated metabolism caused by poor glycemic control in cancer promotion and progression.[46] Although there have been some conflicting results, other than metformin, which seems to reduce cancer risk, many other antidiabetic treatments (i.e., insulin, insulin analogues, and insulin secretagogues) have been associated with increased risk of cancer.[46]

Similar mechanisms are thought to contribute to increased risk of cancers in other organs, including liver, pancreas, colorectal, endometrial, and bladder.[47,48] In addition, hyperglycemia may lead to increased reactive oxygen species (ROS) on tumor cells, which can lead to DNA damage that may give rise to mutations in proto-oncogenes, tumor suppressor genes, and other changes that are favorable for tumor growth.[48]

A meta-analysis of patients with pancreatic cancer showed that risk of mortality seemed higher in patients with resected or resectable tumors than in patients with unresectable tumors.[49] Mortality risk was also higher in patients with new-onset diabetes than in patients with longstanding diabetes. No causative factor for these findings could be identified.[49]

11.4.2 PERIOPERATIVE ISSUES AND WOUND HEALING

The importance of perioperative diabetes control has been continually validated.[50] Poor perioperative diabetes control has been associated with infection, poor wound healing, metabolic derangements, and increased mortality.[50] Stress related to surgery and anesthesia causes release of neuroendocrine hormones that can lead to insulin resistance and hyperglycemia, which can complicate perioperative glucose control.[49] Hyperglycemia can cause endothelial cell dysfunction and impair neutrophil phagocytic function, which increases the risk of infection.[50]

In cardiothoracic surgery, hyperglycemia has been associated with sternal wound infections and other infections.[50] Hemoglobin A_{1c} greater than 8.6% has been associated with increase in mortality, myocardial infarction, and sternal wound infection after coronary artery bypass grafting.[50] In noncardiac surgery, perioperative hyperglycemia has been associated with increased risk of infection, acute renal failure, and increased length of stay.[50] Although not fully elucidated, it seems that the physiologic changes associated with diabetes may cause anti-angiogenic and anti-capillary maturation factors in wounds, which may adversely impact the formation of new vessels and wound and contribute to poor wound healing.[51]

11.4.3 EFFECT OF DIABETES ON BONE FORMATION

Type 1 diabetes has been shown to impact osteoblasts and osteocytes.[52,53] Although controversial, it has been noted in some studies that osteoblast-promoting factors, such as Runt-related transcription factor 2 (a master regulator of bone development) and Wnt/beta catenin pathway (essential for osteoblast differentiation and regulation of bone formation in differentiated osteoblasts) are reduced in diabetes.[52] IGF-1 has been shown to be fundamental for growth and maturation of osteoblasts.[52] It seems to stimulate growth and differentiation of osteoblasts from mesenchymal cells both in vivo and in vitro and is essential for bone mineralization.[52] These actions are thought to be mediated through stimulation of IGF-1 receptors.[52] It has been shown that insulin has the ability to stimulate the IGF-1 receptors in addition to stimulating its own insulin receptors (IR receptors).[52] Absence or decrease of IGF-1 and insulin-signaling cells in cells of the osteoblast lineage could at least in part affect osteoblast activity and bone formation.[52] The oxidative stress present in diabetic bone may also contribute to apoptosis of osteoprogenitor cells, which may affect the survival of osteoblast cells.[52,53] Physiologic factors caused by hyperglycemia, including the upregulation of inflammatory cytokines and production of AGEs, have been shown to affect osteoblasts and contribute to poor bone healing.[51] Osteoclast differentiation also seems to be enhanced by hyperglycemia.[52] Meta-analysis has shown an increased risk of fracture in men and women with diabetes, in Europe and the United States.[53] In addition, the healing of fractures in patients with diabetes is prolonged by 87%, and there is a 3.4-fold higher risk of complications, including delayed union, nonunion, re-dislocation, and pseudoarthrosis.[53]

11.4.4   DIABETES-INDUCED CHANGES IN PREGNANCY

Meta-analysis has shown that poor glycemic control before and during gestation is a relevant factor, affecting obstetrical fetal and neonatal outcomes.[54] Pre-eclampsia is a frequent complication and seems to be related to endothelial dysfunction, insulin resistance, and poor glucose control in early pregnancy.[54] It was observed that in patients with type 1 diabetes without nephropathy, the incidence of eclampsia was 15%–20%; in contrast, the risk of eclampsia in patient with type 1 diabetes and nephropathy was approximately 50%.[54] This suggests that nephropathy, which is more frequent in type 1 diabetes, may be an independent risk factor for onset of pre-eclampsia.[54] Preterm delivery is another common complication that tends to occur in women with pregestational diabetes.[54] The incidence is 33.6% in women with type 1 diabetes and 32% in women with type 2 diabetes.[53] HbA1c higher than 8% and pre-existing nephropathy cause an increased risk of gestational hypertension and pre-eclampsia, which are both independently associated with preterm delivery.[54] Pregestational diabetic women also have an increased risk of preterm pregnancy termination due to impairment of fetal status due to various reasons, including intrauterine death, growth restriction, poor glycemic control, congenital malformation, macrosomia, acute polyhydramnios, and acute fatty liver of pregnancy.[54] It was observed that the mean prevalence of perinatal death was 2.05% in women with type 1 diabetes and 3.36% in women with type 2 diabetes.[54] In addition, the mean prevalence of stillbirth was 2.8% in women with type 1 diabetes and 1.9% in women with type 2 diabetes.[53] The mean prevalence of macrosomia has been noted to be 22.3% in women with type 1 diabetes and 21.7% in women with type 2 diabetes.[54] Newborns from diabetic preterm deliveries were noted to be more susceptible to perinatal complications than non-diabetic preterm neonates, as they have an increased risk of growth retardation, hypoglycemia, hypocalcemia, polycythemia, hyperbilirubinemia, several types of malformations, cardiomyopathy, and asphyxia.[54]

Gestational diabetes causes an increased risk of cesarean section as well as an increased risk of pre-eclampsia.[55] Compared to gestational patients without metabolic abnormalities, there is a 50 times increased risk of mild and severe pre-eclampsia in patients that have gestational diabetes mellitus.[55] Gestational diabetes may also lead to fetal complications including hypoglycemia, hypocalcemia, respiratory distress, stillbirth, and macrosomia that can be associated with birth trauma.[55] Fetal malformation may also occur, especially when gestational diabetes begins early (in the first trimester).[54]

11.5   FINANCIAL IMPACT

As shown above, in addition to being a prevalent and ever-increasing disease, diabetes is a multitentacled disease that can affect many facets of the patient's life. So, even as we discuss its financial impact, our estimations may be falsely minimized, because we may not be able to account for all of its associated costs. One of the main drivers of the high costs associated with diabetes seems to be the associated complications, many of which tend to be sequelae of its related hyperglycemia.[56]

In addition, to the annual progression rate from prediabetes to diabetes mellitus is estimated to be approximately 5%–10%.[57] It is also estimated that, without weight loss and moderate physical activity, approximately 15%–30% of people with prediabetes will develop type 2 diabetes within 5 years.[57] Furthermore, they also have an increased risk for developing heart disease and stroke.[5,57]

In patients with prediabetes, there tends to be an excessive use of ambulatory care services for comorbidities that are associated with diabetes.[57] The annual cost per case for prediabetes in 2007 was estimated to be approximately $443, with the estimated annual global cost for prediabetes in the United States being more than $25 billion.[57] By comparison, the estimated cost per case was estimated to be $2,864 for undiagnosed diabetes and $9,975 for diagnosed type 2 diabetes.[57] The estimated direct medical cost for type 2 diabetes in the United States in 2007 was approximately $176 billion.[57] One study showed that healthcare expenditure increased by $1,429 during the first year, then by $3,621 during the first 3 years in privately insured patients diagnosed with prediabetes that progressed to type 2 diabetes.[57]

Table 11.3 shows results from a study that looked at costs associated with patients diagnosed with prediabetes in the South Carolina Medicaid claims database between January 2009 and December 2013. In addition to the related costs shown in the table, the costs associated with outpatient services accounted for 36%–45% of the total cost over 3 years for all groups of patients.[57] Also, in that study, after they adjusted for demographic and other comorbid conditions, the annual total health care costs related to diabetes in patients who progressed to diabetes were 22.1% (first year), 39.1% (second year), and 47.6% (third year) higher than those who did not progress to diabetes ($P < .001$ for all three groups).[57]

Estimating the lifetime cost of diabetes for individuals is complex, in part because of the impact of lost life-years due to diabetes that varies depending on the age at diagnosis.[58] Table 11.4 shows the estimated lost life-years due to diabetes, based on age of diagnosis.

Table 11.5 shows the mean estimated survival age, depending on the age at time of diagnosis; and Table 11.6 shows the associated incremental lifetime diabetes-related healthcare expenditure based on the age at time of diagnosis.[58]

TABLE 11.3
Annual Costs for Patients Who Progressed from Prediabetes to Diabetes vs Those Who Did Not

	Annual Medical Cost for Patients Who Progressed from Prediabetes to Diabetes	Annual Medical Cost for Patients Who Did Not Progress from Prediabetes to Diabetes	Annual Total Health Care Cost for Patients Who Progressed from Prediabetes to Diabetes	Annual Total Healthcare Cost for Patients Who Did Not Progress from Prediabetes to Diabetes
First year	$14,744	$10,715	$17,506	$12,650
Second year	$10,708	$7,181	$13,428	$9,258
Third year	$12,438	$7,657	$15,151	$9,935

Source: Wu, J. et al., *J. Manag. Care Spec. Pharm.*, 23, 309–316, 2017.
Note: $P < .001$ for all three groups.

TABLE 11.4
Estimated Lost Life-Years Due to Diabetes, Based on Age at Diagnosis

	If Diagnosed at Age 40	If Diagnosed at Age 50	If Diagnosed at Age 60	If Diagnosed at Age 65
Men	7.1	6.0	5.0	4.5
Women	6.2	5.6	4.9	4.4

Source: Zhuo, X. et al., *Diab. Care*, 37, 2557–2564, 2014.

TABLE 11.5
Mean Estimated Survival Age, Depending on Age at Diagnosis

	If Diagnosed at Age 40	If Diagnosed at Age 50	If Diagnosed at Age 60	If Diagnosed at Age 65
Men	72.1	74.5	77.3	79.0
Women	76.5	78.2	80.1	81.4

TABLE 11.6

Associated Incremental Lifetime Diabetes-Related Healthcare Expenditure Depending on Age at Diagnosis

	If Diagnosed at Age 40	If Diagnosed at Age 50	If Diagnosed at Age 60	If Diagnosed at Age 65
Men	$109,000	$79,900	$46,600	$30,800
Women	$138,100	$101,800	$60,800	$40,900

Source: Zhuo, X. et al., *Diab. Care*, 37, 2557–2564, 2014.

For individuals diagnosed after age 65, the excess lifetime spending related to diabetes ranged from $23,900 to $40,900, depending on sex and age at diagnosis.[58] In all age groups, the cost of medical spending was higher in women than men; also, the cost of medical spending was higher in patients with diabetes than patients without diabetes.[58]

A study published in 2013 that reviewed the healthcare costs of diabetes in 2012 showed that the main components of healthcare costs are hospital inpatient care (43% of total medical cost), prescription medications used to treat the complications of diabetes (18%), antidiabetic agents and diabetic supplies (12%), physician office visits (9%), and nursing/residential facility stays (8%).[59] The total estimated cost at that time was $245 billion, which included $176 billion in direct medical costs and $69 billion in reduced productivity.[59]

In addition to direct costs, there are indirect costs associated with diabetes that include increased absenteeism ($5 billion), reduced productivity while at work ($20.8 billion) for employed individuals, reduced productivity for individuals not in the labor force ($2.7 billion), inability to work as a result of disease-related disability ($21.6 billion), and lost productive capacity due to early mortality ($18.5 billion).[59] Other costs that have been more difficult to quantify include intangible cost from patients' pain and suffering, resources from care provided by nonpaid caregivers, and the issues and burdens associated with undiagnosed diabetes.[59]

A recent study looking at the worldwide cost of diabetes in 2014 estimated the total direct global cost of diabetes to be approximately $825 billion, with the highest approximate costs noted in four countries: China, estimated to be $170 billion; United States, $105 billion; India, $73 billion; and Japan, $37 billion.[10] The investigators also noted that approximately 60% of the global costs occur in low- and middle-income countries, where a substantial portion of the treatment costs are paid "out-of-pocket," affecting treatment utilization and adherence, and leading to financial hardship for patients and their families.[10]

11.6 CLOSING THOUGHTS

Diabetes is a significant and global medical problem that has significant complications with both direct and indirect costs. It is crucial that we do what we can to control progression of the disease with diet, exercise, and medical management, as well as continue to increase our awareness of the extent of its potential impact on various aspects of our lives.

REFERENCES

1. Kumar R, Nandhini LP, Kamalanathan S, Sahoo J, Vivekanadan M. Evidence for current diagnostic criteria of diabetes mellitus. *World J Diabetes*. 2016 Sept 15. 7(17): 396–405.
2. De Groot LJ, Chrousos G, Dungan K, et al., editors. *NCBI Bookshelf. Endotext* [Internet]. South Dartmouth (MA): MDText.com; 2000.
3. Chakraborty S, Bhattacharyya R, Banerjee D. Chapter six – Infections: A possible risk factor for type 2 diabetes. *Adv Clin Chem*. 2017. 80: 227–251.

4. Brannick B, Wynn A, Dagogo-Jack S. Prediabetes as a toxic environment for the initiation of microvascular and macrovascular complications. *Exp Biol* Med 2006. 241(12): 1323–1331. doi:10.1177/1535370216654227.

5. Dorcely B, Katz K, Jagannathan R, Chiang SS, Oluwadare B, Goldberg IJ, Bergman M. Novel biomarkers for prediabetes, diabetes, and associated complications. *Diabetes Metab Syndr Obes*. 2017. 10: 345–361.

6. Haring HU. Novel phenotype of prediabetes. *Diabetologia*. 2016. 59: 1806–1818.

7. Dagogo-Jack S. Editorial: The continuum of dysglycemia: Predicting progression from diabetes to type 2 diabetes. *J Diabetes Complications*. 2017. 31: 1249–1251.

8. National Diabetes Statistics Report, 2017. Estimates of diabetes and its burden in the United States. 2017. 1–19.

9. American Diabetes Association. Statistics about Diabetes. Overall numbers, diabetes, and prediabetes. http://www.diabetes.org/diabetes-basics/statistics/.

10. NCD Risk factor collaboration. Worldwide trends in diabetes since 1980: A pooled analysis of 751 population-based studies with 4.4 million participants. *Lancet*. 2016. 387: 1513–1530.

11. The Diabetes Control and Complications Research Group. The effect of intensive treatment of diabetes on the development and progression of long-term complications in insulin-dependent diabetes mellitus. *New Engl J Med*. 1993. 329 (14): 977–986.

12. Geloneck MM, Forbes BJ, Shaffer J, Ying G, Binenbaum G. Ocular complications in children with diabetes mellitus. *Ophthalmology*. 2015. 122 (12): 2457–2464.

13. Borgnakke WS, Ylostalo PV, Taylor GW, Genco RJ. Effect of periodontal disease on diabetes: Systematic review of epidemiological observational evidence. *J Clin Periodontol*. 2013: 40 (Suppl 14): 10.1111.

14. Negrato CA, Tarzia O, Jovanovic L, Montenegro E. Periodontal disease and diabetes mellitus. *J Appl Oral Sci*. 2013. 21 (1): 1–12.

15. Holmstrup P, Damgaard C, Olsen I, Klinge B, Flyvbjerg A, Nielsen CH, Hansen PR. Comorbidity of periodontal disease: Two sides of the same coin? An introduction for the clinician. *J Oral Microbiol*. 2017. Jun 14. 9 (1): 1332710. doi:10.1080/20002297.2017.1332710. eCollection 2017.

16. Hodgson K, Morris J, Bridson T, Govan B, Rush C, Ketheesan N. Immunologic mechanisms contributing to the double burden of diabetes and intracellular bacterial infections. *Immunol*. 2015. Feb. 144(2): 171–185

17. Hardigan T, Ward R, Ergul A. Cerebrovascular complications of diabetes: Focus on cognitive dysfunction. *Clin Sci (Lond)*. 2016. Oct 01. 130 (20): 1807–1822.

18. Zilliox LA, Chadrasekaran K, Kwan JY, Russell JW. Diabetes and cognitive impairment. *Curr Diab Rep*. 2016. Sept. 16(9): 87.

19. De la Monte SM. Relationships between diabetes and cognitive impairment. *Endocrinol Metab Clin North Am*. 2014. Mar. 43(1): 245–267.

20. Riederer P, Korczyn AD, Ali SS, Bajenaru O, Choi MS, Chopp M, Dermanovic-Dobrota V, et al. The diabetic brain and cognition. *J Neural Transm (Vienna)*. 2017. Nov. 124(11): 1431–1454.

21. Heiss WD, Rosenberg GA, Thiel A, Berlot R, De Reuck. Neuroimaging in vascular cognitive impairment: A state-of the-art-review. *BMC Med*. 2016. 14: 174.

22. Holt RIG. Diabetes and depression. *Curr Diab Rep*. 14(6): 491.

23. Badescu SV, Tataru C, Kobylinska L, Georgescu EL, Zahiu DM, Zagrean AM, Zagrean L. The association between diabetes mellitus and depression. *J Med Life*. 2016. Apr-June. 9(2): 120–125.

24. Danna SM, Graham E, Burns RJ, Deschenes SS, Schmitz N. Association between depressive symptoms and cognitive functions in persons with diabetes mellitus: A systematic review. *PLoS One*. 2016. 11(8): e0160809.

25. Beverly EA, Ritholz MD, Shepherd C, Weinger K. The psychosocial challenges and care of older adults with diabetes: "Can't do what I used to do; can't be who I once was". *Curr Diab Rep*. 2016. June. 16(6): 48.

26. Ducat L, Rubenstein A, Philipson LH, Anderson BJ. A review of the mental health issues of diabetes conference. *Diab Care*. 2015. 38: 333–338.

27. Fisher VL, Tahrani AA. Cardiac autonomic neuropathy in patients with diabetes mellitus: Current perspectives. *Diab Metab Synd Obes*. 2017. 10: 419–434.

28. De Ferranti SD, de Boer IH, Fonseca V, Fox CS, Golden SH, Lavie CJ, Magge SN, et al. Type 1 diabetes mellitus and cardiovascular disease: A scientific statement form the American heart association and American diabetes association. *Diab Care*. 2014. 37: 2843–2863.

29. Kittnar O. Electrocardiographic changes in diabetes mellitus. *Physiol Res*. 2015. 64 (Suppl 5): S559–S566.

30. Koektuerk B, Aksoy M, Horlitz M, Bozdag-Turan I, Turan RG. Role of diabetes in heart rhythm disorders. *World J Diab.* 2016. 10; 7(3): 45–49.

31. Foris LA, Bhimji SS. Diabetic gastroparesis. Stat Pearls. Treasure Island FL. StatPearls Publishing. 2017 Jun–2017 Oct. PMID 28613545.

32. Bharucha AE. Epidemiology and natural history of gastroparesis. *Gastroenterol Clin of North Am.* 2015. March. 44 (1): 9–19.

33. Deli G, Bosnyak E, Pusch G, Komoly S, Feher G. Diabetic neuropathies: Diagnosis and management. *Neuroendocrin.* 2013. 8: 267–280.

34. Gheith O, Farouk N, Nampoory N, Halim MA, Al-Otaibi T. Diabetic kidney disease: Worldwide difference of prevalence and risk factors. *J Nephropharmacol.* 2016. 5(1): 49–56.

35. Qi C, Mao X, Zhang Z, Wu H. Classification and differential diagnosis of diabetic nephropathy. *J Diab Res.* Vol 2017 (2017), Article ID 8637138. doi:10.1155/2017/8637138.

36. Haas M. The revised (2013) BANFF classification for antibody-mediated rejection of renal allografts: Update, difficulties, and future considerations. *Am J Transplant.* 2016. 16: 1352–1357.

37. Tervaert TWC, Mooyaart AL, Amann K, Cohen AH, Cook HT, Drachenberg CB, Ferrario F, et al. Pathologic classification of diabetic nephropathy. *J Am Soc Nephrol.* 2010. Apr. 21(4): 556–563. doi:10.1681/ASN.2010010010. Epub 2010 Feb 18.

38. Naidoo P, Liu VJ, Mautone M, Bergin S. Lower limb complications of diabetes mellitus: A comprehensive review with clinicopathological insights form a dedicated high risk diabetic foot multidisciplinary team. *Br J Radiol.* 2015. 88(1053): 20150135 (ISSN: 1748-880X).

39. Bodman MA, Dulebohn SC. Neuropathy, diabetic. StatPearls [Internet}. Treasure Island (FL): StatPearls Publishing. 2017-. 2017 Oct 6.

40. Kucera T, Shaikh HH, Sponer P. Charcot neuropathic arthropathy of the foot: A literature review and single-center experience. *J Diab Res.* 2016. 2016: 1–10. doi:10.1155/2016/3207043.

41. Arellano-Valdez F, Urrutia-Osorio M, Arroyo C, Soto-Vega E. A comprehensive review of urologic complications in patients with diabetes. *Springerplus.* 2014. Sept 23. 3: 549. doi:10.1186/2193-1801-3-549. eCollection 2014.

42. Lue TF, Brant WO, Shindel A, Bella AJ. In: De Groot LJ, Chrousos G, Dungan K, Feingold KR, Grossman A, Hershman JM, Koch C, et al., Editors. Sexual dysfunction in diabetes. Endotext [Internet]. South Dartmouth (MA): MDText.com, 2000.

43. D'Alfonso TM, Ginter PS, Shin SJ. A review of inflammatory processes of the breast with a focus on diagnosis in core biopsy samples. *J Pathol Translat Med.* 2015. 49: 279–287.

44. Akahori H, Kaneko M, Kiyohara K, Terahata S, Sugimoto T. A rare case of diabetic mastopathy in a diabetic man with type 2 diabetes mellitus. *Inter Med.* 2009. 48: 915–919.

45. Honda M, Mori Y, Nishi T, Mizuguchi K, Ishibashi M. diabetic mastopathy in bilateral breasts in an elderly Japanese woman with type 2 diabetes: A case report and a review of the literature in Japan. Intern Med. 2007. 46(18): 1573–6. Epub 2007 Sep 14.

46. Ferroni P, Riondino S, Buonomo O, Palmirotta R, Guadagni F, Roselli M. Type 2 diabetes and breast cancer: The interplay between impaired glucose metabolism and oxidant stress. *Oxidat Med Cellul Longev.* 2015. (2015): 183928. doi:10.1155/2015/183928.

47. Fang H, Yao B, Yan Y, Xu H, Liu Y, Tang H, Zhou J, et al. Diabetes mellitus increases the risk of bladder cancer: An updated meta-analysis of observational studies. *Diab Technol Therap.* 2013. 15 (11): 914–922.

48. Joshi S, Liu M, Turner N. Diabetes and its link with cancer: Providing the fuel and spark to launch an aggressive growth regime. *Biomed Res Int.* 2015. ID 390863.

49. Mao Y, Tao M, Jia X, Xu H, Chen K, Tang H, Li D. Effect of diabetes mellitus on survival in patients with pancreatic cancer: A systematic review and meta-analysis. *Sci Rep.* 5:17102. doi:10.1038.

50. Leung V, Ragbir-Toolsie K. Perioperative management of patients with diabetes. *Health Serv Ins.* 2017. 10: 1–5.

51. Okonkwo UA, DiPietro LA. Diabetes and wound angiogenesis. *Int J Mol Sci.* 2017. 18: 1419. doi:10.3390.

52. Kalaitzoglou E, Popescu I, Bunn RC, Fowlkes JL, Thrailkill KM. Effects of type 1 diabetes on osteoblasts, osteocytes, and osteoclasts. *Curr Osteoporos Rep.* 2016. Dec. 14 (6): 310–319.

53. Jiao H. Diabetes and its effect on bone and fracture healing. *Curr Osteoporos.* 2015. Oct. 13 (5): 327–335.

54. Gizzo S, Patrelli TS, Rossanese M, Noventa M, Berretta R, Di Gangi S, Bertin M, Gangemi M, Nardelli GB. An update on diabetic women obstetrical outcomes linked to preconception and pregnancy glycemic profile: A systematic literature review. *Sci World J.* 2013. Art ID 254901. doi:10.1155/2013/254901.

55. Baz B, Riveline JP, Gautier JF. Endocrinology of pregnancy. Gestational diabetes mellitus: Definition, aetiological and clinical aspects. *Eur J Endocrinol.* 2016. 174: R43–R51.

56. Liebl A, Khunti K, Orozco-Beltran D, Yale JF. Health economic evaluation of type 2 diabetes mellitus: A clinical practice focused review. *Clin Med Ins: Endocrin and Diab.* 2015. 8: 13–19.

57. Wu J, Ward E, Threatt E, Lu ZK. Progression to type 2 diabetes and its effect on health care costs in low income and insured patients with pre-diabetes: A retrospective study using Medicaid claims data. *J Manag Care Spec Pharm.* 2017. 23(3): 309–316.

58. Zhuo X, Zhang P, Barker L, Albright A, Thompson TJ, Gregg E. The lifetime cost of diabetes and its implication for diabetes prevention. *Diab Care.* 2014. 37: 2557–2564.

59. American Diabetes Association. Economic costs of diabetes in the U.S. in 2012. *Diab Care.* 2013. 36: 1033–1046.

12 Nutrient Interactions and Glucose Homeostasis

Emmanuel C. Opara

CONTENTS

12.1 INTRODUCTION

The purpose of this chapter is to present an overview of the metabolism of the key nutrients, glucose, fatty acids, and amino acids in the body, and how the interactions involved in the metabolic processing of these nutrients affect glucose homeostasis. We will pay particular attention to the interplay of the metabolism of fatty acids and glucose, which are the major fuel sources in the postabsorptive state. We will then explore how knowledge of the interrelationships of the metabolism of these nutrients has been used so far and the potential for additional use to design effective treatment strategies for type 2 diabetes. The discussion will be focused on human studies, but results from animal experiments will also be discussed where human data are either limited or not available.

12.2 CHARACTERISTICS OF ENERGY GENERATION FROM NUTRIENTS

The key peripheral tissues whose metabolic activities affect glucose homeostasis are the liver, muscle, adipose tissue, and kidney. These tissues play different roles in blood glucose regulation in the fed and resting post-absorptive states, as well as during extended periods of fasting [1]. Depending on the nutrient and the nutritional status, nutrients are processed primarily to provide the body's energy needs and to replenish or augment body stores of glycogen and fat. In the fed state, excess amino acids not utilized for protein synthesis are preferentially catabolized over glucose and fat for energy, because there are no significant storage sites for amino acids and proteins, while an accumulation of nitrogen products results in toxicity in the body. During fasting, the adipose tissue, muscle, liver, and kidneys work in different capacities to supply, convert, or conserve metabolic fuel for the body [1]. In the resting post-absorptive state, blood glucose homeostasis is achieved by balanced contributions from glycogenolysis by the liver and lipolysis by the adipose tissue. If fasting is continued, proteolysis in the muscle ensues to supply glycogenic amino acids for gluconeogenesis in the liver and kidneys [1,2]. In periods of starvation, defined as 3 or more days of fasting, the body strives to conserve protein and to obtain greater supplies of its energy needs from alternative metabolic fuels, primarily fatty acids and ketone bodies. Under these circumstances, the ability of the kidneys to preserve ketone bodies prevents the loss of this valuable energy source, and the delicate interplay among these key tissues in the regulation of energy needs permits survival for extended periods of caloric deprivation [1].

12.3 BLOOD GLUCOSE REGULATION

Blood glucose regulation is achieved by an intricate balance among many factors, including nutritional status, endocrine and neural mechanisms, and physical activity. However, for the purpose of this discussion, we will focus on the different biochemical processes of glucose utilization and synthesis in the tissues, which maintain normal blood glucose. In the fed state, blood glucose is kept normal by increased utilization of glucose and storage as glycogen. Glucose produced by the catabolism of amino acids not used for protein synthesis is also stored as glycogen. Fatty acids not re-synthesized into triglycerides for storage as lipids are oxidized and, by so doing, generate substrates also used for *de novo* glucose synthesis (gluconeogenesis) and storage as glycogen. In the post-absorptive state, normal blood glucose is maintained by a combination of gluconeogenesis and glycogenolysis. During short-term fasting, blood glucose is primarily maintained by hepatic glycogen breakdown. With extended periods of fasting, fatty acid oxidation and amino acid catabolism become predominant sources of energy, and through these processes, substrates are generated for gluconeogenesis.

As noted earlier, glucose is a major fuel that also occupies a central position in the metabolism of other nutrients in the body. It is a precursor molecule that is capable of providing many metabolic intermediates for various biosynthetic reactions [3]. Therefore, the metabolism of glucose is normally regulated by a well-coordinated system among the different tissues in the body. For instance, in the muscle, glycolytic degradation of glucose produces ATP, and the rate of glycolysis increases as the muscle contracts more intensely thereby demanding more ATP. On the other hand, as previously noted, the liver and the kidneys serve to keep a constant level of glucose in the blood by producing and exporting glucose when the tissues demand it, while the liver takes up and stores glucose when it is available in excess [3]. The turnover of muscle protein occurs slowly, with little or no diurnal changes in the size of the protein pool, in response to feeding and fasting [4].

There are 20 standard amino acids in proteins, with variations in their carbon skeletons. Consequently, there are many different catabolic pathways for the degradation of amino acids for energy production. Altogether, the energy from these pathways accounts for only 10%–15% of the body's energy production [3]. Although much of the catabolism of amino acids takes place in the liver, six amino acids—namely, leucine, isoleucine, valine, asparagine, aspartate, and glutamate— are metabolized in the resting muscle [4]. However, the three branched-chain amino acids (BCAAs), leucine, isoleucine, and valine, are only oxidized as metabolic fuels in the muscle, adipose tissue, kidney, and brain. These extra-hepatic tissues have a single aminotransferase that is not present in the liver and acts on all three BCAAs to produce the corresponding ketoacids [3]. The overwhelming majority of amino acids are glucogenic. Hence their carbon skeleton generates intermediates of the tricarboxylic acid (TCA) cycle that are used for *de novo* glucose synthesis.

The biochemistry of the BCAAs is of particular interest. They are essential amino acids abundant in meats, fish, milk, seafood, and whey protein [5,6]. As with other essential amino acids, they cannot be synthesized by humans and other vertebrates and are primarily used in biosynthesis [3]. The normal degradation products of BCAA are short-chain acylcarnitines C3, C4, and C5 [7]. Under normal conditions, these acylcarnitines are transported into the mitochondria, where they are metabolized into free L-carnitine and acylCoA [8]. The free carnitine, which is water-soluble, is transported back to the cytosol, while the acylCoA undergoes oxidation for ATP generation in the TCA cycle. Recent studies using metabolomics have provided the metabolite profiles of specific amino acids and have revealed perturbations of normal amino acid metabolism that result in abnormalities in blood glucose regulation [9], as discussed in the next section.

12.4 INTERRELATIONSHIPS OF NUTRIENT METABOLISM AND THE EFFECT ON GLUCOSE HOMEOSTASIS

12.4.1 GLUCOSE AND FAT

Competition between nutrients as sources of metabolic fuel has been known for about a century. However, quantitatively, the most important interaction is between glucose and fatty acids [10]. As already mentioned above, if there is a perturbation of the energy supply system in the body, such as an abundance of fatty acids, a competition ensues between glucose and fatty acids as sources of metabolic fuel. This phenomenon came to be historically recognized when Randle and colleagues proposed the glucose–fatty acid cycle to explain the metabolic interactions between glucose and fatty acids and its role in insulin sensitivity and diabetes [10]. Essentially, the Randle hypothesis states that the metabolic relationship between glucose and fatty acids is reciprocal and not dependent [10–12]. Later, to explain this reciprocal relationship, Randle proposed that oversupply of glucose would promote glucose oxidation and glucose and lipid storage, while inhibiting fatty acid oxidation. On the other hand, an abundance of free fatty acids (FFAs) would promote fatty acid oxidation and storage while inhibiting glucose oxidation and may enhance glucose storage if glycogen reserves are incomplete. Randle argued that the evidence for the inhibitory effects of fatty acids on whole-body glucose utilization and oxidation (predominantly muscles) are decisive, and that the enzyme mechanisms mediating these effects are well established. There is also much evidence that fatty acid oxidation inhibits glucose oxidation and stimulates glucose formation in the liver; again, the enzyme reactions are known [11].

According to the original Randle hypothesis, an increase in fatty acid availability results in increased fatty acid oxidation with concomitant inhibition of glucose oxidation. Various mechanisms are involved in the inhibition of glucose oxidation during increased fatty acid supply and oxidation, as illustrated in Figure 12.1. The accumulation of acetyl-CoA would result in the inhibition of pyruvate dehydrogenase (PDH), while the abundance of citrate would inhibit phosphofructokinase (PFK), and excess levels of glucose-6-phosphate (G-6-P) would inhibit the activity of hexokinase (HK) [12,13]. There has also been an accumulation of evidence to show that increases in the glycolytic flux during glucose metabolism may decrease fatty acid oxidation. It has been proposed that the potential sites of fatty acid metabolism affected include the transport of fatty acid into the sarcoplasma, lipolysis of intramuscular triacylglycerol by hormone-sensitive lipase, and transport of fatty acids across the mitochondrial membrane [12]. One scenario among the possible mechanisms of regulation of fatty acid metabolism is an increase in malonyl-CoA concentration, which is formed from acetyl-CoA in a reaction catalyzed by acetyl-CoA carboxylase (ACC). Increased levels of malonyl-CoA will inhibit carnitine palmitoyl transferase 1 (CPT1) [14]. Indeed, using muscle biopsies obtained from obese subjects for lipid analysis and reverse transcription-competitive polymerase chain reaction, it has been shown that down-regulation of ACC2 mRNA, induced by lowering plasma insulin levels, caused improvement in insulin sensitivity [15].

Another possibility is that increased levels of acetyl moiety will result in acetylation of the carnitine pool, decreasing the free carnitine concentration and thereby reducing fatty acid transport into the mitochondria. It has also been suggested in some studies that CPT1 may be inhibited by small reductions in pH that may occur during glycolysis [12]. Moreover, it has been shown that long-chain acyl-CoAs accumulate in the muscle during chronic glucose infusion, an observation that is consistent with malonyl-CoA-induced inhibition of fatty acid oxidation. This phenomenon, by which glucose oxidation yields products that may regulate fatty acid oxidation, has been referred to

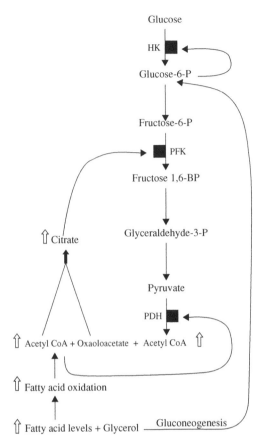

FIGURE 12.1 Illustration of the original Randle hypothesis. Oversupply of lipids will lead to increased fatty-acid oxidation, the products of which include increased levels of acetyl CoA, which inhibits pyruvate dehydrogenase (PDH), and citrate, which inhibits phosphofructose kinase. Simultaneously, other products of fatty-acid oxidation, such as glycerol, are converted to glucose in a pathway that generates an abundance of Glucose-6-P (G-6-P), which inhibits hexokinase, and further impairs glucose utilization.

by some investigators as the *reverse glucose-fatty acid cycle* [16,17], in distinction from the original Randle hypothesis, which proposed that products of fatty acid oxidation affect glucose metabolism.

Studies performed after the original Randle hypothesis was proposed have identified other mechanisms by which oversupply of fatty acids would affect glucose utilization. First, it has been shown that, with adequate insulinization, increased fatty acid levels effectively compete with glucose for uptake into peripheral tissues, regardless of the presence of hyperglycemia [18]. Second, it has been reported that increased fatty acid oxidation may inhibit glucose storage [19]. Third, it has been suggested that the metabolic interactions between FFA and glucose also involve impaired suppression of hepatic glucose production by insulin [20]. In addition, in a situation of enhanced lipolysis, increased levels of glycerol would promote gluconeogenesis [21]. Furthermore, it has been shown that lipid-derived molecules, including diacylglycerol and ceramide, can inhibit glucose disposal by interfering with more than one pathway of insulin signal transduction system, depending on the prevailing species of fatty acids. These pathways include alteration of insulin action via chronic activation of protein kinase C (PKC) isoenzymes by long-chain acyl-CoA [22,23]. Putting together available information from the literature on the various mechanisms by which oversupply of lipids may impair glucose utilization and result in increased blood glucose, the glucose fatty acid cycle at the present time can be summarized by the various pathways shown in Figure 12.2.

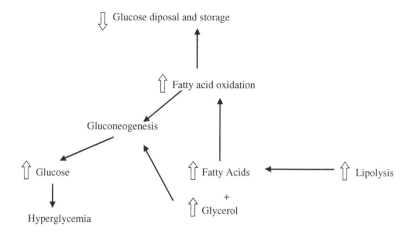

FIGURE 12.2 Summary of pathways of the glucose–fatty-acid cycle. Increased fatty-acid utilization generates intermediate substrates that impair glucose utilization while enhancing *de novo* glucose synthesis and storage, resulting in blood-glucose overload or hyperglycemia.

In trying to explore a cause-and-effect relationship between obesity and type 2 diabetes on the one hand, and insulin resistance on the other, McGarry had proposed a scenario in which hyperinsulinemia and insulin resistance arise either simultaneously or sequentially from some preexisting defect within the leptin signaling pathway. In either case, a central component of his model is that the breakdown of glucose homeostasis that is characteristic of the condition of obesity with type 2 diabetes is secondary to disturbances in lipid dynamics. He raised the possibility that abnormally high concentrations of malonyl-CoA in the liver and skeletal muscle suppress the activity of mitochondrial CPT1 and thus fatty acid oxidation at both sites. He further suggested that the buildup of fat within the muscle cell (caused in part by excessive delivery of VLDLs from the liver) interferes with glucose transport or metabolism, or both, producing insulin resistance. In addition, he proposed that elevated circulating concentrations of fatty acids are also implicated in the etiology of type 2 diabetes by virtue of (1) their powerful acute insulinotropic effect, (2) their ability to exacerbate insulin resistance in muscle, and (3) their long-term detrimental action on pancreatic beta-cell function [24].

12.4.2 Amino Acids and Fat

Recent research has raised the possibility that blood glucose regulation may be affected by the interconnecting intermediary metabolism of fats and amino acids. Although BCAA have been reported to mediate antiobesity effects [9], circulating levels of BCAA are invariably increased in obese individuals and are associated with abnormal levels of metabolic parameters that lead to insulin resistance or type 2 diabetes mellitus [25]. Indeed, obesity, insulin resistance, and type 2 diabetes are commonly associated with elevated concentrations of one or more BCAA, branched-chain α-ketoacid, and/or carnitine esters derived from partial BCAA catabolism in humans [9]. One mechanism that has been proposed linking increased levels of BCAAs and type 2 diabetes involves leucine-mediated activation of the mammalian target of rapamycin complex 1 (mTOR1), which results in uncoupling of insulin signaling at an early stage. Also, as mentioned earlier, acylcarnitines are products of BCAA catabolism, and after acylcarnitines enter the mitochondria, they are metabolized into free carnitine and acylCoA. In normal states, insulin promotes cellular uptake and use of carnitine. However, in obese and insulin-resistant conditions, the level of free carnitine is lower than normal because of increased utilization in excessive fatty acid oxidation and/or impaired cellular uptake induced by insulin resistance. As a consequence of the lower carnitine level, there is reduced ability to transport acylcarnitines into the mitochondria, and the accumulation of these

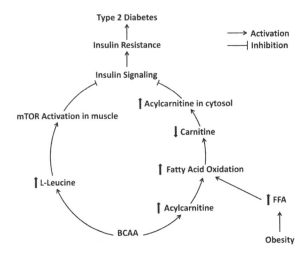

FIGURE 12.3 Branched-chain amino acid (BCAA) metabolism and relationship to insulin resistance and type 2 diabetes. (FFA, free fatty acid; mTOR, mammalian target for rapamycin.)

BCAA metabolites in the cytosol may then exacerbate insulin resistance via impairment of insulin signaling [25], as illustrated in Figure 12.3.

However, definitive evidence to show that elevated levels of leucine or BCAA contribute to insulin resistance often associated with obesity remains elusive. On the one hand, studies in which leucine- or BCAA-rich protein sources (e.g., whey protein isolate, nonfat dry milk) have been administered to rodents in drinking water or food under high-fat, obesogenic conditions have consistently shown a positive effect on metabolic outcomes, including lower adiposity, improved glucose tolerance, and reduced feed efficiency [9]. Also, in subjects with type 2 diabetes, protein-rich diets (i.e., 30% of dietary energy) have resulted in improved metabolic parameters, including reduced fasting glucose and HbA1c levels, even during weight maintenance periods ranging from 5 weeks to 1 year [26–28]. On the other hand, some studies have shown no effect of high-protein diets on indices of glucose control or no difference in metabolic profiles compared to high-carbohydrate controlled diets [29–31]. It is thus unclear whether there are differential effects of specific types of dietary protein on glucose metabolism [9].

From these findings, an emerging concept is that conditions of impaired insulin action, increased FFA oxidation, and concomitant changes in mitochondrial redox status attenuate specific catabolic pathways that in turn affect tissue and blood concentrations of BCAA, as well as sulfur amino acids, tyrosine/phenylalanine, and related derivatives [9]. However, Newgard et al. have suggested that the obese, insulin-resistant state is one of robust BCAA oxidation due to increased BCAA levels, a notion that is supported by their findings of increased blood carnitine derivatives of branched-chain α-ketoacid oxidation [32,33].

Other studies have shown that meat intake is associated with disordered blood glucose regulation, and the mechanism by which processed meat intake affects glucose regulation appears to be complex. The human diet is an important exogenous source of reactive precursor and terminal advanced glycation end products (AGEs) and lipooxidation end products (ALEs), including a-β-dicarbonyl–containing derivatives [34]. Thus, nitrosoamines and AGEs present in processed meats during preparation or formed by interactions of amino acids and nitrates within the body have been shown to have a toxic effect on β-cells and to promote the development of impaired glucose tolerance and insulin resistance [34,35]. In particular, it has been proposed that common methods of food processing, including heating, sterilizing, and ionizing, all of which tend to accelerate the non-enzymatic addition of non-reducing sugars to free NH$_2$-groups of the amino acids in proteins, a chemical process known as the *Maillard reaction*, plays a significant role in this scenario.

It has therefore been suggested that dietary glycoxidation products may represent an important link between increased animal fat and meat consumption and subsequent perturbation in blood glucose regulation [34].

12.5 DESIGN OF TREATMENT FOR TYPE 2 DIABETES BASED ON NUTRIENT INTERACTIONS

It is perhaps apparent by now that increased lipid availability can impair glucose utilization through many different mechanisms and result in the hyperglycemia of type 2 diabetes. Consequently, there are many different approaches that can used to design effective treatment strategies for the disease, on the basis of the competition of nutrients as substrates for metabolic reactions. These strategies include limiting the availability of lipids as metabolic fuels, inhibition of fatty acid uptake and oxidation, inhibition of gluconeogenesis, and uncoupling the energy obtained during fatty acid oxidation, with concomitant manipulation of the fatty acid oxidation gene transcription factors and peroxisome proliferator-activated receptors (PPARs) [36–40].

12.5.1 LIMITING THE AVAILABILITY OF FATTY ACIDS

As pointed out earlier, fatty acid oxidation affects glycemic control not only by decreasing peripheral glucose utilization, but also by enhancing gluconeogenesis. Hence, inhibition of lipolysis is an effective strategy to reduce the availability of FFAs for oxidation and thus enhance glucose oxidation and decrease blood glucose levels [36,38]. One of the early attempts to use antilipolytic agent to limit fatty acid availability and treat type 2 diabetes was made with nicotinic acid. It was found that its inhibitory effect on lipolysis was accompanied by a stimulation of the glucose disposal. It was disappointing, however, to see that although nicotinic acid initially reduced FFA levels in type 2 diabetes, it was followed by a rebound in FFA levels that was associated with hyperglycemia and glucosuria [36]. Subsequently, an analogue of nicotinic acid, acipimox, was developed that was more potent and had less of the rebound effect than nicotinic acid [36]. To date, acipimox remains an active research interest in the treatment of type 2 diabetes. In a recent experimental study with obese Zucker rats, oral administration of 150 mg/kg of acipimox significantly reduced plasma FFA, glucose, and insulin levels and thus improved glucose tolerance while reducing insulin response [41]. Clinically, trials with acipimox have also yielded positive effects in the management of type 2 diabetes. In an early double-blind, placebo-controlled trial, hepatic glucose output (HGO) and fuel use, assessed by indirect calorimetry, were measured in the basal state and during the last 30 minutes of a hyperglycemic clamp in patients with obesity and type 2 diabetes. In these patients, a complete overnight suppression of FFA was achieved by oral administration of 250 mg thrice during 12 hours. It was found that this protocol of prolonged suppression of lipolysis caused a reduction of fasting blood glucose and HGO while increasing peripheral hepatic sensitivity to insulin in the study subjects [42]. The data from this early study were consistent with those from another overnight, placebo-controlled study with acipimox [43]. In the later study, 250 mg acipimox was administered three times in 12 hours to four different groups of individuals—namely, lean control subjects, obese non-diabetic individuals, obese subjects with impaired glucose tolerance, and patients with type 2 diabetes. It was found that lowering plasma FFA levels reduced insulin resistance/hyperinsulinemia and improved oral glucose tolerance in all groups of the study subjects [43]. The observations from these studies of short-term use of acipimox have been confirmed in a randomized, double-blind, placebo-controlled study in which 25 individuals with type 2 diabetes were given 250 mg four times daily, and another 25 received a placebo for 1 week. The study showed that the treatment with acipimox lowered plasma FFA levels and improved acute insulin response and insulin-mediated glucose uptake [44]. However, in one of the earlier studies, acipimox gave mixed results on suppression of plasma FFA levels and had no effect on hepatic glucose production [45]. The reason for this discrepant observation with acipimox is not clear.

12.5.2 INHIBITION OF FATTY ACID OXIDATION

One strategy that has received significant attention is the use of fatty acid oxidation inhibitors in the management of type 2 diabetes. As can be predicted from the glucose-fatty acid cycle, the rationale in the use of this approach is that inhibiting fatty acid oxidation would enhance peripheral tissue glucose utilization, while inhibiting gluconeogenesis. Hence, there has been significant interest in the development of drugs to inhibit fatty acid oxidation and improve glycemic control in individuals with type 2 diabetes. Long-chain fatty acids are converted to fatty acyl-CoA esters in the outer mitochondrial membrane and require carnitine to get across the inner mitochondrial membrane for oxidation in the mitochondrial matrix. The rate-limiting enzyme that catalyzes the transesterification of the fatty acyl group from Co-A to carnitine is carnitine acyltransferase 1, the predominant form being the carnitine palmitoyl transferase 1 (CPT-1). It is therefore not surprising that the first generation of fatty acid oxidation inhibitors developed as therapeutic agents for type 2 diabetes were inhibitors of the CPT-1 enzyme [36,38]. CPT-1 inhibitors like etomoxir and tetradecylglycidic acid (TDGA), have the ability to decrease blood glucose levels. However, enthusiasm for the use of this class of inhibitors of fatty acid oxidation waned because of observations that they induced cardiac hypertrophy in rodents treated with the drugs. The next generation of CPT-1 inhibitors developed were drugs, such as SDZ and CPI 975, whose action on the liver-specific enzyme is reversible and might therefore be less toxic to the heart. Also, some monoamine oxidase inhibitors have been shown to inhibit the acylcarnitine translocase/CPT-2 enzyme and cause reductions in blood glucose levels [38]. Further studies are required to assess both the long-term efficacy and safety of these newer compounds in human subjects.

12.5.3 INHIBITION OF GLUCONEOGENESIS

As discussed earlier, one consequence of the catabolism of amino acids and fatty acids is the generation of metabolic substrates that are used for *de novo* glucose synthesis. It has been shown that hepatic insulin resistance in type 2 diabetes causes overproduction of glucose. Therefore, direct inhibition of gluconeogenesis by blocking a key enzyme in glucose synthesis, pyruvate carboxylase, or by limiting the availability of gluconeogenic substrates, is an attractive target for drug development. However, direct inhibition of pyruvate carboxylase is prone to unwanted side effects, because the enzyme has dual functions in both gluconeogenesis and in the TCA cycle. Indeed, it has been recently proposed that no one individual current medication acts directly to reduce gluconeogenesis [46]. The alternative approach to use indirect inhibitors of pyruvate carboxylase that act by sequestering acetyl-CoA, thereby making it unavailable for the action of the enzyme, has shown promising results in experimental studies with animals [38]. Fructose-1,6-bisphosphatase (FBPase), a well-recognized rate-limiting enzyme in gluconeogenesis, has emerged as a valid molecular level target to control gluconeogenesis-mediated glucose overproduction, and its inhibitors are likely to fulfill an unmet medical need. A class of these FBPase inhibitors has been recently reviewed and mainly acts through non-competitive pathways [46].

Another class of oral antidiabetic drugs, which are derivatives of acetic acid that reduce blood glucose and lipid levels without stimulating insulin secretion, has been developed. One member of this class of drugs being investigated is dichoroacetate (DCA), which inhibits hepatic glucose synthesis and stimulates glucose disposal by peripheral tissues [38,47]. A major effect of DCA is stimulation of the action of PDH, the rate-limiting enzyme in aerobic glucose oxidation, resulting in increased peripheral catabolism of alanine and lactate, thereby disrupting the Cori and alanine cycles and reducing availability of substrates for gluconeogenesis [47].

Metformin hydrochloride, a biguanide, is currently the only clinically available antidiabetic oral agent whose mechanism of action involves suppression of hepatic glucose release through inhibition of gluconeogenesis and glycogenolysis, although other metabolic parameters may also be affected [38,48,49]. For instance, it has been shown that metformin enhances insulin sensitivity at the muscle by promoting glucose transport and glycogen synthesis. It may also enhance peripheral glucose utilization by suppression of FFA release and oxidation [38]. Body weight reduction, as well as significant decreases in plasma levels of LDL-cholesterol, triglycerides, and FFA, has also been reported in patients treated with metformin [38,49]. Based on these metabolic actions of metformin treatment, its use has actually been recommended as a possible strategy to prevent type 2 diabetes in individuals at high risk for developing the disease [50].

Novel pharmacologic actions of metformin have recently been described. In one study, it has been shown that the drug, in combination with a dipeptidyl peptidase IV (DPPIV) inhibitor, caused reductions in food intake and body weight while enhancing the release of GLP-1, an incretin hormone that stimulates insulin secretion and also appears to reduce appetite [51]. In another study, it was shown that metformin caused a significant decrease in mitochondrial permeability and aerobic respiration [52]. However, the clinical significance of this latter *in vitro* observation remains to be determined.

As with any drug, the safety of metformin use has been a subject of investigation. An earlier biguanide, phenformin hydrochloride, was withdrawn from clinical use because it was associated with lactic acidosis in some patients treated with the drug. Thus far, it does not appear that lactic acidosis is a significant side effect in the treatment of uncomplicated type 2 diabetes with metformin [53–55], although it could become a rare but life-threatening problem when used to treat patients with renal failure [55]. A few cases of hypoglycemia have been reported in a combination therapy of metformin and nateglinide [56].

12.5.4 UNCOUPLING OF ENERGY DURING FATTY ACID OXIDATION

A new concept in drug development for type 2 diabetes has emerged with the introduction of therapeutic agents that may enhance lipolysis while promoting fatty acid oxidation in a futile cycle that does not yield metabolic energy, and thus decreases circulating FFA levels while stimulating peripheral tissue glucose utilization [37,41]. One class of these new therapeutic agents is beta-3 agonists, which activate beta3-adrenergic receptors. An example of the beta-3 agonists currently under investigation is Trecadrine, which has been reported to induce lipolysis in adipocytes, with increased oxygen consumption in white adipose tissue, while FFA levels decreased because of their utilization in non-energy-generating tissue, such as the brown adipose tissue [57]. It has also been shown that another beta-3 agonist, CL-316243, may indirectly stimulate glucose uptake in the muscle of type 2 diabetic rats by stimulating the brown adipose tissue to increase uncoupling protein content and fatty acid oxidation, thus progressively decreasing the levels of circulating FFA [41].

The next class of agents involved in this approach of uncoupled oxidation of fatty acids is the peroxisome proliferator-activated receptors (PPARs). This is a group of three nuclear receptor isoforms encoded by different genes, PPAR-α, PPAR-δ, and PPAR-γ. Each of these isoforms appears to be expressed in a specific tissue because of its binding to a specific consensus DNA sequence of the peroxisome proliferator response elements (PPREs) [39,40,58–60]. PPAR-α is highly expressed in the liver and relatively expressed in the heart, kidney, skeletal muscle, intestinal mucosa, and brown adipose tissue [40,60]. It is the most characterized of the three PPAR subtypes and has been shown to play a prominent role in the regulation of nutrient metabolism, including fatty acid oxidation, gluconeogenesis, and amino acid metabolism [39,40,58,60]. PPAR-δ is expressed ubiquitously and has been shown to be effective in the treatment of dyslipidemia and cardiovascular disease [39]. PPAR-γ is mainly expressed in the brown adipose tissue, where it stimulates adipogenesis and lipogenesis [39,60].

Clinically, PPAR-α and PPAR-γ agonists have been used to treat hypertriglyceridemia and insulin resistance. Thiazolidinediones are PPAR-γ agonists, which enhance insulin sensitivity mainly at the skeletal muscle and adipose tissue, with some effect at the liver, where they increase insulin-stimulated glucose disposal [38]. These drugs increase triglyceride uptake into the adipose tissue, thereby reducing circulating FFA levels. One member of the PPAR-γ agonists group of drugs that had been previously used clinically is troglitazone. In one study, a randomized, placebo-controlled trial was performed with troglitazone to determine its effect on whole-body insulin sensitivity, pancreatic β-cell function, and glucose tolerance in Latino women with impaired glucose tolerance and a history of gestational diabetes [61]. After baseline oral glucose tolerance test (OGTT) and intravenous glucose tolerance test (IVGTT), each of three groups (14 participants per group) of subjects was assigned to receive one of three treatments, a placebo, 200 mg, or 400 mg troglitazone daily for 12 weeks. It was found that insulin sensitivity, assessed by the minimal model analysis of IVGTT results, changed by only 4% in the placebo group but was increased by 40% and 88% above basal in the groups treated with 200 mg and 400 mg troglitazone, respectively. Troglitazone treatment was also associated with a dose-dependent reduction in the total insulin output during the glucose tolerance tests [61]. Another PPAR-γ agonist that is still clinically available is pioglitazone, whose potency has been compared with that of troglitazone in regards to their effects as inhibitors of fatty oxidation, esterification, and gluconeogenesis [62]. It was concluded that, at similar concentration, troglitazone was more effective than pioglitazone in inhibiting fatty acid oxidation and gluconeogenesis, and that the inhibition of gluconeogenesis by troglitazone may be the result of its inhibition of fatty acid oxidation [62]. Unfortunately, troglitazone has been withdrawn from clinical use because of its hepatotoxicity, leaving pioglitazone and rosiglitazone as the only two thiazolidinediones currently available for clinical use [38].

The PPAR-α agonist group of drugs includes those synthetic therapeutic agents that are molecular targets for fibrates, such as gemfibrozil, bezafibrate, clofibrate, and fenofibrate, which are used to treat dyslipidemia and cardiovascular disease. PPAR-α promotes fatty acid transport across cell membranes and converts them into a metabolic form that precedes their subsequent metabolism. These drugs have gained popularity in combination treatment with the statins [40].

12.5.5 Nutritionally Based Therapeutic Approach

It is clear that the macronutrient composition of diets has a major effect on glucose homeostasis, and the list of foods and nutrients associated with an increased or reduced incidence of diabetes mellitus is growing [63]. For instance, it has been shown that meat intake is associated with diabetes-related phenotypes [35]. Another recent study has reported that a short-term vegan diet that is nutritionally balanced in macronutrient content was found to improve metabolic parameters of blood glucose regulation, blood lipids, and amino acid metabolism, when compared to an omnivorous diet [64]. This observation is consistent with a view recently expressed by Elmadfa and Meyer, who had concluded that although high protein intake is associated with increased type 2 diabetes risk, milk and seafood are good sources of BCAAs and taurine, which act beneficially on glucose metabolism and blood pressure [5]. In another study, it has been suggested that lipid replacement therapy, administered as a nutritional supplement with antioxidants, can prevent excess oxidative membrane damage and restore mitochondrial and other cellular damage and reduce fatigue prevalent in the metabolic syndrome [65].

A nutritional therapy for type 2 diabetes based on nutrient competition as metabolic substrates is an approach that has been examined in studies performed by our group and others. In a series of studies, it had been shown that fatty acids stimulate insulin secretion through a mechanism involving fatty acid oxidation [66–70], while the amino acid L-glutamine inhibits insulin secretion [71]. It had also been previously shown that L-glutamine inhibits fatty acid oxidation by islets, because it is a preferred fuel source for these cells [72]. We subsequently showed that addition of L-glutamine to a fatty acid perifusate inhibited fatty acid oxidation and prevented fatty acid–induced desensitization of islet response to glucose stimulation [73]. Based on these *in vitro* observations, we hypothesized that L-glutamine supplementation during high-fat feeding would prevent insulin resistance characterized by hyperinsulinemia and hyperglycemia, as seen in C57BL/6J (B/6J) mice. In the B/6J mice, high-fat feeding causes obesity associated with type 2 diabetes [74,75].

In our L-glutamine supplementation studies, the effect of L-alanine on glucose dysregulation induced by high-fat feeding was also examined. Each of four groups of 10 age- and weight-matched male B/6J was raised on one of four diets: (1) low fat, low sucrose (LL); (2) high fat, low sucrose alone (HL); (3) high fat, low sucrose supplemented with L-glutamine; and (4) high fat, low sucrose supplemented with L-alanine. Food intake, body weight, and plasma glucose and insulin levels were monitored over time. We found no difference in food intake per unit body weight between the groups after the first 2 weeks of feeding. However, the mean body weight of the LL group measured at 16 weeks was significantly lower than that of the HL group, as shown in Figure 12.4. Although supplementation with each of the amino acids caused 10% reduction in body weight compared with HL feeding, only L-glutamine supplementation resulted in persistent reductions in plasma glucose and insulin levels during the 5.5-month duration of study. We also found that, when L-glutamine was added to the HL diet of obese hyperglycemic and hyperinsulinemic animals for 2 months, body weight gain shown in Figure 12.5,

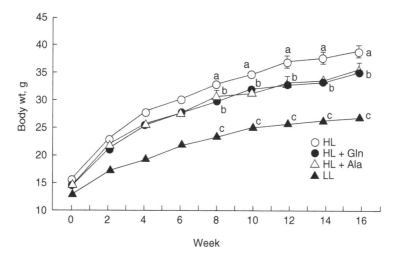

FIGURE 12.4 Body weights of B/6J mice fed a low-fat diet or a high-fat diet with or without supplemental Gln or Ala. Values are means ± SEM, n = 10. The error bars were so small that they are invisible in most data points. Means at a particular time point with different letters are significantly different, p < 0.05. Abbreviations used: HL, high fat, low sucrose; HL + Gln, high fat, low sucrose with L-glutamine supplementation; HL + Ala, high fat, low sucrose with L-alanine supplementation; LL, low fat, low sucrose. (Reprinted with permission from Mallick, S., *Postgrad. Med. J.*, 80, 239–240, 2004, Figure 2.)

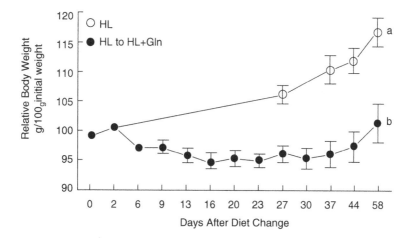

FIGURE 12.5 Effect of supplemental glutamine on relative body weight in heavy, hyperglycemic adult mice switched from the high-fat (HL) to the HL + Gln diet. The gap in the x-axis denotes an alteration in the scale because of the different intervals of determination. Two groups of mice (n = 10/group) were fed the HL diet for 4 months before one group was switched to the HL + Gln diet for 2 months, during which time the other continued being fed the HL diet. Different letters indicate significant differences between groups. Values are mean ± SEM, n = 10. (Reprinted with permission from Mallick, S., *Postgrad. Med. J.*, 80, 239–240, 2004, Figure 5.)

as well as hyperglycemia and hyperinsulinemia, were all significantly attenuated [76]. In another study, we also found that L-glutamine supplementation prevents impaired glucose regulation associated with hyperlipidemia induced by intravenous lipid administration [77]. These observations have been confirmed in a study by other investigators, who found that parenteral glutamine supplementation augmented whole-body insulin stimulation of whole-body glucose utilization, thus suggesting improved insulin sensitivity [78].

It is of interest that glycogen synthesis is stimulated by L-glutamine [79–82], which, as previously noted, inhibits fatty acid oxidation [72] and lipolysis [83,84] while stimulating lipogenesis [85]. The enhancement of glycogen synthesis by glutamine would imply an increase in gluconeogenic fluxes that is associated with an increased rate of non-oxidative glucose clearance [86] that may result in near-normal blood glucose levels during high-fat feeding, as seen in our studies. The clinical applicability of this nutritionally based therapeutic approach remains to be evaluated, although the clinical implication of our observations using this approach is discussed in the chapter by Dr. Lakey et al.

At the micronutrient level, vitamins D and E, as well as magnesium, have been associated with lower diabetes incidence, although the studies in this area need to be properly designed and adequately powered [63]. The potential mechanisms to explain the vitamin D effects on glucose homeostasis include improvements in pancreatic β-cell function, insulin resistance, and inflammation. The effect of vitamin D on insulin sensitivity may be mediated through calcium metabolism, because calcium is important in promoting glucose transport activity in muscle contraction [63]. In other studies, it has been observed that omega-3 fatty acids and vitamin E supplementation might influence glycemic status and lipid concentrations through their increased effects on the AMP-activated protein kinase (AMPK) and inhibition of activation of the nuclear factor kappa-light-chain enhancer of activated B cells (NF-kB). [87]. While some studies have shown an inverse association between magnesium intake and risk of type 2 diabetes, others have not shown this link. The underlying cellular and molecular pathways by which magnesium may affect glucose metabolism are presently unclear. Potential mechanisms include the utilization of high-energy phosphate bonds induced by magnesium, which acts as an enzyme co-factor, and the requirement of magnesium to maintain intracellular calcium levels and tyrosine kinase activity in insulin receptors necessary for both insulin signaling activity and glucose-stimulated insulin secretion [63].

12.6 CONCLUSION

It is clear that the processing of metabolic nutrients is intertwined through intermediary metabolism in the body. Consequently, it is imperative that there is a natural competition among the key nutrients, carbohydrate, fatty acids, and amino acids as sources of biological energy. The specific nutrient that becomes a primary source of energy is regulated by the nutritional status (fed or fasted state) with the concomitant hormonal balance. The convergence of the metabolism of nutrients in the tricarboxylic acid cycle has obvious implications for the utilization of each nutrient as a substrate for the generation of expendable energy, synthesis of macromolecules as storage forms of energy, or tissue maintenance.

Depending on the nutritional status, various studies have shown that the predominant energy-yielding sources are glucose and fatty acids, which compete with each other as the source of metabolic energy. There is overwhelming evidence to show that the converging metabolism of these two nutrients in the glucose–fatty acid cycle plays a predominant role in the pathogenesis of type 2 diabetes, although some studies have challenged the view that this cycle contributes to insulin resistance [88,89]. However, based on the hypothesis of the glucose–fatty acid cycle, it is possible to design effective therapeutic strategies for type 2 diabetes mellitus. These strategies for drug development could involve inhibitions of fatty acid oxidation and/or gluconeogenesis, manipulation of the enzymatic processes involved in nutrient processing, molecular targets for metabolic engineering, or a simple nutritional approach. A significant number of effective therapeutic agents have been developed, but there is still enormous potential for drug development for diabetes treatment on the basis of metabolic interactions of nutrients. This review, which has summarized current understanding of nutrient interactions, thus provides a valid scientific basis for effective strategies in designing new therapeutic approaches for type 2 diabetes.

REFERENCES

1. Owen OE, Reichard Jr. GA, Boden G, Patel MS, Trapp VE. Interelationships among key tissues in the utilization of metabolic substrates. In: *Diabetes, Obesity, and Vascular Disease. Metabolic and Molecular Interrelationships Part 2*, Katzen HM and Mahler RJ (Eds). Advances in Modern Nutrition, Volume 2, Halsted Press, John Wiley & Sons, NY, 1978.
2. Meyer C, Stumvoll M, Dostou J, Welle S, Haymond M, Gerich J. Renal substrate exchange and gluconeogenesis in normal postabsorptive humans. *Am J Physiol* 282: E428–E434, 2002.
3. Lehninger AL, Nelson DL, Cox MM (Eds.). *Principles of Biochemistry*. 2nd Edition, New York, Worth Publishers, 1993.
4. Wagenmakers AJ. Protein and amino acid metabolism in human muscle. *Adv Exp Med Biol* 441: 307–319, 1998.
5. Elmadfa I, Meyer AL. Animal proteins as important contributors to a healthy human diet. *Annu Rev Anim Biosci* 5: 111–131, 2017.
6. Tosukhowong P, Boonla C, Dissayabutra T, et al. Biochemical and clinical effects of Whey protein supplementation in Parkinson's disease: A pilot study. *J Neurol Sci* 367: 162–170, 2016.
7. Kirchberg FF, Harder U, Weber M, et al. *J Clin Endocrinol Metab* 100(1): 149–158, 2015.
8. Adeya-Andany MM, Calvo-Castro I, Fernández-Fernández C, Donapetry-García C, Pedre-Piñeiro AM. Significance of l-carnitine for human health. *IUBMB Life* 69(8): 578–594, 2017.
9. Adams SH. Emerging perspectives on essential amino acid metabolism in obesity and the insulin-resistant state. *Adv Nutr* 2(6): 445–456, 2011.
10. Randle PJ, Garland PB, Hales CN, Newsholme EA. The glucose fatty-acid cycle. Its role in insulin sensitivity and the metabolic disturbances of diabetes mellitus. *Lancet* 1: 785–789, 1963.
11. Randle PJ. Regulatory interactions between lipids and carbohydrates: The glucose fatty acid cycle after 35 years. *Diabetes Metab Rev* 14: 263–283, 1998.
12. Jeukendrup AE. Regulation of fat metabolism in skeletal muscle. *Ann NY Acad Sci* 967: 217–235, 2002.
13. Liu YQ, Tornheim K, Leahy JL. Glucose-fatty acid cycle to inhibit glucose utilization and oxidation is not operative in fatty acid cultured islets. *Diabetes* 48: 1747–1753, 1999.
14. Ruderman NB, Saha AK, Vavvas D, Witters LA. Malonyl-CoA, fuel sensing, and insulin resistance. *Am J Physiol* 276: E1–E18, 1999.
15. Rosa G, Manco M, Vega N, et al. Decreased muscle acetyl-coenzyme A carboxylase 2 mRNA and insulin resistance in formerly obese subjects. *Obes Res* 11: 1306–1312, 2003.
16. Laybutt DR, Schmitz-Peiffer C, Saha AK, et al. Muscle accumulation and protein kinase C activation in the insulin-resistant chronically glucose-infused rat. *Am J Physiol* 277: E1070–E1076, 1999.
17. Jequier E. Effect of lipid oxidation on glucose utilization in humans. *Am J Clin Nutr* 67: 527S–530lS, 1998.
18. Ferrannini E, Barrett EJ, Bevilacqua S, DeFronzo RA. Effect of fatty acids on glucose production and utilization in man. *J Clin Invest* 72: 1737–1747, 1983.
19. Felber JP. Significance of the Randle-mechanism in the etiology of diabetes type II. *Hormone Metab Res – Suppl* 22: 11–17, 1990.
20. Saloranta C, Koivisto V, Widen E, et al. Contribution of muscle and liver to glucose-fatty acid cycle in humans. *Am J Physiol* 264: E599–E605, 1993.
21. Wolfe RR. Metabolic interactions between glucose and fatty acids in humans. *Am J Clin Nutr* 67 (suppl 3): 515S–526S, 1998.
22. Schmitz-Peiffer C. Signalling aspects of insulin resistance in skeletal muscle: Mechanisms induced by lipid oversupply. *Cell Signal* 12: 583–594, 2000.
23. Kraegen EW, Cooney GJ, Ye JM, Thompson AL, Furler SM. The role of lipids in the pathogenesis of muscle insulin resistance and beta cell failure in type II diabetes mellitus and obesity. *Exp Clin Endocrinol Diabetes* 109 (suppl 2): S189–S201, 2001.
24. McGarry JD. Glucose-fatty acid interactions in health and disease. *Am J Clin Nutr* 67(3 Suppl): 500S–504S, 1998.

25. Lynch CJ, Adams SH. Branched-chain amino acids in metabolic signalling and insulin resistance. *Nat Rev Endocrinol* 10(12): 723–736, 2014.

26. Gannon MC, Nuttall FQ, Saeed A, Jordan K, Hoover H. An increase in dietary protein improves the blood glucose response in persons with type 2 diabetes. *Am J Clin Nutr* 78(4): 734–741, 2003.

27. Nuttall FQ, Schweim K, Hoover H, Gannon MC. Effect of the LoBAG30 diet on blood glucose control in people with type 2 diabetes. *Br J Nutr* 99(3): 511–519, 2008.

28. Gannon MC, Hoover H, Nuttall FQ. Further decrease in glycated hemoglobin following ingestion of a LoBAG30 diet for 10 weeks compared to 5 weeks in people with untreated type 2 diabetes. *Nutr Metab (Lond)* 7: 64, 2010 Jul.

29. Brinkworth GD, Noakes M, Parker B, Foster P, Clifton PM. Long-term effects of advice to consume a high-protein, low-fat diet, rather than a conventional weight-loss diet, in obese adults with type 2 diabetes: One-year follow-up of a randomised trial. *Diabetologia* 47(10): 1677–1686, 2004 Oct.

30. Sargrad KR, Homko C, Mozzoli M, Boden G. Effect of high protein vs high carbohydrate intake on insulin sensitivity, body weight, hemoglobin A1c, and blood pressure in patients with type 2 diabetes mellitus. *J Am Diet Assoc* 105(4): 573–580, 2005.

31. Larsen RN, Mann NJ, Maclean E, Shaw JE. The effect of high-protein, low-carbohydrate diets in the treatment of type 2 diabetes: A 12 month randomised controlled trial. *Diabetologia* 54(4): 731–740, 2011.

32. Newgard CB, An J, Bain JR, Muehlbauer MJ, et al. A branched-chain amino acid-related metabolic signature that differentiates obese and lean humans and contributes to insulin resistance. *Cell Metab* 9(4): 311–326, 2009. doi:10.1016/j.cmet.2009.02.002

33. Laferrère B, Reilly D, Arias S, et al. Differential metabolic impact of gastric bypass surgery versus dietary intervention in obese diabetic subjects despite identical weight loss. *Sci Transl Med* 3(80): 80re2, 2011 Apr.

34. Peppa M, Goldberg T, Cai W, Rayfield E, Vlassara H. Glycotoxins: A missing link in the "relationship of dietary fat and meat intake in relation to risk of type 2 diabetes in men". *Diabetes Care* 25(10): 1898–1899, 2002.

35. Fretts AM, Follis JL, Nettleton JA, et al. Consumption of meat is associated with higher fasting glucose and insulin concentrations regardless of glucose and insulin genetic risk scores: A meta-analysis of 50,345 Caucasians. *Am J Clin Nutr* 102(5): 1266–1278, 2015 Nov.

36. Foley JE. Rationale and application of fatty acid oxidation inhibitors in treatment of diabetes mellitus. *Diabetes Care* 15: 773–784, 1992.

37. Bebernitz GR, Schuster HF. The impact of fatty acid oxidation on energy utilization: Targets and therapy. *Curr Pharm Des* 8: 1199–1227, 2002.

38. Moneva MH, Dagogo-Jack S. Multiple targets in the management of Type 2 diabetes. *Curr Drug Targets* 3: 203–221, 2002.

39. Ram VJ. Therapeutic significance of peroxisome proliferator-activated receptor modulators in diabetes. *Drugs Today* 39: 609–632, 2003.

40. Mandard S, Muller M, Kersten S. Peroxisome proliferator-activated receptor alpha target genes. *Cell Mol Life Sci* 61: 393–416, 2004.

41. Blachere JC, Perusse F, Bukowiecki LJ. Lowering plasma fatty acids with Acipimox mimics the antidiabetic effects of the beta 3-adrenergic agonist CL-316243 in obese Zucker diabetic rats. *Metabolism* 50: 945–951, 2001.

42. Fulcher GR, Walker M, Catalano C, Agius L, Alberti KG. Metabolic effects of suppression of non-esterified fatty acid levels with acipimox in obese NIDDM subjects. *Diabetes* 41: 1400–1408, 1992.

43. Santomauro ATMG, Boden G, Silva MER, et al. Overnight lowering of free fatty acids with Acipimox improves insulin resistance and glucose tolerance in obese diabetic and non-diabetic subjects. *Diabetes* 48: 1836–1841, 1991.

44. Paolisso G, Tagliamonte MR, Rizzo MR, et al. Lowering fatty acids potentiates acute insulin response in first degree relatives of people with type II diabetes. *Diabetologia* 41: 1127–1132, 1998.

45. Saloranta C, Taskinen MR, Widen E, et al. Metabolic consequences of sustained suppression of free fatty acids by Acipimox in patients with NIDDM. *Diabetes* 42: 1559–1566, 1993.

46. Kaur R, Dahiya L, Kumar M. Fructose-1,6-bisphosphatase inhibitors: A new valid approach for management of type 2 diabetes mellitus. *Eur J Med Chem* 141: 473–505, 2017 Dec.

47. Stacpoole PW, Greene YJ. Dichloroacetate. *Diabetes Care* 15: 785–791, 1992.

48. Stumvoll M, Nurjhan N, Perriello G, Dailey G, Gerich JE. Metabolic effects of metformin in non-insulin-dependent diabetes mellitus. *N Engl J Med* 333: 550–554, 1995.

49. Setter SM, Iltz JL, Thams J, Campbell RK. Metformin hydrochloride in the treatment of type 2 diabetes mellitus: A clinical review with a focus on dual therapy. *Clin Ther* 12: 2991–3026, 2003.

50. Hess AM, Sullivan DL. Metformin for prevention of type 2 diabetes. *Ann Pharmacother* 38: 1283–1285, 2004.
51. Yasuda N, Inoue T, Nagakura T, et al. Metformin causes reduction of food intake and body weight gain and improvement of glucose intolerance in combination with dipeptidyl peptidase IV inhibitor in Zucker fa/fa rats. *J Pharmacol Exp Ther* 310: 614–619, 2004.
52. Guigas B, Detaille D, Chauvin C, et al. Metformin inhibits mitochondrial permeability transition and cell death: A pharmacological in vitro study. *Biochem J* 382(3): 877–884, 2004.
53. Salpeter SR, Greyber E, Paternak GA, Salpeter EE. Risk of fatal and nonfatal lactic acidosis with metformin use in Type 2 diabetes mellitus. Systematic review and meta-analysis. *Arch Intern Med* 163: 2594–2602, 2003.
54. Stades AM, Heikens JT, Erkelens DW, Holleman F, Hoekstra JB. Metformin and lactic acidosis: Cause or coincidence? A review to case reports. *J Intern Med* 255: 179–187, 2004.
55. Mallick S. Metformin induced acute pancreatitis precipitated by renal failure. *Postgrad Med J* 80: 239–240, 2004.
56. Horton ES, Foley JE, Shen SG, Baron MA. Efficacy and tolerability of initial combination therapy with nateglinide and metformin in treatment – Naïve patients with type 2 diabetes. *Curr Med Res Opin* 20: 883–889, 2004.
57. Milagro FI, Martinez JA. Effects of the oral administration of beta3-adrenergic agonist on lipid metabolism in alloxan-diabetic rats. *J Pharm Pharmacol* 52: 851–856, 2000.
58. Edvardsson U, von Lowenhielm HB, Panfilov O, Nystrom AC, Nilsson F, Dahllof B. Hepatic protein expression of lean mice and obese diabetic mice treated with peroxisome proliferator-activated receptor activators. *Proteomics* 3: 468–478, 2003.
59. Sanchez JC, Converset V, Nolan A, et al. Effect of rosiglitazone on the differential expression of obesity and insulin resistance associated proteins in lep/lep mice. *Proteomics* 3: 1500–1520, 2003.
60. Kersten S. Peroxisome proliferator activated receptors and obesity. *Eur J Pharmacol* 440: 223–234, 2002.
61. Berkowitz K, Peters R, Kjos SL, et al. Effect of Troglitazone on insulin sensitivity and pancreatic β-cell function in women at high risk for NIDDM. *Diabetes* 45: 1572–1579, 1996.
62. Fulgencio JP, Kohl C, Girad J, Pegorier JP. Troglitazone inhibits fatty acid oxidation and esterification, and gluconeogenesis in isolated hepatocytes from starved rats. *Diabetes* 45: 1556–1562, 1996.
63. Thomas T, Pfeiffer AFH. Foods for the prevention of diabetes: How do they work? *Diabetes/Metab Res Rev* 28: 25–49, 2012.
64. Fogarty DC, Vassalo I, Di Cara A, et al. A 48-hour Vegan diet challenge in healthy women and men induces a branch-chain amino acid related, health associated, metabolic signature. *Mol Nutr Food Res* 2017 Oct. doi:10.1002/mnfr.201700703.
65. Nicolson GL. Metabolic syndrome and mitochondrial function: Molecular replacement and antioxidant supplements to prevent membrane peroxidation and restore mitochondrial function. *J Cell Biochem* 100(6): 1352–1369, 2007 Apr.
66. Sako Y, Grill VE. A 48-hour lipid infusion in the rat time-dependently inhibits glucose-induced insulin secretion and B cell oxidation through a process likely coupled to fatty acid oxidation. *Endocrinology* 127: 1580–1589, 1990.
67. Opara EC, Hubbard VS, Burch W, et al. Characterization of the insulinotropic potency of polyunsaturated fatty acids. *Endocrinology* 130: 657–662, 1992.
68. Elks ML. Chronic perifusion of rat islets with palmitate suppresses glucose-stimulated insulin release. *Endocrinology* 133: 208–214, 1993.
69. Zhou YP, Grill VE. Long-term exposure of rat pancreatic islets to fatty acids inhibits glucose-induced insulin secretion and biosynthesis through a glucose fatty acid cycle. *J Clin Invest* 93: 870–876, 1994.
70. Opara EC, Garfinkel M, Hubbard VS, et al. Effect of fatty acids on insulin release: Role of chain length and degree of unsaturation. *Am J Physiol* 266 (Endocrinol. Metab. 29): E635–E639, 1994.
71. Opara EC, Burch W, et al. Characterization of glutamine-regulated pancreatic hormone release. *Surg Forum* 41: 16–19, 1990.
72. Malaisse WJ, Sener A, Carpinelli AR. The stimulus-secretion coupling of glucose-induced insulin release. XLVI. Physiological role of L-glutamine as a fuel for pancreatic islets. *Mol Cell Endocrinol* 20: 171–189, 1980.
73. Opara EC, Hubbard VS, Burch WM, et al. Addition of L-glutamine to a linoleate perifusate prevents the fatty acid-induced desensitization of pancreatic islet response to glucose. *J Nutr Biochem* 4: 357–361, 1993.
74. Surwit RS, Kuhn CM, Cochrane C, Feinglos MN. Diet-induced type 2 diabetes in C57BL/6J mice. *Diabetes* 40: 82–87, 1988.

75. Surwit RS, Feinglos MN, Rodin J, et al. Differential effects of fat and sucrose on the development of obesity and diabetes in C57BL/6J mice. *Metabolism* 44: 645–651, 1995.

76. Opara EC, Petro A, Tevrizian A, Feinglos MN, Surwit RS. L-Glutamine supplementation of a high fat diet reduces body weight and attenuates hyperglycemia and hyperinsulinemia in C57BL/6J mice. *J Nutr* 126: 273–279, 1996.

77. Ballard TC, Farag A, Branum GD, et al. Effect of L-glutamine on impaired glucose regulation during intravenous lipid administration. *Nutrition* 12: 349–354, 1996.

78. Borel MJ, Williams PE, Jabbour K, et al. Parenteral glutamine infusion alters insulin-mediated glucose metabolism. *J Parent Ent Nutr* 22: 280–285, 1998.

79. Katz J, Golden S, Wals PA. Stimulation of hepatic glycogen synthesis by amino acids. *Proc Natl Acad Sci USA* 73: 3433–3437, 1976.

80. Katz J, Golden S, Wals PA. Glycogen synthesis by rat hepatocytes. *Biochem J* 180: 389–402, 1979.

81. Varnier M, Leese GP, Thompson J, et al. Stimulatory effect of glutamine on glycogen accumulation in human skeletal muscle. *Am J Physiol* 269: E309–E315, 1995.

82. Kraus U, Bertrand L, Maisin L, Rosa M, Hue L. Signalling pathways and combinatory effects of insulin and amino acids in isolated rat hepatocytes. *Eur J Biochem* 269: 3742–3750, 2002.

83. Cersosimo E, William P, Hoxworth B. Glutamine blocks lipolysis and ketogenesis of fasting. *Am J Physiol* 250: E248–E252, 1986.

84. Dechelotte P, Damaun D, Rongier, et al. Absorption and metabolic effects of enterally administered glutamine in humans. *Am J Physiol* 260: G677–G682, 1991.

85. Lavoinne A, Baquet A, Hue L. Stimulation of glycogen synthesis and lipogenesis by glutamine in isolated rat hepatocytes. *Biochem J* 248: 429–437, 1987.

86. Chan C, Berthiaume F, Lee K, Yarmush ML. Metabolic flux analysis of hepatocyte function in hormone- and amino acid-supplemented plasma. *Metab Eng* 5: 1–15, 2003.

87. Taghizadeh M, Jamilian M, Mazloomi M, Sanami M, Asemi Z. A randomized-controlled clinical trial investigating the effect of omega-3 fatty acids and vitamin E co-supplementation on markers of insulin metabolism and lipid profiles in gestational diabetes. *J Clin Lipidol* 10(2): 386–393, 2016.

88. Eriksson J, Saloranta C, Widen E, et al. Non-esterified fatty acids do not contribute to insulin resistance in persons at risk of developing Type 2 (non-insulin-dependent) diabetes mellitus. *Diabetologia* 34: 192–197, 1991.

89. Kelley DE, Mandarino LJ. Fuel selection in human skeletal muscle in insulin resistance: A re-examination. *Diabetes* 49: 677–683, 2000.

13 Management of Obesity-Associated Type 2 Diabetes

Wanda C. Lakey, Lillian F. Lien, and Mark N. Feinglos

CONTENTS

13.1 PATHOPHYSIOLOGY: DIETARY EFFECTS ON SUBJECTS AT RISK FOR THE DEVELOPMENT OF OBESITY-INDUCED DIABETES MELLITUS TYPE 2

13.1.1 ANIMAL STUDIES

The impact of dietary factors on metabolism in general and glycemia in particular is well established in animal models [1–4]. For example, Surwit et al. in 1988 noted that the obese (C57BL/6J ob/ob) mouse only develops significant hyperglycemia in the presence of stress [5]. Initially, the background strain (C57BL/6J) was used as a normal control animal. However, when data using both the C57BL/6J animal and another strain (A/J) were compared, it became clear that the former mouse strain was always mildly hyperglycemic and hyperinsulinemic compared to the latter. This raised the possibility that the ob/ob mutation was an obesity mutation, exacerbating the genetic predilection to hyperglycemia already present in the background strain. Thus, Surwit and Feinglos developed a nutritional experiment to explore the effect of a high-fat, high-calorie diet on the development of obesity and hyperglycemia in these mice. This would serve as a model of the development of type 2 diabetes induced by diet in human populations with a similar genetic predisposition. Both A/J and C57BL/6J mice were studied. For each strain, 10 mice were fed a control diet of ad libitum water and Purina Rodent Chow, whereas 10 mice were fed a high-fat, high-simple-carbohydrate diet *ad libitum.* (For more detailed nutrient composition of the diets, please see Table 13.1). The control diet and the high-fat, high-simple-carbohydrate diet were administered for 6 months. Both strains of mice developed obesity after 16 weeks, but the C57BL/6J mice were significantly more obese. Furthermore, the diet-induced obesity led to moderate glucose intolerance and insulin resistance in the A/J mice, but obesity in the C57BL/6J mice led to clear-cut diabetes with markedly increased fasting glucose and insulin levels: glucose 248 ± 8 mg/dL versus 162 ± 6 mg/dL in C57BL/6J mice versus A/J mice, respectively. The authors concluded that, on this "diabetogenic" diet, C57BL/6J

TABLE 13.1
Nutrient Composition of Mice Diets in Surwit et al.

Nutrient	High-Fat, High–Simple Carbohydrate Diet (%)	Control Diet (Purina Rodent Chow and Water) (%)
Protein	20.5	23
Fat	35.8	4.5
Fiber	0.4	6.0
Ash	3.6	8.0
Moisture	3.1	—
Carbohydrate	36.8 (mostly disaccharides)	56 (complex carbohydrate)

Source: Surwit, R.S. et al., *Diabetes*, 37, 1163–1167, 1988.

---

mice appear to develop diabetes in a manner that is analogous to most cases of human type 2 diabetes in predisposed individuals [5].

Several subsequent studies addressed factors that could attenuate the progression to insulin resistance in the diet-induced diabetes mouse model. Bray et al. studied Zucker lean (Fa/?) and obese fatty (fa/fa) rats, which were placed on a control stock diet or a high-fat diet. At 10 weeks of age, the rats were either adrenalectomized or received a sham operation [6]. The dietary interventions began at 15 weeks of age. Among the many parameters analyzed in the study were plasma insulin concentrations in the rats at 32 weeks of age. Results showed that diet affected the insulin levels in the sham-operated rats: Insulin levels were higher in the rats fed a high-fat diet than in those fed the control diet (Table 13.2). This difference was not statistically significant in the fatty rats but was significant in the lean rats. Furthermore, adrenalectomy drastically reduced insulin levels and eliminated the dietary effects. Insulin levels were almost identical in adrenalectomized fatty rats fed a high-fat diet vs fatty rats fed the control diet, and this was the case with adrenalectomized lean rats as well (Table 13.3). After studying the effects of adrenalectomy on other parameters, such as body composition and lipoprotein lipase activity in the rats, the authors concluded that "adrenalectomy ameliorates but does not cure the [genetic and dietary obesity] syndrome" [6]. Nonetheless, the authors concluded that high-fat feeding to animals with obesity (whether caused by hypothalamic injury or by genetic defects) does accelerate the further development of obesity.

Opara et al. also investigated methods of ameliorating diet-induced obesity and diabetes in animal models by analyzing the effects of amino acid supplementation during high-fat feeding. The authors studied C57BL/6J mice on four diets: (1) a low-fat, low-sucrose diet (LL); (2) a high-fat, low-sucrose diet (HL); (3) a high-fat, low-sucrose diet supplemented with L-glutamine (HL + Gln); and (4) a high-fat, low-sucrose diet supplemented with L-alanine (HL + Ala) [7]. For each dietary regimen, 10 age- and weight-matched male mice were maintained on the diet for 5.5 months. As expected, the mice who received a high-fat diet were significantly heavier than those who received a low-fat diet. Yet, at 8 weeks, it was noted that the HL + Gln and HL + Ala mice had gained significantly less weight than the HL mice. With regard to glucose metabolism, it was found that HL mice had higher plasma glucose levels than LL mice, as expected, and this difference persisted for more than

TABLE 13.2

Plasma Insulin Levels in Bray et al.—Sham-Operated Animals

Sham-Operation Rats	High-Fat Diet	Control Stock Diet
Fatty	344.1 ± 53 U/mL	300.3 ± 38.7 U/mL
Lean	99.6 ± 18.7 U/mL	54.6 ± 6.5 U/mL

Source: Bray, G.A. et al., *Am. J. Physiol.*, 262, E32–E39, 1992.

TABLE 13.3

Plasma Insulin Levels in Bray et al.—Adrenalectomized Animals [6]

Adrenalectomized Rats	High-Fat Diet	Control Stock Diet
Fatty	97.5 ± 14.2 U/mL	99.5 ± 128 U/mL
Lean	26.1 ± 3.3 U/mL	25.2 ± 1.9 U/mL

Source: Bray, G.A. et al., *Am. J. Physiol.*, 262, E32–E39, 1992.

5 months. However, both alanine and glutamine supplementation of the high-fat diet were effective in reducing plasma glucose concentrations for the first 3 months, and glutamine supplementation helped maintain normoglycemia for more than 5 months. Hyperinsulinemia was also attenuated by amino acid supplementation. Thus, the authors concluded that the supplementation of a high-fat diet with glutamine reduces body weight and attenuates hyperglycemia and hyperinsulinemia [7]. These findings in mice are particularly intriguing given the recent interest in high-protein diets in human studies (see section 13.2.4, High-Protein Diets).

13.1.2   HUMAN STUDIES—MACRONUTRIENTS: DIETARY FAT

Numerous studies have attempted to address the impact of dietary patterns on the development of type 2 diabetes in humans, but these studies are very heterogeneous in design and are thus difficult to compare. In 2001, Hu et al. performed a literature search of metabolic studies examining dietary intake and hyperglycemia. With regard to the effect of dietary fat, they noted that the impact of fatty acids on the development of insulin resistance could arise from mechanisms independent of obesity, such as direct effects of fatty acids on insulin receptor binding, ion permeability, and cell signaling [8].

In their review of the literature, Hu et al. found that human studies were far less consistent than animal studies in demonstrating adverse effects of high-fat diets on insulin sensitivity, but they cited a number of weaknesses of some of the early studies including diets administered in non-randomized order and studies of very short duration (less than 1 month). Among the major studies investigating total fat intake and insulin sensitivity was the Insulin Resistance and Atherosclerosis (IRAS) study. IRAS was a large, cross-sectional investigation of insulin sensitivity (assessed using intravenous glucose tolerance test [IVGTT] data subjected to minimal model analysis) in more than 1,000 subjects. In multivariate analyses adjusting for variables such as body mass index (BMI), the study could not demonstrate a statistically significant association between dietary fat intake and insulin sensitivity [8,9]. Alternatively, there have been other studies demonstrating positive associations between total fat and diabetes development (i.e., the San Luis Valley Diabetes Study [10]) and especially between saturated fat and hyperglycemia (i.e., the Netherlands Zutphen Study [11]). At the time, Hu et al. reached a tentative conclusion that total dietary fat intake may not be predictive of the risk of developing human type 2 diabetes. However, they noted that available data did suggest a possible beneficial effect of polyunsaturated fat and a possible adverse effect of saturated fat, although the data on types of dietary fat were not consistent [8]. In addition, they pointed out that analyses of monounsaturated fat may have been confounded by its usual correlation with saturated fat intake in the typical Western diet.

Subsequently, Hu et al. collaborated in further investigations of the influence of dietary fat on risk of type 2 diabetes. In the Nurses' Health Study, Hu et al. followed 84,941 women from 1980 to 1996 who, at baseline, were free of diagnosed cardiovascular disease (CVD), diabetes, and cancer [12]. Information about the macronutrient composition of the diet and lifestyle of the subjects was collected over 16 years of follow-up. The authors found that lack of exercise, smoking, and a "poor diet" significantly increased the risk of diabetes, even after adjustment for BMI. Specifically, trans-fat intake was quantified (in terms of ascending quintiles of intake), as was the ratio of polyunsaturated-to-saturated fat intake. As the ratio of polyunsaturated-to-saturated fat increased, the relative risk of type 2 diabetes decreased significantly. From the first to fifth quintile of trans-fat intake, the relative risk trended upward significantly, implying a positive association of trans-fat, and an inverse association of polyunsaturated fat, with risk of type 2 diabetes in women [12]. Furthermore, the argument supporting the role of saturated fat in the development of type 2 diabetes appears to be bolstered by multiple interventional studies demonstrating improvements in insulin sensitivity in healthy, overweight, and diabetic cohorts with increased unsaturated dietary fat compared to saturated fat [13–16].

Van Dam et al. studied dietary fat intake and risk of type 2 diabetes in men [17]. Men who, at baseline, were free of diagnosed diabetes, CVD, and cancer were followed in the Health Professionals Follow-Up study (n = 42,504) for 12 years, during which 1,321 incident cases of type 2 diabetes were documented. The authors found that both total and saturated fat intake were associated with a significantly increased risk of developing type 2 diabetes. The relative risk (and 95% confidence interval [CI]) for extreme quintiles was 1.27 (1.04–1.55) for total fat and 1.34 (1.09–1.66) for saturated fat, although, on additional adjustment for BMI, the associations lost statistical significance. However, in an accompanying editorial, Marshall and Bessesen pointed out that, although adjusting for BMI eliminated the effect, that fact does not imply that dietary fat is not important at all; they emphasized that any dietary factor that leads to weight gain will likely lead to the development of diabetes as well [18]. In addition, they cited the major randomized, controlled trials that have shown that lifestyle change, including dietary modifications, can reduce the risk of type 2 diabetes (i.e., Finnish Diabetes Prevention Study [19], Diabetes Prevention Program [20]).

A 2016 systematic review and meta-analysis of 102 randomized, controlled feeding trials evaluating the effects of macronutrient intake on the homeostasis of glucose and insulin provides additional evidence regarding dietary fat subtypes to consider. Reductions in hemoglobin A1c (HbA1c), 2-hour postchallenge insulin, and homeostasis model assessment for insulin resistance (HOMA-IR) occurred after replacing carbohydrates with monounsaturated fatty acids (MUFAs). HbA1c and fasting insulin were decreased after replacing carbohydrate with polyunsaturated fatty acid (PUFA). Reductions in glucose, HbA1c, c-peptide, and HOMA-IR were observed when PUFA replaced saturated fatty acids (SFAs). Additionally, improved insulin secretion occurred when PUFA replaced carbohydrates, SFAs, and MUFAs [21].

Thus, although debate continues as to the extent to which dietary fat contributes to the development of obesity-associated diabetes, it is clear that attention to not only total fat intake, but also fat subtypes, is warranted in human nutrition analyses.

13.1.3 HUMAN STUDIES—MACRONUTRIENTS: DIETARY CARBOHYDRATE

In a similar manner to the debate regarding the effect of total dietary fat or fat subtypes on the risk of developing type 2 diabetes, studies of the effect of total dietary carbohydrate consumption on diabetes risk are likewise inconsistent. Metabolic derangements may be the consequence of both quantity and quality of the carbohydrates consumed [13]. With regard to the issue of dietary carbohydrate and risk of development of diabetes, Hu et al. proposed in 2001 that the traditional notions of "simple versus complex" carbohydrates are not that helpful in predicting the risk of type 2 diabetes [8]. Rather, the authors addressed use of the concepts of glycemic index (GI) and glycemic load (GL). The GI of a particular ingested carbohydrate refers to its effect on plasma glucose (i.e., how much 50 g of the particular carbohydrate causes the plasma glucose [area under the curve] concentration to increase, as compared with 50 g of a reference carbohydrate such as white bread or glucose) [8,22]. The GL is an attempt to account for both the glycemic effect and quantity of carbohydrate simultaneously (i.e., GL = product of the GI and the carbohydrate content) [8]. Although some studies showed lower plasma insulin levels, fructosamine, and urinary C-peptide concentrations in response to low-GI versus high-GI diets, and others showed a higher incidence of diabetes in association with higher GI and GL, not all data have been consistent [8,13,23–25]. The risk of diabetes associated with dietary GI, GL, and digestible carbohydrates was evaluated in a large, prospective, case-cohort study, the European Prospective Investigation into Cancer and Nutrition (EPIC)-InterAct study [26]. Analyses of dietary data from eight participating European countries comparing the highest and lowest quartiles of consumption did not demonstrate an increased incident rate of diabetes associated with dietary GI (1.05; 95% CI: 0.96, 1.16), GL (1.07; 95% CI: 0.95, 1.20), or digestible carbohydrates (0.98; 95% CI: 0.86, 1.10) after being adjusted for confounders. Thus, the significance of GI and GL on progression to diabetes continues to be a subject of debate.

More recent data from three large cohorts swing the pendulum again toward the relevance of GI and GL in the development of diabetes. Follow-up from Hu et al. in 2014 on US participants in the Nurses' Health Study, the Nurses' Health Study II, and the Health Professionals Follow-Up Study demonstrated the deleterious metabolic effects of high GI and GL, with a subsequent increase in the risk of developing type 2 diabetes [27]. There were 15,027 cases of incident type 2 diabetes over 3,800,618 person-years of follow-up. The risk of developing type 2 diabetes was 33% (95% CI: 26%, 41%) higher for individuals in the highest quintile of energy-adjusted GI compared to those in the lowest quintile and 10% (95% CI: 2%, 18%) higher for participants in the highest quintile of energy-adjusted GL compared to those in the lowest quintile with pooled multivariable analyses. Additionally, Hu et al. performed an updated meta-analysis that included the results of their three cohort studies, along with prior studies evaluating the association of GI and GL and the risk of developing type 2 diabetes. The updated meta-analysis supported the findings from their three cohort studies. The summary relative risks (RRs) for the development of type 2 diabetes for the highest GI category compared to the lowest was 1.19 (95% CI, 1.14–1.24), while the highest GL category compared to the lowest was 1.13 (95% CI, 1.08–1.17). The authors noted several limitations of the prior studies that did not find an association between GI and GL and the development of type 2 diabetes: the sole use of a baseline dietary assessment, differences in GI values found in multiple databases, and difficulty in assigning GI values to foods not in a database. Hu et al. also found a 50% increase in the risk of developing type 2 diabetes when a diet low in cereal fiber was combined with a high-GI or GL diet [27]. Additional epidemiologic cohort studies also found an association between diabetes risk and consumption of whole grains and cereal fiber, although this has not been consistently observed in all studies [13]. The improvements in insulin sensitivity and glucose metabolism associated with whole grains may be partially mediated by the weight loss associated with a higher consumption rate of whole grains and the lower GI of whole grains compared to refined grains [13]. In light of the recent data, despite the inconsistencies, there seems to be a continued role for food choices with a lower GI or GL in the reduction of insulin resistance.

13.1.4 HUMAN STUDIES—FOODS AND FOOD GROUPS

Consumption of individual foods and food groups can influence the risk of developing type 2 diabetes; however, BMI is often a confounding variable in the analyses, because obesity is a risk factor for diabetes [12,13,17,28–40]. When considered separately, long-term weight control has been observed with consumption of food associated with decreased rates of chronic diseases, such as type 2 diabetes [41]. Conversely, long-term weight gain has been observed with the consumption of food associated with increased rates of chronic diseases [41].

13.1.4.1 Fruits and Vegetables

Consumption of three servings of whole fruit per day was associated with a decreased incident risk of type 2 diabetes (multivariate-adjusted hazard ratio [HR], 0.82 [95% CI, 0.72–0.94]) in the Nurses' Health Study, although a similar consumption of total fruits and vegetables per day was not associated with a decreased risk (HR, 0.99 [95% CI, 0.94–1.050]) [29]. In the same cohort, a decreased risk of incident diabetes was associated with an increase in consumption of one serving per day of green, leafy vegetables (HR 0.91 [95% CI, 0.84–0.98]). A meta-analysis demonstrated a similar association with consumption of green, leafy vegetables and a reduction in incident risk of type 2 diabetes [30]. A 14% diabetes risk reduction was associated with consumption of 1.35 servings per day of green leafy vegetables compared to 0.2 servings per day (HR, 0.86; 95% CI, 0.77–0.96). Pooled HRs from the Nurses' Health Study, Nurses' Health Study II, and Health Professionals Follow-Up Study were associated with a decreased risk of incident diabetes for every three servings consumed per week of total fruit (HR, 0.98; 95% CI, 0.96–0.99) [31]. Heterogeneity was observed in the pooled HRs of individual fruits that was not accounted for by the GI of the individual fruits.

A separate study was conducted in these three cohorts that evaluated the relationships between changes in diet and weight at 4-year intervals over the course of the 20-year study [41]. Participants gained an average of 3.35 lbs within each 4-year period. Pooled, multivariate-adjusted analyses of the effects of increased daily servings of individual food groups demonstrated an inverse relationship between weight and increased daily servings of vegetables (–0.22 lbs; 95% CI, –0.34 to –0.11; $P < .001$) and fruits (–0.49 lbs; 95% CI, –0.63 to –0.35; $P < .001$) within each 4-year period. The authors surmised that an increase in dietary fruits and vegetables likely resulted in a reduction in caloric intake from other types of food, with an overall reduction in energy consumption and subsequent weight loss. In addition to consumption of fruits and vegetables, weight changes in these cohorts were also independently associated with other lifestyle factors, such as physical activity, alcohol, smoking, sleep, and watching television. Aggregate data demonstrated greater changes in weight (5.93 lbs; 95% CI, 4.35–7.52) within each 4-year period for participants in the lowest versus highest quintiles of dietary and lifestyle changes.

13.1.4.2 Whole Grains and Cereal Fiber

Consumption of whole grains and cereal fiber has an inverse association with incident diabetes risk in several, but not all, prospective cohort studies [13]. Comparison of whole-grain consumption in the highest quintile compared to the lowest from male participants in the Health Professionals Follow-Up Study was associated with a decreased RR of type 2 diabetes after adjustment for BMI (RR, 0.70; 95% CI, 0.57–0.85) [40]. After additional multivariate adjustments, including cereal fiber, the association was no longer significant. The authors propose that cereal fiber may be a mediating factor in the diabetes risk reduction observed with increased whole-grain consumption. Diabetes risk was not associated with increased consumption of refined grains in this study, although other studies found an association between higher consumption of white rice and an increased risk of diabetes [35,36]. Similar reductions in diabetes risk related to whole-grain consumption, after adjustments for potential confounders and BMI, were observed in the Nurses' Health Study I (RR, 0.75; 95% CI, 0.68–0.83) and Nurses' Health Study II (RR, 0.86; 95% CI, 0.72–1.02) [32]. A decreased association with diabetes risk was also observed with higher consumption rates of bran. Additional prospective cohort studies support the association of diabetes risk reduction with the consumption of cereal fiber [12,33,34], with the suggestion that one mechanism may improve whole-body insulin sensitivity [42].

In the previously cited study conducted with the cohorts from the Nurses' Health Study, Nurses' Health Study II, and Health Professionals Follow-Up, the relationships between changes in diet and weight at 4-year intervals over the course of the 20-year study were evaluated [41]. Pooled, multivariate-adjusted analyses demonstrated an inverse relationship between weight and increased daily servings of whole grains (–0.37 lbs; 95% CI, –0.48 to –0.25; $P < .001$) within each 4-year interval, with greater changes in weight noted with aggregate data combining dietary and lifestyle changes.

13.1.4.3 Red and Processed Meats

An association between consumption of red and processed meats and incident diabetes has been observed in several cohort studies [17,37,38,39]. Female participants in the Nurses' Health Study II who consumed processed meat at least five times per week compared to consumption fewer than one time per week had an increased risk of incident diabetes after adjustments for nondietary confounders (RR, 1.91; 95% CI, 1.42–2.57) [37]. Male participants in the Health Professionals Follow-Up Study also had an increased risk of incident diabetes with consumption of processed meat at least five times per week compared to consumption fewer than one time per month after adjustments for confounding variables (RR, 1.46; 95% CI, 1.14–1.86) [17]. Incident diabetes risk for the male participants was also increased with extreme quintiles of total fat and saturated fat from meat consumption, but this association was not independent of BMI. A systematic review and meta-analysis in 2009 of cohort studies on meat consumption and associated incident diabetes suggests an increased risk with high consumption rates of red meat and processed meat compared to low consumption: total meat (RR, 1.17; 95% CI 0.92–1.48), red meat (RR, 1.21; 95% CI, 1.07–1.38), and processed meat (RR, 1.41; 95% CI, 1.25–1.60) [38]. However, the authors noted considerable heterogeneity and could not discount the possibility of confounding in their conclusion. Pan et al. performed a pooled analysis of the cohorts from the Nurses' Health Study, Nurses' Health Study II, and Health Professionals Follow-Up Study and an updated meta-analysis in 2011 to examine the association further [39]. Each cohort demonstrated a positive association between consumption of unprocessed and processed red meats and incident diabetes risk (all P-trend < .001). This finding remained significant after adjustment for BMI, age, lifestyle factors, and other dietary factors. For a one-serving-per-day increase, the pooled HRs were 1.12 (95% CI, 1.08–1.16) for unprocessed red meat, 1.32 (95% CI, 1.25–1.40) for processed red meat, and 1.14 (95% CI, 1.10–1.18) for total red meat. The authors' updated meta-analysis confirmed the association observed in the three pooled cohort studies.

In the pooled analysis from the Nurses' Health Study, Nurses' Health Study II, and Health Professionals Follow-Up cohorts evaluating the relationship between changes in diet and weight at 4-year intervals over the course of the 20-year study, multivariate-adjusted analyses demonstrated an association between weight gain and increased daily servings of processed meats (0.93 lbs; 95% CI, 0.79–1.08; P < .001), unprocessed meats (0.95 lbs; 95% CI, 0.55–1.34; P < .001), and trans-fat (0.65 lbs; 95% CI, 0.41–0.89; P < .001) within each 4-year interval [41]. Similar findings were observed in the 459 healthy adult participants in the Baltimore Longitudinal Study of Aging [43]. The annual mean change in BMI was 0.30 ± 0.06 kg/m² for participants consuming a meat-and-potatoes dietary pattern, consisting predominantly of red and processed meat.

13.1.4.4 Dairy Products

The Coronary Artery Risk Development in Young Adults (CARDIA) study evaluated the association between dairy consumption and the 10-year incidence of insulin resistance syndrome (obesity, glucose intolerance, hypertension, and dyslipidemia) in a population-based prospective cohort [44]. Among baseline overweight (BMI $\geq$ 25 kg/m²) participants, there was an inverse relationship between dairy consumption and insulin resistance syndrome. Overweight participants with the highest weekly dairy consumption ($\geq$ 35 times) had a 72% lower adjusted odds of developing two or more components of the insulin resistance syndrome compared to participants with the lowest weekly dairy consumption (<10 times). Race and sex analyses did not attenuate these findings. Low-fat dairy consumption in additional prospective cohort studies was significantly associated with a lower risk of incident diabetes when compared with high-fat dairy consumption in men [45] and women [46].

13.1.4.5 Nuts

Increased consumption of nuts and peanut butter was inversely associated with incident diabetes risk in the Nurses' Health Study [47]. BMI, a significant risk factor for type 2 diabetes, was a strong confounder in the analyses. In general, women who consumed more nuts weighed less at baseline compared to women who consumed fewer nuts. Women with a higher weekly consumption of nuts ($\geq$5 times) compared to women who never or almost never consumed nuts had an age-adjusted RR for diabetes of 0.55 (95% CI, 0.45–0.66) and an attenuated RR of 0.73 (95% CI, 0.60–0.89) after multivariate adjustments including BMI. Similar results were also seen with women who had higher weekly peanut butter consumption ($\geq$5 times) compared to women who never or almost never consumed peanut butter with an age-adjusted RR of 0.78 (95% CI, 0.68–0.90) and a slightly attenuated RR of 0.79 (95% CI, 0.68–0.91) after multivariate adjustments including BMI. Although nuts contain a high fat content, women with higher nut consumption at baseline did not gain more weight compared to women who consumed fewer nuts. Weight change over the 16 years of follow-up was not significantly different between the different categories of nut consumption.

In a separate analysis of women in the Nurses' Health Study and Nurses' Health Study II who consumed walnuts and other nuts, BMI was also a significant confounding variable [48].

Women who consumed two or more servings per week of walnuts compared to women who never or rarely consumed walnuts had a reduction in incident diabetes with an age-adjusted pooled HR of 0.61 (95% CI, 0.49–0.75) and an attenuated HR of 0.76 (95% CI, 0.62–0.94) after multivariable adjustments including BMI. The age-adjusted HR for women consuming two or more servings per week of other tree nuts was 0.78 (95% CI, 0.69–0.88), with a null association after multivariable adjustment including BMI. The authors concluded that body weight was possibly mediating the association between a decreased incidence of type 2 diabetes and increased nut consumption. This conclusion was supported by findings from multiple studies [49,50].

In a prior study by the authors of healthy, middle-aged women in the Nurses' Health Study II, women who consumed nuts two or more times per week had less mean weight gain (5.04 ± 0.12 kg) over 8 years of follow-up compared to women who never or rarely ate nuts (5.55 ± 0.04 kg) (P for trend < .001) [49]. A similar association was observed with peanuts and tree nuts. These results were independent of BMI categories. The risk of obesity was slightly lower in women who consumed nuts two or more times per week compared to women who never or rarely consumed nuts (P for trend < .03). Additionally, epidemiologic data from the 1999–2004 National Health and Nutrition Examination Survey (NHANES) demonstrated an association between nut consumption and a reduction in risk factors for type 2 diabetes and CVD [50]. Individuals who consumed at least 0.25 ounces per day of peanuts, peanut butter, or tree nuts had an associated decrease in BMI (27.7 kg/m^2 ± 0.2 vs 28.1 ± 0.1 kg/m^2; P < .05) and waist circumference (95.6 ± 0.4 cm vs 96.4 ± 0.3 cm; P < .05) when compared to individuals who did not consume nuts. Several mechanisms have been proposed for the inverse relationship between nut consumption and weight gain. Nuts are high in protein and fiber, which may increase satiety [49]. An increase in diet-induced thermogenesis and resting energy expenditure may account for weight maintenance associated with nut consumption secondary to the high fiber, protein, and saturated fat content of nuts [49].

13.1.4.6 Sugar-Sweetened Beverages

Consumption of sugar-sweetened beverages has been associated with an increased risk of developing type 2 diabetes in several studies [29,51–57], but not all [58]. A prospective study of 91,249 women without diabetes at baseline in the Nurses' Health Study II identified 741 incident cases of type 2 diabetes over 716,300 person-years [53]. An increased consumption of sugar-sweetened beverages was associated with a significant increase in weight compared to decreased consumption. The RR of type 2 diabetes was 1.83% (95% CI, 1.42–2.36) for women consuming one or more sugar-sweetened beverages per day compared to women consuming less than one per month after adjustment for potential confounders. A prospective cohort of 43,960 African American women without diabetes at baseline and with complete food diary and weight data demonstrated an association between consumption of two or more soft drinks per day (incident rate ratio 1.24; 95% CI, 1.13–1.52) and fruit juices (incident rate ratio 1.31; 95% CI, 1.13–1.52) with incident type 2 diabetes after adjustment for confounding variables [52]. Imamura et al. performed a systematic review and meta-analysis of prospective studies of adults in the United States and United Kingdom without diabetes to examine the association between type 2 diabetes and consumption of sugar-sweetened beverages, artificially sweetened beverages, and fruit juice. They found that 38,253 incident cases of type 2 diabetes were reported over 10,126,754 person-years. After adjustment for adiposity, the incidence of type 2 diabetes was increased by 13% per serving of sugar-sweetened beverages per day (95% CI, 5.8%–21.0%; I^2 = 79%). The evidence for sugar-sweetened beverages was of moderate quality. The incidence risk for type 2 diabetes was 8% per serving of an artificially sweetened beverage per day (95% CI, 2.1%–15.0%; I^2 = 64%) and 7% per serving of fruit juice per day (95% CI, 0.8%–14%; I^2 = 51%) after adjustment for adiposity. The evidence for artificially sweetened beverages and fruit juice was of low quality. Publication bias and residual confounding likely contributed to the findings for artificially sweetened beverages. An association with fruit juice consumption and incident type 2 diabetes was unstable on contour-enhanced funnel plots and was highly dependent on study design. Estimated 10-year absolute event rates of incident type 2 diabetes were 11% (20.9 million events) in the United States and 5.8% (2.6 million events) in the United Kingdom. Adiposity-adjusted analyses assuming a causal association of incident type 2 diabetes and sugar-sweetened beverage consumption estimated 1.8 million excess events in the United States and 79,000 excess events in the United Kingdom would be attributable to sugar-sweetened beverages [51].

13.1.4.7 Coffee and Caffeinated Beverages

Type 2 diabetes risk reduction may be associated with long-term coffee consumption.

Increasing amounts of data support the possible association of long-term coffee consumption and a reduced risk of type 2 diabetes [58–66]. A 2014 systematic review and meta-analysis of 28 prospective cohort studies reported an inverse dose-response association between coffee consumption and incident diabetes [59]. The RR (95% CI) for diabetes associated with daily coffee consumption compared to no or rare coffee consumption was 0.92 (0.90–0.94) for one cup, 0.85 (0.82–0.88) for two cups, 0.79 (0.75–0.83) for three cups, 0.75 (0.71–0.80) for four cups, 0.71 (0.65–0.76) for five cups, and 0.67 (0.61–0.74) for six cups. Both caffeinated and decaffeinated coffee consumption were associated with an inverse relationship with diabetes risk in the meta-analysis. A proposed mechanism for the beneficial effect of coffee includes the role of a phenolic compound found in coffee, chlorogenic acid (CGA), which serves as an antioxidant, reduces liver output, inhibits glucose-6-phosphate translocase, and reduces sodium-dependent glucose transport of brush border membrane vesicles [44–46,59]. Lignans, trigonelline, and quinides are additional coffee components that may contribute to the glycemic benefits [47,48,59]. On the other hand, in patients with established type 2 diabetes, there is evidence that caffeine can aggravate postprandial hyperglycemia, indicating that the use of decaffeinated coffee and other beverages might be more desirable [67].

Cohort studies demonstrating an inverse association between tea consumption and incident diabetes have been inconsistent [60,62,68]. The teas consumed in these studies were presumably caffeinated, although this was not always explicitly stated. Tea consumption in more than 88,000 women in the Nurses' Health Study II did not significantly decrease the risk of incident diabetes [60], whereas an inverse association was observed with total tea consumption (green and black) in a systematic review and meta-analysis conducted several years later [62]. Conversely, green tea, but not black or oolong tea, was associated with a reduced risk of incident diabetes in a study of Japanese adults [68].

Coffee and tea consumption have been associated with protection against weight gain in some studies [69,70]. In a cross-sectional survey study of 8,821 Polish subjects, an inverse relationship was observed between BMI and waist circumference and high consumption (three or more cups per day) of coffee or tea compared to individuals who consumed less than one cup of coffee or tea per day [70]. The proposed mechanisms for this protective effect against weight gain are multifactorial [69,70]. Caffeine in the coffee and tea produces both a thermogenic and ergogenic effect, with subsequent weight loss [69,70]. Phenolic compounds in coffee, such as CGAs, exert a positive effect on glucose metabolism via several mechanisms: effect on GI absorption of glucose, effects on glucose storage (skeletal muscle, adipose tissue, and liver), and effect on hormonal regulation of glucose by the pancreas. CGAs also impact lipid metabolism. The combined effect from CGAs on glucose and lipid metabolism increases insulin secretion, while reducing cholesterol, free fatty acids, insulin resistance, and glucose levels. This can potentially lead to a reduction in obesity, metabolic syndrome, type 2 diabetes, and CVD. The polyphenols found in tea likely contribute in a similar manner to reduce the risk of developing the components of metabolic syndrome, such as insulin resistance [70].

13.1.5 Human Studies—Dietary Patterns

Initial observations demonstrating the benefit of nutrient repletion for the treatment and prevention of diseases attributed to nutrient deficiencies, such as vitamin C for scurvy, were the impetus for initial dietary recommendations focused on a single-nutrient model for the management of chronic disease [71]. However, diets consist of multiple food groups instead of a single nutrient in isolation. More recent research has shifted the paradigm of dietary recommendations to reflect the greater role of dietary patterns compared to a single-nutrient model in the development and prevention of chronic diseases [71]. Dietary patterns are defined by the quantity and frequency of consumption of food groups and nutrients. Two of the largest dietary trials with the longest duration provide evidence to support the recent shift in dietary recommendations [72,73]. After an average 8 years of follow-up, the Women's Health Initiative Dietary Modification Trial did not demonstrate a reduction in CVD in postmenopausal women randomized to a single-nutrient model with a low-fat diet (20% of calories) consisting of five daily servings of fruits/vegetables and six daily servings of grains compared to women receiving diet-related education materials [72]. In contrast, primary prevention of major cardiovascular events occurred in the PREDIMED Study after a median follow-up of 4.8 years in subjects randomized to a dietary pattern consisting of a Mediterranean diet (high in olive oil, fruits, nuts, vegetables, and whole grains) supplemented with extra-virgin olive oil (EVOO) or mixed nuts versus a control diet (recommended low-fat) [73]. Numerous studies provide additional evidence supporting the associated effect of dietary patterns on cardiovascular risk factors, such as weight [17,74–76] and incident type 2 diabetes [17,28,74–85].

13.1.5.1 Mediterranean Diet

The PREDIMED study demonstrated a reduction in major cardiovascular events in subjects with high cardiovascular risk randomized to Mediterranean diets supplemented with EVOO or mixed nuts versus a control diet after median follow-up of 4.8 years [73]. Adherence to the Mediterranean diet study arms in the PREDIMED study was also associated with a reduction in incident diabetes [81,82]. A subanalysis of the PREDIMED study assessed the efficacy of the Mediterranean diet without caloric restriction for the prevention of type 2 diabetes [81]. Compared to the control diet, multivariate-adjusted HRs were 0.60 (95% CI, 0.43–0.85) for subjects randomized to the Mediterranean diet supplemented with EVOO and 0.82 (95% CI, 0.61–1.10) for subjects randomized to the Mediterranean diet supplemented with mixed nuts. Interestingly, the reduction in incident type 2 diabetes occurred in the absence of significant changes in weight or waist circumference among the three dietary study arms, which may indicate an anti-inflammatory or antioxidant effect of the Mediterranean diet itself that contributes to the risk reduction [86]. The metabolic benefits associated with the Mediterranean diet do not appear to be associated with complete adherence. High adherence [84,85] and moderate adherence [85] to the Mediterranean diet were associated with a significant reduction in incident diabetes risk compared to low adherence in two cohort studies.

In another secondary analysis of the PREDIMED study data evaluating the long-term effects of the calorically unrestricted Mediterranean diet on the metabolic syndrome after a median follow-up of 4.8 years, there was no difference in the risk of developing metabolic syndrome between the control group and the two Mediterranean dietary groups [87]. However, when compared to the control group, reversion of metabolic syndrome was more likely to occur with consumption of the Mediterranean diet with olive oil (HR, 1.35; 95% CI, 1.15–1.58; $P < .001$) and the Mediterranean diet with nuts (HR, 1.28; 95% CI, 1.08–1.51; $P < .001$) [87]. In particular, the prevalence of central obesity was significantly reduced for individuals randomized to the two Mediterranean diets compared to the control diet ($P < .001$ for both). Consumption of the Mediterranean diet with olive oil was also associated with significant decreases in fasting glucose ($P = .02$).

13.1.5.2 Dietary Approaches to Stop Hypertension Diet

The Dietary Approaches to Stop Hypertension (DASH) diet was created as an intervention to prevent or treat hypertension through an emphasis on lower sodium intake and an increased consumption of fruits, vegetables, beans, nuts, whole grains, low-fat dairy products, and fish. There is a lower emphasis on consumption of red meats, sweets, and sugar-sweetened beverages. The macronutrient composition of the original DASH diet consisted of carbohydrates as the primary energy source (55%) with lower energy contribution from fat (27%). Modified versions of the DASH diet include replacing 10% of energy from carbohydrates with monounsaturated fat or with protein. Multiple intervention studies have demonstrated improvements in cardiovascular risk factors associated with adherence to the original DASH diet and modified DASH diets, including improvements in blood pressure, lipid parameters, and weight [80,88–90]. In addition, the DASH dietary patterns have been associated with improved insulin sensitivity in subjects without baseline diabetes [91,92] and a reduction in diabetes risk [80]. An inverse association was observed between adherence to the DASH diet in white participants of the Insulin Resistance Atherosclerosis Study (IRAS) and the incidence of type 2 diabetes [80]. This association was not observed with black or Hispanic participants; however, the authors felt this may be attributed to the relatively small sample size of the study and inaccuracy of food assessments among the different racial/ethnicity cohorts. For male participants in the Health Professionals Follow-Up Study, a measure of dietary quality was assessed with a DASH score calculated from food-frequency questionnaires [93]. The DASH score was associated with a significant reduction in incident diabetes after multivariate adjustments. A stratified analysis of the DASH score demonstrated that the absolute risk reduction for type 2 diabetes was greatest in overweight and obese subjects (BMI $\geq$ 25 kg/m^2).

13.1.5.3 Western Diet

Incident diabetes is increased with long-term consumption of a Western diet, which typically consists of red and processed meats, refined grains, white potatoes, high-fat dairy products, sugar-sweetened beverages, and desserts [17,77,79]. An increased risk of incident diabetes was associated with high intakes of total fat and saturated fat in male participants in the Health Professionals Follow-Up Study, although this association was no longer significant after adjustment for BMI [17]. Within the same cohort, an increased risk of diabetes was associated with an increased consumption frequency of processed meat five or more times per week (RR, 1.46; 95% CI, 1.14–1.86) compared to less than once per month. Analysis of the dietary patterns in the Health Professionals Follow-Up Study demonstrated an increased risk of incident diabetes with consumption of a Western diet (RR, 1.59; 95% CI, 1.32–1.93) [17]. Additionally, the risk of diabetes was substantially increased in subjects who consumed a Western diet with low physical activity levels (RR, 1.96; 95% CI, 1.35–2.84) and obese subjects who consumed a Western diet (RR, 11.2; 95% CI, 8.07–15.60). In contrast, consumption of a prudent diet (high consumption of whole grains, vegetables, fruit, poultry, and fish) was associated with a reduction in incident diabetes (RR, 0.84; 95% CI, 0.70–1.00). A Western diet was also associated with an increased risk of diabetes among female subjects in the Nurses' Health Study when comparing the highest and lowest quintiles of consumption (RR, 1.49; 95% CI, 1.26–1.76) [79].

13.1.5.4 Vegetarian

Vegetarian diets are similar to the Mediterranean and DASH diets with an increased consumption of fruits, vegetables, nuts, and legumes. Given the similarities in the composition of these diets, it is conceivable that a vegetarian diet may also demonstrate significant improvements in metabolic parameters, as seen with the Mediterranean and DASH diets. Although not as extensively studied in randomized, controlled trials as the Mediterranean or DASH diets, there are data from observational studies demonstrating an association between consumption of a vegetarian diet and a reduction in diabetes incidence [94,95]. The Adventist Health Study-2, a long-term observational study with more than 60,000 participants, evaluated the relationship between diet and incident diabetes in adult Adventist church members throughout the United States and Canada [94,95]. Subjects were categorized by their reported consumption of animal-based food items. Based on cross-sectional analyses of baseline data, the multivariate adjusted odds ratio (OR) for type 2 diabetes incidence was reduced for vegans (0.51; 95% CI, 0.40–0.66), lacto-ovo vegetarians (0.54; 95% CI, 0.49–0.60), pescovegetarians (0.70; 95% CI, 0.61–0.80), and semi-vegetarians

(0.76; 95% CI, 0.65–0.90)] compared to nonvegetarians [94]. Additionally, mean BMI followed a similar pattern, with the lowest values for vegans (23.6 kg/m^2) and highest values for nonvegetarians (28.8 kg/m^2). In multivariate logistic regression analyses on data from the 2-year follow-up study to the Adventist Health Study-2, the association between a vegetarian diet and a reduction in diabetes incidence remained for vegans (OR, 0.381; 95% CI, 0.236–0.617), lacto-ovo vegetarians (OR, 0.618; 95% CI, 0.503–0.760), and semi-vegetarians (OR, 0.486; 95% CI, 0.312–0.755) when compared to nonvegetarians [95].

13.2 NUTRITIONAL MANAGEMENT OF PATIENTS WITH OBESITY-ASSOCIATED TYPE 2 DIABETES: MACRONUTRIENT COMPOSITION

Medical nutrition therapy prescribes specific diets to treat medical conditions. Evidence from randomized, controlled trials and observational studies demonstrates an improvement in metabolic abnormalities with modest weight loss through lifestyle interventions, including nutritional management of obesity-associated type 2 diabetes [96–99]. Associated beneficial effects on metabolic parameters include reductions in fasting plasma glucose, HbA1c, cholesterol, and blood pressure. Improvements in glycemic control from dietary interventions are greater earlier in the disease course of type 2 diabetes, when β-cell dysfunction is still reversible; however, modest reductions in fasting plasma glucose and HbA1c still occur in individuals with a longer disease duration [97,100]. Sustained weight loss is recommended for continued improvement in metabolic abnormalities. The feasibility of long-term lifestyle modifications, including dietary interventions, for maintenance of weight loss as a treatment modality for obesity-associated type 2 diabetes was demonstrated in a large, multicenter, randomized controlled trial, Action for Health in Diabetes (LOOK AHEAD) [96,99]. Participants in the intensive lifestyle intervention (ILI) cohort were prescribed group and individual counseling sessions, at least 175 minutes per week of moderate intensity physical activity, and diets with caloric restrictions consisting of no more than 30% of calories from fat (<10% from saturated fat) and at least 15% of calories from protein. The ILI cohort achieved greater weight loss compared to the control cohort, with 50% achieving at least a 5% loss of initial weight and 26.9% achieving at least a 10% loss of initial weight after 8 years of ILI. Although the sustained weight loss through ILI did not demonstrate a reduction in cardiovascular morbidity and mortality, the ILI participants required fewer medications for control of type 2 diabetes, hypertension, and hyperlipidemia compared to the control cohort.

Dietary interventions for obesity-associated type 2 diabetes should involve caloric restriction to create an energy deficit, while employing an individualized diet plan [97,101,102]. Optimal benefits are seen with dietary interventions that can achieve and sustain significant weight loss of at least 5%–7% of initial body weight [19,20,97,101,102]. The current guidelines recommend achieving this with a daily caloric deficit of 500–750 kcal or restricting daily calories to 1,200–1,500 kcal for women and 1,500–1,800 kcal for men [97,101,102]. The American Diabetes Association (ADA) does not endorse specific dietary content (macronutrients, food groups) or a dietary pattern, as many options are effective in achieving weight loss goals if coupled with caloric restriction. Furthermore, a meta-analysis of five randomized, controlled trials comparing lifestyle interventions for weight loss did not demonstrate significant differences in HbA1c, lipids, and blood pressure based on the macronutrient composition of the dietary interventions [103]. Thus, nutritional interventions should be individualized for a patient's dietary preferences while also accounting for the patient's lipid parameters, as well as kidney and liver function [86,97]. The quality of the food consumed should also be considered. Reduced caloric intake induces weight loss initially; however, the quality of the diet consumed maintains long-term weight reduction. A healthy eating pattern consists of a high-quality diet consisting of a variety of nutrient-dense foods and beverages across all food groups while maintaining an appropriate individualized caloric intake restriction. A healthy dietary pattern also limits the intake of added sugars, saturated fats and trans-fats, and sodium [71,83].

13.2.1 Low-Fat Diets

For many years, the general public and scientific community have suggested dietary choices for patients with diabetes based on the concept that lowering fat intake is crucial to achieving health benefits. The origin of this impression derives in large part from the abundant animal and human data noted above, which lead to the conclusion that high-fat dietary regimens can induce obesity and diabetes in at-risk subjects. Additionally, the low-fat recommendation recognizes the importance of lowering serum low-density lipoprotein (LDL) cholesterol levels to help prevent coronary disease, an issue of particular importance to the diabetic population. The Institute of Medicine recommends total fat consumption for all adults to be 20%–35% of daily calorie consumption [104]. However, the ADA notes that the data are inconclusive regarding the ideal total dietary fat for individuals with diabetes, but do indicate that the type of fat consumed is more important than the total amount [105]. Diets high in monounsaturated fats demonstrate improvements in glycemic control, whereas saturated fat consumption is associated with an increased risk of CVD [83,105]. Therefore, the goal for patients with diabetes remains the same as for the general population: to reduce saturated fat intake to less than 10% of energy intake [83]. It is important to note that, in the older literature, the reduction in dietary fat was often assumed to be predominantly replaced by a corresponding increase in dietary carbohydrate intake. Thus, questions about the effects of this dietary modification in the overtly diabetic population have arisen and generated a fair amount of controversy.

In 1973, Brunzell et al. studied 15 subjects with untreated fasting hyperglycemia (defined as fasting plasma glucose [FPG] over 115 mg/dL) [106]. Two diets were administered to all patients for 7–10 days each: a "basal" diet with 40% fat, 45% carbohydrate, and 15% protein, or a "fat-free, high-carbohydrate" diet with 0% fat, 85% carbohydrate, and 15% protein. All patients were hospitalized in a metabolic ward and received five equal feedings at 8:00 a.m. and 11:00 a.m., 2:00 p.m., 5:00 p.m., and 8:00 p.m. The authors estimated the calories required to maintain body weight in relation to the degree of obesity. Specifically, they stated that a mean of 32 calories/kg was given for all subjects with a mean ideal body weight of 130%. At this time, before point-of-care glucose testing, FPGs were measured three times per week, and daily 24-hour urine glucose levels were measured over the dietary period; these values were used to calculate mean glucose values for each dietary period. Results showed a mean increase of 15 mg/dL in FPG on the fat-free, high-carbohydrate diet, but this increase was not statistically significant. However, 24-hour urine glucose excretion was increased significantly on the fat-free, high-carbohydrate diet (56 g/24 hr). The authors concluded that glucose tolerance might deteriorate in untreated patients with fasting hyperglycemia on a fat-free, high-carbohydrate diet.

Interestingly, as this paper was written at a time when the lower-fat, higher-carbohydrate diet was increasing in popularity, the value of the fat-free, high-carbohydrate diet was re-examined by the authors in a small cohort of five subjects. They were restudied after institution of insulin or oral sulfonylurea therapy and in four subjects who were studied only while on therapy. In these subjects, FPGs were indeed decreased on the fat-free, high-carbohydrate diet, but the effects of the insulin and oral agent therapy are obvious confounding factors in this analysis [106].

Reaven et al. have long been concerned about the high-carbohydrate, low-fat diet with regard to its effects on triglyceride concentrations in diabetic patients [107–110]. This issue was addressed directly in an examination of the accentuation of postprandial lipemia by such diets in a group of patients with type 2 diabetes [111]. The authors studied a low-fat, high-carbohydrate diet consisting of 55% carbohydrate, 30% fat, and 15% protein versus a diet of 40% carbohydrate, 45% fat, and 15% protein for 6 weeks in nine patients with type 2 diabetes using sulfonylurea monotherapy. Diets were equicaloric and consumed in random order. Results showed that mean hourly concentrations of glucose, insulin, and triglycerides, as well as chylomicron and chylomicron remnant fractions, were significantly higher after the low-fat, high-carbohydrate diet. The very low-density lipoprotein–triglyceride (VLDL-TG) production rate was higher, but the fractional catabolic rate was lower, after the low-fat, high-carbohydrate diet, which the authors speculate was secondary to higher circulating insulin concentrations. Lipoprotein lipase activity was significantly increased as well. The authors concluded that their data provide a mechanism for the hypertriglyceridemic effect of higher-carbohydrate diets in patients with type 2 diabetes. Thus, they believed that multiple risk factors for CVD can actually be exacerbated when such patients ingest these diets, which are recommended by some to reduce this risk [111].

A subsequent meta-analysis was performed on data from randomized, controlled trials published between 1980 and 2005 comparing the effect of low-fat diets versus low-carbohydrate diets without caloric restrictions on individuals with a BMI of at least 25 kg/m^2 [112]. Five trials were included in the analyses, with data from 447 study participants. Greater weight loss was observed after 6 months with the low-carbohydrate diets compared to the low-fat diets (weighted mean difference, –3.3 kg; 95% CI, –5.3 to –1.4 kg), but the difference was no longer significant between the two diets after 12 months (weighted mean difference, –1.0 kg; 95% CI, –3.5 to 1.5 kg). After 6 months, individuals on the low-carbohydrate diet had a significant decrease in triglycerides (weighted mean difference, –22.1 mg/dL; 95% CI, –38.1 to –5.3 mg/dL) and increase in high-density lipoprotein (HDL) cholesterol (weighted mean difference, 4.6 mg/dL; 95% CI, 1.5–8.1 mg/dL) compared to individuals on the low-fat diet. However, individuals on the low-fat diet for 6 months had more favorable changes in total cholesterol (weighted mean difference, 8.9 mg/dL; 95% CI, 3.1–14.3 mg/dL) and LDL cholesterol (weighted mean difference, 5.4 mg/dL; 95% CI, 1.2–10.1 mg/dL) compared to individuals on a low-carbohydrate diet. There were no differences in blood pressure between the two diets. Methodologic differences in the three studies evaluating changes in glucose and insulin prevented their inclusion in a pooled analysis for those parameters. However, none of these individual studies favored the low-fat diet over the low-carbohydrate diet for beneficial effects on glucose or insulin sensitivity. Additionally, a subgroup analysis of patients with diabetes in one of the trials demonstrated greater reductions in HbA1c with a low-carbohydrate diet compared to a low-fat diet at 12 months (–0.7% ± 1% vs –0.1% ± 1.6%; $P = .02$).

13.2.2 Modified Fat/High-Monounsaturated Fatty Acid Diets

Given the controversy surrounding low-fat diets in the diabetic population in terms of glycemic and triglyceridemic effects, along with concerns about patient adherence to such regimens, there has been increasing focus for diabetic patients on modified fat diets and those that stress the use of MUFAs. As previously discussed, the PREDIMED study demonstrated a reduction in major cardiovascular events in high-risk participants randomized to a Mediterranean diet (high in monounsaturated fat) supplemented with EVOO or nuts compared to the control diet [73,81,82]. There was also a decrease in the incidence of diabetes associated with the Mediterranean diets. In another study, 124 overweight/obese participants with type 2 diabetes were randomized to a high-MUFA diet or a high-carbohydrate diet [113,114]. After 1 year, both dietary groups had similar weight loss and improvement in metabolic parameters, including fasting glucose, HbA1c, insulin, HDL cholesterol, diastolic blood pressure, body fat, and waist circumference. The authors concluded that replacing a low-fat, high-carbohydrate diet with a diet high in MUFAs produced comparable beneficial metabolic effects. Furthermore, another randomized, controlled trial compared the effects of a Mediterranean diet with a low-fat diet in overweight/obese participants with type 2 diabetes [114]. At 3 years, there was a statistically significant increase in the number of participants on the Mediterranean diet who met all three ADA goals for HbA1c, blood pressure, and LDL cholesterol, compared to the low-fat diet. After 4 years, a significant reduction was noted in the proportion of subjects on the Mediterranean diet requiring antihyperglycemic medications compared to the low-fat diet (HR adjusted for weight change, 0.70; 95% CI, 0.59–0.90).

Thus, the formerly strict low-fat (and correspondingly higher carbohydrate) recommendations for patients with diabetes have undergone re-evaluation. It seems that patients already diagnosed with diabetes should attend not only to total fat intake, but to fat subtypes as well, when designing a dietary regimen.

13.2.3 Low-Carbohydrate Diets

As noted above, much of the nutrition literature of the last 50 years emphasized decreases in dietary fat intake. However, that recommendation has long been a subject of scientific debate. At the present time, the public's attention has actually shifted to low-carbohydrate diets, which has generated renewed interest in low-carbohydrate diets within the nutrition, endocrine, and cardiovascular literature as well.

Golay et al. directly addressed the issue of macronutrient composition in a study of 43 obese patients (BMI >30), who all received the same level of calorie restriction (1,000 kcal/day), with 22 patients randomly assigned to a diet that had 15% of energy intake as carbohydrate, and 21 patients given a diet that had 45% intake as carbohydrate [115]. The authors found no significant difference between groups in the amount of weight loss at 6 weeks or the magnitude of the decrease in body fat content (as measured by skinfold thickness and bioelectrical impedance analysis). However, the 15% carbohydrate intake group had significant decreases in FPG and insulin levels compared to baseline, while the 45% carbohydrate intake group had less improvement (smaller corresponding decreases) in FPG and no significant change in plasma insulin. This study demonstrates an attempt to limit the influence of potential confounding factors: All patients participated in structured programs including nutritional education, behavioral teaching, and a prescribed physical activity program. Furthermore, all patients were hospitalized during the entire 6-week period, received standardized menus, had a dietitian present at each meal to ensure compliance, and completed a food record. However, this structured environment limits the applicability of the results, and the percentage of patients who had comorbidities, such as impaired glucose tolerance, is unclear (although the authors do note that there were no significant between-group differences in FPG and insulin levels at baseline) [115].

Many other studies have attempted to assess the effects of low-carbohydrate diets in less-structured (i.e., free-living) settings. Samaha et al. performed a randomized study of 132 adult subjects with a BMI of at least 35 kg/m^2 [116]. Subjects were randomized to a low-fat diet (68 subjects) or a low-carbohydrate diet (64 subjects). The low-fat diet guideline included caloric restriction with a goal deficit of 500 calories daily, with 30% or less of the total calories derived from fat. The low-carbohydrate diet restricted subjects to no more than 30 g of carbohydrate daily. Compliance was assessed by 24-hour dietary recall. Although not part of the specific inclusion criteria, diabetes or metabolic syndrome without diabetes was highly prevalent at baseline in the study subjects (prevalence of 39% and 43%, respectively), and randomization was stratified. The primary endpoint was weight loss at 6 months, and patients on the low-carbohydrate diet lost significantly more weight than those on the low-fat diet (mean, −5.8 ± 8.6 kg vs −1.9 ± 4.2 kg) [116]. In addition, the mean FPG was decreased more in the low-carbohydrate group than the low-fat group at 6 months (−9 ± 19% vs −2 ± 17%). In subgroup analyses adjusted for baseline variables, this difference was significant for subjects with diabetes but not for those without the diagnosis. The statistical significance also was eliminated by analyses adjusting for the amount of weight lost. Insulin levels were also reduced more in the low-carbohydrate group as compared to the low-fat group, but this was only significant for subjects not taking diabetes medications. Insulin sensitivity was measured (by QUICK Index) only in subjects without diabetes. In that subgroup, there was a significantly larger increase in insulin sensitivity in those subjects eating the low-carbohydrate diet than the low-fat diet. However, limitations of this study included a significant dropout rate, which exceeded 33% in both groups at 6 months, the unblinded design, and unclear effects of confounding factors, such as physical activity and diabetes medications. The low-carbohydrate diet group also had a greater reduction in caloric intake, though not statistically significant when compared to the low-fat group.

Stern et al. published a follow-up to the above study, which reported the results of the same randomized trial at 1 year [117]. They found that, in contrast to the 6-month data, weight loss at 1 year was not statistically different between the diet groups. Furthermore, 1-year changes in glucose and insulin levels (in subjects with or without diabetes) were not significantly different between groups, nor were there significant differences in insulin sensitivity (as assessed by the QUICK Index in subjects without diabetes). However, in subgroup analyses of the 54 subjects who had diabetes, the HbA1c decreased more in the low-carbohydrate compared to the conventional diet group, although this finding did not remain significant when baseline values were carried forward for missing persons. Findings at 1 year that did remain significant between diet groups in all analyses were a smaller decrease in HDL levels and a larger decrease in triglyceride levels in the low-carbohydrate group than in the conventional diet group. Nonetheless, this study at 1 year is subject to the same limitations as noted above in the description of the 6-month results.

Yancy et al. performed a randomized, controlled trial of 120 obese (BMI between 30 and 60 kg/m^2) and hyperlipidemic, but otherwise healthy, individuals who were prescribed either a low-carbohydrate diet or a low-fat diet [118]. The low-carbohydrate diet restricted carbohydrate consumption to initially less than 20 g daily with nutritional supplementation to simulate the Atkins diet program [119]. Data collected with food records from a sub-sample of subjects showed the following mean macronutrient consumption: The low-carbohydrate group consumed 8% of daily energy intake as carbohydrate, 26% as protein, and 68% as fat, whereas the low-fat diet group consumed 52% carbohydrate, 19% protein, and 29% fat daily. Total estimated daily energy intake was 1,461 ± 325.7 kcal in the low-carbohydrate group and 1,502 ± 162.1 kcal in the low-fat group. Key findings included larger decreases in triglyceride levels and higher HDL levels in the low-carbohydrate group than the low-fat diet group, as well as significantly increased weight loss in the low-carbohydrate group at 24 weeks (mean weight change, –12.9% low-carbohydrate vs –6.7% low-fat). However, the authors caution that LDL should be monitored closely on the low-carbohydrate (higher-fat) diet, because although mean LDL levels were stable in both groups, LDL did increase by more than 10% from baseline in 30% of the low-carbohydrate subjects who completed the study. Other cautions included a higher frequency of minor adverse events in the low-carbohydrate group, such as headache, weakness, and a greater increase in mean BUN than in the low-fat group. Again, the generalizability of this study is limited by several important factors: the lack of data regarding insulin sensitivity, the complete exclusion of subjects using any form of prescription medication in the 2 months prior to the study (presumably eliminating any patients with pharmacologically treated type 2 diabetes), the significant dropout rate in both diet groups, and the effect of confounders, such as the "daily nutritional supplement" consumed by the low-carbohydrate groups and the variation in protein intake between the diet groups [118].

It should be noted that the above studies addressed weight loss as the primary outcome, with only a minor focus on cardiovascular or specific endocrine outcomes, such as insulin resistance. In addition, the number of patients with abnormal glucose metabolism in these studies is unclear.

To further examine the effect of macronutrient dietary composition on metabolic parameters, Hu et al. performed a meta-analysis on randomized, controlled studies published from 1966 to 2011, comparing the effect of a low-carbohydrate diet with a low-fat diet on weight and metabolic risk factors in adults [120]. To be included, these studies had to have an intervention period of 6 months or longer and include a dietary intervention with a low-carbohydrate diet (≤ 45% of calories) or a low-fat diet (≤ 30% of calories). Twenty-three studies were included in the meta-analysis, which included data from 2,788 study subjects. The meta-analysis demonstrated a similar reduction in weight, waist circumference, and blood pressure between subjects on the low-carbohydrate versus low-fat diets. Subjects randomized to a low-carbohydrate arm had significantly less reduction in total cholesterol (2.7 mg/dL; 95% CI, 0.8–4.6) and LDL cholesterol (3.7 mg/dL; 95% CI, 1.0–6.4) compared to the low-fat arm. However, individuals in the low-carbohydrate arm did have a statistically significant improvement in triglycerides (–14.0 mg/dL; 95% CI, –19.4 to –8.7) and HDL cholesterol (3.3 mg/dL; 95% CI, 1.9–4.7). The authors concluded that low-carbohydrate diets may be beneficial for weight loss in obese individuals with metabolic risk factors, but additional studies examining the long-term cardiovascular effects of low-carbohydrate diets are needed.

The effect of a low-carbohydrate diet on glycemic control in adults with type 2 diabetes was examined via a meta-analysis of studies published from 1980 to 2006 [121]. The low-carbohydrate dietary intervention was defined as 45% or less of total calories from carbohydrates. Studies were restricted to the United States and Canada to extrapolate the conclusions to diets in North America. Thirteen studies, including nine randomized, controlled trials, were included in the analysis. Compared to high-carbohydrate diets, participants consuming low-carbohydrate diets had a greater mean reduction in glucose compared to baseline. In 9 of the 11 studies reporting HbA1c, either a decrease in HbA1c or a more robust decrease in HbA1c was demonstrated on the low-carbohydrate diet compared to the high-carbohydrate diet. An association between low-carbohydrate diets and reductions in triglycerides was observed. Weight loss was not statistically significant between the low-carbohydrate and high-carbohydrate diets. The authors noted that several factors likely contributed to the null effect on weight: differences in study designs and the wide range (4%–45%) of carbohydrate composition in the low-carbohydrate diets. Of particular note is the fact that some of the studies promoted weight maintenance with isocaloric diets; however, weight loss was observed in participants on hypocaloric diets independent of the carbohydrate composition. Additional limitations included the small number of studies included, short-term follow-up (< 120 days), heterogeneous inclusion criteria for study populations, and high dropout rates. Nevertheless, the authors concluded that short-term use of low-carbohydrate diets can improve glycemic control and triglycerides in patients with type 2 diabetes, but additional research is needed to determine the sustainability of improvements in metabolic parameters and long-term cardiovascular safety.

Wolever et al. performed a randomized study that focused on endocrine outcomes in a population with impaired glucose tolerance [122]. Furthermore, the study extended the discussion of carbohydrate effects on glycemia, because rather than focusing solely on a low quantity of carbohydrates in the diet, the authors chose to re-explore the concepts of GI and GL. The study included men and nonpregnant women from 30 to 65 years old with BMIs lower than 40 kg/m^2 and serum triacylglycerols below 10 mmol/L; impaired glucose tolerance (IGT) was proven by a 75-g oral glucose tolerance test (OGTT) (using old World Health Organization criteria of FPG less than 7.8 mmol/L but 2-hour glucose > 7.8 and < 11.1). Thirty-four patients were randomized to a 4-month trial of one of three different diets: (1) high-carbohydrate (60% of total energy), high-GI (GI, 61; GL, 63); (2) high-carbohydrate (60% of total energy), low-GI (GI, 53; GL, 55); and (3) low-carbohydrate (49% of total energy; GI, 61; GL, 52), high-MUFA. Results showed that the "low-GI" diet and the "high-MUFA" diet both led to reductions in mean plasma glucose levels compared to baseline, whereas the "high-GI" diet led to a nonsignificant increase from baseline. Thus, the authors concluded that, in subjects with impaired glucose tolerance who consumed normal mixed meals, a reduction in GL by either an alteration of carbohydrate source or diminished intake had the same effect on postprandial blood glucose [122]. However, the study found no significant difference in HbA1c between the low-GI and high-GI diets. Furthermore, the changes in insulin levels were not so well-correlated with the GIs. Whereas the mean 0- to 8-hour plasma insulin levels were significantly reduced from baseline in the high-GI and high-MUFA groups, the decrease was nonsignificant in the low-GI group.

Subsequently, a meta-analysis was conducted to assess the effects of high- and low-GI diets on glycemic control in patients with type 1 or type 2 diabetes [123]. Eleven randomized, controlled trials with at least 4 weeks of follow-up were included in the analyses with data from 402 participants. A significant reduction in HbA1c (weighted mean difference, –0.5%; 95% CI, –0.8 to –0.2) was observed in participants following the low-GI diet. One study reported significantly fewer hypoglycemic events in the low-GI arm compared to the high-GI arm (–0.8 episodes per patient per month) [124]. In another study, a significantly lower proportion of participants on the low-GI diet had 15 or more episodes of hyperglycemia per patient per month compared to those on a higher GI diet [125]. Additionally, one study demonstrated a significant increase in insulin sensitivity within the low-GI arm compared to the high-GI arm, as measured by a euglycemic-hyperinsulinemic clamp (glucose disposal: 7 ± 1.3 vs 4.8 ± 0.9 mg glucose/kg/min; $P < .001$) [126]. Although these findings appear to favor the use of low-GI diets, the authors noted methodologic limitations in the studies, including failure to conceal allocation and the absence of blinding of outcome assessors.

In summary, low-carbohydrate studies have been associated with weight loss, reductions in glucose and HbA1c, a reduction in triglycerides, and an increase in HDL cholesterol. These beneficial effects are seen primarily within the first 6 months after initiating a low-carbohydrate diet. The long-term sustainability of these effects is not well-established. There is also a suggestion from available studies that GI may be an important dietary factor to consider. Large trials evaluating cardiovascular morbidity and mortality associated with low-carbohydrate diets and GI are lacking, and such research is needed before specific recommendations can be made.

13.2.4   HIGH-PROTEIN DIETS

Much of the interest in high-protein diets stems from theories regarding the interrelationships between glucose and amino acid metabolism. Layman et al. describe the hypothesis wherein amino acids provide a major fuel and carbon source for hepatic gluconeogenesis [127]. To elucidate high-protein dietary effects on glucose and insulin homeostasis, Layman et al. performed a study of 24 adult women who were over 15% above ideal body weight. For 10 weeks, 12 women were assigned to a moderate-protein diet (protein group) containing protein as 30% of dietary energy, carbohydrate as 40%, and fats as 30%. The other 12 women formed a control high-carbohydrate group whose diet consisted of protein as 15%, carbohydrate as 55%, and fats as 30% of dietary energy. In all cases, the two diets were designed to produce the same daily energy deficit and matching weight loss (0.6 kg/week). FPG and insulin levels were measured. After the patients were fed test meals designed to be similar to a standard OGTT, postprandial plasma glucose and insulin levels were drawn. Ten weeks later, both groups had lost weight (protein group, 7.53 ± 1.44 kg; carbohydrate group, 6.96 ± 1.36 kg), but the carbohydrate group had FPG levels that were 11% *lower* than the protein group levels. However, after the test meal, plasma insulin was 42% higher than fasting insulin levels in the protein group but 115% higher in the carbohydrate control group. The authors note the apparent contradiction in these results: If the protein diet led to better peripheral insulin sensitivity, as perhaps indicated by the lower postprandial insulin levels, then the finding of higher FPG in the protein group seems inconsistent. However, the authors believe that this finding actually implies a separate advantage of the protein diet: enhancement of hepatic gluconeogenesis, hence protection against episodes of fasting hypoglycemia through increased production and availability of the substrates alanine and glutamine [127]. Yet, it is not clear that this finding would be an advantage in all circumstances, and, as in other cases, the generalizability of this study is limited by the fact that the patient population studied was so restricted (patients with chronic medical conditions, routine medication use, or tobacco use were all excluded), the subjects had minimal daily physical activity, and all subjects received food prepared entirely in the food research lab for the first 4 weeks.

Because Layman et al. showed a higher FPG from eating a higher-protein diet in a group of patients who had *no* known medical conditions and were actively losing weight, it seems reasonable to inquire whether increased protein intake could have adverse effects on glucose control in patients with overt diabetes. Surprisingly, data have actually shown either minimal or even beneficial glycemic effects of a high-protein diet in patients with type 2 diabetes. Parker et al. performed a study in which 54 obese men and women with type 2 diabetes underwent the same level of dietary energy restriction (1,600 kcal/day) for 8 weeks, followed by 4 weeks of dietary energy balance [128]. The subjects were randomly assigned to a high-protein diet (28% protein, 42% carbohydrate, 28% fat) or a low-protein diet (16% protein, 55% carbohydrate, 26% fat). The percentages of fats from saturated, monounsaturated, and polyunsaturated fatty acids were similar in both groups. Nineteen of the subjects were men, 35 women; 25 managed their diabetes with diet only, 26 were on oral agents, and four used insulin. At baseline and at the conclusion of the study, weights were measured, along with FPG and insulin levels, and all subjects underwent a 75-g, 3-hour OGTT, as well as dual-energy x-ray absorptiometry (DEXA) scanning for body composition measurements. The 25 subjects who were not using oral agents or insulin also underwent a continuous low-dose insulin and glucose infusion test (LDIGIT) to determine steady-state plasma glucose and insulin concentrations.

Although both diets led to comparable weight loss (5.2 ± 1.8 kg), there were some diet-specific gender effects on body composition: women lost significantly more total and abdominal fat on the high-protein diet. Interestingly, despite the increased total and abdominal fat mass reduction found in women on the high-protein diet, there were no significant differences between diets on the levels of reduction in plasma glucose or insulin concentrations measured via OGTT, HbA1c, or steady-state plasma glucose or insulin concentrations by LDIGIT. With regard to validity of the study findings, although objective data were reported to support good dietary compliance, there were still a number of potentially confounding factors, including the effects of the oral hypoglycemic agents or insulin, used by many patients, and exercise (patients were told to maintain exercise programs at levels that had been established prior to the study) [128].

Thus, the Parker study showed no difference between high- or low-protein diets in effects on glycemic parameters in patients with type 2 diabetes. If the hypothesis that amino acids provide a major fuel and carbon source for hepatic gluconeogenesis is true, why would this be so? Gannon et al. have addressed this question through a number of studies of both acute and chronic increases in dietary protein ingestion. To investigate acute effects, the authors studied 10 males with untreated type 2 diabetes who were given 50 g of protein versus only water to ingest [129]. During the 8 hours immediately following ingestion, samples were drawn for measurement of glucose, insulin, and other parameters. From the amount of protein ingested, the authors calculated the expected net amount of glucose that would be produced from amino acid deamination (approximately 11–13 g). However, the amount of glucose actually appearing due to protein ingestion was found to be only 2.6 g. The authors thought that ingested protein had such a modest effect on circulating glucose because of intracellular "fuel switching," in which the ingested protein-derived amino acid actually *replaced* the endogenous gluconeogenic substrates that would have otherwise been used [129].

To investigate chronic high-protein ingestion effects, Gannon et al. subsequently performed a study of 12 subjects with untreated type 2 diabetes, in which diets were ingested for 5 weeks [130]. Subjects consumed a high-protein diet (protein:carbohydrate:fat = 30:40:30) and a control diet (15:55:30), with a washout period of 2–5 weeks between diets. Plasma glucose was measured at time points throughout a 24-hour period to allow calculation of a 24-hour net glucose area response, and glycated hemoglobin levels were measured as well. The high-protein diet led to a 40% decrease in the mean 24-hour net glucose area response and a significantly greater reduction in glycated hemoglobin when compared to the control diet [130]. A recent meta-analysis supports the finding that a high-protein diet is associated with improvement in glycemic control in patients with diabetes [131]. Twenty randomized, controlled trials of at least 6 months' duration evaluating the effect of diet on glycemic control demonstrated a reduction in HbA1c of –28% ($P < .00001$) for individuals on the high-protein diet compared to the control diet.

As the studies above have shown possible glycemic benefits of high-protein diets, the question of the effect of a high-protein diet on weight has arisen as well. Johnston et al. reported that higher-protein diets can be advantageous from an energy-cost perspective. In their study of 10 healthy volunteers, it was found that a high-protein diet nearly doubled the level of postprandial thermogenesis (at 2.5 hours post meal) in comparison to a high-carbohydrate diet [132]. The authors suggested that the apparent thermogenesis benefit of the high-protein diet supports its use in dietary regimens designed for weight loss.

Critical appraisal of the high-protein data leads to the following cautions as well: It is quite difficult to separate the effects of increasing protein in the diet from the effects of lowering carbohydrate intake or changing fat subtype (i.e., MUFA) intake, as these are often done concurrently. Further, the long-term systemic effects of increased protein ingestion (such as impact on renal physiology) require further exploration before a firm recommendation for use of these diets can be made. Therefore, the ADA recommends an individualized diet plan that determines the dietary protein composition based on a patient's metabolic risk factors and renal function. For individuals without diabetic kidney disease, a diet that obtains 15%–20% of the total daily calories from protein is recommended [105]. The ADA recommends a daily protein allowance of 0.8 g/kg body weight per day for individuals with diabetic kidney disease.

Finally, the type of protein consumed is another important concept to consider when investigating the glycemic effects of protein. Specifically, recent metabolomics studies have intensified the focus on the effect of branched-chain amino acids (BCAAs) on metabolism. Leucine, isoleucine, and valine are the essential amino acids that comprise the BCAAs. They are vital in protein synthesis, glucose metabolism, and signaling pathways. The level of BCAAs is tightly regulated by enzymatic pathways [133]. A BCAA-rich diet has been positively associated with glucose metabolism, weight maintenance, and synthesis of muscle protein [134]. Despite the known beneficial effects of BCAAs on metabolic health, elevated serum levels of BCAAs have been associated with insulin resistance and incident type 2 diabetes in rodent models and humans [133–137]. In a study with 73 obese and 67 lean individuals, a principal component analysis was performed on the metabolites measured by mass spectrometry [135]. The principal component with the largest variance for the obese and lean cohorts included a combination of BCAAs, Glx (glutamate/glutamine), methionine, aromatic amino acids (phenylalanine, tyrosine), and C3 and C5 acylcarnitines. A significant linear relationship was observed between the metabolite component related to BCAAs and insulin resistance. The association between BCAAs and insulin resistance is supported by additional metabolomics profiling studies [136,137]. Detrimental increases in BCAAs may be mediated by an alteration in the catabolic pathway in obese individuals [133]. Insulin resistance associated with increased circulating BCAAs may occur secondary to insulin receptor substrate 1 (IRS-1) serine phosphorylation via BCAA-mediated activation of the mammalian target of rapamycin complex 1 (mTORC1), which regulates protein and lipid synthesis, cell growth and survival, and gene transcription [133,134]. Despite these proposed mechanisms, further research is still warranted on the glycemic effects of BCAAs. Uncertainty remains regarding whether BCAAs directly contribute to the development of insulin resistance or if BCAAs serve as a marker of insulin resistance [133,134].

13.2.5 Very-Low-Calorie Diets

Very-low-calorie diets (VLCDs) were popular in the 1970s, but interest waned over increasing concerns for patient safety, including death, with the original formulations that included only one protein source, hydrolyzed collagen, and were insufficient in electrolytes, minerals, and vitamins [138]. Current formulations of VLCDs, defined as a maximum of 800 kcal/day, typically consist of commercial meal replacement programs to provide high-quality protein, carbohydrates, and adequate supplementation of minerals, vitamins, and trace elements [86]. The goal is to induce weight loss without inducing a severe nitrogen imbalance or electrolyte imbalance. Mild physiologic ketosis is induced with a reduction in carbohydrate intake to approximately 50 g [138]. Rapid weight loss occurs with VLCDs, followed by rapid weight regain if not followed with a long-term weight maintenance management plan [97]. Close monitoring by medical professionals is required for safety with VLCD.

Several questions remain to be addressed with VLCDs: (1) whether the weight loss observed is greater than what is observed with other diets, and (2) whether weight regain is larger with VLCDs compared with other diets. The answer does not appear to be clear-cut. Saris performed an analysis on data from nine randomized, controlled trials evaluating weight loss from VLCDs and low-calorie diets (LCDs) ($\leq$ 880 kcal/day in this analysis) [138]. Although weight loss occurred in both the VLCDs and LCDs arms, differences in short-term weight loss were not statistically different between the two arms in the first 4–6 weeks or 16–26 weeks. When Saris analyzed initial weight loss regain percentages among participants on VLCDs, a regain percentage of –7% to 122% was observed at the 1-year follow-up data, and 26%–121% at the 5-year follow-up. The author noted lower regain percentages in some, but not all, studies among participants who consumed a VLCD in combination with exercise and behavioral therapy. The author notes the deficiency in numbers of RCTs evaluating the effects of VLCDs and inconsistencies in the methodologies utilized in the available RCTs, which makes it difficult to ascertain any conclusions regarding VLCDs with certainty. Conversely, a subsequent meta-analysis was performed by Tsai on data from RCTs comparing the long-term efficacy of VLCDs and LCDs [139]. Short-term weight loss from initial weight was significantly greater with VLCDs compared to LCDs ($16.1 \pm 1.6\%$ vs $9.7 \pm 2.4\%$, respectively; $P = .0001$); however, long-term weight loss was not significantly different between the two diets ($6.3 \pm 3.2\%$ vs $5 \pm 4\%$, respectively; $P > .2$). Additionally, participants on the VLCDs had a greater weight regain percentage (62%) compared to participants on LCDs (41%).

13.2.6 PROTEIN-SPARING MODIFIED FAST

A protein-sparing modified fast diet combines a very low-carbohydrate ketogenic diet with a VLCD. To meet macronutrient and caloric requirements of the diet, an individual must consume high-to-moderate protein amounts, minimal fat, and utilize meal replacement formulations [86]. During the 6-month initial phase, fewer than 800 calories are consumed per day, with a carbohydrate restriction to 20–50 g per day and a daily protein restriction of 1.2–1.5 g/kg of ideal body weight [140]. A refeeding phase, consisting of a gradual increase in calories, occurs after the initial phase. Rapid weight loss occurs with this diet. Unfortunately, weight regain to baseline is common among individuals on a protein-sparing modified fast diet [86,141].

A study of 668 obese participants placed on the protein-sparing modified fast diet demonstrated a mean weight loss from baseline of 21 ± 13 kg during the initial phase and 19 ± 13 kg during the refeeding phase [142]. Another study evaluated the effects of caloric restriction and weight loss on glycemic control and insulin resistance in obese patients with type 2 diabetes [143]. Six patients were placed on a protein-sparing modified fast diet for up to 6 months until a weight goal of less than 120% of ideal body weight was achieved, or cessation of further weight loss occurred. Six patients were assigned to the gastric bypass arm. Among the six patients in the diet arm, significant decreases occurred over the intervention period in the mean steady-state plasma glucose (from 377 to 208 mg/dL; $P < .008$) and the mean fasting insulin levels (from 31 to 17 µU/mL; $P < .004$).

13.2.7 VEGETARIAN AND VEGAN DIETS

Conclusive data regarding the effects of vegetarian and vegan diets on glycemic control and cardiovascular data are lacking. Studies to date have been of short duration and include multiple combinations of dietary interventions (low fat, vegetarian, or vegan) on obese and nonobese study participants, making it difficult to extrapolate the data to clinical practice. Another important factor to consider is potential nutritional deficiencies that may occur with vegetarian and vegan diets, which may negate possible benefits attributed to these diets [86]. There are some encouraging studies supporting the beneficial effects of vegetarian and vegan diets. One such example is a multicenter study that randomized 291 obese participants with type 2 diabetes to a low-fat vegan diet (no animal products) with weekly group support, or a control diet, for 18 weeks [144]. Weight was significantly decreased with the low-fat vegan diet compared to the control diet (2.9 kg vs 0.06 kg, respectively; $P < .001$). Significant reductions in HbA1c occurred with the low-fat vegan diet compared to the control diet (0.6% vs 0.08%, respectively; $P < .01$). Additionally, the low-fat vegan diet compared to the control diet demonstrated significant reductions in the total cholesterol (8 vs 0.01 mg/dL, respectively; $P < .01$) and LDL cholesterol (8.1 vs 0.9 mg/dL, respectively; $P < .01$).

13.3 PHARMACOLOGIC MANAGEMENT OPTIONS FOR HYPERGLYCEMIA: FROM DIET WITH EXERCISE TO ORAL AGENTS TO INSULIN

Attention to nutrition, as discussed above, is important at all times in the proper management of type 2 diabetes mellitus. Just as lifestyle changes are beneficial in reducing the risk of type 2 diabetes, as demonstrated in the Finnish Diabetes Prevention Study [19] and Diabetes Prevention Program [20], so diet with exercise is a highly effective therapy for patients already diagnosed with type 2 diabetes mellitus. However, the stress of acute illness or progression of diabetes over time may render life-style changes insufficient as monotherapy. As shown in Figure 13.1, indications for the addition of pharmacologic therapy can include progressive fasting or postprandial hyperglycemia on diet and exercise alone, a rising HbA1c, or development of microvascular or macrovascular complications of diabetes. Intensification of treatment can be accomplished with oral agents alone or in combination with noninsulin injectable agents and/or insulin.

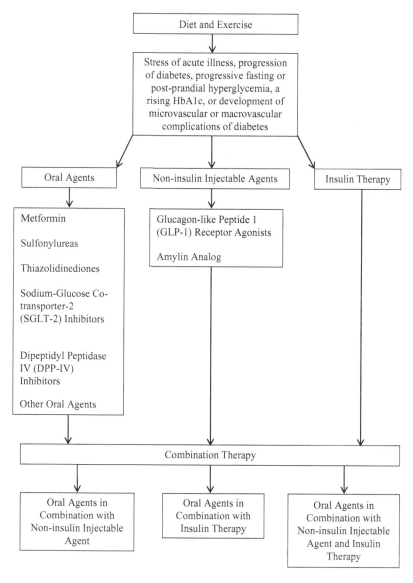

FIGURE 13.1 Pharmacologic hyperglycemia management options schematic. When diet with exercise is insufficient as monotherapy, intensification of treatment can be accomplished with oral antidiabetic agents alone or in combination with noninsulin injectable agents or insulin therapy.

13.3.1 ORAL ANTIDIABETIC MEDICATIONS

13.3.1.1 Biguanides

Metformin is presently the only biguanide available for use in the United States. Metformin acts primarily by reducing hepatic glucose output and increasing peripheral glucose uptake [145]. This agent is considered a first-line medication in the treatment of obese patients with type 2 diabetes, because it does not promote weight gain, and because it may facilitate weight loss. Additionally, it has the advantage of not causing hypoglycemia. The most feared complication of metformin use is the development of lactic acidosis. In patients who have conditions predisposing to hypoxia, such as congestive heart failure requiring medical therapy, cardiovascular collapse, acute myocardial infarction, renal insufficiency, and septicemia, the incidence of lactic acidosis is presumably higher. According to the product labeling, metformin is contraindicated in these patients. Caution should also be used in patients older than 80 years, those with hepatic disease, and those with chronic obstructive pulmonary disease associated with hypoxemia; metformin should also be stopped before and for 48 hours after contrast-media administration [146,147].

13.3.1.2 Sulfonylureas

Sulfonylureas function by binding to and closing an ATP-dependent potassium (K-ATP) channel. In the pancreatic beta-cell, this action results in sustained membrane depolarization, activation of voltage-dependent calcium channels, calcium influx, and migration of insulin-containing vesicles to the cell surface, leading to insulin release. Sulfonylureas also increase insulin sensitivity. In the United States, the most commonly used sulfonylureas are glyburide, glipizide, and glimepiride. Unlike the biguanides, sulfonylureas can be associated with hypoglycemic episodes, particularly if food intake is poor or variable. Thus, the lowest effective dose should be used, and these agents should be used with caution in patients with erratic food intake, such as some elderly individuals. Furthermore, the kinetics of sulfonylureas may be changed with renal or hepatic dysfunction. Thus, these agents should be avoided in patients with significant impairment of these organs [147].

13.3.1.3 Thiazolidinediones

Thiazolidinediones bind to peroxisome proliferator-activator receptors (PPARs). These agents enhance peripheral insulin sensitivity through a series of mechanisms that result in transcription of insulin-responsive genes [148]. In the United States, both pioglitazone and rosiglitazone are presently available for use. The first thiazolidinedione originally released was troglitazone; however, this agent was removed from the market due to reports of liver failure after use of this medication. The presently available thiazolidinediones should not be used in patients with active liver disease or in those with transaminases increased more than 2.5 times normal [147]. It is also worth noting that the thiazolidinediones have been implicated in the exacerbation of fluid retention, a particular concern in patients with congestive heart failure. Additionally, despite the value of increasing insulin sensitivity in insulin-resistant patients, thiazolidinediones may not be ideal drugs to use as the initial choice of an oral antidiabetic agent in patients with significant obesity, given their propensity to increase adiposity, particularly when used in combination with insulin.

13.3.1.4 Sodium-Glucose Cotransporter-2 Inhibitors

Inhibition of sodium-glucose cotransporter-2 (SGLT2) decreases renal reabsorption of filtered glucose and increases urinary excretion of glucose. Available SGLT-2 inhibitors include canagliflozin, dapagliflozin, and empagliflozin. In addition to improving glycemic control, SGLT-2 inhibitors also decrease blood pressure and weight [149]. Empagliflozin is the sole SGLT-2 inhibitor with the approved indication for reduction of cardiovascular death in adults with type 2 diabetes and established cardiovascular disease [150,151]. Hypoglycemia can occur with SGLT-2 inhibitor use if combined with sulfonylureas or insulin. Dehydration, acute kidney injury, and hypotension may also occur with use. SGLT-2 inhibitors have been associated with an increased risk of genitourinary infections. Diabetic ketoacidosis has been reported with SGLT-2 inhibitors [150]. Increased risks associated with SGLT-2 inhibitor use have also been reported for amputations (canagliflozin), fractures (canagliflozin), and bladder cancer (dapagliflozin) [152,153].

13.3.1.5 Other Antidiabetic Agents

Other oral antidiabetic medications include the meglitinides (repaglinide, nateglinide) and alpha-glucosidase inhibitors (acarbose, miglitol). Although the potential for hypoglycemia in both classes is limited, their major role is in modifying postprandial hyperglycemia. Therefore, in patients with erratic food intake, there is no clear role for these agents. In that case, these agents should be discontinued in favor of a scheduled insulin regimen [147]. Colesevelam, a bile acid sequestrant, binds bile acids in the intestinal tract and prevents their reabsorption. The mechanism by which colesevelam improves hyperglycemia is not completely understood. Colesevelam is weight-neutral [149]. Bromocriptine (quick release), a dopamine-2 agonist, improves glycemic control by increasing insulin sensitivity and altering hypothalamic control of metabolism. Bromocriptine is weight-neutral [149].

13.3.2 Other Secretagogue Therapies

Glycemic control is tightly regulated through multiple hormonal interactions: insulin and amylin from the pancreatic β-cells, glucagon from the pancreatic α-cells, and GLP-1 and glucose-dependent insulinotropic polypeptide (GIP) from gastrointestinal cells. Insulin secretion is greater after stimulation from orally ingested glucose compared to intravenous glucose. This incretin effect is mediated by the incretin hormones, GLP-1 and GIP. GLP-1 is produced by the L-cells in the small intestine. GLP-1 affects glycemic control via multiple mechanisms: glucose-dependent increase in insulin secretion, delayed gastric emptying, glucose-dependent suppression of glucagon secretion, and increased satiety. GLP-1 has a short half-life with degradation within minutes by the enzyme dipeptidyl peptidase-4 (DPP-IV) [154].

Patients with type 2 diabetes have impaired endogenous GLP-1 function, which contributes to reduced prandial insulin secretion [155].

13.3.2.1 Oral Incretin Therapy—Dipeptidyl Peptidase-IV Inhibitors

DPP-IV inhibitors slow the action of endogenous DPP-IV enzymes and subsequently prolong the effects of endogenous GLP-1. Thus, DPP-IV inhibitors promote glucose-dependent increases in insulin secretion and glucose-dependent suppression of glucagon secretion. Available DPP-IV inhibitors include sitagliptin, saxagliptin, linagliptin, and alogliptin. DPP-IV inhibitors are weight-neutral. Hypoglycemia can occur with DPP-IV inhibitors when combined with agents known to cause hypoglycemia, such as sulfonylureas or insulin. An increased risk of infections, such as upper respiratory infections and nasopharyngitis, has been reported with DPP-IV inhibitor use. Post-marketing reports of acute pancreatitis, including fatal and nonfatal hemorrhagic and necrotizing pancreatitis, have also been reported [149]. Dose adjustments are required with renal impairment, with the exception of linagliptin. An increase in hospitalizations for heart failure has been observed with patients receiving saxagliptin [156] and alogliptin [157]. Caution should be utilized when prescribing these medications to individuals at risk for heart failure.

13.3.2.2 Injectable Incretin Hormone Therapy—Glucagon-Like Peptide 1 (GLP-1) Receptor Agonists

GLP-1 receptor agonists mimic the actions of endogenous GLP-1. Synthetic GLP-1 receptor agonists are designed to resist degradation from endogenous DPP-IV, which allows them to be clinically useful as a treatment option for patients with type 2 diabetes. In the United States, the available GLP-1 receptor agonists are exenatide, liraglutide, albiglutide, lixisenatide, and dulaglutide. GLP-1 receptor agonists improve hyperglycemia and are not typically associated with hypoglycemia unless paired with other agents that may induce hypoglycemia. GLP-1 receptor agonists are also associated with weight loss, which is advantageous to overweight or obese patients with type 2 diabetes. In addition, liraglutide is the sole GLP-1 receptor agonist with the FDA-approved indication to reduce major cardiovascular events, myocardial infarction, cerebrovascular accident, and cardiovascular death in adult patients with type 2 diabetes and established cardiovascular disease [158,159]. Gastrointestinal side effects are common with GLP-1 receptor agonists and include nausea, vomiting, diarrhea, and exacerbation of gastroparesis. There have been postmarketing reports of pancreatitis associated with GLP-1 receptor agonist use. Individuals with a known history of, or who are at risk for, medullary thyroid carcinoma should not receive therapy with GLP-1 receptor agonists [158].

13.3.2.3   Injectable Hormone Therapy—Amylin Analog

The pancreatic beta-cells co-secrete amylin and insulin in response to food intake. Secretion of both amylin and insulin are impaired in patients with diabetes. The normal physiologic activity of amylin modulates postprandial glucose excursions by slowing gastric emptying and suppressing glucagon secretion. Appetite suppression also occurs with amylin via a centrally-mediated mechanism. The FDA-approved amylin analogue pramlintide can be used by patients with poor glycemic control in conjunction with prandial insulin. Weight loss due to pramlintide's mechanisms of action is particularly advantageous for overweight and obese patients with type 2 diabetes. A decrease in prandial insulin is required upon initiating pramlintide to avoid hypoglycemia induced by a reduction in food consumption. This aids in further weight loss [160].

13.3.3   Insulin Therapy

One of the first steps in determining an appropriate insulin regimen for a patient with type 2 diabetes consists of gathering important baseline data on the diabetes history. Crucial data items include the following: the patient's usual weight; dietary habits; oral agent regimen, if any; presence and severity of diabetic complications; and an assessment of home glucose control, including frequency and severity of any hypoglycemic episodes.

For individuals with type 2 diabetes, the total daily insulin dose can be estimated at 0.3 units/kg/day to 0.6 units/kg/day [147]. This range reflects varying degrees of insulin sensitivity in this patient population. Very insulin-resistant patients may require doses as high as 0.6–1.0 units/kg/day [161], but in contrast, a patient who is insulin naive may be more insulin sensitive and benefit from a lower starting dose.

After estimating the total daily insulin dose, the next step is to determine the frequency of standing-dose insulin administration. Several options are available. Of note, once-daily insulin injection alone rarely provides adequate glucose control but may be used in combination with oral hypoglycemic agents. Other options include two, three, or four injections daily, or the use of a subcutaneous insulin infusion pump, which is the most intensive alternative.

There is a propensity for weight gain while receiving insulin therapy. Patients should be encouraged to incorporate individualized dietary and lifestyle modifications to mitigate this risk.

Education regarding management of potential hypoglycemia is important for patients taking oral hypoglycemic medications and/or insulin. Patients should be counseled to maintain a supply of glucose tablets or gel at home or in the car for treatment of hypoglycemia. For those at risk of significant hypoglycemia, a Glucagon Emergency Kit may be useful; this kit consists of an intramuscular injection of glucagon to be used emergently for the unconscious patient with hypoglycemia. However, effective use of this device requires that the patient has adequate hepatic function, as well as a caregiver to administer the injection. Finally, all patients taking hypoglycemic medications should obtain a Medic-Alert bracelet [147].

13.4 PHARMACOLOGIC MANAGEMENT OPTIONS FOR OVERWEIGHT AND OBESITY

In patients with modifiable weight-related complications, such as type 2 diabetes, pharmacotherapy for overweight and obesity should be considered in conjunction with lifestyle modifications [97,101,102]. This includes patients with a BMI $\geq$ 27 kg/m^2 and one or more complications from obesity or patients with a BMI $\geq$ 30 kg/m^2 who desire weight loss [97].

Weight loss of 5% or greater from baseline after 3–6 months of pharmacologic therapy and maintenance of the lower weight is considered a success, as this degree of weight loss can significantly improve metabolic parameters. Five pharmacologic agents have been approved by the US Food and Drug Administration (FDA) for long-term management of overweight and obese patients.

Liraglutide, at a lower 3-mg daily subcutaneous injection than the dose prescribed for glycemic control, induces weight loss as an agonist of the GLP-1 receptor. In one study, overweight and obese nondiabetic patients randomized to liraglutide lost significantly more weight compared to the placebo cohort (8.4 ± 7.3 kg vs 2.8 ± 6.5 kg, respectively; $P < .001$) over 1 year [162]. In addition, a greater proportion of patients receiving liraglutide compared to placebo lost at least 5% (63.2% vs 27.1%, respectively; $P < .001$) and 10% (33.1% vs 10.6%, respectively; $P < .001$) of their body weight. Similar weight loss was also observed in overweight and obese patients with type 2 diabetes who were randomized to liraglutide 1.8 mg, 3.0 mg, or placebo over 1 year in combination with increased physical activity and a caloric deficit of 500 kcal/day [163]. Gastrointestinal side effects are common with liraglutide, including nausea, vomiting, diarrhea, and constipation. Caution should be used in patients with hepatic or renal impairment. Patients receiving liraglutide should be monitored for symptoms of pancreatitis and should not initiate therapy with a prior history of pancreatitis. A potential increased risk of medullary thyroid carcinoma may be associated with liraglutide use [97,102].

Lorcaserin is a serotonin 2C receptor agonist associated with weight loss when combined with lifestyle modifications. After randomization to lorcaserin (10 mg twice daily or 10 mg daily) or placebo in one study, overweight and obese patients with an obesity-related condition, including impaired glucose tolerance, lost significantly more weight in the lorcaserin cohorts compared to placebo [164]. The proportion of patients randomized to lorcaserin achieving 5% loss of baseline body weight was dose-dependent at 47.2% for the twice-daily cohort and 40.2% for the daily cohort (40.2%). A greater proportion of patients randomized to lorcaserin twice daily attained 5% loss of baseline body weight compared to placebo (25%, $P < .001$). The proportion of patients achieving at least 10% loss of baseline body weight was 22.6% and 17.4% in the lorcaserin twice-daily cohort and lorcaserin daily cohort, respectively. Fewer patients in the placebo arm achieved 10% loss of body weight (9.7%; $P < .001$) compared to lorcaserin twice daily. The BLOOM-DM (Behavioral Modification and Lorcaserin for Obesity and Overweight Management in Diabetes Mellitus) study demonstrated similar findings when overweight and obese patients with type 2 diabetes were randomized to lorcaserin 10 mg twice daily, 10 mg daily, or placebo [165]. A greater proportion of subjects receiving lorcaserin twice daily (37.5%; $P < .001$) and lorcaserin daily (44.7%; $P < .001$) lost 5% or greater body weight from baseline compared to patients receiving placebo (16.1%). In addition, patients randomized to lorcaserin had significant improvements in HbA1c and fasting glucose compared to the placebo arm. HbA1c was reduced by -0.9 ± 0.6 with lorcaserin twice daily, -1.0 ± 0.09 with lorcaserin daily, and -0.4 ± 0.06 with placebo ($P < .001$ for each). Fasting glucose was reduced by -27.4 ± 2.5 mg/dL with lorcaserin twice daily, -28.4 ± 3.8 mg/dL with lorcaserin daily, and -11.9 ± 2.5 with placebo ($P < .001$ for each). Headache, nausea, and dizziness are common side effects associated with lorcaserin. Heart valve disorders and bradycardia have been reported. Serotonin syndrome is also a potential risk associated with lorcaserin use [97,102].

Combination drug therapy with naltrexone, an opioid receptor antagonist, and bupropion, a nor-epinephrine and dopamine reuptake inhibitor, works synergistically to suppress appetite in the hypothalamus and stimulate the reward system via the mesolimbic dopamine circuit to achieve significant weight loss [166]. In a randomized, controlled trial, overweight and obese adults were prescribed a calorically restricted diet with exercise and randomized to 32 mg naltrexone/360 mg bupropion, 16 mg naltrexone/360 mg bupropion, or placebo for 56 weeks [167]. A greater proportion of patients receiving 32 mg naltrexone/ bupropion (48%; $P < .0001$) and 16 mg naltrexone/360 mg bupropion (39%; $P < .0001$) achieved 5% or greater weight loss from baseline compared to placebo (16%). Although patients with diabetes were excluded from the study, there were significant improvements in fasting insulin and glucose associated with 56 weeks of naltrexone 32 mg/bupropion compared to placebo. Nausea, vomiting, constipation, and headache are common side effects associated with naltrexone/bupropion use [97,167]. Naltrexone/bupropion is contraindicated in patients with uncontrolled hypertension and should be used with caution in patients with CVD, as it can raise blood pressure and heart rate [166]. It should also be avoided in patients with seizure disorders, given that bupropion lowers the seizure threshold [97,102,166]. It is contraindicated in patients on long-term opioid therapy [166]. Post-marketing reports of neuropsychiatric adverse events have been reported with naltrexone/bupropion [97,102,166].

Orlistat inhibits pancreatic lipases and alters fat absorption. Orlistat can induce significant weight loss with a subsequent reduction in cardiovascular risk factors [168,169]. In the XENDOS (XENical in the prevention of Diabetes in Obese Subjects) study, obese patients were randomized to lifestyle modifications and orlistat or placebo [169]. Impaired glucose tolerance was present in 21% of the patients at baseline. After 4 years, the patients randomized to orlistat lost more weight than those on placebo (5.8 kg vs 3 kg, $P < .0001$). In addition, the incidence of type 2 diabetes was significantly reduced by 37.3% in the orlistat arm compared to placebo. Patients randomized to orlistat also had significantly greater reductions in blood pressure, total cholesterol, LDL cholesterol, and waist circumference compared to the placebo arm. Gastrointestinal side effects are the most common, including cramps, flatus, oily discharge, and fecal incontinence [97,168]. These side effects may be mitigated for some patients by altering their dietary fat intake. Malabsorption of fat-soluble vitamins and medications may occur [97,168]. Oxalate nephropathy and liver failure are more rare and have serious adverse effects [97,168].

A combination drug therapy with phentermine and topiramate has been approved by the FDA for long-term weight management. Phentermine, a sympathomimetic amine, decreases appetite and food consumption by stimulating catecholamine release from the hypothalamus [170]. The exact mechanism for appetite suppression associated with topiramate, an antiepileptic, is not entirely understood [170]. In a randomized, controlled trial, obese adults were assigned a calorically restricted diet and randomized to phentermine/topiramate (3.75/23 mg or 15/92 mg) or placebo for 56 weeks [171]. A greater proportion of patients receiving phentermine/topiramate 3.75/23 mg (44.9%) and 15/92 mg (66.7%) lost 5% or greater of their baseline weight compared to placebo (17.3%) ($P < .0001$). In addition, patients receiving phentermine/topiramate 15/92 mg had significantly greater changes in fasting glucose, lipid parameters, systolic blood pressure, and waist circumference compared to placebo. Common side effects with phentermine/topiramate include paresthesias, xerostomia, dysgeusia, insomnia, and constipation [97,102,170,171]. Tachycardia may occur and heart rate should be monitored. Pregnancy is a contraindication for phentermine/topiramate use [97,102,170].

Although these pharmacologic management options have been approved for long-term management of overweight and obese patients, there are several caveats to consider.

Given the potential benefits and risks associated with these therapies, selection of a specific pharmacologic agent should be individualized. The clinician and patient should also have realistic expectations regarding the benefits of these therapies. The effect on weight loss is modest, and long-term adherence to these therapies is often poor. In addition, weight regain is frequent after discontinuation of therapy [97].

13.5 SURGICAL MANAGEMENT OPTIONS FOR OBESITY

The term *metabolic surgery* encompasses multiple gastrointestinal surgical procedures that significantly alter normal gastrointestinal anatomy. The etiology of weight loss and improvements in glycemic control after metabolic surgery are multifactorial: malabsorption of nutrients, gastrointestinal volume restriction, enhanced BCAA metabolism, and alteration of gut hormone and glucose homeostasis [172,173]. Multiple national and international societies recognize the significant improvements in glycemic control and cardiovascular risk factors associated with metabolic surgery compared to medical and lifestyle interventions in obese patients, particularly those with type 2 diabetes [97,101,102,172]. Metabolic surgery is recommended for obese adults with type 2 diabetes and a BMI of at least 40 kg/m^2 (or BMI $\geq$ 37.5 kg/m^2 in Asian Americans), irrespective of glycemic control [97,101,102,172]. In obese adults with a BMI between 35 and 39.9 kg/m^2 (or 32.5–37.4 kg/m^2 in Asian Americans), metabolic surgery should be recommended in the setting of persistent hyperglycemia despite optimal medical therapy and adherence to lifestyle modifications [97,101,102,172]. Metabolic surgical referral should be considered for obese adults with a BMI between 30 and 34.9 kg/m^2 (27.5–32.4 kg/m^2 in Asian Americans) with uncontrolled hyperglycemia who are receiving optimal medical therapy and adhering to lifestyle modifications [97,102,172]. Metabolic surgery should occur at high-volume surgical centers with multidisciplinary teams. A comprehensive assessment of mental health is required prior to surgery and may be necessary long-term in the postoperative period. Long-term monitoring of a patient's nutritional status is required for optimal postoperative health.

13.6 CONCLUSION

The debate regarding specific guidelines for the optimal intake of carbohydrate, dietary fat, and protein in the diet of patients with obesity and abnormal glucose metabolism will undoubtedly continue. Although there is now considerable controversy regarding the relative importance of the quantity or the quality of a particular dietary macronutrient, perhaps the best recommendation at present is to consider *both* amounts and subtypes when designing nutrition regimens for prevention or management of obesity-associated diabetes mellitus. Even as evidence may build in support of individual macronutrient effects on glycemia or weight loss, it is important to emphasize the overarching principle of caloric restriction. Finally, one should be vigilant for the time at which diet therapy alone has failed and the addition of pharmacologic or surgical intervention is necessary.

REFERENCES

1. Schmidt-Nielsen, K., Harnes, H.B., and Hackel, D.B. 1964. Diabetes mellitus in the sand rat induced by the standard laboratory diets. *Science* 143:689–90.
2. Reaven, G.M., Risser, T.R., Chen, Y.D., and Reaver, E.P. 1979. Characterization of a model of dietary-induced hypertriglyceridemia in young nonobese rats. *J Lipid Res* 20:3718.
3. Storlien, L.H., James, D.E., Burleigh, K.M., Chisholm, D.J., and Kraegen, E.W. 1986. Fat feeding causes widespread in vivo insulin resistance, decreased energy expenditure, and obesity in rats. *Am J Physiol* 251:E576–83.
4. Kraegen E.W., James, D.E., Storlien, L.H., Burleigh, K.M., and Chisholm, D.J. 1986. In vivo insulin resistance in individual peripheral tissues of the high fat fed rat: Assessment by euglycaemic clamp plus deoxyglucose administration. *Diabetologia* 29:192–8.
5. Surwit, R.S., Kuhn, C.M., Cochrane, C., McCubbin, J.A., and Feinglos, M.N. 1988. Diet-induced type II diabetes in C57BL/6J mice. *Diabetes* 37:1163–7.
6. Bray, G.A., Stern, J.S., and Castonguay, T.W. 1992. Effect of adrenalectomy and high-fat diet on the fatty Zucker rat. *Am J Physiol* 262: E32–9.
7. Opara, E.C., Petro, A., Tevrizian, A., Feinglos, M.N., and Surwit, R.S. 1996. L-Glutamine supplementation of a high fat diet reduces body weight and attenuates hyperglycemia and hyperinsulinemia in C57BL/6J mice. *J Nutr* 126:273–9.

8. Hu, F.B., Van Dam, R.M., and Liu, S. 2001. Diet and risk of type II diabetes: The role of types of fat and carbohydrate. *Diabetologia* 44:805–17.

9. Mayer-Davis, E.J., Monaco, J.H., Hoen, H.M., Carmichael, S., Vitolins, M.Z., Rewers, M.J., Haffner, S.M., Ayad, M.F., Bergman, R.N., and Karter, A.J. 1997. Dietary fat and insulin sensitivity in a triethnic population: The role of obesity. The Insulin Resistance Atherosclerosis Study (IRAS). *Am J Clin Nutr* 65:79–87.

10. Marshall, J.A., Hoag, S., Shetterly, S., and Hamman, R.F. 1994. Dietary fat predicts conversion from impaired glucose tolerance to NIDDM. The San Luis Valley Diabetes Study. *Diabetes Care* 17:50–6.

11. Feskens, E.J. and Kromhout, D. 1990. Habitual dietary intake and glucose tolerance in euglycaemic men: The Zutphen Study. *Int J Epidemiol* 19:953–9.

12. Hu, F.B., Manson, J.E., Stampfer, M.J., Colditz, G., Liu, S., Solomon, C.G., and Willett, W.C. 2001. Diet, lifestyle, and the risk of type 2 diabetes mellitus in women. *N Engl J Med* 345:790–7.

13. Schulze, M.B. and Hu, F.B. 2005. Primary prevention of diabetes: What can be done and how much can be prevented? *Annu Rev Public Health* 26:445–67.

14. Summers, L.K., Fielding, B.A., Bradshaw, H.A., Ilic, V., Beysen, C., Clark, M.L., Moore, N.R., and Frayn, K.N. 2002. Substituting dietary saturated fat with polyunsaturated fat changes abdominal fat distribution and improves insulin sensitivity. *Diabetologia* 45:369–77.

15. Lovejoy, J.C., Smith, S.R., Champagne, C.M., Most, M.M., Lefevre, M., DeLany, J.P., Denkins, Y.M., Rood, J.C., Veldhuis, J., and Bray, G.A. 2002. Effects of diets enriched in saturated (palmitic), mono-unsaturated (oleic), or trans (elaidic) fatty acids on insulin sensitivity and substrate oxidation in healthy adults. *Diabetes Care* 25:1283–88.

16. Vessby, B., Uusitupa, M., Hermansen, K., Riccardi, G., Rivellese, A.A., Tapsell, L.C., Nalsen, C., et al. 2001. Substituting dietary saturated for monounsaturated fat impairs insulin sensitivity in healthy men and women: The KANWU Study. *Diabetologia* 44:312–19.

17. Van Dam, R.M., Willett, W.C., Rimm, E.B., Stampfer, M.J., and Hu, F.B. 2002. Dietary fat and meat intake in relation to risk of type 2 diabetes in men. *Diabetes Care* 25:417–24.

18. Marshall, J.A. and Bessesen, D.H. 2002. Dietary fat and the development of type 2 diabetes. *Diabetes Care* 25:620–2.

19. Tuomilehto, J., Lindstrom, J., Eriksson, J.G., Valle, T.T., Hamalainem, H., Ilanne-Parikka, P., et al. 2001. Finnish Diabetes Prevention Study Group: Prevention of type 2 diabetes mellitus by changes in lifestyle among subjects with impaired glucose tolerance. *N Engl J Med* 344:1343–50.

20. Diabetes Prevention Program Research Group. 2002. Reduction in the incidence of type 2 diabetes with lifestyle intervention or metformin. *N Engl J Med* 346:393–403.

21. Imamura, F., Micha, R., Wu, J.H., deOliveira Otto, M.C., Otite, F.O., Abioye, A.I., and Mozaffarian, D. 2016. Effects of saturated fat, polyunsaturated fat, monounsaturated fat, and carbohydrate on glucose-insulin homeostasis: A systematic review and meta-analysis of randomized controlled feeding trials. *PLoS Med.* 13:e1002087.

22. Jenkins, D.J., Wolever, T.M., Taylor, R.H., Barker, H., Fielden, H., Baldwin, J.M., Bowling, A.C., Newman, H.C., Jenkins, A.L., and Goff, D.V. 1981. Glycemic index of foods: A physiological basis for carbohydrate exchange. *Am J Clin Nutr* 34:362–6.

23. Livesey, G., Taylor, R., Livesey, H., and Liu, S. 2013. Is there a dose-response relation of dietary gly-cemic load to risk of type 2 diabetes? Meta-analysis of prospective cohort studies. *Am J Clin Nutr* 97:584–96.

24. Barclay, A.W., Petocz, P., McMillan-Price, J., Flood, V.M., Prvan, T., Mitchell, P., and Brand-Miller, J.C. 2008. Glycemic index, glycemic load, and chronic disease risk—A meta-analysis of observational studies. *Am J Clin Nutr* 87:627–37.

25. Dong, J.Y., Zhang, L., Zhang, Y.H., and Qin, L.Q. 2011. Dietary glycaemic index and glycaemic load in relation to the risk of type 2 diabetes: A meta-analysis of prospective cohort studies. *Br J Nutr* 106:1649–54.

26. Sluijs, I., Beulens, J.W., van der Schouw, Y.T., van der A, D.L., Buckland, G., Kuijsten, A., Schulze, M.B., et al. 2013. Dietary glycemic index, glycemic load, and digestible carbohydrate intake are not associated with risk of type 2 diabetes in eight European countries. *J Nutr* 143:93–9.

27. Bhupathiraju, S.N., Tobias, D.K., Malik, V.S., Pan, A., Hruby, A., Manson, J.E., Willett, W.C., and Hu, F.B. 2014. Glycemic index, glycemic load, and risk of type 2 diabetes: Results from 3 large US cohorts and an updated meta-analysis. *Am J Clin Nutr* 100:218–32.

28. Ardisson Korat, A.V., Willett, W.C., and Hu, F.B. 2014. Diet, lifestyle, and genetic risk factors for type 2 diabetes: A review from the Nurses' Health Study, Nurses' Health Study II, and Health Professionals' Follow-Up Study. *Curr Nutr Rep* 3:345–54.

29. Bazzano, L.A., Li, T.Y., Joshipura, K.J., and Hu, F.B. 2008. Intake of fruit, vegetables, and fruit juices and risk of diabetes in women. *Diabetes Care* 31:1311–17.

30. Carter, P., Gray, L.J., Troughton, J., Khunti, K., and Davies, M.J. 2010. Fruit and vegetable intake and incidence of type 2 diabetes mellitus: Systematic review and meta-analysis. *BMJ* 341:c4229.

31. Muraki, I., Imamura, F., Manson, J.E., Hu, F.B., Willett, W.C., van Dam, R.M., and Sun, Q. 2013. Fruit consumption and risk of type 2 diabetes: Results from three prospective longitudinal cohort studies. *BMJ* 347:f5001.

32. de Munter, J.S., Hu, F.B., Spiegelman, D., Franz, M., and van Dam, R.M. 2007. Whole grain, bran, and germ intake and risk of type 2 diabetes: A prospective cohort study and systematic review. *PLoS Med* 4:e261.

33. Schulze, M.B., Schulz, M., Heidemann, C., Schienkiewitz, A., Hoffman, K., and Boeing, H. 2007. Fiber and magnesium intake and incidence of type 2 diabetes: A prospective study and meta-analysis. *Arch Intern Med* 167:956–65.

34. Krishnan, S., Rosenberg, L., Singer, M., Hu, F.B., Djousse, L., Cupples, L.A., and Palmer, J.R. 2007. Glycemic index, glycemic load, and cereal fiber intake and risk of type 2 diabetes in US black women. *Arch Intern Med* 167:2304–9.

35. Hu, E.A., Pan, A., Malik, V., and Sun, Q. 2012. White rice consumption and risk of type 2 diabetes: Meta-analysis and systematic review. *BMJ* 344:e1454.

36. Sun, Q., Spiegelman, D., van Dam, R.M., Holmes, M.D., Malik, V.S., Willett, W.C., and Hu, F.B. 2010. White rice, brown rice, and risk of type 2 diabetes in US men and women. *Arch Intern Med* 170:961–9.

37. Schulze, M.B., Manson, J.E., Willett, W.C., and Hu, F.B. 2003. Processed meat intake and incidence of type 2 diabetes in younger and middle-aged women. *Diabetologia* 46:1465–73.

38. Aune, D., Ursin, G., and Veierod, M.B. 2009. Meat consumption and the risk of type 2 diabetes: A systematic review and meta-analysis of cohort studies. *Diabetologia* 52:2277–87.

39. Pan, A., Sun, Q., Bernstein, A.M., Schulze, M.B., Manson, J.E., Willett, W.C., and Hu, F.B. 2011. Red meat consumption and risk of type 2 diabetes: 3 cohorts of US adults and an updated meta-analysis. *Am J Clin Nutr* 94:1088–96.

40. Fung, T.T., Hu, F.B., Pereira, M.A., Liu, S., Stampfer, M.J., Colditz, G.A., and Willett, W.C. 2002. Whole-grain intake and the risk of type 2 diabetes: A prospective study in men. *Am J Clin Nutr* 76:535–40.

41. Mozaffarian, D., Hao, T., Rimm, E.B., Willett, W.C., and Hu, F.B. 2011. Changes in diet and lifestyle and long-term weight gain in women and men. *N Engl J Med* 364:2392–404.

42. Weickert, M.O., Mohlig, M., Schofl, C., Arafat, A.M., Otto, B., Viehoff, H., Koebnick, C., Kohl, A., Spranger, J., and Pfeiffer, A.F. 2006. Cereal fiber improves whole-body insulin sensitivity in overweight and obese women. *Diabetes Care* 29:775–80.

43. Newby, N.K., Muller, D., Hallfrisch, J., Qiao, N., Andres, R., and Tucker, K.L. 2003. Dietary patterns and changes in body mass index and waist circumference in adults. *Am J Clin Nutr* 77:1417–25.

44. Pereira, M.A., Jacobs, D.R. Jr, Van Horn, L., Slattery, M.L., Kartashov, A.I., and Ludwig, D.S. 2002. Dairy consumption, obesity, and the insulin resistance syndrome in young adults: The CARDIA Study. *JAMA* 287:2081–9.

45. Choi, H.K., Willett, W.C., Stampfer, M.J., Rimm, E., and Hu, F.B. 2005. Dairy consumption and risk of type 2 diabetes mellitus in men: A prospective study. *Arch Intern Med* 165:997–1003.

46. Liu, S., Choi, H.K., Ford, E., Song, Y., Klevak, A., Buring, J.E., and Manson, J.E. 2006. A prospective study of dairy intake and risk of type 2 diabetes in women. *Diabetes Care* 29:1579–84.

47. Jiang, R., Manson, J.E., Stampfer, M.J., Liu, S., Willett, W.C., and Hu, F.B. 2002. Nut and peanut butter consumption and risk of type 2 diabetes in women. *JAMA* 288:2554–60.

48. Pan, A., Sun, Q., Manson, J.E., Willett, W.C., and Hu, F.B. 2013. Walnut consumption is associated with lower risk of type 2 diabetes in women. *J Nutr* 143:512–8.

49. Bes-Rastrollo, M., Wedick, N.M., Martinez-Gonzalez, M.A., Li, T.Y., Sampson, L., and Hu, F.B. 2009. Prospective study of nut consumption, long-term weight change, and obesity risk in women. *Am J Clin Nutr* 89:1913–9.

50. O'Neil, C.E., Keast, D.R., Nicklas, T.A., and Fulgoni, V.L. 3rd. 2011. Nut consumption is associated with decreased health risk factors for cardiovascular disease and metabolic syndrome in U.S. adults: NHANES 199-2004. *J Am Coll Nutr* 30:502–10.

51. Imamura, F., O'Connor, L., Ye, Z., Mursu, J., Hayashino, Y., Bhuparthiraju, S.N., and Forouhi, N.G. 2015. Consumption of sugar sweetened beverages, artificially sweetened beverages, and fruit juice and incidence of type 2 diabetes: Systematic review, meta-analysis, and estimation of population attributable fraction. *BMJ* 351:h3576.

52. Palmer, J.R., Boggs, D.A., Krishnan, S., Hu, F.B., Singer, M., and Rosenberg, L. 2008. Sugar-sweetened beverages and incidence of type 2 diabetes mellitus in African American women. *Arch Intern Med* 168:1487–92.

53. Schulze, M.B., Manson, J.E., Ludwig, D.S., Colditz, G.A., Stampfer, M.J., Willett, W.C., and Hu, F.B. 2004. Sugar-sweetened beverages, weight gain, and incidence of type 2 diabetes in young and middle-aged women. *JAMA* 292:927–34.

54. Montonen, J., Jarvinen, R., Knekt, P., Heliovaara, M., and Reunanen, A. 2007. Consumption of sweetened beverages and intakes of fructose and glucose predict type 2 diabetes occurrence. *J Nutr* 137:1447–54.

55. Odegaard, A.O., Koh, W.P., Arakawa, K., Yu, M.C., and Pereira, M.A. 2010. Soft drink and juice consumption and risk of physician-diagnosed incident type 2 diabetes: The Singapore Chinese Health Study. *Am J Epidemiol* 171:701–8.

56. Malik, V.S., Pan, A., Willett, W.C., and Hu, F.B. 2013. Sugar-sweetened beverages and weight gain in children and adults: A systematic review and meta-analysis. *Am J Clin Nutr* 98:1084–102.

57. Romaguera, D., Norat, T., Wark, P.A., Vergnaud, A.C., Schulze, M.B., van Woudenbergh, G.J., Drogan, D., et al. 2013. Consumption of sweet beverages and type 2 diabetes incidence in European adults: Results from EPIC-InterAct. *Diabetologia* 56:1520–30.

58. Paynter, N.P., Yeh, H.C., Voutilainen, S., Schmidt, M.I., Heiss, G., Folsom, A.R., Brancati, F.L., and Kao, W.H. 2006. Coffee and sweetened beverage consumption and the risk of type 2 diabetes mellitus. *Am J Epidemiol* 164:1075–1084.

59. Ding, M., Bhupathiraju, S.N., Chen, M., van Dam, R.M., and Hu, F.B. 2014. Caffeinated and decaffeinated coffee consumption and risk of type 2 diabetes: A systematic review and meta-analysis and a dose-response meta-analysis. *Diabetes Care* 37:569–86.

60. van Dam, R.M., Willett, W.C., Manson, J.E., and Hu, F.B. 2006. Coffee, caffeine, and risk of type 2 diabetes: A prospective cohort study in younger and middle-aged U.S. women. *Diabetes Care* 29:398–403.

61. van Dam, R.M. and Hu, F.B. 2005. Coffee consumption and risk of type 2 diabetes: A systematic review. *JAMA* 294:97–104.

62. Huxley, R., Lee, C.M., Barzi, F., Timmermeister, L., Czernichow, S., Perovic, V., Grobbee, D.E., Batty, D., and Woodward, M. 2009. Coffee, decaffeinated coffee, and tea consumption in relation to incident type 2 diabetes mellitus. *Arch Intern Med* 169:2053–63.

63. Bhupathiraju, S.N., Pan, A., Manson, J.E., Willett, W.C., van Dam, R.M., and Hu, F.B. 2014. Changes in coffee intake and subsequent risk of type 2 diabetes: Three large cohorts of US men and women. *Diabetologia* 57:1346–54.

64. Salazar-Martinez, E., Willett, W.C., Ascherio, A., Manson, J.E., Leitzmann, M.F., Stampfer, M.J., and Hu, F.B. 2004. Coffee consumption and risk of type 2 diabetes mellitus. *Ann Intern Med* 140:1–8.

65. Tuomilehto, J., Hu, J., Bidel, S., Lindstrom, J., and Jousilahti, P. 2004. Coffee consumption and risk of type 2 diabetes mellitus among middle-aged Finnish men and women. *JAMA* 291:1213–9.

66. Pereira, M.A., Parker, E.D., and Folsom, A.R. 2006. Coffee consumption and risk of type 2 diabetes mellitus: An 11-year prospective study of 28812 postmenopausal women. *Arch Intern Med* 166:1311–6.

67. Lane, J., Hwang, A., Feinglos, M., and Surwit, R. 2007. Exaggeration of postprandial hyperglycemia in patients with type 2 diabetes by administration of caffeine in coffee. *Endoc Pract* 13:239–43.

68. Iso, H., Date, C., Wakai, K., Fukui, M., Tamakoshi, A., and JACC Study Group. 2006. The relationship between green tea and total caffeine intake and risk for self-reported type 2 diabetes among Japanese adults. *Ann Intern Med* 144:554–62.

69. Santos, R.M. and Lima, D.R. 2016. Coffee consumption, obesity, and type 2 diabetes: A min-review. *Eur J Nutr* 55:1345–58.

70. Grosso, G., Stepaniak, U., Micek, A., Topor-Madry, R., Pikhart, H., Szafraniec, K., and Pajak, A. 2015. Association of daily coffee and tea consumption and metabolic syndrome: Results from the Polish arm of the HAPIEE study. *Eur J Nutr* 54:1129–37.

71. Mozaffarian, D. 2016. Dietary and policy priorities for cardiovascular disease, diabetes, and obesity. *Circulation* 133:187–225.

72. Howard, B.V., Van Horn, L., Hsia, J., Manson, J.E., Stefanick, M.L., Wassertheil-Smoller, S., Kuller, L.H., et al. 2006. Low-fat dietary pattern and risk of cardiovascular disease. The Women's Health Initiative Randomized Controlled Dietary Modification Trial. *JAMA* 295:655–66.

73. Estruch, R., Ros, E., Salas-Salvado, J., Covas, M.I., Corella, D., Aros, F., Gomez-Gracia, E., et al. 2013. Primary prevention of cardiovascular disease with a Mediterranean diet. *N Engl J Med* 368:1279–90.

74. Pan, A.N., Sun, Q., Bernstein, A.M., Manson, J.E., Willett, W.C., and Hu, F.B. 2013. Changes in red meat consumption and subsequent risk of type 2 diabetes: Three cohorts of US men and women. *JAMA Intern Med* 173:1328–35.

75. Song, Y., Manson, J.E., Buring, J.E., and Liu, S. 2004. A prospective study of red meat consumption and type 2 diabetes in middle-aged and elderly women. *Diabetes Care* 27:2108–15.

76. Bendinelli, B., Palli, D., Masala, G., Sharp, S.J., Schulze, M.B., Guevara, M., van Der, A.D., et al. 2013. Association between dietary meat consumption and incident type 2 diabetes: The EPIC-InterAct study. *Diabetologia* 56:47–59.

77. van Dam, R.M., Rimm, E.B., Willett, W.C., Stampfer, M.J., and Hu, F.B. 2002. Dietary patterns and risk of type 2 diabetes mellitus in U.S. men. *Ann Intern Med* 136:201–9.

78. Ley, S.H., Hamdy, O., Mohan, V., and Hu, F.B. 2014. Prevention and management of type 2 diabetes: Dietary components and nutritional strategies. *Lancet* 383:1999–2007.

79. Fung, T.T., Schulze, M., Manson, J.E., Willett, W.C., and Hu, F.B. 2004. Dietary patterns, meat intake, and the risk of type 2 diabetes in women. *Arch Intern Med* 164:2235–40.

80. Liese, A.D., Nichols, M., Sun, X., D'Agostino, R.B., and Haffner, S.M. 2009. Adherence to the DASH diet is inversely associated with incidence of type 2 diabetes: The Insulin Resistnace Atherosclerosis Study. *Diabetes Care* 32:1434–6.

81. Salas-Salvado, J., Bullo, M., Estruch, R., Ros, E., Covas, M.I., Ibarrola-Jurado, N., Corella, D., et al. 2014. Prevention of diabetes with Mediterranean diets. *Ann Intern Med* 160:1–10.

82. Salas-Salvado, J., Bullo, M., Babio, N., Martinez-Gonzalez, M.A., Ibarrola-Jurado, N., Basora, J., Estruch, R., et al. 2011. Reduction in the incidence of type 2 diabetes with the Mediterranean diet: Results of the PREDIMED-Reus nutrition intervention randomized trial. *Diabetes Care* 34:14–9.

83. Office of Disease Prevention and Health Promotion, U.S. Department of Health and Human Services. 2015. *Dietary Guidelines for Americans: 2015–2020*. 8th Ed. Available from https://health.gov/dietaryguidelines/2015/guidelines/. Accessed 15 August 2017.

84. The InterAct Consortium. 2011. Mediterranean diet and type 2 diabetes risk in the European Prospective Investigation into Cancer and Nutrition (EPIC) Study. *Diabetes Care* 34:1913–8.

85. Martinez-Gonzalez, M.A., de la Fuente-Arrilaga, C., Nunez-Cordoba, J.M., Basterra-Gortari, F.J., Beunza, J.J., Vazquez, Z., Benito, S., Tortosa, A., Bes-Rastrollo, M. 2008. Adherence to Mediterranean diet and risk of developing diabetes: Prospective cohort study. *BMJ* 336:1348–51.

86. Sandouk, Z. and Lansang, M.C. 2017. Diabetes with obesity – Is there an ideal diet? *Cleve Clin J Med* 84:S4–14.

87. Babio, N., Toledo, E., Estruch, R., Ros, E., Martinez-Gonzalez, M.A., Castaner, O., Bullo, M., et al. 2014. Mediterranean diets and metabolic syndrome status in the PREDIMED randomized trial. *CMAJ* 186:E649–57.

88. Appel, L.J., Sacks, F.M., Carey, V.J., Obarzanek, E., Swain, J.F., Miller, ER 3rd, Conlin, P.R., et al. 2005. Effects of protein, monounsaturated fat, and carbohydrate intake on blood pressure and serum lipids. *JAMA* 294:2455–64.

89. Haring, B., von Ballmoos, M.C., Appel, L.J., and Sacks, F.M. 2014. Healthy dietary interventions and lipoprotein(a) plasma levels: Results from the Omni Heart Trial. *PLoS One* 9:e114859.

90. Hollis, J.F., Gullion, C.M., Stevens, V.J., Brantley, P.J., Appel, L.J., Ard, J.D., Champagne, C.M., et al. 2008. Weight loss during the intensive intervention phase of the weight-loss maintenance trial. *Am J Prev Med* 35:118–26.

91. Ard, J.D., Grambow, S.C., Slentz, C.A., Kraus, W.E., and Svetkey, L.P. 2004. The effect of the PREMIER interventions on insulin sensitivity. *Diabetes Care* 27:340–7.

92. Gadgil, M.D., Appel, L.J., Yeung, E., Anderson, C.A., Sacks, F.M., and Miller, E.R. 3rd. 2013. The effects of carbohydrate, unsaturated fat, and protein intake on measures of insulin sensitivity. *Diabetes Care* 36:1132–7.

93. De Koning, L., Chiuve, S.E., Fung, T.T., Willett, W.C., Rimm, E.B., and Hu, F.B. 2011. Diet-quality scores and the risk of type 2 diabetes in men. *Diabetes Care* 34:1150–6.

94. Tonstad, S., Butler, T., Yan, R., and Fraser, G.E. 2009. Type of vegetarian diet, body weight, and prevalence of type 2 diabetes. *Diabetes Care* 32:791–6.

95. Tonstad, S., Stewart, K., Oda, K., Batech, M., Herring, R.P., and Fraser, G.E. 2013. Vegetarian diets and incidence of diabetes in the Adventist Health Study-2. *Nutr Metab Cardiovasc Dis* 23:292–9.

96. Wing, R.R., Bolin, P., Brancati, F.L., Bray, G.A., Clark, J.M., Coday, M., Crow, R.S., et al. 2013. Cardiovascular effects of intensive lifestyle intervention in type 2 diabetes. *N Engl J Med* 369:145–54.

97. American Diabetes Association. 2017. Obesity management for the treatment of type 2 diabetes. Sec. 7. *In* Standards of Medical Care in Diabetes—2017. *Diabetes Care* 40(Suppl. 1):S57–63.

98. Pastors, J.G., Warshaw, H., Daly, A., Franz, M., and Kulkarni, K. 2002. The evidence for the effective-ness of medical nutrition therapy in diabetes management. *Diabetes Care* 25:608–13.

99. Look AHEAD Research Group. 2014. Eight-year weight losses with an intensive lifestyle intervention: The Look AHEAD Study. *Obesity* 22:5–13.

100. Franz, M.J., Monk, A., Barry, B., McClain, K., Weaver, T., Cooper, N., Upham, P., Bergenstal, R., and Mazze, R.S. 1995. Effectiveness of medical nutrition therapy provided by dieticians in the management of non-insulin-dependent diabetes mellitus: A randomized, controlled clinical trial. *J Am Diet Assoc* 95:1009–17.

101. Jensen, M.D., Ryan, D.H., Apovian, C.M., Ard, J.D., Comuzzie, A.G., Donato, K.A., Hu, F.B., et al. 2014. 2013 AHA/ACC/TOS guideline for the management of overweight and obesity in adults. *J Am Coll Cardiol* 63 (25 Part B):2985–3023.

102. Garvey, T.W., Machanick, J.I., Brett, E.M., Garber, A.J., Hurley, D.L., Jastreboff, A.M., Nadolsky, K., et al. 2016. American Association of Clinical Endocrinologists and American College of Endocrinology clinical practice guidelines for comprehensive medical care of patients with obesity-executive summary. *Endoc Pract* 22:1–203.

103. Franz, M.J., Boucher, J.L., Rutten-Ramos, S., and VanWormer, J.J. 2015. Lifestyle weight-loss inter-vention outcomes in overweight and obese adults with type 2 diabetes: A systematic review and meta-analysis of randomized clinical trials. *J Acad Nutr Diet* 115:1447–63.

104. Institute of Medicine. *Dietary Reference Intakes for Energy, Carbohydrate, Fiber, Fat, Fatty Acids, Cholesterol Protein, and Amino Acids [Internet].* Washington, DC, National Academies Press, 2005. Available from http://www.iom.edu/Reports/2002/Dietary-Reference-Intakes-for-Energy-Carbohydrate-Fiber-Fat-Fatty-Acids-Cholesterol-Protein-and-Amino-Acids.aspx. Accessed 19 August 2017.

105. American Diabetes Association. 2017. Lifestyle management. Sec. 4. *In* Standards of medical care in diabetes—2017. *Diabetes Care* 40(Suppl 1):S33–43.

106. Brunzell, J.D., Lerner, R.L., Porte, D. Jr., and Bierman, E.L. 1974. Effect of a fat free, high carbohydrate diet on diabetic subjects with fasting hyperglycemia. *Diabetes* 23:139–42.

107. Farquhar, J.W., Frank, A., Gross, R.C., and Reaven, G.M. Glucose, insulin, and triglyceride responses to high and low carbohydrate diets in man. *J Clin Invest* 45:1648–56.

108. Ginsberg, H., Olefsky, J.M., Kimmerling, G., Crapo, P., and Reaven, G.M. 1976. Induction of hypertri-glyceridemia by a low-fat diet. *J Clin Endocrinol Metab* 42, 729–35.

109. Coulston A., Hollenbeck, C.B., Swislocki, A.L., and Reaven, G.M. 1989. Persistence of the hypertri-glyceridemic effect of high-carbohydrate, low-fat diets in patients with non-insulin-dependent diabetes mellitus (NIDDM). *Diabetes Care* 12:94–101.

110. Chen Y.D., Swami, S., Skowronski, R., Coulston, A.M., and Reaven, G.M. 1993. Effect of variations in dietary fat and carbohydrate intake on postprandial lipemia in patients with non-insulin-dependent diabetes mellitus. *J Clin Endocrinol Metab* 76:347–51.

111. Chen, Y.D., Coulston, A.M., Zhou, M.Y., Hollenbeck, C.B., and Reaven, G.M. 1995. Why do low-fat high-carbohydrate diets accentuate postprandial lipemia in patients with NIDDM? *Diabetes Care* 18:10–6.

112. Nordmann, A.J., Nordmann, A., Briel, M., Keller, U., Yancy, W.S. Jr., Brehm, B.J., and Bucher, H.C. 2006. Effects of low-carbohydrate vs low-fat diets on weight loss and cardiovascular risk factors. *Arch Intern Med* 166:285–93.

113. Brehm, B.J., Lattin, B.L., Summer, S.S., Boback, J.A., Gilchrist, G.M., Jandacek, R. J., and D'Alessio, D.A. 2009. One-year comparison of a high-monounsaturated fat diet with a high-carbohydrate diet in type 2 diabetes. *Diabetes Care* 32:115–20.

114. Esposito, K., Maiorino, M.I., Ciotola, M., Di Palo, C., Scognamiglio, P., Gicchino, M., Ptetrizzo, M., et al. 2009. Effects of a Mediterranean-style diet on the need for antihyperglycemic drug therapy in patients with newly diagnosed type 2 diabetes: A randomized trial. *Ann Intern Med* 151:306–14.

115. Golay, A., Allaz, A.F., Morel, Y., de Tonnac, N., Tankova, S., and Reaven G. 1996. Similar weight loss with low-or high-carbohydrate diets, *Am J Clin Nutr* 63:174–8.

116. Samaha, F.F., Iqbal, N., Seshadri, P., Chicano, K.L., Daily, D.A., McGrory, J., Williams, T., Williams, M., Gracely, E.J., and Stern, L. 2003. A low-carbohydrate as compared with a low-fat diet in severe obesity. *N Engl J Med* 348:2074–81.

117. Stern, L., Iqbal, N., Seshadri, P., Chicano, K.L., Daily, D.A., McGrory, J., Williams, M., Gracely, E.J., and Samaha, F.F. 2004. The effects of low-carbohydrate versus conventional weight loss diets in severely obese adults: One-year follow-up of a randomized trial. *Ann Intern Med* 140:778–85.

118. Yancy, W. Jr, Olsen, M.K., Guyton, J.R., Bakst, R.P., and Westman, E.C. 2004. A low-carbohydrate, ketogenic diet versus a low-fat diet to treat obesity and hyperlipidemia. *Ann Intern Med* 140:769–77.

119. Atkins, R.C., *Dr. Atkins' New Diet Revolution*. New York: Simon & Schuster; 1998.

120. Hu, T., Mills, K.T., Yao, L., Demanelis, K., Eloustaz, M., Yancy, W.S. Jr., Kelly, T.N., He, J., and Bazzano, L.A. 2012. Effects of low-carbohydrate diets versus low-fat diets on metabolic risk factors: A meta-analysis of randomized controlled clinical trials. *Am J Epidemiol* 176(Suppl):S44–54.

121. Kirk, J.K., graves, D.E., Craven, T.E., Lipkin, E.W., Austin, M., and Margolis, K.L. 2008. Restricted-carbohydrate diets in patients with type 2 diabetes: A meta-analysis. *J Am Diet Assoc* 108:91–100.

122. Wolever, T. and Mehling, C. 2003. Long-term effect of varying the source or amount of dietary carbohydrate on postprandial plasma glucose, insulin, tracylglycerol, and free fatty acid concentrations in subjects with impaired glucose tolerance. *Am J Clin Nutr* 77:61221.

123. Thomas. D. and Elliott, E.J. 2009. Low glycaemic index, or low glycaemic load, diets for diabetes mellitus. *Cochrane Database Syst Rev* 1:CD006296.

124. Giacco, R., Parillo, M., Riellese, A.A., Lasorella, G., Giacco, A., D'Episcopo, and Riccardi, G. 2000. Long-term dietary treatment with increased amounts of fiber-rich low-glycemic index natural foods improves blood glucose control and reduces the number of hypoglycemic events in type 1 diabetic patients. *Diabetes Care* 23:1461–6.

125. Gilbertson, H.R., Brand-Miller, J.C., Thorburn, A.W., Evans, S., Chondros, P., and Werther, G.A. 2001. The effect of flexible low glycemic index dietary advice versus measured carbohydrate exchange on glycemic control in children with type 1 diabetes. *Diabetes Care* 24:1137–43.

126. Rizkalla, S.W., Taghrid, L., Laromiquiere, M., Huet, D., Boillot, J., Riqoir, A., Elgrably, F., and Slama, G. 2004. Improved plasma glucose control, whole-body glucose utilization, and lipid profile on a low-glycemic index diet in type 2 diabetic men: A randomized controlled trial. *Diabetes Care* 27:1866–72.

127. Layman, D.K., Shiue, H., Sather, C., Erickson, D.J., and Baum, J. 2003. Increased dietary protein modifies glucose and insulin homeostasis in adult women during weight loss. *J Nutr* 133:405–10.

128. Parker, B., Noakes, M., Luscombe, N., and Clifton, P. 2002. Effect of a high-protein, high-monounsaturated fat weight loss diet on glycemic control and lipid levels in type 2 diabetes. *Diabetes Care* 25:425–30.

129. Gannon, M.C., Nutall, J.A., Damberg, G., Gupta, V., and Nuttall, F.Q. 2001. Effect of protein ingestion on the glucose appearance rate in people with type 2 diabetes. *J Clin Endocrinol Metab* 86:1040–7.

130. Gannon, M.C., Nutall, F.Q., Saeed, A., Jordan, K., and Hoover, H. 2003 An increase in dietary protein improves the blood glucose response in persons with type 2 diabetes. *Am J Clin Nutr* 78:734–41.

131. Ajala, O., English, P., and Pinkney, J. 2013. Systematic review and meta-analysis of different dietary approaches to the management of type 2 diabetes. *Am J Clin Nutr* 97:505–16.

132. Johnston, C.S., Day, C.S., and Swan, P.D. 2002. Postprandial thermogenesis is increased 100% on a high-protein, low-fat diet versus a high-carbohydrate, low-fat diet in healthy, young women. *J Am Coll Nutr* 21:55–61.

133. O'Connell, T.M. 2013. The complex role of the branched chain amino acids in diabetes and cancer. *Metabolites* 3:931–45.

134. Yoon, M. 2016. The emerging role of the branched-chain amino acids in insulin resistance and metabolism. *Nutrients* 8:405.

135. Newgard, C.B., An, J., Bain, J.R., Muehlbauer, M.J., Stevens, R.D., Lien, L.F., Haqq, A.M., et al. 2009. A branched-chain amino acid-related metabolic signature that differentiates obese and lean humans and contributes to insulin resistance. *Cell Metab* 9:311–26.

136. Tai, E.S., Tan, M.L., Stevens, R.D., Low, Y.L., Muehlbauer, M.J., Goh, D.L., Ilkayeva, O.R., et al. 2010. Insulin resistance is associated with a metabolic profile of altered protein metabolism in Chinese and Asian-Indian men. *Diabetologia* 53:757–67.

137. Huffman, K.M., Shah, S.H., Stevens, R.D., Bain, J.R., Muehlbauer, M., Slentz, C.A., Tanner, C.J., et al. 2009. Relationships between circulating metabolic intermediates and insulin action in overweight to obese, inactive men and women. *Diabetes Care* 32:1678–83.

138. Saris, W.H.M. 2001. Very-low-calorie diets and sustained weight loss. *Obes Res* 9(Suppl 4):295S–301S.

139. Tsai, A.G. and Walden, T.A. 2006. The evolution of very-low-calorie diets: An update and meta-analysis. *Obesity* 14:1283–93.

140. Chang, J. and Kashyap, S.R. 2014. The protein-sparing modified fast for obese patients with type 2 diabetes: What to expect. *Cleve Clin J Med* 81:557–65.

141. Paisey, R.B., Frost, J., Harvey, P., Paisey, A., Bower, L., Paisey, R.M., Taylor, P., and Belka, I. 2002. Five year results of a prospective very low calorie diet or conventional weight loss programme in type 2 diabetes. *J Hum Nutr Diet* 15:121–7.

142. Palgi, A., Read, J.L., Greenberg, I., Hoefer, M.A., Bistrian, B.R., and Blackburn, G.L. 1985. Multidisciplinary treatment of obesity with a protein-sparing modified fast: Results in 668 outpatients. *AJPH* 75:1190–4.

143. Hughes, T.A., Gwynne, J.T., Switzer, B.R., Herbst, C., and White, G. 1984. Effects of caloric restriction and weight loss on glycemic control. Insulin release and resistance, and atherosclerotic risk in obese patients with type II diabetes mellitus. *Am J Med* 77:7–17.

144. Mishra, S., Xu, J., Agarwal, U., Gonzales, J., Levin, S., and Barnard, N.D. 2013. A multicenter randomized controlled trial of a plant-based nutrition program to reduce body weight and cardiovascular risk in the corporate setting: The GEICO study. *Eur J Clin Nutr* 67:718–24.

145. Bailey, C.J. and Turner, R.C. 1996. Drug therapy: Metformin. *N Engl J Med* 334:574–9.

146. Glucophage (metformin hydrochloride){package insert}, Princeton, NF: Bristol-Myers Squibb, December, 1998.

147. Lien, L.F., Bethel, M.A., and Feinglos, M.N. 2004. In-hospital management of type 2 diabetes mellitus. *Med Clin N Am* 88:1085–105.

148. Saltiel, A.R. and Olefsky, J.M. 1996. Thiazolidinediones in the treatment of insulin resistance and type II diabetes. *Diabetes* 45:1661–9.

149. American Diabetes Association. 2017. Pharmacologic approaches to glycemic treatment. Sec. 8 *In* Standards of medical care in diabetes – 2017. *Diabetes Care* 40(Suppl. 1):S64–74.

150. http://docs.boehringer-ingelheim.com/Prescribing%20Information/PIs/Jardiance/jardiance.pdf. Accessed 9/2/17.

151. Zinman, B., Wanner, C., Lachin, J.M., Fitchett, D., Blumki, E., Hantel, S., Mattheus, M., et al. 2015. Empagliflozin, cardiovascular outcomes, and mortality in type 2 diabetes. *N Engl J Med* 373:2117–28.

152. https://www.invokanahcp.com/sites/www.invokanahcp.com/files/prescribing-information-invokana.pdf. Accessed 9/2/17.

153. https://www.azpicentral.com/farxiga/pi_farxiga.pdf#page=1. Accessed 9/2/17.

154. Lee, Y. and Jun, H. 2014. Anti-diabetic actions of glucagon-like peptide-1 on pancreatic beta-cells. *Metabolism* 63:9–19.

155. Vilsboll, T., Krarup, T., Deacon, C.F., Madsbad, S., and Holst, J.J. 2001. Reduced postprandial concentrations of intact biologically active glucagon-like peptide 1 in type 2 diabetic patients. *Diabetes* 50:609–13.

156. Scirica, B.M., Bhatt, D.L., Braunwald, E., Steq, P.G., Davidson, J., Hirshberg, B., Ohman, P., et al. 2013. Saxagliptin and cardiovascular outcomes in patients with type 2 diabetes mellitus. *N Engl J Med* 369:1317–26.

157. Zannad, F., Cannon, C.P., Cushman, W.C., Bakris, G.L., Menon, V., Perez, A.T., Fleck, P.R., et al. 2015. Heart failure and mortality outcomes in patients with type 2 diabetes taking alogliptin versus placebo in EXAMINE: A multicentre, randomized, double-blind trial. *Lancet* 385:2067–76.

158. http://www.novo-pi.com/victoza.pdf#guide. Accessed 9/2/17.

159. Marso, S.P., Daniels, G.H., Brown-Frandsen, K., Kristensen, P., Mann, J.F., Nauck, M.A., Nissen, S.E., et al. 2016. Liraglutide and cardiovascular outcomes in type 2 diabetes. *N Engl J Med* 375:311–22.

160. https://www.azpicentral.com/symlin/pi_symlin.pdf#page=1. Accessed 9/1/17.

161. Nathan D. Insulin treatment of type 2 diabetes mellitus. In: Porte D, Sherwin R, Baron A, editors. *Ellenberg & Rifkin's Diabetes Mellitus*, 6th edition. New York: McGraw-Hill; 2003. p. 515–22.

162. Pi-Sunyer, X., Astrup, A., Fujioka, K., Greenway, F., Halpem, A. Krempf, M., Lau, D.C., et al. 2015. A randomized, controlled trial of 3.0 mg of liraglutide in weight management. *N Engl J Med* 373:11–22.

163. Davies, M.J., Bergenstal, R., Bode, B., Kushner, R.F., Lewin, A., Skjoth, T.V., Andreasen, A.H., Jensen, C.B., and DeFronzo, R.A. 2015. Efficacy of liraglutide for weight loss among patients with type 2 diabetes: The SCALE diabetes randomized clinical trial. *JAMA* 314:687–99.

164. Fidler, M.C., Sanchez, M., Raether, B., Weissman, N.J., Smith, S.R., Shanahan, W.R., Anderson, C.M., and BLOSSOM Clinical Trial Group. 2011. A one-year randomized trial of lorcaserin for weight loss in obese and overweight adults: The BLOSSOM Trial. *J Clin Endocrinol Metab* 96:3067–77.

165. O'Neill, P.M., Smith, S.R., Weissman, N.J., Fidler, M.C., Sanchez, M., Zhang, J., Raether, B., Anderson, C.M., and Shanahan, W.R. 2012. Randomized placebo-controlled clinical trial of lorcaserin for weight loss in type 2 diabetes mellitus: The BLOOM-DM Study. *Obesity* 20:1426–36.

166. https://contravehcp.com/wp-content/uploads/2017/05/CONTRAVE_LBL-00033.3_PI_May2017.pdf. Accessed 9/17/17.

167. Greenway, F.L., Fujioka, K., Plodkowski, R.A., Mudaliar, S., Guttadauria, M., Erickson, J., Kim, D.D., Dunayevich, E., COR-I Study Group. 2010. Effect of naltrexone plus bupropion on weight loss in over-weight and obese adults (COR-I): A multicenter, randomized, double-blind, placebo-controlled, phase 3 trial. *Lancet* 376:595–605.

168. LeBlanc, E.S., O'Connor, E., Whitlock, E.P., Patnode, C.D., and Kapka, T. 2011. Effectiveness of pri-mary care-relevant treatments for obesity in adults: A systematic evidence review for the U.S. Preventive Services Task Force. *Ann Intern Med* 155:434–47.

169. Torgerson, J.S., Hauptman, J., Boldrin, M.N., and Sjostrom, L. 2004. Xenical in the prevention of dia-betes in obese subjects (XENDOS) study. *Diabetes Care* 27:155–61.

170. https://qsymia.com/patient/include/media/pdf/prescribing-information.pdf. Accessed 9/1/17.

171. Allison, D. B., Gadde, K.M., Garvey, W.T., Peterson, C.A., Schwiers, M.L., Najarian, T., Tam, P.Y., Troupin, B., and Day, W.W. 2011. Controlled-release phentermine/topiramate in severely obese adults: A randomized controlled trial (EQUIP). *Obesity* 20:330–42.

172. Rubino, F., Nathan, D.M., Eckel, R.H., Schauer, P.R., Alberti, K.G., Zimmet, P.Z., Del Prato, S., et al. 2016. Metabolic surgery in the treatment algorithm for type 2 diabetes: A joint statement by interna-tional diabetes organizations. *Diabetes Care* 39:861–77.

173. Laferrere, B., Reilly, D., Arias, S., Swerdlow, N., Gorroochurn, P., Bawa, B., Bose, M., et al. 2011. Differential metabolic impact of gastric bypass surgery versus dietary intervention in obese diabetic subjects despite identical weight loss. *Sci Transl Med* 3:80re2.

14 Type 2 Diabetes in Childhood
Diagnosis, Pathogenesis, Prevention, and Treatment

Robert Benjamin

CONTENTS

14.1 INTRODUCTION

In 1936, Sir Harold Himsworth, professor of medicine at the University of London, distinguished type 1 diabetes ("insulin-sensitive") and type 2 diabetes ("insulin-insensitive"). Type 2 diabetes (T2D) was thought to only affect adults and was not included in many pediatric textbooks until the 1990s.

Over the past 30 years, there has been an alarming increase in the incidence of T2D in American teenagers. In the United States, it is estimated that there are 5,000 new diagnoses of T2D per year, and current projections are that 30,000 children will be affected by T2D by the year 2020. There are many causes ascribed to this epidemic, including obesity, genetic predisposition, and environmental and lifestyle factors. Youth-onset T2D differs from adult-onset T2D in its rapid rate of pancreatic beta-cell decline and progression of complications, yet there has been a paucity of literature on the subject.

The objectives of this chapter are to discuss the diagnosis, epidemiology, risk factors, pathogenesis, and complications of T2D in pediatrics and to review current management strategies. Special emphasis will be placed on the role of nutrition in all of these areas.

14.1.1 DIAGNOSIS

Criteria for diagnosing diabetes were established by the American Diabetes Association in the 1990s and do not distinguish between T1D and T2D (Table 14.1) [1]. A patient is diagnosed with diabetes with fasting plasma glucose at least 126 mg/dl, plasma glucose at least 200 mg/dl drawn randomly or after oral glucose tolerance testing (OGTT), or hemoglobin A1c (HbA1c) of at least 6.5%. Isolated fasting hyperglycemia must be confirmed on a subsequent day, while post-glucose tolerance challenge hyperglycemia must be accompanied by diabetic symptoms, such as polyuria or polydipsia. Patients are considered prediabetic or at increased risk of diabetes if they have impaired fasting glucose (IFG; glucose at least 100 mg/dl), impaired glucose tolerance (IGT; glucose at least 140 mg/dl after OGTT), or HbA1c values ranging from 5.7% to 6.4%. Patients with transient hyperglycemia accompanied by stress, infection, or medication use should not be diagnosed with diabetes unless diabetes persists after their stressor resolves.

Historically, distinguishing between T1D and T2D was thought to be straightforward. Children with T1D often presented at an early age and were more likely to have a thin body habitus. They often presented emergently with ketoacidosis and had evidence of insulin deficiency (low C-peptide) and of islet autoimmunity, with seropositivity to islet antigens including glutamic acid decarboxylase, tyrosine phosphatase, insulin, and a zinc transporter. In contrast, children

---

TABLE 14.1
Diagnostic Criteria for Diabetes Mellitus

Criteria for Diagnosis of Diabetes Mellitus	Notes
Fasting plasma glucose ≥ 126 mg/dl (7.0 mmol/l)[a]	Fasting = no caloric intake for at least 8 hours
Random plasma glucose ≥ 200 mg/dl (11.1 mmol/l)	In patient with classic symptoms of hyperglycemia or hyperglycemic crisis
2-hr OGTT plasma glucose ≥ 200 mg/dl (11.1 mmol/l)[a]	Using 75 g anhydrous glucose dissolved in water
HbA1c ≥ 6.5%[a]	Using method that is NGSP certified and standardized to DCCT assay

Source: Association, A.D., *Diabetes Care*, 40, S4–S5, 2017.

[a] In absence of hyperglycemia, repeat testing.

(DCCT, diabetes control and complications trial; NGSP, national glycohemoglobin standardization program; OGTT, oral glucose tolerance test.)

with T2D presented at an older age, had a more protracted course, and did not present in diabetic ketoacidosis (DKA). They were thought to be seronegative for diabetes auto-antibodies and had measurable C-peptide levels.

Differentiating between T1D and T2D has become increasingly difficult. Many patients with T1D have a more protracted course and do not present in DKA. The C-peptide may fall in the low-normal range at diagnosis, and some endogenous insulin production may persist for months to years after diagnosis. Markers of seropositivity are not always present, and patients are not uncommonly overweight at diagnosis. Patients with T2D may present in DKA, and may present at an early age. In addition, markers of autoimmunity have been detected in some of patients with the phenotype and family history of T2D.

Their overlapping similarities notwithstanding, T1D and T2D can generally be distinguished by age at diagnosis, family history, physical examination findings, and clinical course after diagnosis. Patients with T1D are often under 8 years of age at diagnosis, while T2D is more commonly diagnosed in the peripubertal period and teenage years. Children and adolescents with T2D are very likely to have first- and second-degree family members with T2D, while pediatric patients with T1D commonly have a negative family history of diabetes. Patients with T1D often have normal body mass index (BMI) and do not show signs of insulin resistance (IR), while those with T2D are usually obese and have acanthosis nigricans (a marker of IR). Lastly, patients with T1D require intensive insulin therapy and are prone to ketosis with prolonged hyperglycemia or other stressors, while many patients with T2D may be controlled with oral hypoglycemic medications and/or less-intensive insulin regimens. They are usually ketone-negative, even with marked hyperglycemia. In contrast to the majority of patients with T1D, T2D patients often have measurable C-peptide 1 year after diagnosis.

14.1.2 EPIDEMIOLOGY

In the past, most studies detailing the incidence and prevalence of diabetes in youth have focused on T1D. In the last decade, more studies have emerged investigating T2D in children.

SEARCH is a population-derived prospective cohort study following US children and adolescents diagnosed with T1D and T2D at younger than 20 years. SEARCH received funding from the US Centers for Disease Control and Prevention and support from the National Institute of Diabetes and Digestive and Kidney Diseases, and has provided invaluable prevalence and longitudinal data. Patients are from diverse racial and ethnic backgrounds and were identified at four geographically defined populations in Ohio, Washington, South Carolina, and Colorado; from health plan enrollees in California; and from American Indian populations in Arizona and New Mexico [2]. Surveillance started in 2001 and is ongoing [3]. Prevalence data was captured for the years 2001 and 2009. Over 3 million children participated in the study, with 7,505 pediatric patients identified as having T1D or T2D. SEARCH estimates from 2009 showed prevalence of T2D to be 4.6% for youths younger than 18 years of age, a 30% increase from 2001. Prevalence rates increased with increasing age, and were highest from 15 to 19 years of age. A SEARCH study published in 2017 detailed incidence data in T1D and T2D from 2002 to 2012. After adjustment for age, sex, and race or ethnic group, the relative annual increase in the incidence of T2D was 4.8%, compared to 1.8% in T1D. Unlike T1D, which affected predominately non-Hispanic white children, T2D prevalence was higher in minority race/ethnic groups. SEARCH estimates suggest that over 20,000 children in the United States were affected by T2D in 2010, and that the number will grow to 30,000 by the year 2020 [3].

The average age of onset of T2D in children is 13 years. In some geographic areas, T2D accounts for more than one-half of all new cases of diabetes in youth. For Asian/Pacific Islander and American Indian youth aged 10 to 19 years, the rate of new cases of T2D is now higher than for T1D. Several factors have been associated with this rapid rise, with obesity as the strongest risk factor.

14.2 PATHOGENESIS OF T2D

T2D is the endpoint of a process of metabolic decompensation that may evolve over a period of months or years. In most cases, in childhood the disease begins with peripheral resistance to insulin action accompanied by hyperinsulinemia. Progression from IR to IFG is accompanied by dysregulation of basal insulin secretion and loss of the first-phase glucose-dependent insulin secretion, which usually occurs within 10–15 minutes of a glucose stimulus and is thought to result from release of pre-formed insulin stored within the beta cell. IGT is characterized by a more pronounced degree of peripheral resistance and more severe deficiency in the first-phase insulin response [4]. Initially, there may be a compensatory increase in the second phase of insulin secretion, which usually occurs from 30 minutes to 2 hours after the glucose stimulus and results in hyperinsulinemia. With progression of disease, the second phase of insulin secretion will decline, and there is relative or absolute hypoinsulinemia, a reduction in beta cell mass, and overt T2D.

14.2.1 Normal Insulin Signaling

In normal states, insulin binds to its receptor, a tetrameric protein that consists of two extracellular α subunits and two transmembrane β subunits that are joined by disulfide bonds. Binding to the extracellular receptor induces a conformational change and leads to increased tyrosine kinase activity of the β subunits. Increased kinase activity of the receptor enables recruitment and activation of intracellular substrates, with the insulin receptor substrate (IRS) family of proteins the most well described (Figure 14.1). IRS proteins act as scaffolds to bind other intracellular substrates involved in insulin-mediated activity, including PI3-kinase (PI3K). Recruitment and activation of PI3K leads to generation of phosphatidylinositol (3,4,5)-triphosphate (PIP_3), which then recruits Akt to the plasma membrane [5]. Activated Akt is involved in multiple downstream processes and is thought to be the major mediator of insulin action.

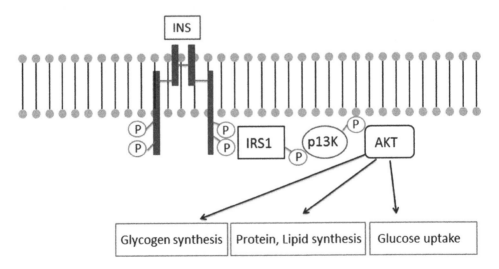

FIGURE 14.1 Intracellular insulin signaling: Insulin binds to its receptor, increasing intracellular tyrosine kinase activity and phosphorylating IRS proteins. IRS proteins phosphorylate p13K, which recruits and activates AKT. AKT is involved in multiple cellular processes.

14.2.2 INSULIN RESISTANCE

Reduced insulin action may result from alteration or inhibition of the insulin receptor or through suppression of intracellular processes downstream of the receptor. This is primarily accomplished through inhibition of IRS proteins, PI3K or Akt. In contrast to the activating effects of *tyrosine* phosphorylation, *serine* and *threonine* phosphorylation of the insulin receptor or IRS proteins down-regulates their actions [5]. In particular, phosphorylation of serine residues on IRS proteins appears to play a prominent role. Multiple stimuli may inhibit insulin action through serine phosphorylation of IRS, including hyperglycemia, cytokine exposure, mitochondrial dysfunction, endoplasmic reticulum (ER) stress, and accumulation of free fatty acids (FFAs) in muscle and liver. Hyperglycemia may inhibit insulin action in skeletal muscle and adipose tissue and impair insulin release from the beta cell. This is thought to result from oxidative stress, accumulation of advanced glycation end (AGE) products and subsequent serine phosphorylation of IRS-1. Caloric overload is associated with expansion of adipose tissue and with infiltration of inflammatory cytokines. Macrophages and adipocytes are capable of secreting cytokines, including tumor necrosis factor-alpha (TNF-α), interleukin-1-beta (IL1β), or interleukin-6 (IL-6), which may lead to serine-phosphorylation of IRS proteins or work downstream of these proteins to inhibit insulin action. Mitochondrial dysfunction may lead to IR through accumulation of high levels of reactive oxygen species (ROS). ROS are by-products of the electron transport chain but may become elevated in obese subjects, possibly due to increased metabolite flux into the mitochondria. This may induce stress kinases, which will lead to Ser-phosphorylation of IRS-1. The ER stress response, also known as the *unfolded protein response* (UPR) is an adaptive process used to protect the ER from damage. It is often triggered in obesity and will lead to many changes within the cell, including serine phosphorylation of IRS-1 [5].

14.2.3 ECTOPIC FAT AND TYPE 2 DIABETES

Significant insight into the progression from IR to T2D has been gained in the last several years. A link between obesity and T2D has clearly been established. In addition to body fat percentage, body fat distribution appears to play a crucial role in the development of T2D. Intraperitoneal (visceral) and abdominal fat accumulation has been associated with higher levels of IR than femoral or gluteal subcutaneous fat. Adipose tissue resistance and partitioning of excess adipose tissue into other organs, including skeletal muscle and especially the liver, may play the most important role in the development of IR and progression to T2D [6].

Adipose uptake of glucose and FFA is reduced in patients with IR. Rates of lipolysis are increased, and triglyceride clearance impaired because of the down-regulation of lipoprotein lipase. The resistance to insulin appears to be mediated by changes in the expression of adipocyte cytokines. Storage of surplus fuel in peripheral tissues is facilitated by a resistance to leptin, which normally stimulates tissue fatty acid oxidation and inhibits lipogenesis [7]. TNF-α, IL-6, and resistin are overexpressed in adipose tissue of obese subjects, while adiponectin expression is reduced. TNF-α and resistin inhibit insulin-mediated glucose and FFA uptake and triglyceride synthesis in fat and, like the catecholamines, induce lipolysis and the release of FFA from adipose stores. The lipolytic effects are potentiated by IL-6, which inhibits lipoprotein lipase and triglyceride (TG) deposition in adipose tissue. Interestingly, IL-6 and TNF-α reduce expression of adiponectin in cultured preadipocytes, explaining in part the downregulation of adiponectin in obesity. Plasma adiponectin concentrations are inversely related to BMI, waist circumference, and abdominal fat mass and are higher in females than in males. Adiponectin levels correlate with insulin sensitivity in children as well as adults, and targeted deletion of adiponectin causes diet-dependent resistance to insulin action in skeletal muscle and liver.

The elevations in plasma FFAs, TG, and circulating adipocytokines in the setting of leptin resistance have profound effects on insulin action in skeletal muscle. Analysis of muscle biopsies from insulin-resistant adults shows reductions in tyrosine phosphorylation of the insulin receptor and insulin receptor substrate (IRS)-1, decreased IRS-1–associated PI-3 kinase activity, and impaired threonine- and serine-phosphorylation of Akt. The defects in insulin signaling are thought to be induced by intramyocellular accumulation of TG (IMCL) or other lipid species. High intramyocellular lipid content (IMCL) in skeletal muscle has been associated with IGT in obese youth. Nondiabetic, nonobese adult patients with high IMCL have also been shown to have greater IR in skeletal muscle than adults with normal IMCL [6]. The myocellular lipid accumulation may reflect in part an inherited defect in mitochondrial oxidative phosphorylation [7]. Inhibition of Akt phosphorylation impairs skeletal muscle glucose uptake by reducing glucose transporter 4 (GLUT-4) expression, translocation, and/or activity [8,9]. The result is a progressive decrease in insulin-stimulated nonoxidative glucose disposal.

Ectopic fat deposition in the liver is also thought to play a major role in the progression from IR to T2D. Fat synthesis in the liver is accomplished through *de novo* synthesis and through fatty acid esterification. *De novo* lipid synthesis is driven by delivery of glucose from other insulin-resistant tissues (including skeletal muscle) and from the compensatory hyperinsulinemia that accompanies the IR [10]. The major source of intrahepatic lipid synthesis comes from esterification of FFAs. Rates of FFA flux are increased in patients with upper-body abdominal obesity compared to those with lower-body obesity or lean subjects. FFAs derived from visceral fat are transported through the portal vein to the liver and are used for TG synthesis; portal flux of FFA increases in proportion to the mass of visceral fat.

Hepatic steatosis is the first step in the development of nonalcoholic fatty liver disease (NAFLD). NAFLD is defined as the presence of macrovesicular steatosis in at least 5% of hepatocytes in the absence of exposure to alcohol, drugs of abuse, or other medications known to cause liver disease [11]. NAFLD may resolve, may progress to steatohepatitis (NASH), or, in the most severe cases, may lead to cirrhosis of the liver. NAFLD is the most common pediatric and adult chronic liver disease in the United States [11] and is projected to affect 50% of all adults by 2030. NAFLD is strongly associated with IR in animal and human studies, independent of obesity. In rats, NAFLD was induced after 3 days of being fed a high-fat diet. This led to dampened insulin suppression of hepatic gluconeogenesis without inducing significant changes in body weight, adiposity, or skeletal muscle resistance to insulin [12]. Studies in humans with lipodystrophy, a condition characterized by reduced subcutaneous and visceral adipose tissue and a high degree of ectopic fat deposition, have confirmed a link between the degree of hepatic steatosis and severity of IR in nonobese patients. With medical treatment directed at improving hepatic steatosis, these patients have resolution of their IR. A recent study investigating the role of hepatic steatosis on IR in obese adolescents demonstrated that, despite no differences in their BMI, IMCL, or visceral fat content, the group of patients with hepatic steatosis had increased IR compared to the group without liver disease [13]. Another study showed that, in obese children with NAFLD, increased markers of liver damage were correlated with greater IR in Hispanic and Caucasian children, but not in African American children and adults, who appear to manifest a dissociation between their extent of liver injury and degree of IR [10].

While the mechanism for the IR induced by ectopic fat deposition has not been fully elucidated, diacylglycerol (DAG) has been implicated. DAG is a signaling intermediate for protein kinase-C (PKC) and appears to be increased in the intracellular compartment of patients with higher IMCL and in patients with NAFLD. DAG appears to promote IR through novel PKC pathways involved in glucose uptake and in nonoxidative glucose metabolism. Hepatic DAG levels were elevated in rats with diet-induced NAFLD and IR. There was increased translocation of the primary novel PKC isoform in liver, protein kinase-Cε (PKCε) to the plasma membrane, where it bound and inhibited the intracellular tyrosine kinase activity of the insulin receptor. This led to reduced insulin-mediated glycogenesis and suppression of gluconeogenesis (Figure 14.2) [12]. In rats with NAFLD and chemically induced downregulation of PKC, hepatic insulin activity was normal despite high DAG levels and hepatic lipid content [12].

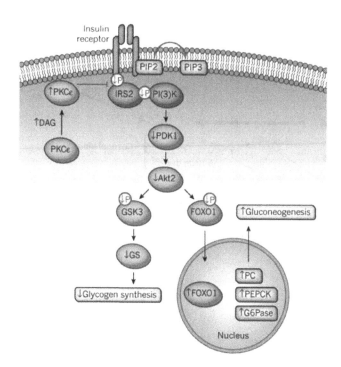

FIGURE 14.2 Molecular mechanism by which excess diacylglycerol leads to hepatic insulin resistance and hyperglycemia. Increases in liver diacylglycerol (DAG) cause protein kinase Cε (PKCε) activation and translocation to the cell membrane, which results in inhibition of insulin signaling. Reduced phosphorylation of insulin receptor substrate-2 (IRS2) and PI(3)K impairs Akt2 activity by reductions in 3-phosphoinositide-dependent protein kinase 1 (PDK1) activity, suppressing glycogen synthase kinase-3 (GSK3) phosphorylation and reducing insulin-stimulated liver glycogen synthesis through reduced glycogen synthase (GS) activity. Impaired Akt2 activity also reduces insulin suppression of hepatic gluconeogenesis by promoting Forkhead box protein O1 (FOXO1) translocation to the nucleus due to reduced phosphorylation and increasing expression of the gluconeogenic proteins pyruvate carboxylase (PC), phosphoenolpyruvate carboxykinase (PEPCK), glucose-6-phosphatase (G6Pase). (PIP3, phosphatidylinositol (3,4,5)-triphosphate.)

14.2.4 METABOLOMICS, BRANCHED-CHAIN AMINO ACIDS, AND TYPE 2 DIABETES

Metabolomics describes the detection and quantification of the spectrum of small-molecule metabolites measured in a biological sample. Approximately 2,000 measurable metabolites have been registered in the Human Metabolome Database to date [14]. Analysis of metabolites in the presence of disease allows generation of hypotheses about mechanisms involved in disease. Recent metabolomics studies have consistently shown a disturbance in amino acid profiles, including branched-chain amino acids (BCAAs), in rodents and in humans with obesity, IR, and T2D. The BCCA valine, leucine, and isoleucine comprise approximately 40% of the free essential amino acids in blood. They cannot be synthesized *de novo* and, therefore, when measured, reflect protein degradation or dietary intake. BCAAs are found in many foods considered rich in protein, including meats, chicken, fish, dairy products, and eggs. Despite their link to obesity and an apparent predictive role for progression to metabolic disease and T2D, the role of BCAA in the *development of IR* remains controversial. It is presently unknown whether BCAA accumulation is damaging to cellular processes, or if it is merely one measure of obesity and IR.

In normal states, BCAAs serve an anabolic function and are involved in the synthesis of proteins. BCAA are taken into mammalian cells through a large neutral amino acid transporter (LAT1) that is involved in transport of other amino acids as well. Overload of BCAA and other amino acids due

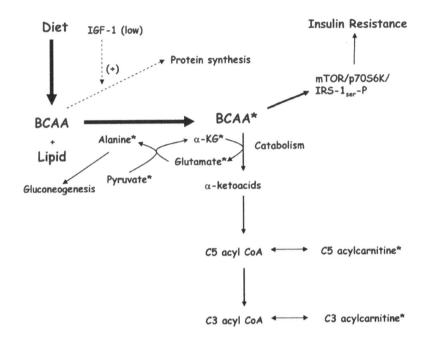

FIGURE 14.3 Schematic summary of branched-chain amino acids (BCAA) overload hypothesis. In the physiological context of overnutrition and low IGF-1 levels, as found in our obese subjects, circulating BCAAs rise, leading to increased flux of these amino acids through their catabolic pathways. We detected changes in several of the intermediary metabolites of the BCAA catabolic pathway in obese subjects, as indicated by the symbol *. A consequence of increased BCAA levels is the activation of the mTOR/S6K1 kinase pathway and phosphorylation of insulin receptor substrate-1 (IRS-1) on multiple serines, contributing to insulin resistance. In addition, increased BCAA catabolic flux may contribute to increased gluconeogenesis and glucose intolerance via glutamate transamination to alanine.

to exogenous intake or altered metabolism may lead to competition of this transporter and excessive levels of BCAAs (Figure 14.3) [13]. Accumulation of C3-acylcarnitine from metabolism of valine and isoleucine and accumulation of C5-acylcarnitine from metabolism of isoleucine and leucine suggest that altered flux through the BCAA catabolic pathway may be responsible for IR. In normal states, acylcarnitines are transported into the mitochondria, where they are metabolized into free carnitine and a long-chain acyl-CoA. Free carnitine returns to the cytosol, and the acyl-Coa undergoes fatty acid oxidation (FAO) for ATP production via the tricarboxylic acid (TCA) cycle and respiratory chain. In normal states, insulin enables cellular uptake and use of carnitine. In obese and IR states, free carnitine is lower because of increased use (from excess of substrate and higher FAO relative to TCA activity) or because of IR (from impaired cellular uptake). With lower carnitine, there is reduced ability to transport acylcarnitines into the mitochondria, and cystosolic acylcarnitines may compound the IR through impairment of insulin signaling [15].

Another proposed mechanism for BCAA to cause IR involves persistent activation of mechanistic target of rapamycin (mTOR). mTOR is a serine/threonine kinase enzyme involved in multiple critical cellular processes, including insulin signaling, and has been shown to be persistently activated by BCAA and other amino acids. mTOR exists as two distinct complexes, mTORC1 and mTORC2. When activated, mTORC1 increases phosphorylation of serine residues of IRS-1, thus downregulating insulin action [15,16]. This would imply that states of BCAA accumulation, as seen with exogenous obesity and excessive caloric intake, would lead to IR in part through mTORC1 activation. It should be noted, however, that BCAA activation of mTOR has usually been examined in experimental conditions with supraphysiologic BCAA levels. It is unclear if *physiologic* levels of BCAAs can induce mTOR activation and the subsequent serine phosphorylation of IRS1. In addition, it is unclear if BCAA elevation over the long term affects mTOR and IR, or if this is a transient effect. Weickert et al. showed that patients following a high-protein diet had evidence of mTOR activation in the short term, but that this effect was lessened over the long term [17]. Animal studies have also cast doubt on the BCAA and IR relationship. Deletion of mitochondrial branched-chain amino-transferase (BCATm), the enzyme involved in the first step of BCAA catabolism, leads to marked elevation in BCAA levels, up to 10-fold higher than controls. Despite this and evidence of mTOR activation, these mice lost weight and remained insulin sensitive [18]. Lastly, it is clear that BCAA is not the only factor involved in mTOR activation. Case studies in obese patients undergoing bypass surgery have shown mTOR elevation despite a marked fall in BCAA levels [19].

Several human studies have linked BCAA with IR. Newgard et al. looked at analytes in plasma samples from obese (BMI 37) and insulin-resistant versus lean (BMI 23) and insulin-sensitive adult subjects [13].They found that BCAA metabolites were strongly correlated with IR in obese subjects, particularly when associated with increased lipid metabolites, and that the elevation in BCAAs could be seen without a marked difference in protein intake [13]. Similar elevations in BCAAs (despite no dietary differences) were seen in adult patients with T2D compared to nondiabetic adults in the Framingham cohort. This suggests that altered BCAA catabolism may contribute to BCAA elevation in those at risk.

Studies with BCAA in obese children have been limited to date. In 2013, 69 healthy pediatric subjects, ages 8–18 years, were enrolled in a cross-sectional cohort study. They were healthy, with no personal history of diabetes or diabetes in a first-degree relative, had no history of smoking, and had never taken a medication for obesity or for prevention of diabetes. By design, 50% of the cross-sectional cohort was overweight or obese [20]. A subset of children ages 8–13 were enrolled to participate in a longitudinal study (n = 25) lasting 18 months. Sixty-four percent of these subjects were obese. At baseline, obese children had higher concentrations of the BCAAs. Elevations in the BCAAs were also positively associated with BMI Z-score in all subjects, though they were not correlated with markers of IR. In the longitudinal cohort, the fasting concentrations of BCAAs at baseline were strongly associated with impaired insulin sensitivity at 12 months and with IR at 18 months (Figure 14.4) [20].

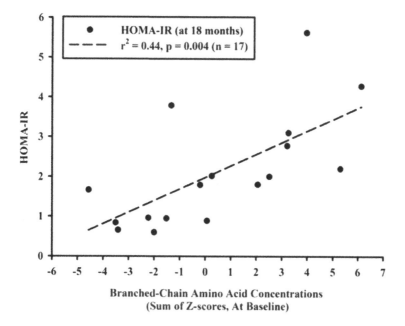

FIGURE 14.4 Concentrations of branched-chain amino acids measured at baseline (expressed as the sum of the cohort-specific Z-scores for each of leucine, isoleucine, and valine) and Homeostatic model assessment – Insulin Resistance (HOMA-IR) measured at 18 months.

14.3 RISK FACTORS FOR TYPE 2 DIABETES

14.3.1 Obesity

In SEARCH, the prevalence of overweight among youth with T2D was approximately 90%, and 80% of subjects were obese. The average BMI of pediatric patients with T2D in published reports ranges from 35 to 39 kg/m². Abdominal obesity was present in 90% of females and 68% of males [21].

The link between obesity and the development of T2D in adults has been established for several years. In the Nurses' Health Study, approximately 17,000 adult women were followed prospectively for 16 years [22]. The risk of developing T2D was nearly 40-fold higher among those with the highest BMI, while smoking, intake of saturated fats, and sedentary lifestyle increased diabetes risk approximately twofold.

The dramatic increase in pediatric T2D has paralleled the meteoric rise in rates of pediatric obesity. Since the late 1970s, the prevalence of overweight has doubled among children 6–11 years of age and tripled among those 12–17 years of age [23]. Recent estimates from the National Health and Nutrition Examination Survey are that approximately one-third of US children are overweight, and 17% are obese. Obesity rates have increased significantly in younger children. A national longitudinal study found that 27% of children in kindergarten were overweight, and that 12% were obese. Worldwide, it is estimated that 43 million preschool children are currently overweight or obese [23]. This has important implications for adolescence and adulthood, as children overweight by age 5 are at a fourfold increase of being overweight during their teenage years. Obesity in adolescence is a primary risk factor for obesity in adulthood. The odds of developing obesity in adulthood increase to 17-fold in overweight adolescents aged 15–17 years [24].

There are many risk factors ascribed to pediatric obesity, including ethnicity, genetic background, socioeconomic status, and the living environment. There is significant overlap between these risk factors for obesity and for T2D. Children from African American and Hispanic backgrounds are at the highest risk of obesity. A child born to an overweight mother is much more likely to be overweight or obese by 4 years of age than a child born to a mother with normal BMI. Girls born to parents who are both overweight have an eightfold increase of being overweight by their teenage years. The family environment is also an important predictor of childhood obesity. Children living in a single-parent home, with lower socioeconomic status, higher family stress, and less parental knowledge about healthy dietary choices are at increased risk of overweight [24]. Lifestyle also plays a strong role, with overweight children less likely to be following a healthy diet or participating in daily exercise. A 2011 youth behavior risk study showed that 15% of overweight children ate vegetables regularly, 22% consumed fruit three or more times daily, and fewer than one-half of the participants exercised for at least 1 hour per day, five times per week.

Insulin sensitivity in prepubertal and pubertal children correlates inversely with BMI and percentage of body fat, and severe obesity in prepubertal American children and adolescents is commonly associated with IGT and T2D [24].

14.3.2 Ethnicity and Genetics

T2D disproportionally affects disadvantaged families of minority, migrant, or indigenous communities. It occurs more commonly among African Americans, Hispanic Americans, Native Americans, Pacific Islanders, and Asian Americans than among those of Caucasian background. American Indians have the highest rate of onset of pediatric T2D. In children more than 10 years of age, T2D is now responsible for 3% of all cases of diabetes among Caucasians, 23% in Hispanics, 25% in African Americans, and 64% in American Indians [25]. Globally, data indicate marked variation in incidence and prevalence of T2D, depending on geographic region and on ethnicity.

T2D in youth is far more common in subjects with a family history of the disease. By some estimates, 75%–100% of pediatric patients diagnosed with T2D have a first- or second-degree family member with T2D. The high concordance rate among monozygotic twins also supports the strong influence of genetic factors. Extrapolating genetic data for pediatric T2D has been challenging owing to a lack of research on the topic. With the advent of genome-wide association studies (GWAS), however, much information has been gained in recent years. GWAS data suggest that the same susceptibility genes involved in progression to T2D in adults are involved in pediatrics [26]. Currently, over 800 genes have been implicated. Progression to T2D involves genetic dysregulation in weight gain, IR, and beta-cell growth, survival, and function. GWAS have highlighted 40 loci in particular. The transcription factor 7-like 2 (*TCF7L2*) gene appears to be the most important T2D susceptibility gene identified to date, with linkage to all ethnicities affected by T2D, with the exception of Native Americans. *TCF7L2* is thought to affect beta-cell function and insulin release. Individuals with prediabetes and a variant in *TCF7L2* have up to 70% risk of progressing to T2D within 5 years [26]. Despite the improved technology involved in GWAS, much remains unknown about the genetics involved in T2D. Rare genetic variants are not picked up by GWAS and may be responsible. Epigenetic phenomena, characterized by chemical alteration of gene expression without change in gene sequence, may also contribute.

14.3.3 BIRTH AND PUBERTY

The prevalence of T2D increases with age, but risk is modified by events that transpire before birth: The disease occurs more frequently in those born to diabetic mothers and those born small for gestational age (SGA), particularly if there is rapid catch-up growth in early childhood. The increased risk of T2D in children born SGA may reflect reductions in skeletal muscle insulin sensitivity and diminished beta-cell mass.

Children who are born large for gestational age (LGA) are also at increased risk for overweight and T2D. Intrauterine overnutrition may lead to adverse metabolic programming in the fetus, with accumulation of adipose tissue and pathologic changes in appetite and energy regulation. In a nutrient-rich environment postnatally, the LGA child may soon become obese. Maternal risk factors for having an LGA child include overweight and pregestational and gestational diabetes. LGA children born to overweight parents are more likely to be overweight themselves due to genetic, environmental, and lifestyle factors. Maternal diabetes leads to compensatory fetal hyperinsulinism, which may contribute to adverse fetal programming and predispose to early obesity and risk for IR and T2D [27].

The vast majority of pediatric patients diagnosed with T2D are in puberty at diagnosis. Puberty is characterized by marked changes in physiology, including a transient reduction in insulin sensitivity in all subjects, including healthy, lean individuals. This demands a compensatory increase in insulin release, which may lead to hyperglycemia in those with more severe IR or reduced beta-cell reserve. Thus, puberty is a high-risk time for diabetes development in susceptible individuals. Many have resolution of IFG due to the transient nature of IR, and testing should therefore be repeated in those with abnormal results. A higher risk of permanent dysfunction occurs in those prediabetic patients with higher HbA1c at diagnosis.

14.3.4 DIET

The critical role of diet in the pathogenesis of IR and T2D is unquestioned, although the precise mechanisms have remained unknown. Historically, it has been thought that diets high in fat and carbohydrate have been responsible for the greatest weight gain and for the greatest risk of diabetes. Diets high in saturated fat are typically calorie-rich; many, but not all, studies in adults and children demonstrate that such diets predispose to weight gain and IR [28]. Conversely, intake of polyunsaturated and monounsaturated fat and long-chain omega-3 fatty acids is associated with improved insulin sensitivity or glucose tolerance. Diets low in saturated fats reduce total energy intake, improve insulin sensitivity, and, in combination with exercise, can reduce significantly the risks of T2D and cardiovascular disease in adults with IGT [29–32].

Yet some investigations have shown that obese men and women lost more weight in the short term and had more significant reductions in plasma triglyceride concentrations on low-carbohydrate diets than on conventional low-fat diets [33,34]. A review of adult studies suggests that the efficacy of low-carbohydrate diets may be related to decreased caloric intake rather than to reduction in carbohydrate intake *per se* [35]. The effect of a low-carbohydrate diet may diminish with time.

Limited evidence suggests that the nature or quality of ingested carbohydrate may modulate weight gain in childhood. The insulin secretory response to foods containing rapidly absorbed, concentrated carbohydrates (high glycemic index) exceeds the response to foods containing protein, fat and fiber; the postprandial hyperinsulinemia may facilitate weight gain and reduce resting energy expenditure. The rapid rise and subsequent fall in blood glucose following ingestion of sucrose may precipitate hunger [36], while fructose is lipogenic and delays the oxidation of fatty acids, facilitating fat storage [37].

Comprehensive metabolic profiling, also known as *metabolomics*, has shed light onto the role of other macronutrients on the development of IR and T2D. In particular, BCAAs appear to be linked with risk for IR and T2D. The link between BCAAs and IR was described decades ago, but current metabolic profiling has shed further insight into their possible mechanism of action. BCAAs have been associated with reduced food intake and body weight, improved muscle synthesis, and improved glucose homeostasis. Despite these positive effects, BCAAs have also been linked to obesity, IR, and T2D in multiple human and animal studies.

To investigate the possible combined role of BCAAs and lipids in IR, Newgard et al. fed rats diets consisting of standard chow (SC), high fat (HF), and HF with BCAA. They found that rats fed HF with BCAA had the highest IR despite less food intake than the SC and HF groups and less weight gain than the HF group. When the SC group were supplemented with BCAAs, their markers of IR did not change. When the HF group had their consumption reduced to match the HF-with-BCAA group, their markers of IR improved [13]. These findings suggest that a diet high in fat that also includes BCAAs predisposes rats to IR.

Other macronutrients, vitamins, and trace elements may contribute to diabetes risk. For example, intake of fiber (particularly whole grains and cereal) correlates inversely with the risks of T2D and cardiovascular disease [38]. Insoluble and soluble fiber may limit fat absorption and thereby improve glucose tolerance. The intake of magnesium (from whole grains, nuts, and green leafy vegetables) and dairy products containing vitamin D and calcium may also correlate inversely with diabetes risk in young adults [39,40].

14.3.5 EXERCISE

A sedentary lifestyle increases the risk of T2D, while exercise, in combination with caloric and fat restriction, reduces the rate of progression to diabetes in adults with IGT [29–32]. The mechanisms by which exercise improves insulin sensitivity and glucose tolerance are complex, involving metabolic adaptations in adipose tissue, liver, and skeletal muscle. Exercise has beneficial effects on fat storage and distribution, with losses of visceral fat depots exceeding those of subcutaneous fat stores. Lean body mass increases, thereby augmenting resting energy expenditure. A reduction in abdominal fat mass increases adipose tissue sensitivity to insulin; this explains in part the reductions in fasting and postprandial FFA, LDL and triglyceride concentrations, and the increase in plasma HDL levels in adults who adhere to a rigorous diet and exercise regimen. The effect of exercise on plasma triglyceride is mediated through induction of lipoprotein lipase and reduction in triglyceride production.

Exercise increases hepatic glucose uptake and glycogen synthesis and decreases hepatic glucose production, thereby reducing fasting glucose and insulin concentrations. In skeletal muscle, exercise stimulates insulin-dependent glucose uptake and thereby reduces postprandial glucose levels; this action is mediated by increases in muscle GLUT-4 synthesis and induction of GLUT-4 translocation from intracellular pools to the plasma membrane [41]. The induction of GLUT-4 activity may be mediated in turn by an increase in cellular levels of AMP-activated protein kinase (AMPK) [42]. Activation of AMPK after an acute bout of exercise promotes increased cycling of existing GLUT-4 transporters in skeletal muscle, as well as enhanced expression of hexokinase II and mitochondrial enzymes.

Several studies suggest that insulin action is related to the oxidative capacity of skeletal muscle. Insulin-resistant individuals (including those with T2D) have reduced activities of muscle oxidative enzymes; aerobic exercise training increases muscle oxidative enzyme activity and improves insulin sensitivity by 26%–46%. The effect of exercise on oxidative enzyme activity may reflect in part an increase in mitochondrial size [43]. Interestingly, weight loss alone may improve insulin sensitivity but may not alter fasting rates of lipid oxidation. In contrast, weight loss coupled with exercise increases fat oxidation.

14.4 COMPLICATIONS OF TYPE 2 DIABETES

14.4.1 PRESENTING MANIFESTATIONS AND ACUTE COMPLICATIONS

As noted previously, children with T2D may be asymptomatic when first identified. On the other hand, many have longstanding polyuria and polydipsia, and some have lost weight prior to diagnosis. Presenting manifestations may include vaginal candidiasis, superficial bacterial and urinary tract infections, cervical adenitis, or Bartholin gland abscess. Mild ketoacidosis occurs in 30%–40% of African American and Hispanic American children with T2D; less commonly, the child presents with nonketotic hyperosmolarity associated with severe hyperglycemia.

Obese diabetic children commonly develop fatty liver, which may progress to cirrhosis. Other complications in obese children may include cholecystitis, pancreatitis, and pseudotumor cerebri. Many patients have a history of asthma and/or sleep apnea, which results from upper airway obstruction (possibly from fat deposition in pharyngeal tissues) and/or decreased residual lung volume (caused by increased intra-abdominal pressure). Menstrual irregularity and mild hirsutism are common in adolescent girls, many of whom may have polycystic ovary syndrome. Microalbuminuria may be detected within a short time after diagnosis, particularly in obese hypertensive adolescents.

14.4.2 MICROVASCULAR AND MACROVASCULAR DISEASE IN OBESITY AND TYPE 2 DIABETES

The development of IR and T2D have ominous implications for long-term cardiovascular health; microvascular complications including neuropathy, retinopathy, and microalbuminuria, and macrovascular complications including hypertension, myocardial infarction, and stroke all occur with increased frequency in patients with T2D. Pediatric T2D patients appear to have a more rapid progression of many diabetes-related microvascular and macrovascular complications than T1D and adult T2D patients, for reasons that are not entirely clear.

In a SEARCH study examining risk of complications in youth diabetes, 2,018 patients (1,746 with T1D, 272 with T2D) were evaluated for microvascular complications and for other comorbidities including hypertension, arterial stiffness, and cardiovascular autonomic neuropathy. Duration of disease was the same in both groups (7.9 years) [44]. T2D patients were diagnosed at an older age than T1D (14 years of age vs 10 years of age) and had a similar average HbA1c (7.2% vs 7.4%). Participants with T2D had significantly higher odds of having diabetic kidney disease, retinopathy, and peripheral neuropathy compared to patients with T1D, even after correcting for glycemic control, blood pressure, and obesity, and had a higher prevalence of hypertension and arterial stiffness [44]. In another SEARCH study, 258 youth patients with T2D and 1,700 youth with T1D were screened for peripheral neuropathy [2]. Average duration of diabetes was 7.9 years in T2D study subjects and 7.2 years in the T1D group. Average HbA1c was similar in T2D and T1D (9.4 ± 2.3% and 9.1 ± 1.9%, respectively). Twenty-two percent of T2D subjects had findings concerning for peripheral neuropathy, compared to 7% in the T1D patients. Risk factors included older age, male sex, longer diabetes duration, smoking, and lower high-density lipoprotein cholesterol (HDL-c) [2]. Glycemic control was not worse in the T2D cohort affected by neuropathy compared to those unaffected.

Alarmingly, 72% of T2D patients had at least one microvascular complication or comorbidity at the time of these studies. Also, these complications disproportionately affected teenagers and young adults with T2D. Cardiovascular disease and mortality rates are higher in young-onset T2D than in T1D or later-onset T2D [45], implying that the presence of obesity, arterial stiffness, and hypertension are involved in the increased risk for subsequent cardiovascular events [46,47].

The pathogenesis of vascular disease involves a complex web of hormones, growth factors, vasoactive agents, cytokines, oxygen radicals, and cellular adhesion molecules [48,49]. Under normal conditions, insulin stimulates vasodilatation through induction of nitric oxide synthase (NOS) and generation of NO in vascular endothelial cells. In obesity and other states associated with IR, the production of NO is disrupted, leading to vasoconstriction and tissue ischemia. Hyperglycemia contributes to endothelial dysfunction and vascular insufficiency through production of superoxide radicals; reactive oxygen species cause direct endothelial damage and deplete endothelial NO, reducing vascular reactivity. Oxygen radicals also activate poly(ADP ribose) polymerase (PARP), which inhibits glyceraldehyde phosphate dehydrogenase activity and thereby promotes the formation of polyols, glucosamine, and advanced glycation end products and the activation of protein kinase C [50]. These end products promote the development of microvascular and macrovascular disease. Glucose-dependent expression of growth factors (such as vascular endothelial growth factor [vEGF], endothelial growth factor [EGF], and insulin-like growth factor-1 [IGF-1]) and cytokines (IL-1, IL-6, and TNF-α), and a reduction in plasma adiponectin concentrations aggravate these effects by stimulating migration and proliferation of smooth muscle cells and increasing leukocyte adhesion to endothelial surfaces. Reduction in NO availability enhances platelet aggregation and limits fibrinolysis, promoting the progression of atheromatous clots. Increases in the concentrations of the prothrombotic plasminogen activator-1, which is also overexpressed by adipose tissue in obesity, may contribute to fibrin deposition on luminal walls, and production of endothelin-1 in terminal blood vessels is increased, promoting vasoconstriction [48]. These effects are exacerbated by dyslipidemia and hypertension; increases in blood pressure may reflect insulin-dependent increases in sodium and water reabsorption and activation of the sympathetic nervous system [51]. Reductions in tissue perfusion limit insulin-mediated glucose disposal and may increase circulating glucose concentrations, creating a vicious cycle.

14.5 PREVENTION OF TYPE 2 DIABETES IN HIGH-RISK SUBJECTS

14.5.1 LIFESTYLE INTERVENTION

The first objective in preventing T2D is to assess the family history in detail. Particular attention should be focused on those with first- or second-degree family members with T2D, hypertension, or early-onset cardiovascular disease or stroke. In such cases, early intervention to prevent metabolic complications is essential. Given the risks of adult T2D and cardiovascular disease among infants born to diabetic mothers and children born SGA, it is best for a prospective mother to be healthy and lean even before she gets pregnant and to remain healthy and well-nourished during pregnancy. If at all possible, her newborn baby should be breast-fed.

The American Diabetes Association recommends that patients with prediabetes (and with T2D) focus on losing a minimum of 7% of body weight and that they perform physical activity at least 150 minutes per week. These recommendations come from insight gained in the Diabetes Prevention Program (DPP) and the Look AHEAD trial, two adult studies investigating lifestyle modification in prediabetic and T2D subjects [52].

The DPP was a randomized, controlled trial conducted in 27 centers in the United States aimed at preventing T2D in high-risk subjects. Over 3,000 eligible participants with IGT were randomly assigned to one of three groups: placebo, metformin given at a dose of 850 mg twice per day, or lifestyle modification aimed at 7% weight loss and 150 minutes per week of exercise. A fourth, troglitazone-treated group was disbanded after the development of severe hepatotoxicity in a small number of subjects. The experimental groups were studied for 1.8–4.6 years. The lifestyle group kept fat intake at 25% of daily intake and targeted total calorie intake between 1,200 and 2,000 calories (based on initial weight) [52]. Subjects in this group received supervised exercise sessions two times per week. When compared to placebo, the lifestyle group achieved a 58% reduction in risk of developing diabetes, compared to 31% decrease in the metformin group. The lifestyle intervention group had 7.2% weight loss at 6 months, and 7% at 1 year. The benefits were sustained, with the lifestyle group having a 27% reduction in diabetes risk 15 years after the conclusion of the study. This group also sustained lower HbA1c, lower blood pressure, lower lipid levels, and less-frequent use of medications to treat these comorbidities. This was the first time that lifestyle intervention has been shown to be more effective than medication in reducing diabetes risk [52].

The Look AHEAD trial also investigated weight loss efficacy in adult patients. This was an 11-year randomized, clinical trial involving 5,000 patients aged 45–74 years with T2D and BMI of at least 25 kg/m^2. Study groups were divided into a lifestyle modification group and a diabetes support and education (DSE) group [52]. Lifestyle modification had goals of 7% weight loss and 175 minutes of exercise per week, with calorie intake of 1,200–1,800 calories and 30% of calories from fat. Exercise sessions were supervised, as in the DPP trial. After the first year of the study, the lifestyle group had 8.6% weight loss, 20% improvement in fitness levels, and a greater percentage of subjects meeting goals for A1c and blood pressure than the DSE group. After 4 years of intervention, the lifestyle group had 4.7% weight loss compared to 1.1% weight loss with DSE. The improvements in weight tracked with improved HbA1c, blood pressure, and TG levels and were significantly better than with DSE. In addition, patients in the lifestyle group had greater reduction in c-reactive protein (marker of inflammation), less self-reported retinopathy, 31% reduction in nephropathy, less sleep apnea, and decreased incidence of fatty liver disease. Remission of diabetes occurred in 11.5% of lifestyle patients compared to 2% of DSE patients [52].

Pediatric studies investigating weight loss with lifestyle modification have also been promising. A randomized, modified crossover study [50] of 79 obese children (age 7–11 years) demonstrated that 4 months of exercise training (40 minutes of activity 5 days a week) decreased fasting insulin (10%) and triglyceride (17%) concentrations and reduced percent body fat (5%), even in the absence of dietary intervention. The effects on plasma insulin and body fat were reversed when training was discontinued. An 8-week trial of cycle ergometry and resistance training in obese adolescents reduced abdominal (7%) and trunk (3.7%) fat mass and normalized flow-mediated dilation of the brachial artery [53]. Exercise exerts beneficial effects on general cardiovascular health and, in combination with a low-saturated-fat diet, may reverse hepatic steatosis. The capacity for voluntary exercise declines as BMI rises. It is therefore critical to begin regular exercise before the child becomes morbidly obese and functionally immobile.

In obese subjects, moderate reductions in body fat mass can reduce the risks of type 2 diabetes and cardiovascular complications if weight loss is accompanied by negative energy balance. Mild caloric restriction is safe for obese children and can be effective when families are motivated and encouraged to change longstanding feeding behaviors. Avoidance of sugar-sweetened beverages, reduction of saturated fat to less than 10% of calories, and minimizing trans-fat are also recommended.

Significant reductions in weight are unusual and often transient unless caloric restriction is accompanied by increased energy expenditure. Nevertheless, even relatively small reductions (5%–10%) in BMI Z-score may increase insulin sensitivity, enhance glucose tolerance, improve measures of cardiovascular health, and reduce the risk of progression to T2D [54].

Diets severely restricted in calories produce more dramatic weight loss but cannot be sustained under free-living conditions. Very low-calorie, low-protein diets are potentially dangerous and may precipitate recurrent and futile cycles of dieting and binge eating.

The child should be encouraged to remain active, and prolonged sedentary activities (television, computer games) should be discouraged. Family and communal pursuits, such as walking, hiking, bike-riding, and ball play are best for young people; the "exercise" should be fun and participatory. More intensive and directed exercise may be useful in the setting of obesity.

Benefits from lifestyle intervention are most likely to be reaped when diet and exercise programs are coordinated with individual and family counseling and behavior modification. School-based programs, supported by community groups and by state and federal agencies, may assist families and reduce the child's sense of isolation, frustration, and guilt.

14.5.2 PHARMACOTHERAPY IN DIABETES PREVENTION

Unfortunately, the long-term success of lifestyle intervention has been disappointing; rates of obesity and IR in children and adults continue to increase despite widespread recognition of the dangers of dietary indiscretion and a sedentary existence. This may reflect in part the resistance of complex feeding and activity behaviors to change, as well as the power of social and economic forces that shape lifestyles in the modern, industrialized world. Metabolic and hormonal adaptations to initial weight loss may also create barriers to long-term success; for example, reductions in food intake and body weight decrease the circulating concentrations of tri-iodothyronine (T3) and leptin and increase circulating concentrations of ghrelin. The fall in T3 and leptin levels limits energy expenditure and sympathetic nervous system activity and may facilitate rebound food intake. Hunger may be intensified by the rise in plasma ghrelin, which stimulates food intake [55]. Food restriction also causes a secondary resistance to growth hormone (GH) action and an increase in insulin sensitivity that may reduce the rates of lipolysis and fat breakdown [56,53]. The obstacles to success with lifestyle intervention have stimulated interest in pharmacologic approaches to diabetes prevention in obese children.

The FDA requires that medications targeted for weight loss meet the following criteria: (1) they must produce weight loss of at least 5% of the loss experienced by those taking placebo over the course of 1 year, (2) they must demonstrate that at least 35% of treated individuals achieved the at least 5% weight loss and that this was statistically significant compared to controls, and (3) they must show improvements in lipid, blood pressure, and blood glucose profiles [57]. These guidelines have significantly limited the number of FDA-approved medications available in the United States (Table 14.2) [57]. In addition, weight loss is usually minimal on these medications. Despite these factors, there may be considerable clinical benefit to even modest weight reduction on medication. Unfortunately, there are few medications that are FDA approved for those under 18 years of age.

14.5.2.1 Metformin

Metformin is an oral antihyperglycemic medication approved by the FDA to treat T2D in adults and in children over 10 years of age. Metformin derives from a natural product used in herbal medicine. It is a biguanide derivative that has been in clinical use since the 1950s [58]. It was not targeted for a particular disease or disorder, and much is still unknown about its mechanism of action. Human pharmacokinetic data point to the liver and intestines as major sites of its action. Metformin increases hepatic glucose uptake and decreases hepatic gluconeogenesis [58]. The latter effect results from accumulation of metformin in mitochondria (at a concentration 1,000-fold greater than extracellular medium) and inhibition of ATP production through effects on the respiratory chain. Increased AMP activates AMPK. AMPK has multiple cellular effects in the liver, including inhibiting lipogenesis, activating fatty acid oxidation, and increasing insulin sensitivity. Increased AMP also works in an AMPK-independent manner through inhibition of enzymes involved in gluconeogenesis [58].

TABLE 14.2

US Food and Drug Administration-Approved Medications for Weight Loss

Anorectics/Appetite Suppressants

Generic Name (Brand Name[s])	Dosage Forms	Max Daily Dose
Phentermine (Adipex-P, Suprenza)	15 mg, 30 mg, 37.5 mg	37.5 mg
Phendimetrazine (Bontril PDM, Bontril SR)	35 mg, 150 mg	210 mg
Methamphetamine (Desoxyn)	5 mg	15 mg
Benzphetamine (Didrex, Regimex)	25 mg, 50 mg	50 mg
Diethylproprion (Tenuate)	25 mg, 75 mg	75 mg

Lipase Inhibitor

Generic Name (Brand Name[s])	Dosage Forms	Max Daily Dose
Orlistat (Zenical, Alli)	120 mg	360 mg

Selective Serotonin 2CR Agonist

Generic Name (Brand Name[s])	Dosage Forms	Max Daily Dose
Locaserin (Belviq, Belviq XR)	10 mg, 20 mg	20 mg

GLP-1 Agonist

Generic Name (Brand Name)	Dosage Forms	Max Daily Dose
Liraglutide (Saxenda)	6 mg/ml pen	3 mg

Combination Medications

Generic Name (Brand Name[s])	Dosage Forms	Max Daily Dose
Phentermine/Topiramate ER (Qsymia)	3.75 mg/23 mg, 7.5 mg/46 mg, 11.25 mg/69 mg, 15 mg/92 mg	15 mg/92 mg
Naltrexone HCL/Bupropion HCL ER (Contrave)	8 mg/90 mg	32 mg/360 mg

Source: Leahy, L.G., *J Psychosoc Nurs Ment Health Serv.*, 55, 21–26, 2017.
2CR, 2C receptor; GLP-1, glucagon-like peptide 1.

Metformin also has important glucose-lowering effects in the intestines. Long-term use of metformin has been shown to increase glucose utilization in the gut, with decreased glucose uptake, increased anaerobic glucose metabolism in enterocytes, and increased production of lactate. Extended-release forms of metformin have been developed to improve tolerability of the drug. They are spread along the gut and thereby reduce local concentrations of the drug. Patients using the extended-release form of metformin have very little systemic absorption of the medicine, yet have equivalent reductions in blood sugar compared to patients using the standard immediate-release form. Also, metformin treatment has been shown to increase the GLP-1 concentration in human and animal studies. GLP-1 is secreted from L cells, which are distributed throughout the intestine but are highly concentrated in the ileum [59]. The GLP-1 increase is likely a direct stimulatory effect of metformin on L-cells but also may be indirect through inhibition of ileal bile acid absorption, in a similar manner to the effects of bile-acid sequestrants [59]. Lastly, metformin may have important effects on microbacteria in the gastrointestinal tract. Alteration of the gut microbiome has been implicated in the development of obesity, IR, and T2D, with a shift shown toward increased opportunistic pathogens and increased gut inflammation in affected patients. Studies in mice and humans have shown a marked increase in the bacterium *Akkermansia muciniphila* with metformin use [60]. *A. muciniphila* has been demonstrated to reduce gut inflammation, modify gut peptide secretion, and improve thickness of the gut mucous barrier.

Metformin also improves insulin sensitivity in skeletal muscle. Although a minor effect, this may have major implications in weight loss. Through improving insulin sensitivity, metformin may lessen the degree of postprandial hypoglycemia (and food-seeking behaviors) often seen in insulin-resistant patients. Other benefits of the drug include decreased fat stores (subcutaneous > visceral), improved lipid profiles (possibly through its effects on bile acids), and reduced liver enzymes in patients with hepatic steatosis [59]. Of even greater importance, metformin may improve cardiovascular health in obese patients. Burgert et al. showed that short-term treatment of obese adolescents with metformin improved cardiovascular function as assessed by heart rate recovery after exercise [61].

Evidence regarding metformin use in pediatric obesity is limited. A recent meta-analysis showed that metformin use for 3–6 months in obese adolescents, at doses ranging from 1,000 to 2,000 mg/day, was more effective than lifestyle intervention on weight reduction [62], though the effect was modest and short-lived. There were also modest improvements in markers of insulin sensitivity in the metformin-treated children. In a randomized, double-blind, placebo-controlled study conducted at six pediatric centers in the United Kingdom [63], 150 pediatric patients were randomly assigned placebo or metformin use for 6 months. Metformin use was associated with improved BMI-standard deviation score (SDS), fasting glucose, and Alanine aminotransferase (ALT) at 3 months, and with significant BMI-SDS reduction at 6 months.

The Diabetes Prevention Program [30] established the efficacy of metformin in delaying or preventing the onset of T2D in adults (age ≥ 25 years) with IGT. Daily energy and fat intake decreased only in the group randomized to intensive lifestyle modification, and the lifestyle intervention was more effective than metformin in reducing the incidence of T2D. Nevertheless, patients in the metformin group also lost weight, and metformin was as effective as lifestyle change in subjects with BMI exceeding 34.9 and in those with highest fasting glucose concentrations; these subgroups are at greatest risk for progression to type 2 diabetes. Metformin was also as effective as lifestyle intervention in younger adults aged 25–44 years. In addition to reducing the risk of development of T2D, intensive lifestyle intervention and metformin also had favorable, albeit small, effects on blood pressure and serum lipids. Studies performed in nondiabetic subjects 1–2 weeks after the trial's conclusion showed that the protective effect of metformin persisted in three-fourths of the drug-treated subjects, even after discontinuation of medication. The duration of this protective effect is unknown; prolonged treatment with metformin might be necessary to reduce the rate of progression to diabetes in high-risk subjects.

In an open-label extension of the 2,155 subjects randomized to the DPP metformin and placebo arms, the Diabetes Prevention Program Outcome Study (DPPOS) investigated the effects of metformin use after a total of 10 years of treatment. Subjects on metformin had sustained weight loss over the follow-up period [52]. Metformin was well-tolerated by the majority of subjects, though many patients had transient abdominal discomfort, which can be prevented by taking the medication with food. There were no instances of hepatic dysfunction or lactic acidosis; nevertheless, the drug should not be administered to patients with underlying cardiac, hepatic, renal, or gastrointestinal disease.

14.5.2.2 Drugs That Reduce Appetite

14.5.2.2.1 *Appetite Suppressants/Anorectics*

The most common types of prescription weight loss medications are appetite-suppressing anorectic agents, and include phentermine, phendimetrazine, methamphetamine, benzphetamine, and diethylpropion. These are categorized by the FDA as controlled dangerous substances (CDS). They are only approved for short-term use due to their potential for overuse and abuse. Although cleared by the FDA, they are contraindicated in subjects with cardiac disease, hypertension, or hyperthyroidism. Side effects include increased blood pressure, tachycardia, anxiety, restlessness, dry mouth, and constipation. None of these medications is FDA-approved for use in those younger than 18 years, though some have used them in patients as young as 12 years [57].

14.5.2.2.2 Selective Serotonin 2C Receptor Agonist

Locaserin works by increasing satiety and feelings of fullness. It is a selective serotonin receptor 2C agonist, and thus should be used with caution in patients on other medications affecting the serotonin system. The most common side effects include constipation, dry mouth, fatigue, muscular pain, headache, and anxiety. Prescribers must be alert for the high potential for dependency with this medication [57].

14.5.2.2.3 Glucagon-Like Peptide 1 Agonists

Glucagon-like peptide 1 (GLP-1) agonists have been shown to be safe and effective for weight management in adults with obesity. In addition to their incretin effects, GLP-1 agonists at higher doses reduce food intake and body weight in obese adults. The dual mechanisms of action for GLP-1 agonists include targets in the central nervous system and in the gastrointestinal tract. Leptin is an anorexigenic hormone whose secretion increases in response to GLP-1 agonist therapy. This leads to appetite suppression, decreased caloric intake, and delayed gastric emptying (Boland). There are many GLP-1 medications on the market, with twice-daily (exenatide), once-daily (liraglutide, lixisenatide), and once-weekly (exenatide extended release, albiglutide, dulaglutide, semaglutide) injectable options available. Semaglutide is in phase 3 trials in adults and awaiting FDA approval. It has also been formulated as a daily oral medication, with plans to have this available by 2020 [57].

Two studies evaluating exenatide for management of pediatric obesity have been published. In one, 6 months of open-label exenatide therapy (10 μg twice daily) and lifestyle intervention was associated with BMI reduction and reduced fasting insulin levels (Boland) in severely obese children aged 9–16 years. Weight reduction did not result in reduced body fat and there were no significant improvements in cardiovascular risk factors. In a double-blinded, placebo-controlled study, 26 obese adolescents randomized to placebo or exenatide (10 μg bid) also showed weight loss and reduced BMI in the treated group [57].

Liraglutide is a GLP-1 agonist given as a once-daily injection. Studies have been promising in adult patients when dose has been titrated to 3 mg per day. This is higher than the usual diabetes treatment dose of 1.8 mg per day. Studies using liraglutide have been limited in pediatric patients and have shown mixed results, possibly due to administration of the lower 1.8-mg daily dose.

GLP-1 agonists are generally well-tolerated by pediatric and adult patients. Gastrointestinal side effects are most common and include nausea, abdominal pain, vomiting, and diarrhea. Patients are advised to start at a low daily dose (0.6 mg per day) and titrate up to avoid these side effects, which occur most often in the early phases of dose titration. GLP-1 agonists are contraindicated in patients with a family history of endocrine tumors or thyroid cancers [57].

14.5.2.2.4 Combined Agents

Phentermine/topiramate extended release (ER) combines an appetite suppressor (phentermine) with an anticonvulsant (topiramate ER) that contributes to feelings of satiety. This combination should not be used by women who are or may become pregnant due to risk of birth defects. It is also contraindicated in patients with glaucoma or those who have had a heart attack or stroke in the past 6 months. Side effects include headache and dizziness, numbness or tingling in the face or extremities, decreased attention and concentration, dry mouth, and excessive thirst [57].

Naltrexone/bupropion ER combines the opioid antagonistic effects of naltrexone with the dopamine-norepinephrine reuptake inhibition of bupropion ER. This is thought to reduce appetite and cravings for food through an effect on the brain reward center. The medicine is contraindicated in those prescribed opioids or in those with a seizure disorder. Side effects include constipation, headache, increased anxiety, and increased blood pressure [57].

14.5.2.3 Drugs That Limit Nutrient Absorption

Orlistat inhibits pancreatic lipase and thereby increases fecal losses of triglyceride. It is the only long-term agent FDA-approved for use in children 12 years and older. Orlistat reduces body weight and total and LDL cholesterol levels and reduces the risk of T2D in adults with IGT. In obese adolescents, the combination of orlistat with lifestyle intervention reduced weight (-4.4 ± 4.6 kg), BMI, total cholesterol, LDL, fasting insulin, and fasting glucose concentrations and increased insulin sensitivity during a 3-month trial period [64]. There was considerable variability in response to the drug. Variable reductions in body weight (-12.7– $+2.5$ kg) and fat mass were also noted in a study of 11 morbidly obese children age 7–12 years. Side effects include diarrhea, fatty stools, fecal spotting, urgency, flatulence, bloating, and recurrent pain in the upper abdomen. Side effects are tolerable as long as subjects reduce fat intake, but this proves to be very difficult over the long term, and dropout rates are high. Orlistat may impair fat-soluble vitamin absorption; vitamin A, D, E, and K levels may decline despite supplementation [57].

Acarbose, an alpha-glucodase inhibitor, may reduce progression to T2D by limiting gastrointestinal absorption of carbohydrate. The STOP-NIDDM trial demonstrated a 25%–36% reduction in T2D in obese adults (mean age, 55 years; mean BMI, 31) with impaired glucose tolerance. Postprandial glucose and insulin concentrations were reduced, and weight declined slightly in patients treated with acarbose (100 mg three times/day[TID]) for a mean of 3.3 years. In addition, the rate of development of cardiovascular events (coronary heart disease, cardiovascular death, congestive heart failure, stroke, and peripheral vascular disease) was only one-half that in the placebo group. However, the dropout rate in the acarbose group was 24%, and the gastrointestinal side effects of the medication, which include flatulence and diarrhea, limit its acceptability in children and adolescents.

14.6   TREATMENT OF PEDIATRIC TYPE 2 DIABETES

The presentation of T2D in youth is often similar to that of adults, with beta-cell failure and insufficient insulin production. However, the development of comorbidities in youth may be more aggressive than in adults, with high rates of early microalbuminuria, hypertension, and dyslipidemia. This highlights the importance of prevention of T2D through lifestyle change, but also underscores the importance of achieving rapid glycemic control at diagnosis to prolong beta-cell function and to delay the onset of complications.

Clinical practice guidelines on the management of newly diagnosed T2D in children aged 10–18 years were established by a subcommittee convened by the American Academy of Pediatrics in 2013. The subcommittee consisted of representatives from the American Diabetes Association, Pediatric Endocrine Society, the American Academy of Family Physicians, and the Academy of Nutrition and Dietetics. Six action statements were proposed [65]:

1. Insulin should be started in patients presenting with T2D in ketosis or diabetic ketoacidosis and in patients in whom the diagnosis of T1D vs T2D is unclear who have (a) random venous or plasma glucose concentrations of 250 mg/dl or higher, or (b) HbA1c higher than 9%.
2. In all other instances, a lifestyle modification program (including nutrition and physical activity) and metformin therapy should be started. Metformin should be titrated up to 2,000 mg per day.
3. Clinicians should monitor HbA1c concentrations every 3 months and should intensify treatment if goals for blood glucose (BG) and HbA1c are not met.
4. Patients should monitor finger-stick BG concentrations in those who (a) are taking insulin or other hypoglycemic agents, (b) are initiating or changing their diabetes regimen, (c) have not met treatment goals, or (d) have intercurrent illness.
5. Clinicians should incorporate nutritional counseling into the treatment plan at diagnosis and ongoing, utilizing the Academy of Nutrition and Dietetic's *Pediatric Weight Management Evidence-Based Nutrition Practice Guidelines*.
6. Children and adolescents should be encouraged to engage in vigorous physical activity daily and should limit nonacademic screen time to less than 2 hours per day. The exercise should last at least 60 minutes each day, but does not need to be done in one session.

The impact of exercise on T2D can be profound. Recently, a study in Europe investigated the impact of regular physical activity on the management of pediatric T2D. A multicenter survey of 578 patients in 225 centers in Germany and Austria was conducted, with patients ranging in age from 10 to 20 years. Increasing physical activity was associated with a lower HbA1c, a lower BMI-SDS, and a higher HDL-cholesterol [66]. Unfortunately, more than half of the adolescents with T2D did not perform regular physical exercise.

Rapid normalization of blood glucose concentrations generally requires insulin administration, particularly if there is ketosis at diagnosis. Once near-normoglycemia is established, it is useful to begin metformin, increasing the dose gradually until maximal tolerated levels are achieved. The dose of insulin can then be reduced, facilitating weight loss in combination with lifestyle intervention. Insulin corrects the insulin deficiency observed in patients with long-standing disease and can prevent the ketosis that may recur in some children and adolescents with T2D.

Currently, metformin is the only noninsulin, FDA-approved medication for the management of pediatric T2D. SEARCH data published in 2014 revealed that, of the 428 youth with T2D, 40% were on metformin alone and 33% were on insulin therapy [3]. The HbA1c was lowest in subjects with lifestyle management alone (6.8%) compared to metformin monotherapy (7.5%) and insulin monotherapy (9.1%). More than 50% of patients with T2D lasting 2 or more years had HbA1c of 8% or higher. The FDA has recognized the importance of establishing other medical alternatives for patients and has enforced legislation supporting greater pharmaceutical company involvement in pediatric T2D studies.

14.6.1 THIAZOLIDINEDIONES

Metformin is not tolerated in a minority of subjects. In such cases, a thiazolidinedione (TZD) may prove useful. TZDs regulate lipid and carbohydrate metabolism through binding to peroxisome proliferator-activated receptor (PPAR)-γ [67]. When activated by TZDs, PPAR-γ heterodimerizes with the retinoid X receptor and binds to the promoters of target genes, including lipoprotein lipase, fatty acid transport protein, acetyl coA-synthase, and adipocyte protein 2 (aP2). The major effects of the TZDs are exerted in adipose tissue and skeletal muscle. In 2005, pioglitazone was studied in 36 adolescent patients with T2D. This was an open-label, multisite study conducted over 18 days, investigating the safety, tolerance, and pharmacokinetics of three daily doses (15, 30, and 45 mg). Pharmacokinetic profiles and side effects were similar to those seen in adult patients. Side effects included hypoglycemia, nausea, headache, peripheral edema, hepatic dysfunction, and diarrhea [67].

The TODAY (Treatment Options for Type 2 Diabetes in Adolescents and Youth) study was a multisite, randomized parallel-group pediatric T2D study, conducted between 2004 and 2011 [68]. Eligible patients were between the ages of 10 and 17 years, with T2D diagnosed within the last 2 years and with BMI higher than 85%. After a run-in period in which patients were treated with metformin (1,000 mg twice daily), received diabetes education, demonstrated adherence to medications and attendance at visits, and maintained HbA1c levels below 8%, 700 subjects were randomized to one of three treatment regimens, each including continuation of metformin at the same dose: (1) metformin alone, (2) metformin + rosiglitazone 4 mg per day, and (3) metformin + intensive lifestyle intervention. The study investigated time to treatment failure, which was defined as a HbA1c of 8% or more for 6 consecutive months, or the continued need for insulin for 3 months after an acute event. The use of metformin and rosiglitazone was the most successful, with a failure rate of 38.6%, compared to metformin and lifestyle change (46.6% failure rate) and metformin alone (51.7% treatment failure) (Figure 14.5) [68]. Currently, TZDs are not approved for use in children. Ongoing studies will assess the benefits and risks of TZDs and combination therapy (metformin + TZD) in children with T2D [67].

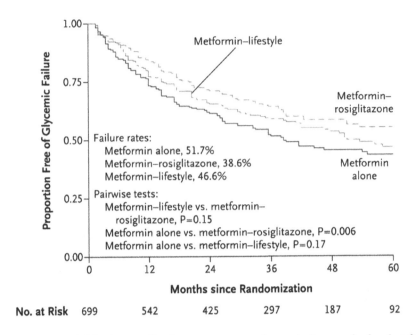

FIGURE 14.5 The TODAY Study: overall primary outcome results survival curves for freedom from glyce-mic failure are shown. Data are for up to 60 months of follow-up (accounting for 98.4% of cases of glycemic failure), although the rates and analysis are based on the complete data set.

14.6.2 SULFONYLUREAS

Sulfonylureas are mainstays of therapy in adults with T2D. Their use as primary agents for treat-ment of T2D in children has not been studied extensively. In a 26-week single-blind, randomized comparative study published in 2007, metformin and glimepiride were used in 263 obese T2D participants between the ages of 8 and 17 years. Participants were given metformin (500–1,000 mg twice daily) or escalating doses of glimepiride (1–8 mg once daily). There was no statistically sig-nificant difference in HbA1c at 12 and 24 weeks, but weight gain was greater in the glimepiride group (1.3 kg vs no difference in metformin group). In addition, the metformin-treated group had less hypoglycemia [69].

14.6.3 GLUCAGON-LIKE PEPTIDE AGONISTS

Use of GLP-1 agonists in adult T2D has increased dramatically in recent years. There have been very few pediatric studies with GLP-1 agonists and T2D, however. In 2009, results were published from a study investigating exenatide use in adolescents currently treated with metformin. Thirteen obese adolescents with T2D with ages ranging from 10 to 16 years were enrolled in the 5-week study. Exenatide was given as a single daily dose (2.5 or 5 μg), and metformin was continued (doses ranged from 250 mg twice daily to 1,000 mg twice daily). Both doses of exenatide were associated with lower postprandial blood glucose levels, reduced glucagon secretion, and increased glucose-mediated insulin release. None of the patients had gastrointestinal side effects [70].

Liraglutide has also been studied in youth T2D. Nineteen T2D subjects aged 10–17 years were studied by Klein et al. in a 5-week placebo-controlled trial. Thirteen of 19 participants were on liraglutide, with dose titration (from 0.3 mg to 1.8 mg once daily) until fasting blood glucose was at goal for at least 3 consecutive days. Six subjects received placebo. Fourteen of the 19 patients were on metformin therapy at baseline and throughout the trial. Mean HbA1c levels decreased in the liraglutide group compared to the placebo group. There were no serious adverse effects during the brief trial, though hypoglycemia was experienced more often in the liraglutide group [67].

Adult studies have shown promising results with GLP-1 medications and cardiovascular outcomes in patients with T2D. In a randomized, double-blind, placebo-controlled parallel group trial at 230 sites in 20 countries, 3,000 adults with T2D were randomized to placebo or to once-weekly injectable semaglutide at doses of either 0.5 mg or 1 mg per week. Patients were followed for 2 years. Mean duration of diabetes was 13.9 years, and mean HbA1c was 8.7% at onset of the study. Fifty-eight percent of patients had established cardiovascular disease. After 2 years, semaglutide-treated patients had significant reduction in HbA1c compared to placebo (1.4% decrease compared to 0.4%) and had 26% lower risk of the primary composite outcome of death from cardiovascular causes, nonfatal myocardial infarction, or nonfatal stroke than did those receiving placebo [71].

14.6.4 Alpha-Glucosidase Inhibitor

Acarbose has been studied in adult patients with T2D [72]. In a meta-analysis of 75 studies comparing metformin and acarbose, Gu et al. found that acarbose was as effective as metformin in lowering HbA1c when used as monotherapy. Metformin was more effective than acarbose when used in combination with other medications. Acarbose has not been studied as therapy for T2D in children, and, as noted above, GI side effects limit its acceptability for long-term use.

14.7 A MULTIFACETED APPROACH TO PREVENTION OF COMPLICATIONS

The major causes of death in adults with T2D are myocardial infarction and stroke. Although cardiovascular risk in patients with T2D varies with glycemic control, other factors play equal or more important roles. These include obesity, hypertension, smoking, dyslipidemia, ethnic background, and family history. In theory, aggressive lifestyle intervention in children and adolescents should include abolition of smoking and reduction in the intake of caffeine, which may raise blood pressure and postprandial glucose concentrations. Pharmacologic therapy may be necessary to reduce blood pressure, control microalbuminuria, and treat dyslipidemia. A multifaceted approach that combined dietary counseling, statins, angiotensin-converting enzyme inhibitors, and low-dose aspirin reduced by 50%–60% the long-term (8-year) risks of nephropathy, retinopathy, autonomic neuropathy, and cardiovascular endpoints (myocardial disease and stroke and amputation) in diabetic adults with microalbuminuria (Gaede et al.). Such an approach may be necessary in the management of obese, insulin-resistant, and glucose-intolerant adolescents, who are commonly hypertensive and hyperlipidemic. The age and intensity of intervention may depend upon the family history of cardiovascular disease as well as the severity of problems in the individual teenager under the physician's care.

14.8 SUMMARY AND CONCLUSION

The twenty-first century has seen a dramatic rise in the incidence of pediatric T2D. Previously described as an adult disease, T2D has been diagnosed in children of all ages and, in some areas, outnumbers T1D diagnoses. The alarming increase in pediatric T2D can be attributed to multiple risk factors, including obesity, diet, ethnicity, genetic predisposition, and lifestyle choices. Obesity is the strongest risk factor for T2D and is rising at a staggering rate in pediatric populations. Predictions are that 60 million children will be overweight by the year 2020. The distribution of adipose tissue in obese patients plays a critical role in the development of IR and T2D. Skeletal and hepatic fat deposition are particularly damaging and appear to adversely affect insulin signaling and glucose disposal.

Emerging data also support a strong role for nutrition in the pathogenesis of T2D. Metabolomic studies have shown that BCAAs are elevated in obese and insulin-resistant subjects. Accumulation of BCAAs and their metabolites through diet and through altered protein metabolism may lead to intracellular stress and impaired insulin secretion, particularly when paired with a high-fat diet. A sedentary lifestyle is also a risk factor for T2D. Increasing daily physical activity can have significant metabolic and cardiovascular benefits for the overweight child. Even slight reductions in weight and fat distribution can have dramatic beneficial effects and may prolong or prevent the progression to T2D.

Diagnosing T2D early in its course is critical for long-term health. Pediatric patients appear to have rapid development of microvascular and macrovascular complications when compared to pediatric patients with T1D and adults with T2D. Achieving glycemic control early after diagnosis is crucial. In the opinion of the author, pharmacologic therapy should be considered for severely resistant or glucose-intolerant (IFG or IGT) children or adolescents who fail to respond to a 6- to 12-month trial of lifestyle intervention despite a "good-faith effort." "Good-faith effort" means that the patient has attempted to follow a low–saturated fat/low-calorie diet recommended by a dietary counselor and has increased his or her energy expenditure through regular exercise. "Unsuccessful" means that the elevations of fasting or postprandial glucose persist or worsen despite lifestyle intervention. The decision to initiate drug therapy relieves neither the child nor the physician of the commitment to long-term lifestyle change; thus diet and exercise regimens should be maintained, even if they had not proven effective in the absence of medication.

Given its proven efficacy in treating insulin-resistant, as well as diabetic adolescents and adults and women with PCOS, its track record of safety in men and women, and its ability to limit weight gain, the author considers metformin the drug of choice for treating the obese child with IR, IFG, or IGT. Though lactic acidosis is extraordinarily rare in pediatric patients, metformin should not be administered to children with underlying cardiac, hepatic, renal, or gastrointestinal disease. Obese subjects with mild elevations in hepatic enzymes (less than threefold higher than established norms) may receive the drug; indeed, some studies suggest that metformin may be useful in treatment of hepatic steatosis. Concurrent use of a multivitamin seems reasonable, because metformin increases urinary excretion of vitamins B_1 and B_6.

It is not possible at this time to provide firm or uniform guidelines regarding the duration of pharmacologic intervention. A trial off medication may be warranted if glucose tolerance is normalized, particularly if there has been a decline in BMI Z-score. If IGT persists despite compliance with the medical/pharmacologic regimen, it may be necessary to intensify lifestyle intervention and/or to increase the dose of medication. If glucose tolerance declines or the patient develops overt diabetes, it may be necessary to add insulin or another pharmacologic agent to the therapeutic regimen.

ACKNOWLEDGEMENT

The author thanks Dr. Michael Freemark, who composed the chapter for the first edition of this book. While some of the original content was preserved, several additions were made to reflect current developments in the field of pediatric T2D.

REFERENCES

1. Association AD. Standards of medical care in diabetes-2017: Summary of revisions. *Diabetes Care.* 2017;40(Suppl 1):S4–5. doi:10.2337/dc17-S003.
2. Jaiswal M, Divers J, Dabelea D, Isom S, Bell RA, Martin CL, et al. Prevalence of and risk factors for diabetic peripheral neuropathy in youth with type 1 and type 2 diabetes: SEARCH for diabetes in youth study. *Diabetes Care.* 2017;40(9):1226–32.
3. Pettitt DJ, Talton J, Dabelea D, Divers J, Imperatore G, Lawrence JM, et al. Prevalence of diabetes in U.S. youth in 2009: The SEARCH for diabetes in youth study. *Diabetes Care.* 2014;37(2):402–8.
4. Samuel VT, Shulman GI. Mechanisms for insulin resistance: Common threads and missing links. *Cell.* 2012;148(5):852–71.
5. Boucher J, Kleinridders A, Kahn CR. Insulin receptor signaling in normal and insulin-resistant states. *Cold Spring Harb Perspect Biol.* 2014;6(1):a009191.

6. Weiss R, Dufour S, Taksali SE, Tamborlane WV, Petersen KF, Bonadonna RC, et al. Prediabetes in obese youth: A syndrome of impaired glucose tolerance, severe insulin resistance, and altered myocellular and abdominal fat partitioning. *Lancet*. 2003;362(9388):951–7.

7. Unger RH. Minireview: Weapons of lean body mass destruction: The role of ectopic lipids in the metabolic syndrome. *Endocrinology*. 2003;144(12):5159–65.

8. Boden G, Shulman GI. Free fatty acids in obesity and type 2 diabetes: Defining their role in the development of insulin resistance and beta-cell dysfunction. *Eur J Clin Invest*. 2002;32 Suppl 3:14–23.

9. Petersen KF, Dufour S, Befroy D, Garcia R, Shulman GI. Impaired mitochondrial activity in the insulin-resistant offspring of patients with type 2 diabetes. *N Engl J Med*. 2004;350(7):664–71.

10. D'Adamo E, Cali AM, Weiss R, Santoro N, Pierpont B, Northrup V, et al. Central role of fatty liver in the pathogenesis of insulin resistance in obese adolescents. *Diabetes Care*. 2010;33(8):1817–22.

11. Van Name M, Santoro N. Type 2 diabetes mellitus in pediatrics: A new challenge. *World J Pediatr*. 2013;9(4):293–9.

12. Perry RJ, Samuel VT, Petersen KF, Shulman GI. The role of hepatic lipids in hepatic insulin resistance and type 2 diabetes. *Nature*. 2014;510(7503):84–91.

13. Newgard CB, An J, Bain JR, Muehlbauer MJ, Stevens RD, Lien LF, et al. A branched-chain amino acid-related metabolic signature that differentiates obese and lean humans and contributes to insulin resistance. *Cell Metab*. 2009;9(4):311–26.

14. Frohnert BI, Rewers MJ. Metabolomics in childhood diabetes. *Pediatr Diabetes*. 2016;17(1):3–14.

15. Lynch CJ, Adams SH. Branched-chain amino acids in metabolic signalling and insulin resistance. *Nat Rev Endocrinol*. 2014;10(12):723–36.

16. Yoon MS. The emerging role of branched-chain amino acids in insulin resistance and metabolism. *Nutrients*. 2016;8(7):405.

17. Weickert MO, Roden M, Isken F, Hoffmann D, Nowotny P, Osterhoff M, et al. Effects of supplemented isoenergetic diets differing in cereal fiber and protein content on insulin sensitivity in overweight humans. *Am J Clin Nutr*. 2011;94(2):459–71.

18. She P, Reid TM, Bronson SK, Vary TC, Hajnal A, Lynch CJ, et al. Disruption of BCATm in mice leads to increased energy expenditure associated with the activation of a futile protein turnover cycle. *Cell Metab*. 2007;6(3):181–94.

19. Magkos F, Bradley D, Schweitzer GG, Finck BN, Eagon JC, Ilkayeva O, et al. Effect of Roux-en-Y gastric bypass and laparoscopic adjustable gastric banding on branched-chain amino acid metabolism. *Diabetes*. 2013;62(8):2757–61.

20. McCormack SE, Shaham O, McCarthy MA, Deik AA, Wang TJ, Gerszten RE, et al. Circulating branched-chain amino acid concentrations are associated with obesity and future insulin resistance in children and adolescents. *Pediatr Obes*. 2013;8(1):52–61.

21. Weiss R, Dziura JD, Burgert TS, Taksali SE, Tamborlane WV, Caprio S. Ethnic differences in beta cell adaptation to insulin resistance in obese children and adolescents. *Diabetologia*. 2006;49(3):571–9.

22. Hu FB, Manson JE, Stampfer MJ, Colditz G, Liu S, Solomon CG, et al. Diet, lifestyle, and the risk of type 2 diabetes mellitus in women. *N Engl J Med*. 2001;345(11):790–7.

23. Cali AM, Caprio S. Prediabetes and type 2 diabetes in youth: An emerging epidemic disease? *Curr Opin Endocrinol Diabetes Obes*. 2008;15(2):123–7.

24. Pulgaron ER, Delamater AM. Obesity and type 2 diabetes in children: Epidemiology and treatment. *Curr Diab Rep*. 2014;14(8):508.

25. Gandica R, Zeitler P. Update on youth-onset type 2 diabetes: Lessons learned from the treatment options for type 2 diabetes in adolescents and youth clinical trial. *Adv Pediatr*. 2016;63(1):195–209.

26. Morgan AR. Determining genetic risk factors for pediatric type 2 diabetes. *Curr Diab Rep*. 2012;12(1):88–92.

27. Hammoud NM, de Valk HW, van Rossem L, Biesma DH, Wit JM, Visser GH. Growth and BMI during the first 14 y of life in offspring from women with type 1 or type 2 diabetes mellitus. *Pediatr Res*. 2017;81(2):342–8.

28. Lovejoy JC. The influence of dietary fat on insulin resistance. *Curr Diab Rep*. 2002;2(5):435–40.

29. Eriksson KF, Lindgarde F. Prevention of type 2 (non-insulin-dependent) diabetes mellitus by diet and physical exercise. The 6-year Malmo feasibility study. *Diabetologia*. 1991;34(12):891–8.

30. Knowler WC, Barrett-Connor E, Fowler SE, Hamman RF, Lachin JM, Walker EA, et al. Reduction in the incidence of type 2 diabetes with lifestyle intervention or metformin. *N Engl J Med*. 2002;346(6):393–403.

31. Pan XR, Li GW, Hu YH, Wang JX, Yang WY, An ZX, et al. Effects of diet and exercise in preventing NIDDM in people with impaired glucose tolerance. The Da Qing IGT and Diabetes Study. *Diabetes Care*. 1997;20(4):537–44.

32. Uusitupa M, Lindi V, Louheranta A, Salopuro T, Lindstrom J, Tuomilehto J. Long-term improvement in insulin sensitivity by changing lifestyles of people with impaired glucose tolerance: 4-year results from the Finnish Diabetes Prevention Study. *Diabetes*. 2003;52(10):2532–8.

33. Foster GD, Wyatt HR, Hill JO, McGuckin BG, Brill C, Mohammed BS, et al. A randomized trial of a low-carbohydrate diet for obesity. *N Engl J Med*. 2003;348(21):2082–90.

34. Samaha FF, Iqbal N, Seshadri P, Chicano KL, Daily DA, McGrory J, et al. A low-carbohydrate as compared with a low-fat diet in severe obesity. *N Engl J Med*. 2003;348(21):2074–81.

35. Bravata DM, Sanders L, Huang J, Krumholz HM, Olkin I, Gardner CD, et al. Efficacy and safety of low-carbohydrate diets: A systematic review. *JAMA*. 2003;289(14):1837–50.

36. Warren JM, Henry CJ, Simonite V. Low glycemic index breakfasts and reduced food intake in preadolescent children. *Pediatrics*. 2003;112(5):e414.

37. Elliott SS, Keim NL, Stern JS, Teff K, Havel PJ. Fructose, weight gain, and the insulin resistance syndrome. *Am J Clin Nutr*. 2002;76(5):911–22.

38. Montonen J, Knekt P, Jarvinen R, Aromaa A, Reunanen A. Whole-grain and fiber intake and the incidence of type 2 diabetes. *Am J Clin Nutr*. 2003;77(3):622–9.

39. Guerrero-Romero F, Simental-Mendia LE, Hernandez-Ronquillo G, Rodriguez-Moran M. Oral magnesium supplementation improves glycaemic status in subjects with prediabetes and hypomagnesaemia: A double-blind placebo-controlled randomized trial. *Diabetes Metab*. 2015;41(3):202–7.

40. Pereira MA, Jacobs DR, Jr., Van Horn L, Slattery ML, Kartashov AI, Ludwig DS. Dairy consumption, obesity, and the insulin resistance syndrome in young adults: The CARDIA Study. *JAMA*. 2002;287(16):2081–9.

41. Spriet LL, Watt MJ. Regulatory mechanisms in the interaction between carbohydrate and lipid oxidation during exercise. *Acta Physiol Scand*. 2003;178(4):443–52.

42. McGee SL, Howlett KF, Starkie RL, Cameron-Smith D, Kemp BE, Hargreaves M. Exercise increases nuclear AMPK alpha2 in human skeletal muscle. *Diabetes*. 2003;52(4):926–8.

43. Santoro C, Cosmas A, Forman D, Morghan A, Bairos L, Levesque S, et al. Exercise training alters skeletal muscle mitochondrial morphometry in heart failure patients. *J Cardiovasc Risk*. 2002;9(6):377–81.

44. Dabelea D, Stafford JM, Mayer-Davis EJ, D'Agostino R, Jr., Dolan L, Imperatore G, et al. Association of type 1 diabetes vs type 2 diabetes diagnosed during childhood and adolescence with complications during teenage years and young adulthood. *JAMA*. 2017;317(8):825–35.

45. Luk AO, Lau ES, So WY, Ma RC, Kong AP, Ozaki R, et al. Prospective study on the incidences of cardiovascular-renal complications in Chinese patients with young-onset type 1 and type 2 diabetes. *Diabetes Care*. 2014;37(1):149–57.

46. Al-Saeed AH, Constantino MI, Molyneaux L, D'Souza M, Limacher-Gisler F, Luo C, et al. An inverse relationship between age of type 2 diabetes onset and complication risk and mortality: The impact of youth-onset type 2 diabetes. *Diabetes Care*. 2016;39(5):823–9.

47. Constantino MI, Molyneaux L, Limacher-Gisler F, Al-Saeed A, Luo C, Wu T, et al. Long-term complications and mortality in young-onset diabetes: Type 2 diabetes is more hazardous and lethal than type 1 diabetes. *Diabetes Care*. 2013;36(12):3863–9.

48. Deedwania PC. Mechanisms of endothelial dysfunction in the metabolic syndrome. *Curr Diab Rep*. 2003;3(4):289–92.

49. Vincent MA, Montagnani M, Quon MJ. Molecular and physiologic actions of insulin related to production of nitric oxide in vascular endothelium. *Curr Diab Rep*. 2003;3(4):279–88.

50. Watts K, Beye P, Siafarikas A, Davis EA, Jones TW, O'Driscoll G, et al. Exercise training normalizes vascular dysfunction and improves central adiposity in obese adolescents. *J Am Coll Cardiol*. 2004;43(10):1823–7.

51. Montani JP, Antic V, Yang Z, Dulloo A. Pathways from obesity to hypertension: From the perspective of a vicious triangle. *Int J Obes Relat Metab Disord*. 2002;26 Suppl 2:S28–38.

52. Delahanty LM. Weight loss in the prevention and treatment of diabetes. *Prev Med*. 2017;11(104):120–123.

53. Kratzsch J, Dehmel B, Pulzer F, Keller E, Englaro P, Blum WF, et al. Increased serum GHBP levels in obese pubertal children and adolescents: Relationship to body composition, leptin and indicators of metabolic disturbances. *Int J Obes Relat Metab Disord*. 1997;21(12):1130–6.

54. Long SD, O'Brien K, MacDonald KG, Jr., Leggett-Frazier N, Swanson MS, Pories WJ, et al. Weight loss in severely obese subjects prevents the progression of impaired glucose tolerance to type II diabetes. A longitudinal interventional study. *Diabetes Care*. 1994;17(5):372–5.

55. Inui A, Asakawa A, Bowers CY, Mantovani G, Laviano A, Meguid MM, et al. Ghrelin, appetite, and gastric motility: The emerging role of the stomach as an endocrine organ. *FASEB J.* 2004;18(3):439–56.

56. Douyon L, Schteingart DE. Effect of obesity and starvation on thyroid hormone, growth hormone, and cortisol secretion. *Endocrinol Metab Clin North Am.* 2002;31(1):173–89.

57. Leahy LG. Medication-assisted weight loss in the age of obesity. *J Psychosoc Nurs Ment Health Serv.* 2017;55(8):21–6. doi:10.3928/02793695-20170718-02.

58. Rena G, Hardie DG, Pearson ER. The mechanisms of action of metformin. *Diabetologia.* 2017;60(9):1577–1585.

59. McCreight LJ, Bailey CJ, Pearson ER. Metformin and the gastrointestinal tract. *Diabetologia.* 2016;59(3):426–35.

60. Karlsson FH, Tremaroli V, Nookaew I, Bergstrom G, Behre CJ, Fagerberg B, et al. Gut metagenome in European women with normal, impaired and diabetic glucose control. *Nature.* 2013;498(7452):99–103.

61. Burgert TS, Duran EJ, Goldberg-Gell R, Dziura J, Yeckel CW, Katz S, et al. Short-term metabolic and cardiovascular effects of metformin in markedly obese adolescents with normal glucose tolerance. *Pediatr Diabetes.* 2008;9(6):567–76.

62. McDonagh MS, Selph S, Ozpinar A, Foley C. Systematic review of the benefits and risks of metformin in treating obesity in children aged 18 years and younger. *JAMA Pediatr.* 2014;168(2):178–84.

63. Kendall D, Vail A, Amin R, Barrett T, Dimitri P, Ivison F, et al. Metformin in obese children and adolescents: The MOCA trial. *J Clin Endocrinol Metab.* 2013;98(1):322–9.

64. Norgren S, Danielsson P, Jurold R, Lotborn M, Marcus C. Orlistat treatment in obese prepubertal children: A pilot study. *Acta Paediatr.* 2003;92(6):666–70.

65. Copeland KC, Silverstein J, Moore KR, Prazar GE, Raymer T, Shiffman RN, et al. Management of newly diagnosed type 2 diabetes mellitus (T2DM) in children and adolescents. *Pediatrics.* 2013;131(2):364–82.

66. Herbst A, Kapellen T, Schober E, Graf C, Meissner T, Holl RW. Impact of regular physical activity on blood glucose control and cardiovascular risk factors in adolescents with type 2 diabetes mellitus—A multicenter study of 578 patients from 225 centres. *Pediatr Diabetes.* 2015;16(3):204–10.

67. Smith JD, Mills E, Carlisle SE. Treatment of pediatric type 2 diabetes. *Ann Pharmacother.* 2016;50(9):768–77.

68. Narasimhan S, Weinstock RS. Youth-onset type 2 diabetes mellitus: Lessons learned from the TODAY study. *Mayo Clin Proc.* 2014;89(6):806–16.

69. Gottschalk M, Danne T, Vlajnic A, Cara JF. Glimepiride versus metformin as monotherapy in pediatric patients with type 2 diabetes: A randomized, single-blind comparative study. *Diabetes Care.* 2007;30(4):790–4.

70. Malloy J, Capparelli E, Gottschalk M, Guan X, Kothare P, Fineman M. Pharmacology and tolerability of a single dose of exenatide in adolescent patients with type 2 diabetes mellitus being treated with metformin: A randomized, placebo-controlled, single-blind, dose-escalation, crossover study. *Clin Ther.* 2009;31(4):806–15.

71. Marso SP, Bain SC, Consoli A, Eliaschewitz FG, Jodar E, Leiter LA, et al. Semaglutide and cardiovascular outcomes in patients with type 2 diabetes. *N Engl J Med.* 2016;375(19):1834–44.

72. Gu S, Shi J, Tang Z, Sawhney M, Hu H, Shi L, et al. Comparison of glucose lowering effect of metformin and acarbose in type 2 diabetes mellitus: A meta-analysis. *PLoS One.* 2015;10(5):e0126704.

15 The Contribution of Iron and Transition Metal Micronutrients to Diabetes and Metabolic Disease

Lipika Salaye, Zhenzhong Bai, and Donald A. McClain

CONTENTS

15.1 INTRODUCTION

Macronutrient excess is the largest single risk factor for type 2 diabetes mellitus (T2DM). Micronutrients also play essential roles in metabolism, however, and emerging data suggest that, within the broad range of average intake for these entities, much narrower optimal levels exist for various cellular functions. This is true for vitamins, minerals, and trace elements, although this chapter will focus on the transition metals, and in particular those with a developed literature relating to diabetes, notably iron, zinc, manganese, copper, and chromium. Surveys of individuals in China reveal diabetes risk is associated with all of these, as well as other metals such as arsenic, cesium, and strontium, some of which may be assumed to be acting as toxins rather than reflecting imbalance of necessary trace elements [1]. We will focus on and begin with a consideration of iron, because of its long historic connection with diabetes in the context of hereditary hemochromatosis, the substantial literature, and the potential significance to the largest numbers of those with diabetes.

15.2 IRON AND METABOLIC DISEASE

15.2.1 INTRODUCTION TO DIABETES AND IRON

In humans, markers of high tissue iron levels are a risk factor for insulin resistance, metabolic syndrome (MetS), T2DM, and the progression of nonalcoholic fatty liver disease (NAFLD) to steatohepatitis (NASH). Importantly, the effects of iron are seen not only in pathologic iron overload, but also across the very broad range of "normal" iron. In this chapter, we will briefly review iron homeostasis, a complex system that has evolved to protect us from iron, a potentially dangerous oxidant, while allowing its use for redox reactions essential for oxidation of glucose and fat. We will then discuss the diseases of pathologic iron overload, such as hereditary hemochromatosis (HH), and how they demonstrated that excess iron could drive diabetes pathogenesis. This led to the recognition that, even within its very broad range of "normal," iron also conferred diabetes risk, causing both insulin resistance and insulin insufficiency. Other conditions associated with excess nutrition, aging, and oxidant stress are also associated with increased risk from high iron, including NASH, Alzheimer's disease, cardiovascular disease, and others. In this chapter, we will concentrate on investigation in human models, although we will also use salient animal studies that have revealed the causal relationships between iron and these conditions and their mechanisms. The clear relation of dietary and pathologic iron overload to diabetes in rodent models has been recently reviewed [2,3]. It should be pointed out that papers and a review [4] also exist challenging the relationship between iron and diabetes, both in HH and T2DM, although one might argue the positive studies in the literature quoted therein are not adequately addressed, and the negative studies are complicated by several factors, such as mixing populations with different background diabetes prevalence, inadequate analyses of glycemia, and including younger individuals who in general have not had time to develop T2DM or HH-associated DM. Readers are encouraged to consult that literature and form their own opinion.

15.2.2 EVOLUTIONARY ASPECTS OF THE REGULATION OF IRON
AND ITS CONTRIBUTION TO METABOLISM

Most organisms evolved under pressure of fuel insufficiency, hence the systems that control energy balance are mainly responsive to that pressure. This may be one reason humans are not as effectively adapted to deal with the relatively recent phenomenon of a surfeit of food, and why they seek out more food even when adequately or overnourished. Another evolutionary pressure in which humans evolved, especially after the agrarian revolution, was insufficient iron [5]. The most common elemental nutritional deficiency on the planet is of iron, affecting an estimated 2 billion humans, mainly in developing countries. Consistent with this pressure, the most common human mutations affecting iron homeostasis are the human hemochromatosis protein (high iron, or *HFE*) mutations that cause HH. As described below, the most common *HFE* mutations arose in northern Europe, where dietary iron intake is low. Based on its high allelic frequency in those populations, approximately 5%–10%, the mutation is presumed to have exerted positive selective pressure. Because it dampens the negative feedback system that controls iron absorption in the gut and iron availability to tissue, it allows carriers to take up excess iron on the presumably rare occasions when an iron-rich meal was available.

The evolutionary pressure of iron deficiency is counterintuitive, given the abundance of iron, which is the earth's most abundant element and comprises 5.6% of the earth's crust. A possible explanation is that lower organisms, exposed directly to that iron, evolved highly controlled systems to limit its uptake as a defense against potential oxidant damage. At the same time, organisms evolved to take advantage of iron—for example, for fuel oxidation, other redox reactions, and oxygen delivery. In fact, the use of iron for cellular processes may not be fully appreciated, insofar as it is estimated that hundreds of proteins may carry iron prosthetic groups, with iron usually bound complexed to heme or iron-sulfur clusters [6]. This need for iron in the face of its potential danger has given rise to a complex system to tightly regulate its tissue levels, tissue distribution, and bioavailability, discussed in Section 15.3. The importance of iron is also manifest in the rapid evolution in primates of systems to prevent the use of iron by invading organisms, and the organisms' equally rapid evolution to neutralize those defenses [7].

A corollary is that there has also arisen in evolution an important link between iron availability and metabolism. Fuel choice in yeast, for example, is tightly and reciprocally coupled to iron: The potentially dangerous atom is not imported unless needed for fuel oxidation, and likewise the complex systems needed for fuel oxidation are not created unless iron is available [8]. The importance and simultaneous dangers of iron are also reflected in the fact that approximately 50 genes in yeast are devoted to importing, chaperoning, and storing iron. Many of these connections are conserved in higher eukaryotes [6].

Although iron deficiency also carries metabolic consequences including obesity, possibly related to limited capacity for fuel oxidation, this review will concentrate on the contribution of iron excess to diabetes and related conditions.

15.2.3 Mechanisms of Iron Homeostasis

Systemic and cellular iron metabolism have been the subject of excellent recent reviews [9–11] and will be only briefly recapitulated here (Figure 15.1). Intestinal free ferric (Fe^{3+}) iron is reduced to ferrous Fe^{2+} by duodenal cytochrome B (DCTB) and enters duodenal enterocytes by way of the divalent metal-ion transporter 1 (DMT1) and possibly other carriers. Dietary heme is directly absorbed into enterocytes, where iron is released by heme oxygenase (HMOX). Ferrous iron exits the enterocytes through the iron export channel ferroportin (FPN). After oxidization by hephaestin (HEPH), Fe^{3+} binds to transferrin (Tf) in the blood, which in turn binds to transferrin receptors (TfR) on the surface of target cells. In most cells (Figure 15.1, lower right), after endocytosis of TfR1 and acidification of the endosome, iron is released, reduced by STEAP (6-transmembrane epithelial antigen of the prostate), and enters the cytosol through DMT1, where it is used (e.g., for heme or Fe-S-cluster synthesis in mitochondria) or, if in excess, sequestered by ferritin. Apoferritin secreted into the circulation is a marker for tissue iron stores, although the trigger for its secretion versus use to sequester more iron is not known. The intracellular trafficking of iron is much more complicated than indicated in the figure. For example, iron is highly controlled and chaperoned to its various targets, as ferrous iron or after iron-sulfur cluster synthesis, by mechanisms that are still under study [6].

The liver is one of the primary organs that regulates systemic iron balance. In the liver, Tf binds TfR2 and the protein HFE, and in concert with signaling via the glycophosphatidylinositol (GPI)-anchored protein hemojuvelin (HJV), bone morphogenic proteins (BMPs), and transducers of TGFβ signaling (SMAD's), the 21mer peptide hepcidin is produced. Hepcidin induces internalization and degradation of FPN in the enterocytes, thus completing a negative feedback regulatory loop. Hepcidin and ferritin are also induced by inflammatory cytokines such as interleukin (IL)-6, complicating the use of those markers as reflections of iron stores, as will be discussed below. Hepcidin is suppressed by erythroferrone, produced by erythroblasts under conditions of

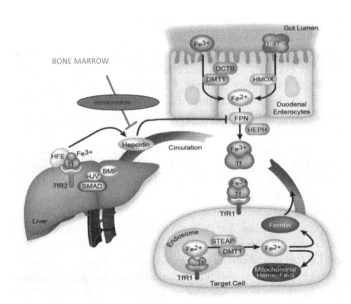

FIGURE 15.1 Iron homeostasis. Iron enters the circulation from gut enterocytes (above right) through the iron channel ferroportin (FPN), where it binds to serum transferrin (Tf). Target cells (lower right) take up the iron through transferrin receptors (TfR) for utilization or storage. Tf-bound iron also interacts with a liver receptor complex to generate the peptide hepcidin that downregulates FPN to complete a negative regulatory loop on iron absorption. (BMP, bone morphogenic protein; DCTB, duodenal cytochrome B; DMT1, divalent metal-ion transporter 1; FE-S, iron sulfur clusters; HEPH, hephaestin; HFE, high iron; HJV, hemojuvelin; HMOX, heme oxygenase; SMAD, *Smalll and Mothers against decapentaplegic* transducers of TGFβ signaling; STEAP, 6-transmembrane epithelial antigen of the prostate.)(From Simcox, J.A. and McClain, D.A., *Cell Metab.*, 17, 329–341, 2013.)

accelerated erythropoiesis such as after blood loss [12], thus facilitating entry of gut iron into the circulation and cycling of iron from macrophages.

An additional level of feedback control exists in the regulation of the mRNAs for many proteins important to iron metabolism. TfR mRNA stability and ferritin mRNA translation, for example, are controlled by iron regulatory proteins (IRPs) that bind these mRNAs in conditions of low iron [13]. In the case of ferritin, translation of its mRNA is blocked by 5′ IRPs, and when there is sufficient iron to bind to the IRPs, they are released and ferritin is produced to sequester excess iron. Conversely, TfR mRNA has IRPs bound to its 3′ end that stabilize it. When iron binds to those IRPs, they are released, destabilizing the message so as to decrease TfR levels and limit further iron entry into cells. This system allows very rapid response to iron fluxes, further emphasizing the importance of tight iron regulation to cell function and health.

A relatively recent discovery in this picture is the recycling of iron from its ferritin-sequestered state. This is accomplished by a specialized form of autophagy, ferritinophagy. Autophagosomes are targeted to ferritin by the protein NCOA4, which is stabilized under conditions of low cytosolic iron [14]. The process thus results in ferritin degradation and release of iron stores when tissue iron levels fall. All of the processes involved in iron trafficking—chaperoning, sequestration by ferritin, ferritinophagy, and incorporation into prosthetic groups—mean that total intracellular iron levels may have very different consequences to cell function, depending on whether the iron is free, safely sequestered in ferritin, or incorporated into heme or iron-sulfur clusters. Thus, understanding the functional intracellular iron status requires knowledge of its flux and compartmentalization [6,15], which can be at least partially inferred from levels of TfR mRNA, NCOA4, ferritin, heme-bound iron, and so on.

15.2.4 Iron Excess and Diabetes

15.2.4.1 Diabetes in Hereditary Hemochromatosis and Other Conditions of Pathologic Iron Overload

It is thought that hemochromatosis mutations arose in response to iron deficiency, but with greater availability of iron in the modern diet, individuals with HH become iron overloaded because of decreased levels of hepcidin and the resulting failure to fully downregulate ferroportin channels in the gut (Figure 15.1). The dangers of excess iron were first manifest in HH, which is associated with diabetes, NASH, and other complications [16]. Originally, HH was termed "bronze diabetes" because of the characteristic discoloration of skin in advanced cases, caused by a combination of jaundice and iron deposition. Thought to be relatively rare, it was determined after identification of the recessive disease mutation in 1996 [17] that, in fact, one of 200 Caucasians were homozygous for the more common C282Y mutation, but with variable disease penetrance.

Although the most common genetic causes of the disease are mutations in the HFE protein that interacts with the TfR2 in the liver to induce hepcidin secretion, hemochromatosis also occurs with mutations in the genes for hepcidin itself (*HAMP*), hemojuvelin (*HFE2*, a coreceptor for bone morphogenic proteins that also induce hepcidin), *TFR2*, and ferroportin (*SLC40A1*), thus validating many of the pathways shown in Figure 15.1. The phenotypes of the latter forms of HH are generally more severe and present earlier in life than *HFE*-associated HH, which generally does not manifest until after the fifth decade and even later in females. The later onset in females is at least partially related to blood and iron loss from parturition and menstruation, although interplay of estrogen with iron metabolism may also play a role. Because of the late onset of its complications and the low penetrance of the full clinical syndrome in *HFE* C282Y homozygotes, the clinical significance of HH has been questioned [18,19]. Two large prospective studies, however, in which severity of disease was assessed by objective criteria including liver biopsy, including in a clinically unselected cohort, revealed the prevalence of at least one disease-related condition was 38% in males and 10% in females [20,21]. In a second study of 203 C282Y homozygotes, iron-overload related disease was found in 28.4% of men and 1.7% of women [22].

The studies above reported a diagnosis of diabetes, but it is known that diabetes is often underdiagnosed. In two recent cross-sectional studies in which subjects received oral glucose tolerance tests (OGTTs), the prevalence of diabetes in HH adults was found to be 13%–23% and impaired glucose tolerance (IGT) 15%–30% [23,24]. The higher prevalence of diabetes and IGT in the second study may be related to their examination of a somewhat older age group (all > 40 years) [24]. Consistent with that, in the former study, younger individuals were overrepresented in the group with normal glucose tolerance. The latter study also included a chart review of over 300 homozygotes ascertained largely by transferrin saturation and, hence, not clinically biased by pre-existing medical diagnoses. Thus, diabetes prevalence is significant in older HH individuals, and it is estimated based on these figures that 1%–2% of Caucasians in a typical T2DM clinic may have HH. Other studies have shown a lower prevalence of diabetes, but they have also included younger subjects and subjects with less pathogenic *HFE* mutations, such as H63D (reviewed in [25]).

Both impaired insulin secretion and insulin resistance have been implicated in the pathophysiology of diabetes in HH. Diminished acute insulin response to glucose and normal insulin sensitivity were observed in patients with HH in the absence of diabetes (though all patients had IGT) and cirrhosis [26]. We also found evidence of impaired insulin secretion without insulin resistance in patients with HH and prediabetes [24]. In fact, a trend toward increased insulin sensitivity was observed in this series, and in a mouse model of HH [27]. Contradicting these findings are those of Hatunic et al., who found increased insulin resistance and no change in measures of insulin secretion in nondiabetic individuals with HH, although that was only assessed with static model indices after OGTT [23].

One possible resolution of these conflicting findings is that our study suggested a two-hit phenomenon, wherein relative insulin deficiency is tolerated because of increased insulin sensitivity in lean HH subjects. When they begin to get overweight, however, that "second hit" induces insulin resistance that cannot be compensated by hyperinsulinemia because of loss of insulin secretory capacity. Thus, depending upon the precise time at which the subject is analyzed, they may be transitioning to an insulin-resistant state based more on caloric intake than iron *per se*. The difference between this situation and that of T2DM is that HH starts with insulin deficiency, and the "second hit" of insulin resistance tips the scale to diabetes, whereas the evolution of T2DM is the opposite—namely, one of insulin resistance with the "second hit" being acquired insulin deficiency as beta-cells lose the capacity to respond adequately to the insulin resistance [28].

The question of why iron decreases insulin secretory capacity has been investigated. Increased iron content of human beta-cells has been observed in iron overload and is toxic to these cells [29]. Mouse models of HH have further contributed to our understanding of the mechanisms underlying diabetes in HH. Hfe$^{-/-}$ mice display increased iron content in the islets of Langerhans, beta-cell apoptosis, and decreased insulin content [27]. Similar to observations in humans reported above [24], these mice have decreased insulin secretory capacity and increased insulin sensitivity. Islet dysfunction is thought to be the result of increased oxidative stress in this model, and iron is known to contribute directly to the generation of free radicals through reaction with hydrogen peroxide. Iron also interferes with trafficking of manganese, which is required for normal activity of manganese-dependent superoxide dismutase [30]. In addition to loss of beta cell mass, however, the mouse model also demonstrates defective coupling of glucose to insulin secretion, perhaps related to mitochondrial dysfunction or other, yet-unknown mechanisms. The mechanism of increased insulin sensitivity is discussed below, in connection with effects of dietary iron on adiponectin.

That iron overload and not some other aspect of HH is responsible for diabetes is supported by two lines of evidence. Firstly, other conditions of iron overload are also associated with diabetes—for example, transfusional iron overload in patients with β-thalassemia. Six percent to 14% of those patients develop diabetes, a number that has decreased with greater implementation of iron chelation therapy [31–33]. A second line of evidence that iron causes diabetes is that the glucose homeostasis abnormalities associated with HH improve with iron reduction, usually accomplished by phlebotomy. Therapeutic phlebotomy remains the mainstay of treatment for HH. Initiation prior to the onset of cirrhosis or diabetes can arrest disease progression. In one study, phlebotomy improved only insulin secretory capacity (Figure 15.2) [34], consistent with the finding that insulin sensitivity may already be high in HH. Hatunic et al. describe similar findings in two studies of patients with HH and abnormal glucose metabolism. Glucose tolerance and insulin secretion, but not insulin sensitivity, assessed either by IVGTT or static measures, improved in most, although improvement was more noticeable in those with prediabetes (IGT) than in those with established diabetes [35]. Hramiak et al. also observed improvement in insulin secretion and glucose tolerance in 14 individuals with hemochromatosis who underwent IVGTT [26]. In participants with IGT, phlebotomy to normalize serum ferritin improved the acute insulin response to glucose by 35% and normalized glucose tolerance. The individuals in this study who had HH complicated by cirrhosis or diabetes did not, however, have an improvement in insulin sensitivity or insulin secretion following phlebotomy. Lastly, following 2 years of routine phlebotomy to achieve a normal serum ferritin and transferrin saturation, Equitani et al. observed a mean increase in insulin secretion of 20% and 33% in HFE carriers with normal glucose tolerance and diabetes, respectively [36]. In sum, all studies suggest a predominant effect of phlebotomy on insulin secretion, although in more advanced disease, damage to beta-cells and insulin secretion may be irreversible.

15.2.4.2   Iron and Typical Type 2 Diabetes Mellitus

15.2.4.2.1   Associations of Type 2 Diabetes Mellitus with Ferritin

Beyond pathologic iron overload, the question has arisen if there is also a relationship between T2DM and tissue iron levels in the broad "normal" range. Epidemiologic evidence demonstrates a clear association between diabetes risk and serum ferritin, a generally reliable biomarker for tissue

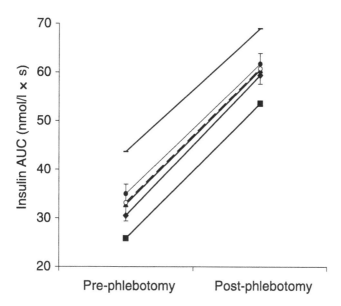

FIGURE 15.2 Improvement in insulin secretion after phlebotomy for HH. Shown are integrated areas under the insulin curves (AUC) after oral glucose tolerance testing. Values for each subject before and after phlebotomy are shown as *solid lines* with *closed symbols*, and the group average as the *dashed line* and *open circles* (±SE). *P* < .0001 for the increase in insulin values. (From Abraham, D. et al., *Diabetologia*, 49, 2546–2551, 2006.)

iron stores. Using Third National Health and Nutrition Examination Survey (NHANES III) data (n = 9,486), Ford et al. found an odds ratio (OR) for newly diagnosed diabetes of 4.94 (CI, 3.05–8.01) for men with a ferritin concentration of 300 ng/mL or higher, compared to those with ferritin concentration below 300, and 3.61 (CI, 2.01–6.48) for women with ferritin concentration of 150 ng/mL of higher, compared to those with ferritin concentration below 150 ng/mL [37].

Similar associations for prediabetes were observed in an analysis of 2,575 participants in the more recent NHANES 1999–2002 data [38]. The upper quartiles of ferritin and lower levels of transferrin saturation were significantly associated with greater odds of prediabetes. Cheung et al. also performed a meta-analysis combining this data with 3,876 participants in NHANES III and found an OR of 1.32 (CI, 1.05–1.66) for each 10 ng/mL increment of ferritin. Using another large database, the Nurses' Health Study cohort, Jiang et al. conducted a prospective nested case-control study examining ferritin in relation to incident cases of type 2 diabetes. With 698 cases and 716 controls, the relative risk of diabetes in the highest quintile of ferritin (≥ 107.2 ng/mL) was 2.61. *Importantly, progressively increasing risk is seen through the entire range of normal ferritin [39].* All of the aforementioned studies observed the positive association of increased ferritin with increased T2DM risk, even after adjustment for obesity, other conventional risk factors for diabetes, and markers of inflammation. One study confirmed ferritin's relation to diabetes, but the association did not hold for transferrin saturation or serum iron, a finding not necessarily surprising given the narrower range of those highly regulated markers, and their higher variability with acute changes in iron intake [40].

The reported ORs for abnormal glucose tolerance as a function of serum ferritin are highly variable in these studies because of differing comparator groups—for example, above or below variable cutoffs at midrange ferritin levels, or highest versus lowest quartile or quintile. However, when ferritin is analyzed as a continuous variable and lowest normal ferritin is compared to highest normal ferritin, the OR of 4–5 approaches the risk of diabetes with obesity [37].

Similar relationships between iron and T2DM risk, insulin resistance, or both are seen in Europeans and African Americans [39,41,42]; several Asian nationalities including Japanese,

Chinese and Koreans [43–45]; gestational DM [46–48]; and prediabetes [49]. The relationship of ferritin with T2DM and gestational DM risk has been confirmed in meta-analyses [50,51]. High ferritin also doubles the risk for MetS, the constellation of impaired glucose tolerance, obesity, hyperlipidemia, and hypertension, after accounting for other risk factors [52].

While high ferritin confers risk for MetS and T2DM, low iron/ferritin is a marker for so-called "healthy obesity"—namely, obesity that does not proceed (or perhaps has not yet proceeded) to MetS and diabetes. In a cohort of individuals with BMI over 40, some with no evidence of MetS other than waist girth, and others that had all elements of MetS (hypertension, glucose intolerance or diabetes, high serum triglycerides, and low high-density lipoprotein [HDL]), we found serum ferritin to be nearly twice as high in the MetS group [53]. Possible mechanistic contributors are the regulation of both adiponectin and leptin by iron discussed below [53,54]. In rodents, it is also possible to maintain healthy obesity simply by decreasing bioavailable iron in adipocytes: Mice on the Ob/Ob background with adipocyte-targeted overexpression of an iron-sulfur cluster binding protein, MitoNEET, *weigh up to 140 g but do not develop diabetes or NAFLD* [55].

15.2.4.2.2   Is Ferritin a Reliable Marker of Tissue Iron?

A key question in the studies above is whether serum ferritin is actually a marker for tissue iron stores in the populations studied. While tissue ferritin is an accepted index of sequestered intracellular iron, serum ferritin is an apoprotein secreted into the circulation, so its relation to tissue iron is less clear. The signal for its rerouting from intracellular iron sequestration to secretion is unknown, although it has been hypothesized to occur in response to falling intracellular iron when synthesis of new ferritin has successfully sequestered iron and further release of ferritin into the cytosol is not needed.

In humans, daily absorption of iron from the diet varies several-fold, and also depends upon bioavailability; heme iron, for example, is absorbed more efficiently than free iron [56]. The recommended daily allowance (RDA) of iron is 8 and 18 mg for adult men and women, and the "tolerable upper intake" is 45 mg, largely based on prevention of extremes of deficiency and excess [57]. Average iron intake has approximately doubled in the United States in the past 20–30 years, a result of improved nutrition but also increased fortification of foods and red meat consumption. All of these variables cause serum ferritin, a reliable indicator of tissue iron stores in the absence of significant systemic inflammation, to have a normal range of approximately 15-fold, much greater than most other serum biomarkers [58].

Because ferritin can also be a marker of systemic inflammation, the relationship of ferritin to diabetes risk was initially attributed to the inflammation associated with diabetes. The magnitude of the contribution of inflammation to ferritin in diabetics is difficult to analyze directly, given the likelihood that there are simultaneous and bidirectional relationships between ferritin and diabetes status. The situation is clearer in obesity, which also has an inflammatory component. Some, but not all, studies have reported an increase in ferritin with obesity (see, e.g., [59]). However, the magnitude of the average increase in ferritin from lean to morbidly obese individuals (approximately 20 ng/mL) is tiny (7%) compared to the normal range in the population (20 to approximately 300 ng/mL). The paper showing the largest difference of ferritin with obesity only reveals a difference when compared to lean individuals (BMI < 25), whereas there is *no change at all* going from the overweight (not obese) group with BMI of 25–30 (average ferritin, 144 ng/mL), to those with BMI of 30–35, 35–40, and more than 40 (ave. ferritin 146 ng/mL) [60]. Thus, the contribution of diabetes and obesity to ferritin in an otherwise healthy individual, ignoring the contribution of excess nutrient intake, is probably small.

More to the point, however, studies have shown that *diabetes risk associated with high ferritin is not accounted for by HH or inflammation but rather by increased dietary intake* [61]. In the analysis, the relation of diabetes and ferritin was corrected for association with markers of systemic inflammation, usually C-reactive protein (CRP). Although there is no disagreement that serum ferritin is not a perfect marker for tissue iron, serum ferritin still correlates well with the number of phlebotomies required to reach a target ferritin in studies reporting the response of diseases like HH to phlebotomy (e.g., in [62], $R^2 = 0.8$; $P < .0001$). Furthermore, in studies of phlebotomy, ferritin falls predictably, though not necessarily monotonically, a result that would not be expected if ferritin were mainly reflecting inflammation.

Studies that measure iron in liver, a primary storage site for total body iron, are a better index of the relation of ferritin to tissue iron. Studies show that hepatic iron is the predominant determinant of serum ferritin levels [63], and in a phlebotomy study, serum ferritin correlated very well with tissue iron as determined by imaging techniques [64]. Finally, biopsy-based studies in NASH reveal that ferritin is an excellent reporter of tissue iron even in the presence of the inflammation accompanying that condition [65].

15.2.4.2.3   Iron Intake and Type 2 Diabetes Mellitus

If ferritin is indeed reporting tissue iron stores that in turn are causing diabetes, there should be a direct correlation of dietary iron intake with ferritin and T2DM. Serum ferritin is associated with increased use of iron supplements and red meat intake in the Framingham Heart Study cohort [61]. Recent studies of gestational diabetes have shown that the increased risk is associated in particular with intake of red meat heme [46], which is more efficiently absorbed than nonheme iron. Those studies suggest that eating as little as 1.5 lbs of red meat per week can raise iron to the levels that are associated with T2DM, while a meta-analysis reports the risk to be 1.38-fold per mg per day of heme iron consumed [50], the equivalent of approximately 1 oz of lean red meat. The relationship of diabetes to taking iron supplements has been less clear and the effects less pronounced, probably related to the low and variable efficiency of gut absorption of elemental iron, which is approximately 5% of that of heme iron.

The studies on heme intake do not rule out the possibility that there is another substance in red meat that is causing diabetes and that iron and ferritin are innocent side effects of the meat ingestion. In rodents, however, it is clear that with all other components of the diet, including total caloric intake, controlled, increased levels of dietary iron are sufficient to cause diabetes, and low levels of iron sufficient to protect from diabetes. This has been shown in wild-type and genetically obese models in mice and rats [66,67]. Importantly, the iron contents of the rodent diets used in these studies lead to tissue iron levels that are good representations of the range resulting from normal human diets, from vegetarians to heavy eaters of red meat. The lower-iron diets, for example, have sufficient iron to maintain normal erythropoiesis, and the higher-iron diets result in levels of hepatic iron well within the fold-increases seen in the upper range of normal humans.

15.2.4.2.4   Improvement of Type 2 Diabetes Mellitus with Iron Reduction Therapy

Surprisingly, despite the extensive data above, clinical trials of iron reduction have been limited. Relatively small studies in humans that demonstrated improvements in fasting glucose, HgbA1c, insulin secretory capacity, and insulin sensitivity after modest phlebotomy to reduce iron from the upper to the lower ranges of normal [53,68,69]. Most of the resistance to such studies has come from the erroneous assumption that ferritin is not a marker of tissue iron, an assumption that flies in the face of considerable data and that can, after all, be relatively easily tested in a simple and safe phlebotomy study.

Demonstrated mechanisms for the beneficial effects of lowering iron in "garden variety" T2DM and MetS include improvements in insulin secretion and insulin sensitivity, the principal determining factors of T2DM. Increased insulin sensitivity is mediated at least in part by adiponectin, which is directly regulated by iron [53].

15.2.4.2.5   Differences between Diabetes in Hereditary Hemochromatosis
and Type 2 Diabetes Mellitus Associated with High Iron

The phenotype of HH-associated diabetes, namely, a primary defect in insulin secretion associated, at least at the stage of prediabetes, with *increased* insulin sensitivity, is distinctly different from the phenotype of typical T2DM that is characterized by insulin resistance and subsequently increased insulin secretion. How might both of these disparate phenotypes be associated with high tissue iron?

One possibility is the differential tissue distribution of iron in the two conditions. In low-hepcidin states like HH, any cell with high expression of ferroportin will have *decreased* cellular iron because ferroportin is not being downregulated, and iron is given free egress from those cells. In addition to gut enterocytes, cells with high ferroportin expression include macrophages, and, as our group discovered, adipocytes [53]. Both cell types are central to the pathogenesis of diabetes: Isolating inflammatory signaling to adipocytes or macrophages is sufficient to cause insulin resistance. Thus, in HH, both cell types would have decreased iron and, from that source, at least, decreased oxidant stress, whereas the opposite would be true in dietary excess, in which high hepcidin will trap that excess iron in those cell types.

In addition to the possible global increase in oxidant stress in those cell types, iron has more specific effects in adipocytes that could explain its association with insulin resistance. One is decreased secretion of the insulin-sensitizing adipokine, adiponectin [53]. In humans, normal-range serum ferritin levels are inversely associated with adiponectin, independent of inflammation assessed by CRP and other cytokines. Ferritin is increased and adiponectin decreased in subjects with type 2 diabetes and in subjects with obesity and diabetes compared to equally obese individuals without MetS. Mice fed a high-iron diet and cultured adipocytes treated with iron exhibited decreased adiponectin mRNA and protein. Iron negatively regulates adiponectin transcription via FOXO1-mediated repression; thus, one of the central transcriptional control points for metabolic processes is affected by iron. Loss of the adipocyte iron export channel, ferroportin, in mice resulted in adipocyte iron loading, decreased adiponectin, and insulin resistance. Conversely, organismal iron overload and increased adipocyte ferroportin expression because of hemochromatosis are associated with decreased adipocyte iron, increased adiponectin, improved glucose tolerance, and increased insulin sensitivity. These findings demonstrate a causal role for iron as a risk factor for MetS and a role for adipocytes in modulating metabolism through adiponectin in response to iron stores.

A potential role of adipose tissue as an iron sensor is suggested by the above findings, that adipocytes use iron levels to determine the levels of secretion of hormones that regulate metabolism in other tissues, such as muscle and liver. This role is consistent with adipose expression of several specialized proteins normally restricted to iron metabolism, such as ferroportin and hepcidin [53]. Further evidence for this role is the regulation by iron of leptin secretion, leptin being another adipokine that regulates central energy and fuel homeostasis [54].

By contrast to cells expressing high levels of ferroportin, cells with little or no ferroportin will accumulate iron when serum iron is high, be that in a low-hepcidin state such as HH or a high-hepcidin state such as dietary iron overload. Beta-cells do not express ferroportin, hence one would expect beta-cell dysfunction in both situations, and that is the case. Why the beta-cell would be especially sensitive to iron is not clear. Iron entry into cells is normally regulated at the level of the transferrin receptor, whose mRNA is downregulated when intracellular iron is high. However, when transferrin has higher levels of saturation, as in HH, there will be levels of free iron in blood that could enter cells through other, less-specific divalent metal transporters. It is reasonable to hypothesize that cells with high levels of such transporters, such as beta-cells that transport high amounts of zinc for condensation of insulin in secretory granules, might be especially vulnerable to high transferrin saturation. This might even explain the relatively increased prominence of beta-cell loss in HH compared to T2DM, due perhaps to the higher levels of Tf saturation in HH compared to dietary excess.

15.2.5 IRON AND DIABETES COMPLICATIONS

15.2.5.1 Iron and Diabetic Vascular Complications

Less is known about the role of iron in typical diabetic complications. Studies are hampered by the fact that, if iron worsens diabetes, the contribution of iron to any complication may be obscured by its contribution to worse diabetes control, which will itself impact the complication. Furthermore, the common diabetic complication of nephropathy is also associated with disturbances in normal iron homeostasis due to anemia, decreased erythropoietin, and possibly other electrolyte changes, such as calcium-phosphate balance. There are some indications of a relationship, however. Vascular endothelial growth factor (VEGF) has been implicated in the microvascular complications of diabetes such as retinopathy, and VEGF levels are positively associated with ferritin [70]. Clearly, more work is needed in this area.

More is known about ferritin and macrovascular disease. While iron is well known to cause dilated cardiomyopathy, a complication of HH and β-thalassemia [71], its potential role in cardiovascular disease has also been recognized [72]. Dietary heme intake is a risk factor for coronary disease in women [73], an association that is also true for stroke risk [70,74], although the potential of other components of red meat to be conferring the risk needs to be acknowledged. Indirectly, the association of iron with MetS also provides a mechanistic link to vascular disease through the risk factors of hypertension and hyperlipidemia [75].

15.2.5.2 Iron and Other Metabolic Complications of Diabetes: Nonalcoholic Fatty Liver Disease

NAFLD, a condition that has been termed the hepatic manifestation of MetS and T2DM, is present in a majority of people with T2DM [76] and is a common reason for liver transplantation. NASH is a complex, multifactorial disease with inputs from many or all cell types in the liver, not to mention other tissues, such as adipose [77,78]. The pathways that lead to NAFLD and NASH are not completely understood. Excess nutrients and disordered lipid homeostasis play important roles, and the contributions of obesity, diabetes and/or insulin resistance, and associated changes in adipokines add risk. Inflammation from multiple sources, including excess or inefficient fat oxidation, cellular damage in adipose and liver tissues, and potentially gut microbiota, also likely play a role. Within hepatocytes, lipotoxicity, endoplasmic reticulum (ER) stress, dysregulated autophagy, transforming growth factor (TGF)-β signaling, mitochondrial dysfunction, and resulting increases in reactive oxygen species (ROS) contribute. The final mediator and *sine qua non* of fibrosis involves activation of hepatic stellate cells (HSCs) [79], with many of the above pathways being involved, both intrinsically in HSC and from paracrine signaling between hepatocytes and other cells.

Just as all obesity does not proceed to T2DM, not all NAFLD proceeds to NASH, and high iron/ferritin is shared as a risk factor for both progressions [80,81]. A link between iron and the progression of NAFLD to NASH has also been noted in genome-wide association studies, wherein increased risk of NASH is seen in individuals with mutations in genes that cause iron overload (thalassemia and HH) [82].

Causality of the relationships among serum ferritin, liver iron, and increased risk of NASH is as germane to this disease as to T2DM. NASH is, by definition, an inflammatory disorder that could increase ferritin by that mechanism and confound the relation of iron to the disease. However, in biopsy-proven NAFLD/NASH, ferritin is more closely related to liver iron than to markers of inflammation [65]. Most importantly, reducing iron by phlebotomy or chelation in humans has been shown to improve NAFLD/NASH [65,83,84]. Other studies are conflicting, and a recent meta-analysis concluded there was no benefit to NASH of iron reduction by phlebotomy [85]. However, at odds with its own conclusion, that same analysis revealed phlebotomy significantly reduces the canonical marker of NASH, serum alanine aminotransferase (ALT). Furthermore, the two most prominent "negative" studies in that analysis were one in which the pretreatment population started with *normal* transaminases (hence, lack of improvement was a foregone conclusion) and the other followed subjects with NASH for only 6 months, a period previously shown in a positive study to be insufficient to demonstrate improvement [86]. Thus, based in part on a seriously flawed analysis, phlebotomy (blood donation), a safe, simple, and promising therapy, has not been widely adopted.

Animal models will no doubt contribute greatly to our understanding of the relation of iron to NAFLD/NASH. Our laboratory has demonstrated, (McClain and Salaye, unpublished data, 2018), that a diet low in iron, but not so low as to result in iron deficiency (i.e., sufficient to maintain

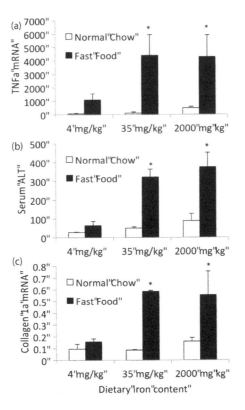

FIGURE 15.3 Effects of low-iron diet to prevent NASH in a mouse model. (a) Liver tumor necrosis factor (TNF)-α mRNA, (b) serum alanine aminotransferase (ALT), and (c) liver collagen 1α mRNA in mice fed the indicated levels of iron (mg/kg or ppm) in either normal chow (open bars) or a "fast food" (black bars) diet for 4 months. *$P < .05$ compared to 4 ppm by analysis of variance (ANOVA).

normal blood hemoglobin), protects from NASH induced by a "fast food" diet (40% fat with fructose supplementation of water, [87]). The low-iron diet protects from induction of the inflammatory response (Figure 15.3a), steatohepatitis (Figure 15.3b), and induction of fibrotic genes (Figure 15.3c). The intermediate (35 mg/kg) diet provided protection in terms of a delay in the rise of ALT, with normal levels seen at 12 weeks on diet (not shown). Protection occurs despite the high-fat diet's not having a significant effect on iron stores, and without the differing levels of dietary iron having an effect on hepatic steatosis (not shown). Thus, as was the case for diabetes, animal models prove a causal role for iron, and pathogenicity of "normal" range iron, in NASH progression

15.2.6 OTHER DISEASES ASSOCIATED WITH HIGH IRON

The detrimental effects of the higher range of "normal" iron levels on glucose homeostasis take on extra importance because of iron's association with a number of other diseases, including NASH [80], Parkinson's and Alzheimer's diseases [88], colon/breast cancer [89], and cardiovascular disease [74]. While this chapter cannot fully address all of these conditions, it is worth pointing out that most also share aging, excess nutrient intake, and even diabetes as risk factors, suggesting common ground for their pathogenesis, with oxidative stress being one reasonable candidate mechanism.

15.2.7   MECHANISMS UNDERLYING THE REGULATION OF FUEL UTILIZATION AND ENERGY HOMEOSTASIS BY IRON

The regulation of metabolism by iron is a rapidly expanding field, and this review will not attempt to explore all of the mechanisms for those connections. Some have been reviewed [2] and will be briefly mentioned here to illustrate how iron sensing and iron levels are integrated into most of the fundamental mechanisms of metabolic regulation. These do not include the simple "toxic" effects of iron in generating free radicals by Fenton chemistry.

- The regulation of leptin and adiponectin, two adipokines that act on multiple tissues to control fuel and energy homeostasis, has been described above [53,54]. Of note, the effect of iron on the transcriptional regulation of these hormones operates through transcription factors that are central to metabolic regulation in multiple tissues and multiple pathways, forkhead box O1 (FoxO1) and cyclic adenosine monophosphate (AMP) response element binding protein (CREB).
- Iron affects the hypoxia-sensing pathway, a pathway that is largely responsible for the protean changes in metabolism observed in cancer [90]. This occurs through the iron-dependent hydroxylases that are responsible for stabilizing and activating the hypoxia inducible factor (HIF) transcription factors. HIF and iron interact, for example, to regulate hepatic gluconeogenesis, an important pathogenic factor in the hyperglycemia of T2DM [91].
- Iron affects the circadian rhythm, and night shift work is a known diabetes risk factor. We showed that high dietary iron exerts this effect through affecting heme synthesis. Stimulated by one of the master transcriptional regulators of metabolism, peroxisome proliferator-activated receptor gamma coactivator 1-alpha (PGC-1α), heme is limiting in nonerythroid cells for activation of several heme-binding proteins, including the metabolic transcriptional repressor RevErbα, a component of the central mechanism that controls the circadian rhythm.
- Iron regulates glucose homeostasis in liver and muscle via AMP-activated protein kinase in mice [92].
- Similar to iron's regulation of the diauxic shift in yeast [8], iron also controls fuel choice in mammals, causing a shift to fatty acid oxidation from glucose metabolism through regulation of pyruvate dehydrogenase kinase [93].
- High iron induces mitochondrial dysfunction [30].

These few examples illustrate iron's impingement on the most central pathways of metabolic regulation and suggest that other effects of iron on glucose and fat metabolism are yet to be uncovered.

15.3   ZINC

Zinc, not strictly a transition metal but often included in that category, has potential ties to diabetes on several fronts. It is a necessary cofactor for thousands of proteins that serve every function imaginable, from catalysis to structure to regulation. Its importance is underlined by the existence of over 30 zinc transporters. Of particular interest to the diabetes field are the roles it plays in antioxidant defenses (e.g., superoxide dismutase [SOD]-1, also known as Cu/Zn SOD, and in normal islet physiology.

The best known function of zinc in insulin secretion is its necessity for the coordination of insulin into the crystalline hexamer that allows efficient packaging in secretory granules. The importance of this process is revealed in the association of mutations in the zinc transporter that transports zinc into the secretory granule (SLC30A8, or ZnT8) with risk for T2DM [94]. SLC30A8 is also an autoantigen in T1DM [95]. Loss of the transporter in mice results in defective insulin packaging and secretion [96] and is associated with impaired conversion of proinsulin to insulin in humans [97]. Several subsequent studies have confirmed insulin secretory defects in these individuals.

There is no system for zinc storage in higher eukaryotes. The RDA ranges from 2 to 11 mg per day in infants to adults, with a tolerable upper limit of intake approximately 2–3 times that. A substantial fraction of older adults in the NHANES had marginal or inadequate zinc intake [98], and a substantial fraction of people with both T1 and T2DM may be zinc deficient [99]. As a result, there have been a number of studies of the effects of zinc supplementation on insulin secretion and diabetes status, both in the general population and in those with SLC30A8 mutations.

A meta-analysis of several studies of zinc supplementation supports a modest benefit to fasting glucose and HgbA1c in individuals with T2DM [100]. In a relatively homogeneous population (old-order Amish), zinc was supplemented at a dose of 50 mg twice daily to approximately 50 individuals each, with homozygotes for the R325W SLC30A8 risk allele (arginine/arginine) compared to arginine/tryptophan and tryptophan/tryptophan [101]. Modest increases in insulin secretion and processing were observed in the anticipated *nonrisk* RW and WW genotypes. Nineteen percent of those taking the zinc reported nausea. Another prospective study showed a positive association of dietary zinc intake with T2DM risk, but a lowered risk in supplement takers [102]. These associations were independent of SLC30A8 genotype, although interactions of genotype with obesity and zinc-to-iron ratios were noted. This study emphasizes the many interacting variables that may dictate response to zinc: insulin demand dictated by obesity and insulin resistance; genotype for zinc transporter polymorphisms; background dietary intake, and the degree to which those levels may also reflect other dietary practices; and interactions with other divalent metals, such as iron, that can share and compete for the many transporters that shepherd the metals among tissues and within cells [30,103].

15.4 MANGANESE

Given the important role of oxidative metabolism in glucose-stimulated insulin secretion, a role of manganese in diabetes risk has been postulated based upon a possible connection between its levels and activity of SOD2 (MnSOD), which serves an antioxidant protective function in mitochondria [104]. There is no RDA for manganese, only reported "adequate intake" levels, and also, given its potential to cause neurotoxicity at higher levels, a recommended upper limit for intake.

Studies of mitochondrial function and insulin secretion in mouse models of HH have revealed important interactions between iron and manganese. Specifically, in iron-overloaded beta-cells in the HH model, it was found that manganese and zinc were present in lower-than-normal levels in the mitochondria, despite normal cytosolic levels [30,103]. This resulted in undermetallation of MnSOD, decreased MnSOD activity, and mitochondrial oxidant stress that was reversible with manganese supplementation. Wild-type mice, on normal rodent chow, also showed less-than-full metallation of MnSOD, whose activity could be increased with manganese supplementation. Thus, there is evidence that biological systems are not necessarily optimized with regard to levels of trace metals such as manganese, and further, that the levels of transition metals may be interrelated and interactive.

Epidemiologic studies support a relation between diabetes and manganese. In China, for example, T2DM rates are lowest in mid-quartile ranges of manganese [105,106]. Unlike the case for zinc, however, trials of manganese supplementation have not been reported, at least in part because of the potential for causing neurotoxicity.

15.5 COPPER, CHROMIUM, AND OTHER METALS

As pointed out in the introduction to this chapter, the levels of several trace metals in serum have been positively and negatively correlated with diabetes risk or prevalence. Few of them have been pursued as avidly as iron or zinc, however. Clinical investigations are hampered by the lack of appropriate and specific tools to manipulate their levels, and in some cases by the risk of toxicity with over supplementation. Hints of importance of a wide variety of metals to diabetes and diabetic complications, however, come from studies of broad-spectrum chelators that reduce the risk of cardiovascular disease in people with diabetes down to levels seen in nondiabetics [107].

A meta-analysis has supported the existence of elevated levels of copper in those with diabetes [108]. Similar to the case for iron, a potentially causal role is suggested by the association of diabetes risk with dietary copper intake [109]. The case for copper in diabetes is also supported by its interaction with iron metabolism. For example, the most common copper-containing protein in serum is the ferroxidase ceruloplasmin. Improvements in insulin resistance and glycemia have been observed with copper chelation [110], and copper chelators have been proposed for human use [111]. Thus, the status of the role of copper in diabetes is reminiscent of that of iron, though it has not been studied as thoroughly.

Studies of chromium were prompted by several reports of an inverse association between chromium levels and diabetes. Its potential actions in augmenting insulin action have been the subject of excellent review [112]. Although some meta-analyses have concluded that chromium supplementation improves glycemia and other markers of MetS [113], other reviews have questioned that conclusion, and the results of studies are not consistent [114].

15.6   IRON AND OTHER TRANSITION METALS IN METABOLIC DISEASE: SUMMARY

We have attempted to show in this chapter that levels of at least some metal ions in cells and tissues, particularly iron, have large and biologically significant effects on metabolic regulation. A key point is that these effects occur not only in pathologic overload, but also across the entire range of levels seen in normal populations. An important corollary to that observation is that there may exist within the broad range of "normal" levels, much narrower "optimal" ranges, if a normal level is even defined for the metal. Those optima may also be dependent on other environmental variables, such as dietary composition, genetic factors, and disease comorbidities. Given the potential ease of manipulating some of these metals' levels, particularly iron and zinc, it seems reasonable to suggest from the data that have been amassed that clinical trials are justified in T2DM and NASH. Attention needs to be given in such trials to stratification for other risk factors, such as age, gender, obesity, and genetic makeup, and to controlling the levels of other metals with which the target may interact.

REFERENCES

1. Li XT, Yu PF, Gao Y, Guo WH, Wang J, Liu X, Gu AH, Ji GX, Dong Q, Wang BS, et al. Association between plasma metal levels and diabetes risk: A case-control study in China. *Biomed Environ Sci.* 2017;30(7):482–91.
2. Simcox JA, and McClain DA. Iron and diabetes risk. *Cell Metab.* 2013;17(3):329–41.
3. Fernandez-Real JM, McClain D, and Manco M. Mechanisms linking glucose homeostasis and iron metabolism toward the onset and progression of type 2 diabetes. *Diabetes Care.* 2015;38(11):2169–76.
4. Barton JC, and Acton RT. Diabetes in HFE hemochromatosis. *J Diabetes Res.* 2017;2017:9826930.
5. Denic S, and Agarwal MM. Nutritional iron deficiency: An evolutionary perspective. *Nutrition.* 2007;23(7–8):603–14.
6. Philpott CC, Ryu MS, Frey A, and Patel S. Cytosolic iron chaperones: Proteins delivering iron cofactors in the cytosol of mammalian cells. *J Biol Chem.* 2017;292(31):12764–71.
7. Barber MF, and Elde NC. Buried treasure: Evolutionary perspectives on microbial iron piracy. *Trends Genet.* 2015;31(11):627–36.
8. Haurie V, Boucherie H, and Sagliocco F. The Snf1 protein kinase controls the induction of genes of the iron uptake pathway at the diauxic shift in *Saccharomyces cerevisiae. J Biol Chem.* 2003;278(46):45391–6.
9. Muckenthaler MU, Rivella S, Hentze MW, and Galy B. A red carpet for iron metabolism. *Cell.* 2017;168(3):344–61.
10. Coffey R, and Ganz T. Iron homeostasis: An anthropocentric perspective. *J Biol Chem.* 2017;292(31):12727–34.

11. Chifman J, Laubenbacher R, and Torti SV. A systems biology approach to iron metabolism. *Adv Exp Med Biol.* 2014;844:201–25.

12. Kautz L, Jung G, Valore EV, Rivella S, Nemeth E, and Ganz T. Identification of erythroferrone as an erythroid regulator of iron metabolism. *Nat Genet.* 2014;46(7):678–84.

13. Muckenthaler MU, Galy B, and Hentze MW. Systemic iron homeostasis and the iron-responsive element/iron-regulatory protein (IRE/IRP) regulatory network. *Annu Rev Nutr.* 2008;28:197–213.

14. Mancias JD, Wang X, Gygi SP, Harper JW, and Kimmelman AC. Quantitative proteomics identifies NCOA4 as the cargo receptor mediating ferritinophagy. *Nature.* 2014;509(7498):105–9.

15. Pantopoulos K, Porwal SK, Tartakoff A, and Devireddy L. Mechanisms of mammalian iron homeostasis. *Biochemistry.* 2012;51(29):5705–24.

16. Buysschaert M, Paris I, Selvais P, and Hermans MP. Clinical aspects of diabetes secondary to idiopathic haemochromatosis in French-speaking Belgium. *Diabetes Metab.* 1997;23(4):308–13.

17. Feder JN, Gnirke A, Thomas W, Tsuchihashi Z, Ruddy DA, Basava A, Dormishian F, Domingo R, Jr., Ellis MC, Fullan A, et al. A novel MHC class I-like gene is mutated in patients with hereditary haemochromatosis. *Nat Genet.* 1996;13(4):399–408.

18. Beutler E, Felitti V, Gelbart T, and Ho N. The effect of HFE genotypes on measurements of iron overload in patients attending a health appraisal clinic. *Ann Intern Med.* 2000;133(5):329–37.

19. Beutler E, Felitti V, Ho NJ, and Gelbart T. Relationship of body iron stores to levels of serum ferritin, serum iron, unsaturated iron binding capacity and transferrin saturation in patients with iron storage disease. *Acta Haematol.* 2002;107(3):145–9.

20. Bulaj ZJ, Ajioka RS, Phillips JD, LaSalle BA, Jorde LB, Griffen LM, Edwards CQ, and Kushner JP. Disease-related conditions in relatives of patients with hemochromatosis. *N Engl J Med.* 2000;343(21):1529–35.

21. Bulaj ZJ, Griffen LM, Jorde LB, Edwards CQ, and Kushner JP. Clinical and biochemical abnormalities in people heterozygous for hemochromatosis. *N Engl J Med.* 1996;335(24):1799–805.

22. Allen KJ, Gurrin LC, Constantine CC, Osborne NJ, Delatycki MB, Nicoll AJ, McLaren CE, Bahlo M, Nisselle AE, Vulpe CD, et al. Iron-overload-related disease in HFE hereditary hemochromatosis. *N Engl J Med.* 2008;358(3):221–30.

23. Hatunic M, Finucane FM, Brennan AM, Norris S, Pacini G, and Nolan JJ. Effect of iron overload on glucose metabolism in patients with hereditary hemochromatosis. *Metabolism.* 2010;59(3):380–4.

24. McClain D, Abraham D, Rogers J, Brady R, Gault P, Ajioka R, and Kushner J. High prevalence of abnormal glucose homeostasis secondary to decreased insulin secretion in individuals with hereditary haemochromatosis. *Diabetologia.* 2006;49(7):1661–9.

25. Creighton Mitchell T, and McClain DA. Diabetes and hemochromatosis. *Curr Diab Rep.* 2014;14(5):488.

26. Hramiak IM, Finegood DT, and Adams PC. Factors affecting glucose tolerance in hereditary hemochromatosis. *Clin Invest Med.* 1997;20(2):110–8.

27. Cooksey RC, Jouihan HA, Ajioka RS, Hazel MW, Jones DL, Kushner JP, and McClain DA. Oxidative stress, beta-cell apoptosis, and decreased insulin secretory capacity in mouse models of hemochromatosis. *Endocrinology.* 2004;145(11):5305–12.

28. Weyer C, Bogardus C, Mott DM, and Pratley RE. The natural history of insulin secretory dysfunction and insulin resistance in the pathogenesis of type 2 diabetes mellitus. *J Clin Invest.* 1999;104(6):787–94.

29. Kishimoto M, Endo H, Hagiwara S, Miwa A, and Noda M. Immunohistochemical findings in the pancreatic islets of a patient with transfusional iron overload and diabetes: Case report. *J Med Invest.* 2010;57(3–4):345–9.

30. Jouihan HA CP, Cooksey RC, Hoagland EA, Boudina S, Abel ED, Winge DR, McClain DA. Iron-mediated inhibition of mitochondrial manganese uptake mediates mitochondrial dysfunction in a mouse model of hemochromatosis. *Mol Med.* 2008;14(3–4):98–108.

31. Borgna-Pignatti C, Rugolotto S, De Stefano P, Piga A, Di Gregorio F, Gamberini MR, Sabato V, Melevendi C, Cappellini MD, and Verlato G. Survival and disease complications in thalassemia major. *Ann N Y Acad Sci.* 1998;850:227–31.

32. Borgna-Pignatti C, Rugolotto S, De Stefano P, Zhao H, Cappellini MD, Del Vecchio GC, Romeo MA, Forni GL, Gamberini MR, Ghilardi R, et al. Survival and complications in patients with thalassemia major treated with transfusion and deferoxamine. *Haematologica.* 2004;89(10):1187–93.

33. Gamberini MR, De Sanctis V, and Gilli G. Hypogonadism, diabetes mellitus, hypothyroidism, hypoparathyroidism: Incidence and prevalence related to iron overload and chelation therapy in patients with thalassaemia major followed from 1980 to 2007 in the Ferrara Centre. *Pediatr Endocrinol Rev.* 2008;6 Suppl 1:158–69.

34. Abraham D, Rogers J, Gault P, Kushner J, and McClain D. Increased insulin secretory capacity but decreased insulin sensitivity after correction of iron overload by phlebotomy in hereditary haemochromatosis. *Diabetologia*. 2006;49(11):2546–51.

35. Hatunic M, Finucane FM, Norris S, Pacini G, and Nolan JJ. Glucose metabolism after normalization of markers of iron overload by venesection in subjects with hereditary hemochromatosis. *Metabolism*. 2010;59(12):1811–5.

36. Equitani F, Fernandez-Real JM, Menichella G, Koch M, Calvani M, Nobili V, Mingrone G, and Manco M. Bloodletting ameliorates insulin sensitivity and secretion in parallel to reducing liver iron in carriers of HFE gene mutations. *Diabetes Care*. 2008;31(1):3–8.

37. Ford ES, and Cogswell ME. Diabetes and serum ferritin concentration among U.S. adults. *Diabetes Care*. 1999;22(12):1978–83.

38. Cheung CL, Cheung TT, Lam KS, and Cheung BM. High ferritin and low transferrin saturation are associated with pre-diabetes among a national representative sample of U.S. adults. *Clin Nutr*. 2013;32(6):1055–60.

39. Jiang R, Manson JE, Meigs JB, Ma J, Rifai N, and Hu FB. Body iron stores in relation to risk of type 2 diabetes in apparently healthy women. *JAMA*. 2004;291(6):711–7.

40. Yeap BB, Divitini ML, Gunton JE, Olynyk JK, Beilby JP, McQuillan B, Hung J, and Knuiman MW. Higher ferritin levels, but not serum iron or transferrin saturation, are associated with Type 2 diabetes mellitus in adult men and women free of genetic haemochromatosis. *Clin Endocrinol (Oxf)*. 2015;82(4):525–32.

41. Aregbesola A, Voutilainen S, Virtanen JK, Mursu J, and Tuomainen TP. Body iron stores and the risk of type 2 diabetes in middle-aged men. *Eur J Endocrinol*. 2013;169(2):247–53.

42. Wilson JG, Lindquist JH, Grambow SC, Crook ED, and Maher JF. Potential role of increased iron stores in diabetes. *Am J Med Sci*. 2003;325(6):332–9.

43. Gao S, Zhao D, Qi Y, Wang M, Zhao F, Sun J, and Liu J. The association between serum ferritin levels and the risk of new-onset type 2 diabetes mellitus: A 10-year follow-up of the Chinese Multi-Provincial Cohort Study. *Diabetes Res Clin Pract*. 2017;130:154–62.

44. Akter S, Nanri A, Kuwahara K, Matsushita Y, Nakagawa T, Konishi M, Honda T, Yamamoto S, Hayashi T, Noda M, et al. Circulating ferritin concentrations and risk of type 2 diabetes in Japanese individuals. *J Diabetes Investig*. 2017;8(4):462–70.

45. Kim S, Park SK, Ryoo JH, Choi JM, Hong HP, Park JH, Suh YJ, and Byoun YS. Incidental risk for diabetes according to serum ferritin concentration in Korean men. *Clin Chim Acta*. 2015;451(Pt B):165–9.

46. Afkhami-Ardekani M, and Rashidi M. Iron status in women with and without gestational diabetes mellitus. *J Diabetes Complications*. 2009;23(3):194–8.

47. Qiu C, Zhang C, Gelaye B, Enquobahrie DA, Frederick IO, and Williams MA. Gestational diabetes mellitus in relation to maternal dietary heme iron and nonheme iron intake. *Diabetes Care*. 2011;34(7):1564–9.

48. Bowers K, Yeung E, Williams MA, Qi L, Tobias DK, Hu FB, and Zhang C. A prospective study of prepregnancy dietary iron intake and risk for gestational diabetes mellitus. *Diabetes Care*. 2011;34(7):1557–63.

49. Sharifi F, Nasab NM, and Zadeh HJ. Elevated serum ferritin concentrations in prediabetic subjects. *Diab Vasc Dis Res*. 2008;5(1):15–8.

50. Zhao L, Lian J, Tian J, Shen Y, Ping Z, Fang X, Min J, and Wang F. Dietary intake of heme iron and body iron status are associated with the risk of gestational diabetes mellitus: A systematic review and meta-analysis. *Asia Pac J Clin Nutr*. 2017;26(6):1092–106.

51. Kunutsor SK, Apekey TA, Walley J, and Kain K. Ferritin levels and risk of type 2 diabetes mellitus: An updated systematic review and meta-analysis of prospective evidence. *Diabetes Metab Res Rev*. 2013;29(4):308–18.

52. Jehn M, Clark JM, and Guallar E. Serum ferritin and risk of the metabolic syndrome in U.S. adults. *Diabetes Care*. 2004;27(10):2422–8.

53. Gabrielsen JS, Gao Y, Simcox JA, Huang J, Thorup D, Jones D, Cooksey RC, Gabrielsen D, Adams TD, Hunt SC, et al. Adipocyte iron regulates adiponectin and insulin sensitivity. *J Clin Invest*. 2012;122(10):3529–40.

54. Gao Y, Li Z, Gabrielsen JS, Simcox JA, Lee SH, Jones D, Cooksey B, Stoddard G, Cefalu WT, and McClain DA. Adipocyte iron regulates leptin and food intake. *J Clin Invest*. 2015;125(9):3681–91.

55. Kusminski CM, Holland WL, Sun K, Park J, Spurgin SB, Lin Y, Askew GR, Simcox JA, McClain DA, Li C, et al. MitoNEET-driven alterations in adipocyte mitochondrial activity reveal a crucial adaptive process that preserves insulin sensitivity in obesity. *Nat Med*. 2012;18(10):1539–49.

56. Hulten L, Gramatkovski E, Gleerup A, and Hallberg L. Iron absorption from the whole diet. Relation to meal composition, iron requirements and iron stores. *Eur J Clin Nutr.* 1995;49(11):794–808.

57. Schumann K, Borch-Iohnsen B, Hentze MW, and Marx JJ. Tolerable upper intakes for dietary iron set by the US Food and Nutrition Board. *Am J Clin Nutr.* 2002;76(3):499–500.

58. Koziol JA, Ho NJ, Felitti VJ, and Beutler E. Reference centiles for serum ferritin and percentage of transferrin saturation, with application to mutations of the HFE gene. *Clin Chem.* 2001;47(10):1804–10.

59. Cheng HL, Bryant C, Cook R, O'Connor H, Rooney K, and Steinbeck K. The relationship between obesity and hypoferraemia in adults: A systematic review. *Obes Rev.* 2012;13(2):150–61.

60. Ausk KJ, and Ioannou GN. Is obesity associated with anemia of chronic disease? A population-based study. *Obesity (Silver Spring).* 2008;16(10):2356–61.

61. Fleming DJ, Tucker KL, Jacques PF, Dallal GE, Wilson PW, and Wood RJ. Dietary factors associated with the risk of high iron stores in the elderly Framingham Heart Study cohort. *Am J Clin Nutr.* 2002;76(6):1375–84.

62. Panch SR, Yau YY, West K, Diggs K, Sweigart T, and Leitman SF. Initial serum ferritin predicts number of therapeutic phlebotomies to iron depletion in secondary iron overload. *Transfusion.* 2015;55(3):611–22.

63. Ryan JD, Armitage AE, Cobbold JF, Banerjee R, Borsani O, Dongiovanni P, Neubauer S, Morovat R, Wang LM, Pasricha SR, et al. Hepatic iron is the major determinant of serum ferritin in NAFLD patients. *Liver Int.* 2017;38(1):164–173.

64. Valenti L, Fracanzani AL, Dongiovanni P, Bugianesi E, Marchesini G, Manzini P, Vanni E, and Fargion S. Iron depletion by phlebotomy improves insulin resistance in patients with nonalcoholic fatty liver disease and hyperferritinemia: Evidence from a case-control study. *Am J Gastroenterol.* 2007;102(6):1251–8.

65. Beaton MD, Chakrabarti S, and Adams PC. Inflammation is not the cause of an elevated serum ferritin in non-alcoholic fatty liver disease. *Ann Hepatol.* 2014;13(3):353–6.

66. Minamiyama Y, Takemura S, Kodai S, Shinkawa H, Tsukioka T, Ichikawa H, Naito Y, Yoshikawa T, and Okada S. Iron restriction improves type 2 diabetes mellitus in Otsuka Long-Evans Tokushima fatty rats. *Am J Physiol Endocrinol Metab.* 2010;298(6):E1140–9.

67. Cooksey RC, Jones D, Gabrielsen S, Huang J, Simcox JA, Luo B, Soesanto Y, Rienhoff H, Abel ED, and McClain DA. Dietary iron restriction or iron chelation protects from diabetes and loss of beta-cell function in the obese (ob/ob lep-/-) mouse. *Am J Physiol Endocrinol Metab.* 2010;298(6):E1236–43.

68. Houschyar KS, Ludtke R, Dobos GJ, Kalus U, Brocker-Preuss M, Rampp T, Brinkhaus B, and Michalsen A. Effects of phlebotomy-induced reduction of body iron stores on metabolic syndrome: Results from a randomized clinical trial. *BMC Med.* 2012;10(1):54.

69. Fernandez-Real JM, Penarroja G, Castro A, Garcia-Bragado F, Hernandez-Aguado I, and Ricart W. Blood letting in high-ferritin type 2 diabetes: Effects on insulin sensitivity and beta-cell function. *Diabetes.* 2002;51(4):1000–4.

70. Feskens EJ, Sluik D, and van Woudenbergh GJ. Meat consumption, diabetes, and its complications. *Curr Diab Rep.* 2013;13(2):298–306.

71. Horwitz LD, and Rosenthal EA. Iron-mediated cardiovascular injury. *Vasc Med.* 1999;4(2):93–9.

72. Pisano G, Lombardi R, and Fracanzani AL. Vascular damage in patients with nonalcoholic fatty liver disease: Possible role of iron and ferritin. *Int J Mol Sci.* 2016;17(5):pii:E675.

73. Qi L, van Dam RM, Rexrode K, and Hu FB. Heme iron from diet as a risk factor for coronary heart disease in women with type 2 diabetes. *Diabetes Care.* 2007;30(1):101–6.

74. Zhang W, Iso H, Ohira T, Date OC, Tanabe N, Kikuchi S, and Tamakoshi A. Associations of dietary iron intake with mortality from cardiovascular disease: The JACC study. *J Epidemiol.* 2012;22(6):484–93.

75. Mojiminiyi OA, Marouf R, and Abdella NA. Body iron stores in relation to the metabolic syndrome, glycemic control and complications in female patients with type 2 diabetes. *Nutr Metab Cardiovasc Dis.* 2008;18(8):559–66.

76. Dai W, Ye L, Liu A, Wen SW, Deng J, Wu X, and Lai Z. Prevalence of nonalcoholic fatty liver disease in patients with type 2 diabetes mellitus: A meta-analysis. *Medicine (Baltimore).* 2017;96(39):e8179.

77. Ganz M, and Szabo G. Immune and inflammatory pathways in NASH. *Hepatol Int.* 2013;7 Suppl 2:771–81.

78. Takaki A, Kawai D, and Yamamoto K. Molecular mechanisms and new treatment strategies for non-alcoholic steatohepatitis (NASH). *Int J Mol Sci.* 2014;15(5):7352–79.

79. Tsuchida T, and Friedman SL. Mechanisms of hepatic stellate cell activation. *Nat Rev Gastroenterol Hepatol.* 2017;14(7):397–411.

80. Fargion S, Mattioli M, Fracanzani AL, Sampietro M, Tavazzi D, Fociani P, Taioli E, Valenti L, and Fiorelli G. Hyperferritinemia, iron overload, and multiple metabolic alterations identify patients at risk for nonalcoholic steatohepatitis. *Am J Gastroenterol.* 2001;96(8):2448–55.

81. Kowdley KV, Belt P, Wilson LA, Yeh MM, Neuschwander-Tetri BA, Chalasani N, Sanyal AJ, Nelson JE, and Network NCR. Serum ferritin is an independent predictor of histologic severity and advanced fibrosis in patients with nonalcoholic fatty liver disease. *Hepatology.* 2012;55(1):77–85.

82. Valenti L, Fracanzani AL, Bugianesi E, Dongiovanni P, Galmozzi E, Vanni E, Canavesi E, Lattuada E, Roviaro G, Marchesini G, et al. HFE genotype, parenchymal iron accumulation, and liver fibrosis in patients with nonalcoholic fatty liver disease. *Gastroenterology.* 2010;138(3):905–12.

83. Valenti L, Fracanzani AL, Dongiovanni P, Rovida S, Rametta R, Fatta E, Pulixi EA, Maggioni M, and Fargion S. A randomized trial of iron depletion in patients with nonalcoholic fatty liver disease and hyperferritinemia. *World J Gastroenterol.* 2014;20(11):3002–10.

84. Dongiovanni P, Fracanzani AL, Fargion S, and Valenti L. Iron in fatty liver and in the metabolic syndrome: A promising therapeutic target. *J Hepatol.* 2011;55(4):920–32.

85. Murali AR, Gupta A, and Brown K. Systematic review and meta-analysis to determine the impact of iron depletion in dysmetabolic iron overload syndrome and non-alcoholic fatty liver disease. *Hepatol Res.* 2017.

86. Adams LA, Crawford DH, Stuart K, House MJ, St Pierre TG, Webb M, Ching HL, Kava J, Bynevelt M, MacQuillan GC, et al. The impact of phlebotomy in nonalcoholic fatty liver disease: A prospective, randomized, controlled trial. *Hepatology.* 2015;61(5):1555–64.

87. Charlton M, Krishnan A, Viker K, Sanderson S, Cazanave S, McConico A, Masuoko H, and Gores G. Fast food diet mouse: Novel small animal model of NASH with ballooning, progressive fibrosis, and high physiological fidelity to the human condition. *Am J Physiol Gastrointest Liver Physiol.* 2011;301(5):G825–34.

88. Altamura S, and Muckenthaler MU. Iron toxicity in diseases of aging: Alzheimer's disease, Parkinson's disease and atherosclerosis. *J Alzheimers Dis.* 2009;16(4):879–95.

89. Toyokuni S. Role of iron in carcinogenesis: Cancer as a ferrotoxic disease. *Cancer Sci.* 2009;100(1):9–16.

90. Majmundar AJ, Wong WJ, and Simon MC. Hypoxia-inducible factors and the response to hypoxic stress. *Mol Cell.* 2010;40(2):294–309.

91. Nam H, Jones D, Cooksey RC, Gao Y, Sink S, Cox J, and McClain DA. Synergistic inhibitory effects of hypoxia and iron deficiency on hepatic glucose response in mouse liver. *Diabetes.* 2016;65(6):1521–33.

92. Huang J, Simcox J, Mitchell TC, Jones D, Cox J, Luo B, Cooksey RC, Boros LG, and McClain DA. Iron regulates glucose homeostasis in liver and muscle via AMP-activated protein kinase in mice. *FASEB J.* 2013;27(7):2845–54.

93. Huang J, Jones D, Luo B, Sanderson M, Soto J, Abel ED, Cooksey RC, and McClain DA. Iron overload and diabetes risk: A shift from glucose to fatty acid oxidation and increased hepatic glucose production in a mouse model of hereditary hemochromatosis. *Diabetes.* 2011;60(1):80–7.

94. Sladek R, Rocheleau G, Rung J, Dina C, Shen L, Serre D, Boutin P, Vincent D, Belisle A, Hadjadj S, et al. A genome-wide association study identifies novel risk loci for type 2 diabetes. *Nature.* 2007;445(7130):881–5.

95. Wenzlau JM, Juhl K, Yu L, Moua O, Sarkar SA, Gottlieb P, Rewers M, Eisenbarth GS, Jensen J, Davidson HW, et al. The cation efflux transporter ZnT8 (Slc30A8) is a major autoantigen in human type 1 diabetes. *Proc Natl Acad Sci U S A.* 2007;104(43):17040–5.

96. Nicolson TJ, Bellomo EA, Wijesekara N, Loder MK, Baldwin JM, Gyulkhandanyan AV, Koshkin V, Tarasov AI, Carzaniga R, Kronenberger K, et al. Insulin storage and glucose homeostasis in mice null for the granule zinc transporter ZnT8 and studies of the type 2 diabetes-associated variants. *Diabetes.* 2009;58(9):2070–83.

97. Kirchhoff K, Machicao F, Haupt A, Schafer SA, Tschritter O, Staiger H, Stefan N, Haring HU, and Fritsche A. Polymorphisms in the TCF7L2, CDKAL1 and SLC30A8 genes are associated with impaired proinsulin conversion. *Diabetologia.* 2008;51(4):597–601.

98. Ervin RB, and Kennedy-Stephenson J. Mineral intakes of elderly adult supplement and non-supplement users in the third national health and nutrition examination survey. *J Nutr.* 2002;132(11):3422–7.

99. Jansen J, Rosenkranz E, Overbeck S, Warmuth S, Mocchegiani E, Giacconi R, Weiskirchen R, Karges W, and Rink L. Disturbed zinc homeostasis in diabetic patients by in vitro and in vivo analysis of insulinomimetic activity of zinc. *J Nutr Biochem.* 2012;23(11):1458–66.

100. Capdor J, Foster M, Petocz P, and Samman S. Zinc and glycemic control: A meta-analysis of randomised placebo controlled supplementation trials in humans. *J Trace Elem Med Biol.* 2013;27(2):137–42.

101. Maruthur NM, Clark JM, Fu M, Linda Kao WH, and Shuldiner AR. Effect of zinc supplementation on insulin secretion: Interaction between zinc and SLC30A8 genotype in Old Order Amish. *Diabetologia.* 2015;58(2):295–303.

102. Drake I, Hindy G, Ericson U, and Orho-Melander M. A prospective study of dietary and supplemental zinc intake and risk of type 2 diabetes depending on genetic variation in SLC30A8. *Genes Nutr.* 2017;12:30.

103. Lee SH, Jouihan HA, Cooksey RC, Jones D, Kim HJ, Winge DR, and McClain DA. Manganese supplementation protects against diet-induced diabetes in wild type mice by enhancing insulin secretion. *Endocrinology.* 2013;154(3):1029–38.

104. Madsen-Bouterse SA, Zhong Q, Mohammad G, Ho YS, and Kowluru RA. Oxidative damage of mitochondrial DNA in diabetes and its protection by manganese superoxide dismutase. *Free Radic Res.* 2010;44(3):313–21.

105. Wang X, Zhang M, Lui G, Chang H, Zhang M, Liu W, Li Z, Liu Y, and Huang G. Associations of serum manganese levels with prediabetes and diabetes among >/=60-year-old Chinese adults: A population-based cross-sectional analysis. *Nutrients.* 2016;8(8).

106. Shan Z, Chen S, Sun T, Luo C, Guo Y, Yu X, Yang W, Hu FB, and Liu L. U-shaped association between plasma manganese levels and type 2 diabetes. *Environ Health Perspect.* 2016;124(12):1876–81.

107. Lamas GA, Goertz C, Boineau R, Mark DB, Rozema T, Nahin RL, Lindblad L, Lewis EF, Drisko J, Lee KL, et al. Effect of disodium EDTA chelation regimen on cardiovascular events in patients with previous myocardial infarction: The TACT randomized trial. *JAMA.* 2013;309(12):1241–50.

108. Qiu Q, Zhang F, Zhu W, Wu J, and Liang M. Copper in diabetes mellitus: A meta-analysis and systematic review of plasma and serum studies. *Biol Trace Elem Res.* 2017;177(1):53–63.

109. Eshak ES, Iso H, Maruyama K, Muraki I, and Tamakoshi A. Associations between dietary intakes of iron, copper and zinc with risk of type 2 diabetes mellitus: A large population-based prospective cohort study. *Clin Nutr.* 2017.

110. Tanaka A, Kaneto H, Miyatsuka T, Yamamoto K, Yoshiuchi K, Yamasaki Y, Shimomura I, Matsuoka TA, and Matsuhisa M. Role of copper ion in the pathogenesis of type 2 diabetes. *Endocr J.* 2009;56(5):699–706.

111. Cooper GJ. Selective divalent copper chelation for the treatment of diabetes mellitus. *Curr Med Chem.* 2012;19(17):2828–60.

112. Cefalu WT, and Hu FB. Role of chromium in human health and in diabetes. *Diabetes Care.* 2004;27(11):2741–51.

113. Huang H, Chen G, Dong Y, Zhu Y, and Chen H. Chromium supplementation for adjuvant treatment of type 2 diabetes mellitus: Results from a pooled analysis. *Mol Nutr Food Res.* 2017.

114. Costello RB, Dwyer JT, and Bailey RL. Chromium supplements for glycemic control in type 2 diabetes: Limited evidence of effectiveness. *Nutr Rev.* 2016;74(7):455–68.

16 The Role of Gut Microbiota in the Pathogenesis and Treatment of Diabetes

Stephen J. Walker and Shaun P. Deveshwar

CONTENTS

16.1 INTRODUCTION

16.1.1 MICROBIOTA: THE IMPORTANCE OF GUT BACTERIA

The microbiota is comprised of an assortment of microorganisms (bacteria, fungi, and viruses) found throughout the body. The *microbiome*, sometimes called the second genome, refers to the genetic component of the human microbiota. For simplicity, the terms *microbiota* and *microbiome* will be used interchangeably in this chapter, and the primary focus will be on the bacterial component found within the gastrointestinal (GI) microbiome and its relationship to the development and pathogenesis of diabetes mellitus.

There are roughly 10 times more microbial cells than host cells within the human body. The gut microbiome is host specific, evolves throughout an individual's lifetime, and is susceptible to both exogenous (e.g., antibiotic use) and endogenous (e.g., systemic disease) factors. Gut bacteria have an important relationship, whether symbiotic or pathogenic, to the host and play a vital role in an individual's GI and systemic health [1]. *Firmicutes*, *Bacteriodetes*, *Actinobacteria*, and *Proteobacteria* comprise the four major bacterial phyla in the human gut [2]. When there is a disruption in the microbiota homeostasis, caused by either an excess or depletion of specific bacterial species, systemic complications and disease may follow. One important condition that has been shown to be associated with an out-of-balance microbiome is diabetes mellitus (DM). The two variations of diabetes mellitus, type 1 (DM-1) and type 2 (DM-2), while differing in their respective etiologies and disease manifestations, have both been linked to alterations in gut microbiota.

16.1.2 DIABETES MELLITUS TYPES 1 AND 2

DM-1 and DM-2 can be most easily differentiated clinically by the patient's age at first presentation. DM-1, formerly known as *juvenile diabetes*, is typically diagnosed in individuals during childhood or young adulthood and can be best understood as an autoimmune disease. Host immune cells destroy beta islet (insulin-secreting) cells in the pancreas, at which point patients can become hyperglycemic and may experience polyuria, polydipsia, weight loss, and mood swings [3].

In contrast, the onset of DM-2 can occur at any age, although it is found to occur more commonly in adults with a high body mass index (BMI). Confounding the ability to diagnose DM-2 is the fact that patients may be asymptomatic at first. While there are certain established risk factors for the development of diabetes, practicing a healthy lifestyle can prevent the onset of DM-2. Once diagnosed with DM-1 or DM-2, it is important for patients to monitor glucose and insulin levels.

Although individuals with either DM-1 or DM-2 will both experience insulin dependence, the prognoses for patients with DM-1 and DM-2 are quite different. Individuals diagnosed with DM-1 must continue to take insulin for the duration of their lifetime, as the pancreatic beta islet cells no longer produce insulin. Patients with DM-2 have a more varied prognosis. Through dietary modifications and lifestyle changes such as exercise and weight loss, these individuals can experience a decrease in insulin dependency and in many cases return to normal pancreatic insulin functioning without insulin resistance.

16.2 MICROBIOTA AND DIABETES

16.2.1 PATHOGENESIS

Individuals with DM-1 have malfunctioning pancreatic beta islet cells, which are unable to secrete insulin into the bloodstream to facilitate storage of excess sugar as glycogen [4,5]. However, pancreatic alpha cells are still able to secrete the antagonist hormone to insulin, glucagon, into the bloodstream and therefore deplete the body of its stored glycogen through glycogenolysis. Individuals with untreated DM-1 will experience severe weight loss and ketoacidosis. Moreover, the body feels the need to urinate more frequently, resulting in the excretion of important nutrients due to the increased glucose concentration in the bloodstream.

The pathogenesis of DM-2 involves a cumulative development of insulin resistance, as opposed to the autoimmune destruction of pancreatic beta islet cells seen in DM-1 [6]. Insulin resistance occurs when these receptors no longer respond to insulin and ignore its message to absorb glucose. Individuals with higher BMIs tend to consume foods rich in carbohydrates and starches. These foods are then broken down into glucose and enter the bloodstream to be used by organs in the body for fuel. However, glucose must be transported from the bloodstream and into the cells of various organs with the aid of insulin. Insulin released from the pancreas enters the bloodstream, where it enables glucose in the blood to be transported into cells via the insulin membrane receptors.

Any imbalance of microbiome homeostasis in the gut (i.e., gut dysbiosis) can be detrimental, and gut dysbiosis has been shown to be associated with the pathogenesis of both DM-1 and DM-2. Much of the research on the influence of the microbiome in DM-1 susceptibility involves investigations into genetic predisposition and autoimmunity. In contrast, in the case of DM-2, metabolic endotoxemia, nonalcoholic fatty acid liver disease (NAFLD), and obesity have been shown to alter the gut microbiome, and each can result in the development of DM-2. Understanding how the accumulation of excess toxins and unhealthy lipopolysaccharides disrupt the normal gut microbiome is critical to understanding how diseases such as NAFLD inhibit normal GI functioning and are risk factors in the development of diabetes.

The human body stores fat in adipose tissue, which contains triglycerides. A triglyceride is composed of a glycerol backbone and three fatty acid chains. Triglycerides travel throughout the bloodstream to any fat-storing tissue in the body, and move into the cytoplasm of the target cells. They then travel into the matrix of the mitochondria, where they become oxidized. Through seven rounds of this cycle in the mitochondrial matrix, the end products are eight acetyl CoA, seven NADH, and seven FADH2 molecules, all of which will be fed into the tricarboxylic acid (TCA) cycle and electron transport chain for the production of ATP.

The TCA cycle becomes disrupted by the accumulation of excess triglycerides within the bloodstream, and, instead of breaking down the fats, the body begins to store fats. Triacylglycerides consumed in our diet are processed into chylomicrons, which then enter the bloodstream, where they can enter capillaries and travel through the lymphatic system. Fats can also be released from adipose tissue cells throughout the body into the circulatory system as well. Several hours after the consumption of food, insulin levels begin to drop, glucagon levels rise, and hydrophobic free fatty acids are pulled into the bloodstream and into the liver.

The liver plays a vital role in the filtration of toxins out of the body but also plays an equally critical role in the regulation of the gut microbiome. The liver has the enzymes alanine aminotransferase (ALT) and aspartate aminotransferase (AST) that package fatty acids into cholesterol, and what will eventually become very low-density lipoproteins (VLDLs). An elevated VLDL level is a precursor of cardiovascular disease and can be an indication of excess and unhealthy fat in one's diet. A buildup of excessive fats in the liver can be attributed to a disruption of the gut microbiome and the development of DM-2 and obesity through gut dysbiosis.

NAFLD has also been associated with metabolic syndrome, liver failure, insulin resistance, obesity, DM-2, and hepatocellular carcinoma [7]. A study conducted in 2010 showed that, out of 70 participants with DM-2, 30% also had NAFLD. DM-2 can manifest identically to alcoholic fatty liver disease, with the only difference being the source of toxins being consumed by an individual [7]. The potential development of DM-2 stems from dietary choices made by the individuals, which can lead to insulin resistance. It is believed that insulin resistance occurs over time, when insulin receptors throughout the body, and particularly in the liver, become less responsive to insulin. This then causes the liver to increase fatty acid synthesis and storage and decrease beta-oxidation. This can lead to systemic steatosis. Steatosis is a process in which there is a decrease in secretion of lipoproteins and an increase in synthesis and storage of fat from the bloodstream. Insulin resistance is a strong indicator of prediabetes and is best defined as a state where muscles, fat cells, and liver cells do not adequately respond to insulin and therefore cannot absorb glucose from the bloodstream into muscle and liver cells. As a result, the body begins to produce more VLDL cholesterol, triglycerides, and fatty acids. The increase of lipogenesis contributes to the disruption of the gut microbiome. However, it is not simply a nutrient-poor diet that contributes to gut dysbiosis and eventually DM-2, stemming from fatty liver disease. Gut dysbiosis also has a direct effect on the development of NAFLD, obesity, and DM-2 [8].

It has been shown that a high-fat diet increases the number of lipopolysaccharides (LPS) in the body and, as a result, affects the metabolism and percent body fat. The consumption of excess LPS and bacterial lipopeptides is strongly associated with metabolic endotoxemia. Metabolic endotoxemia is a state in which there is an elevation in the normal amounts of endotoxins present in the gut epithelium. This is a strong contributing factor to diabetes, obesity, and NAFLD [9]. Inflammatory cytokines and macrophages begin to infiltrate the gut epithelium, which leads to an influx of immune cells in the GI tract.

Generally speaking, individuals with a higher BMI, higher lipopolysaccharides, and higher body fat percentage have a higher *Firmicutes*-to-*Bacteriodetes* ratio in the gut. As people begin to lose weight, this ratio begins to normalize to a more equal distribution [10]. This has caused researchers to look more closely to the *Firmicutes* bacteria, because thousands of *Lactobacilli* are within this family, and *Lactobacilli* are a significant portion of the microbiota found in the digestive, urinary, and reproductive systems. A study by Kasai et al. investigating the distribution of gut microbiota in nonobese and obese individuals found that the percentage of *Firmicutes* was 49.53% in nonobese individuals compared to 48.74% in obese individuals, whereas the percentage of *Bacteriodetes* was found to be 35.44% in nonobese individuals and 23.28% in obese individuals ($P < .05$) [11]. This would suggest that a presence of higher levels of *Bacteriodietes* in the body is an indicator of a healthier gut microbiome and plays a potential role in the preventing the development of obesity, insulin resistance, and ultimately diabetes.

16.2.2 RISK FACTORS

Changes in the composition of the human microbiome can have a dramatic impact on human health and disease. Because of this, there has been significant effort put forth to better understand specifically how this occurs. In the context of diabetes, there are known risk factors for developing DM-1 and DM-2 that are directly associated with the gut microbiome. Several of these risk factors and the supporting research studies in which they were identified are discussed next.

The predominant effector mechanism (although not necessarily the cause) of DM-1 is autoimmunity; therefore, numerous studies investigating the etiology of DM-1 have focused specifically on the immune system function in the gut. The GI tract contains Paneth cells, which secrete antimicrobial peptides in response to foreign pathogens. These proteins disrupt the luminal microbiology, which, in turn, can affect the gut microbiome. Recently there has been interest in the association of the gram-negative bacteria *B. dorei* with normal intestinal function in DM-1, as studies have shown significant differences in *B. dorei* levels in individuals with and without DM-1. These observations have led researchers to hypothesize that elevated levels of *B. dorei* could be a risk factor for the onset of DM-1.

To test this hypothesis, a Finnish research team conducted a study to evaluate the levels of *B. dorei* in infants, specifically investigating the idea that the amount of *B. dorei* in the gut at a very early age may be predictive (i.e., a risk factor) for the development of DM-1 [12]. Stool samples were obtained from 76 high-risk infants and, using high-throughput 16sRNA sequencing, the composition of the microbiome was determined. The stool microbiome composition was evaluated every 4–6 months until the infants reached 2.2 years of age. Of the total 76 infants enrolled in the study, 29 seroconverted to DM-1 related immunity, and 22 of those 29 would go on to develop DM-1. The remaining 47 individuals did not go on to develop DM-1 or DM-1 autoimmune–related illnesses. The 22 children who developed DM-1 cases had significantly elevated levels of *B. dorei* and *B. vulgatus*. Compared to controls, cases showed an increased level of *B. dorei* at every point of study. A sliding window analysis showed that *B. dorei* levels were significantly higher in cases prior to seroconversion at around 7.6 months of age ($P < .05$). These levels remained higher than control infant levels for the remainder of the 2-year window of study. The authors concluded that the relative amount of *B. dorei* early in development may represent an early risk factor for the development of DM-1.

To further explore the relationship between the gut microbiome and genetic risk factors for DM-1, researchers at the University of Queensland studied nonobese diabetic (NOD) mice and also humans from the UK twin cohort study [13]. Previous research had shown that NOD mice harbor a distinct gut microbiota profile that renders them susceptible to the development of DM-1 [14,15]. Manipulation of the microbiome of NOD mice by antibiotic exposure or dietary change revealed that these NOD mice harbored a diabetes-permissive microbiota, and fluctuations in the microbiota could cause a shift, either up or down, in the rate of DM-1.

Previous studies have also highlighted the importance of specific genetic loci associated with autoimmune disease susceptibility in humans that were also shown to influence the gut environment, although these findings were not applied directly to assess DM-1 risk. There have, however, been genome association studies in DM-1 that show a correlation between DM-1 and adaptive and innate immune pathways. While human studies investigating autoimmune diseases (e.g., Crohn's disease) have revealed specific genetic loci associated with disease susceptibility that influenced the gut environment, no human study had been performed specifically to evaluate an association between the gut environment and DM-1. Genetic studies in humans have shown that human leukocyte antigen (HLA)–DQ and HLA-DRB1, the major histocompatibility complex II (MHC II), and the interleukin (IL)-2 pathways have all been linked to genes that could influence the microbiome. Regulatory T cells (Treg), which line the gut, communicate with the IL-2 signaling pathway and are strongly linked to disease pathogenesis in mice.

The Queensland research team designed a study to evaluate the impact of gut inflammation on the gut microbiome in NOD mice and then examined whether results from NOD mice (i.e., these same genetic effects) were present in humans from the UK twins study [13]. NOD mice were found to have a common microbiome independent of their animal facility. In order to show that the mice microbiome was predominantly genetically determined, fecal samples from DM-1–susceptible NOD inbred mice and C57BL/B6 (B6) mice were used to evaluate the microbiome by 16s-RNA gene sequencing. A distinctly different microbiome composition was seen in these two types of mice; a PERMANOVA test showed high levels of *Lactobacillus* in NOD mice, whereas *Allobacterium* was predominant in B6 mice. This showed that the composition of the gut microbiome has a genetically determined component [13].

After showing that genetic determination played a significant role in the gut microbiome of NOD mice, researchers began to manipulate the IL-2 inflammatory pathway. It was found that in these mice, alleles at the *Idd3* locus lead to a deficiency in IL-2 production, which ultimately led to defects in T-reg functioning. To determine whether this could be reversed, NOD mice were treated with IL-2 therapy. IL-2c was administered in mice 4–10 weeks old, and it was found that low-dose treatments of IL-2 led to Treg expansion. The IL-2c treatment was shown to have an effect on the gut microbiome as well. There were significant reductions in *Bacteroidales* and *Oscillospira*, a nonsignificant decrease in *Rikenellacea, Turicbacter,* and *Muscipirillum,* and an increase in *Bifidobacterium*. This suggested a mechanism by which IL-2 expansion could regulate immune system function within the GI tract (i.e., by controlling inflammation and thereby being able to influence the gut microbiome in a positive manner, thus preventing the potential development of DM-1 in NOD mice) [13].

Based on the results of the NOD mice study, the *Idd3* and *IddI5* alleles were studied to see how manipulation of the IL-2 pathway might impact DM-1 susceptibility in humans. This was done using human samples from a cohort twin study, conducted in the United Kingdom, which recruited 1,392 individuals. The twin study previously looked at the stool microbiome and single nucleotide polymorphism (SNP) genotyping of all enrolled subjects. Using these data from the twin study, this research team looked for associations between SNPs and IL-2 pathway interactions and Treg functioning. They calculated a combined risk score, and the analysis suggested a DM-1 susceptibility allele within the IL-2 pathway that could be associated with a decrease in the microbial species of *Clostridiales, Bacteroides, Lachnospiaceae, Ruminoccaceae,* and *Rikenellaceae* [13].

The mice and human studies described here illustrate that variations at the *Idd3* and *Idd5* loci were associated with decreased amounts of *Ruminococus, Lachnospiraceae,* and *Clostridiales* in the gut microbiome and with a higher risk of developing DM-1. Manipulation of the IL-2 pathway could be used therapeutically to increase the amount of Treg cells in the body, which could promote a healthier gut microbiome, thereby decreasing the risk of developing DM-1. Fluctuations in levels of *Ruminococus, Lachnospiraceae,* and *Clostridiales* in the human gut microbiome could be seen as potential genetic risk factors for the future development of DM-1 and show how the microbiome has an impact on the future manifestation of DM-1.

There is an even larger body of research regarding microbiome-related risk factors for the development of DM-2. Much of the evidence in these studies reveal a significant positive correlation between the consumption of foods high in fat, calories, and sugars and the later development of DM-2 in individuals with an elevated BMI. As one begins to consume calorically dense foods rich in sugars and fats, adipose tissue begins to accumulate in the body. One result can be the disruption of the existing *symbionts* (i.e., "healthy gut" bacteria) that line the GI tract in healthy individuals. Symbionts are found in foods consumed in a healthy diet. These foods aid and promote a healthy and balanced gut microbiome.

On the other hand, foods that promote adipose tissue development increase levels of *pathobionts*, or unhealthy gut bacteria. When this happens, inflammatory cytokines such as MyD88 and NF-kB, together with macrophages, begin to infiltrate the GI tract. The immune system is unable to distinguish between pathobionts and healthy gut bacterial species, such as *B. dorei*, and therefore, beneficial bacteria may be eliminated from the GI tract. As this process continues, it can promote the influx of even more inflammatory cytokines, increasing the likelihood of developing gut permeability, endotoxemia, and the infiltration of harmful gut bacteria, such as *B. spp*, *B. phyla*, and *Clostridium difficile* into the GI tract. This ultimately results in gut dysbiosis; gut dysbiosis increases the likelihood of insulin resistance, which can ultimately lead to the development of DM-2 [16].

Another risk factor for the development of diabetes mellitus is premature antibiotic exposure to infants and young children. In a recent study, the microbiota in infants was studied to determine whether exposure to antibiotics, either during pregnancy or early in infancy and childhood, had an effect on the future development of obesity or diabetes. Infants exposed to antibiotics during pregnancy showed twice the risk of developing obesity during childhood. Exposure to antibiotics during infancy and early childhood was also correlated with an increased risk for developing a serious GI disease, such as Crohn's disease or ulcerative colitis, or another systemic health illness, such as diabetes and/or obesity [17]. Although there is a combination of other genetic and environmental risk factors that contribute to an infant's overall future health, the quality of the gut microbiome and nutritional status of the mother are two critical components that can predict future GI health, including risk for developing diabetes.

16.3 TREATMENT OF DIABETES MELLITUS THROUGH MANIPULATION OF THE GUT MICROBIOME

16.3.1 SYNBIOTIC EFFECTS ON THE GUT MICROBIOME

16.3.1.1 Prebiotic and Probiotic Effects on Gastrointestinal and Systemic Health

Probiotics are bacterial supplements administered orally to restore healthy bacterial function within the GI system. These are typically most effective if administered in the form of live cultures. The bacteria act on receptors that actively communicate with both the immune and nervous systems. Probiotics can also be derived from dietary foods that are rich in healthy bacteria (Table 16.1 lists common dietary probiotics). *Prebiotics* are complex sugars containing an oligo-fructose backbone. These are found only in plant-based dietary sources and are used to provide fuel for the bacteria in the GI tract (Table 16.1).

Prebiotics and probiotics are useful in manipulating the gut microbiome, and extensive research has provided evidence for the health benefits in individuals with inflammatory illnesses. Abundant prebiotics and probiotics in the diet can improve the health of the immune system, decrease the chances of developing leaky gut syndrome, improve bone density, and even help with weight loss. They can also be taken simultaneously or individually to target the gut microbiome of a patient suffering from a GI ailment, diabetes, or obesity. Probiotics act to replenish the healthy gut bacteria in the presence of unhealthy gut bacteria, whereas prebiotics are used to promote and enrich the health of the existing beneficial gut microbiota.

16.3.1.2 Synbiotic Treatment for Diabetes Mellitus

One way to combat an unhealthy gut microbiota and poor health is through diet and supplementation, or synbiotics. *Synbiotics* refers to the combination of using both probiotics and prebiotics to treat individuals with ailments of the GI tract and flora by bringing the bacteria present in the gut back to a

TABLE 16.1

Common Dietary Sources of Prebiotics and Probiotics

Common Probiotic-Rich Foods	Common Prebiotic-Rich Foods
Yogurt	Raw chicory root
Kefir	Raw Jerusalem artichoke
Cheeses	Raw dandelion greens
Any naturally fermented food	Raw garlic
	Raw leeks
	Raw/cooked onion
	Raw asparagus
	Baked wheat flour
	Raw banana

Source: Jackson, F.W., Foods containing prebiotics, *Prebiotin Prebiotic*, https://www.prebiotin.com/foods-containing-prebiotics/, 2015.

healthy balance. Studies have shown that probiotics are most efficacious in treating GI diseases such as irritable bowel syndrome, colitis, gas bloating, abdominal pain, and chronic constipation.

Many probiotics are commonly used in treating DM-2 and obese patients, including *L. rhaminosis, L. lantarum, L. gasser, and L. fermentum*. *L. rhaminosis* is a standard probotic ingested by most individuals and *L. rhaminosis* plus inulin, a prebiotic fiber designed to provide nutrients to already present healthy gut microbiota, is typically given to people who take synbiotic supplements for imbalances in their GI health [18].

Results from human studies have demonstrated the benefits of synbiotics on GI health, obesity, and DM-2, and weight loss in children. Prebiotics have been found to lower fasting and postprandial glucose levels, as well as to increase glucose sensitivity and improve lipid profiles. Probiotics have been shown to provide a significant benefit in DM-2 patients through weight loss via consumption of fermented milk and dairy products. Prebiotics have also been shown to stimulate the production of glucagon-like peptide 1 (GLP-1), a hormone used to regulate metabolism. One prebiotic in particular, inulin, has been studied and is a popular way to aid a nutrient supply to healthy gut microbiota. Inulin is a type of fiber found in plants, consisting of chains of fructose molecules. The nutrients from inulin are broken down into short fatty acid chains, which nourish the gut microbiota. A randomized, controlled study was conducted in which 46 participants with metabolic syndrome were given either a placebo or probiotic supplement capsule consisting of 1.2×10^{10} colony-forming cells, together with an inulin fiber prebiotic. Participants were instructed to take this probiotic capsule twice a day for 12 weeks. At 12 weeks, those participants in the experimental group had a lower blood pressure and greater weight loss compared to controls. The placebo group also experienced weight loss, but only during the first 6 weeks of the study [19].

A similar study consisting of 60 participants examined the effects of synbiotics on DM-2 patients who were overweight but not clinically obese. All study participants were also diagnosed with cardiovascular disease and were given an amount of synbiotics equaling 2×10^9 colony-forming units (CFUs) per day for 12 weeks. After 12 weeks, all individuals in the experimental group showed a significant decrease in weight, an increase in insulin sensitivity, an increase in high-density lipoprotein (HDL), and a decrease in fasting blood glucose and serum insulin levels. The differences in the benefits of synbiotics on the men and women in this study were also evaluated independently. Obese and prediabetic men and women were studied for 24 weeks while on a dosage of probiotics at 1×10^9 CFU per day. After 24 weeks, women experienced significantly more weight loss than men, suggesting that a combination of synbiotics may provide more weight loss benefit to women than men [20].

Metformin, a drug commonly used to control blood glucose levels in individuals with DM-2, was tested in mice to study its effectiveness as a potential prebiotic. Control mice were fed a standard diet for 6 weeks, whereas experimental mice were given a high-fat diet for the same period of time. The high-fat diet group was also given metformin for the 6 weeks and were found to have a higher abundance of *Akkermansia*, a mucin-degrading bacterium, along with improved glucose tolerance compared to the control group [21]. This demonstrated the ability of metformin to alter the composition of the gut microbiota in these mice. The researchers concluded that metformin mimics the role of a prebiotic, which may explain its effectiveness in treating individuals with DM-2 (i.e., by altering the microbiome).

16.3.2 Nutrition and Lifestyle

16.3.2.1 Dietary Modifications

Balancing of gut microbiota is accomplished and maintained largely through the foods we consume. Research studies have consistently shown that the ratio of *Bacteriodiotes* to *Firmicutes* bacterium is related to the risk for development of diabetes and obesity during one's lifetime. Table 16.2 provides a list of the top bacterial species (by abundance) found in those (both male and female) with a low versus high BMI.

Many prebiotics and probiotics can be derived from foods that we eat. These foods can exert both positive and negative effects on gut microbiota. For example, individuals with diabetes are instructed to stay away from foods that have a high glycemic index, meaning anything that is high in sugar or lipopolysaccharides, as these foods can cause a spike in blood sugar levels. Unfortunately, much of the food consumed in the Western world has little, if any, beneficial components for the gut microbiota. For individuals with diabetes or gut microbial illness, it is important to regulate the types of carbohydrates consumed in their daily diet. Traditionally, individuals with diabetes have been advised to refrain from consuming lots of carbohydrates. However, based on the research in mice that showed metformin's prebiotic effects, researchers have investigated whether manipulating the types of foods in one's diet may be equally effective. In one study, patients with diabetes or GI ailments were instructed to go on a high–complex carbohydrate diet that consisted of 40–60 g of fiber consumed daily. In addition, they were also given many servings of legumes, fruits, vegetables, and whole grains. The results showed that these individuals were equally effective at controlling and managing their blood sugar as individuals who were micromanaging and restricting the amount of carbohydrates in their diet. These findings suggest that foods such as the legumes played a prebiotic role in establishing a healthier gut microbiome. Table 16.1 provides examples of common dietary prebiotic and probiotic-rich foods.

TABLE 16.2

Top Gut Bacterial Microbiota Found in High- and Low-Body Mass Index Individuals

Low Body Fat	High Body Fat
Bacteroidetes	*Firmicutes*
Bacteroides	*Enterobacteriaecae*
Lactobacillus plantarum	*Staphylococcus aureus*
Bifidobacterium animalis	*Lactobacillus reuteri*

Source: Million, M. et al., *Clin. Microbiol. Infect.*, 19, 305–313, 2013.

16.3.2.2   Bariatric Surgery for Diabetic and Obese Patients

Surgical treatments have been used to treat patients with diabetes and obesity. Malabsorptive bariatric surgery is a surgical procedure that is used to reverse the effects of DM-2 and obesity in patients and includes removing portions of the stomach or creating an alternate route for food to travel and be digested in the GI tract. The Roux-en-Y gastric bypass (RYGB), vertical banded gastroplasty (VBG), and laparoscopic adjustable gastric banding procedure (LAGP) have all been found to induce long-term changes in the gut microbiome [22–24].

When these procedures were first used to treat diabetic and obese patients, it was anticipated that there would eventually be long-term alterations in the gut microbiome. What was observed, however, was that within just a few days post procedure, long before their bodies could adjust to the procedure (and prior to them losing a substantial amount of weight), some of patients with diabetes no longer needed insulin and medication to manage their diabetes.

To further explore this concept, one research study collected stool samples from adult women and gave them to mice. Afterward, the change in weight and in gut microbial composition of these mice was assessed. Three groups of women were selected for the study. In the first, the women were diabetic and obese. The second group was comprised of women who were clinically obese and diabetic but had undergone the RYGP and lost weight since the procedure. The third group of women had undergone the VBG and had lost weight post procedure as well. The fecal samples of these women were given to germ-free mice to eat, and the BMI and behavioral changes were noted. Mice who had consumed the stool from the first group became obese and had a decreased number of *Bacteriodetes* present in their gut microbiota. The mice who had consumed stool from the women who had undergone either the RYGP or VGP procedures did not experience any weight gain and showed no decrease in the number of *Bacteriodetes* in their gut microbiota [22].

The effects of bariatric (malabsorptive) surgery have also been studied in patients with DM-2. Results have shown significant effects of the RYGP bypass in diabetic patients with a BMI of at least 35 kg/m^2. In a case series study involving 330 patients, there was an observed decrease in mean fasting blood glucose levels. In 89% of the patients, blood glucose levels dropped to within normal range ($\approx$117 mg/dL), and glycolated hemoglobin levels were also within normal range at 6.6%, without the use of any diabetic medications. Patients who had undergone the procedure achieved a better control of their diabetes and also experienced a mean weight loss of 97 lbs [23].

Additional studies have also found beneficial effects of RYGP and LAGB procedures related to glycemic control, weight loss, and post-treatment diabetic risk in patients who had the surgery. The gastric bypass procedure showed an average of 16.1% in weight loss post procedure, whereas control subjects experienced a slight weight gain. The risk of developing diabetes was found to be three times lower in surgically treated patients in comparison to the controls. The LAGB method, in particular, resulted in significantly larger reductions in fasting blood glucose and glycolated hemoglobin levels [25].

To investigate the impact of gastric surgery on the gut microbiome, a research team in Japan recently conducted a study wherein they evaluated two alternative forms of bariatric surgery. In this study, 44 obese individuals were treated for metabolic disorders with one of the three following procedures: the duodenojejunal bypass (DJB; an alternative to the RYGP), the laparoscopic sleeve gastrectomy (LSG), or the LAGB. A total of 22 patients underwent the LSG procedure, 18 underwent the DJB, and four underwent the LAGB to treat their obesity. Patients' stool samples were collected just prior to having the procedure and then 6 months post operation to study the effects of the procedure on the gut microbiota. It was found that the LSG and DJB procedures significantly improved metabolic disorders in these obese patients and that the proportion of *Bacteroidetes* and *Lactobacillales* increased significantly in the DJB group. While the two types of bariatric surgeries had differing effects on the gut microbiota, both the DJB and LSG procedures were shown to improve DM-2 and obesity [25].

16.4   CONCLUSIONS

It is evident from the recent literature that the gut microbiota has a significant impact on the pathogenesis and development of DM-1 and DM-2. Human and murine studies have shown that variations in gut microbiota composition can be indicative of genetic risk factors for the development of DM-1 or DM-2. The NOD mice studies demonstrate that a manipulation in the *Idd3* and *Idd5* loci along the IL-2 pathway can increase or decrease rates of DM-1 by impacting the gut microbiome, while elevated levels of *B. dorei* can also be a risk factor for the future development of DM-1. Individuals with DM-2 should be educated about lifestyle and dietary modifications that may be beneficial. The importance of a balanced diet with added natural probiotics and prebiotics has been shown to promote a healthy ratio of *Firmicutes* to *Bacteriodetes*, which has been associated with a lower BMI and overall improved health. Surgical RYGP, VGP, and LAGP gastric bypass procedures have also been shown to provide significant improvement for DM-2 and obese individuals and also facilitate restoration of the gut microbiota to a healthy balanced state.

REFERENCES

1. Guianane C and Cotter PD, Role of the gut microbiota in health and chronic gastrointestinal disease: Understanding a hidden metabolic organ, *Therap Adv Gastroenterol.*, 6, 295, 2013.
2. Khanna S and Tosh PK, A clinician's primer on the role of the microbiome in human health and disease, *Mayo Clin Proc.*, 89, 107, 2014.
3. Yi B, Huang G, and Zhou Z, Different role of zinc transporter 8 between type 1 diabetes mellitus and type 2 diabetes mellitus, *J Diabetes Investig.*, 7, 459, 2016.
4. Dunne JL, Triplett EW, Gevers D, et al., The intestinal microbiome in Type 1 diabetes, *Clin Exp Immunol.*, 177, 30, 2014.
5. Gülden E, Wong FS, and Wen L, The gut microbiota and type 1 diabetes, *Clin Immunol.*, 159, 143, 2015.
6. Zhang Y and Zhang H, Type 2 diabetes microbiota associated with type 2 diabetes and its related complications, *Food Sci Hum Wellness,* 2, 167, 2013.
7. Tilg H and Moschen AR, Evolution of inflammation in nonalcoholic fatty liver disease: The multiple parallel hits hypothesis, *Hepatology,* 52, 1836, 2010.
8. Lau E, Carvalho D, and Freitas P, Gut microbiota: Association with NAFLD and metabolic disturbances, *BioMed Res Int.*, 2015, 979515, 2015.
9. Rial SA, Kareli AD, Bergeron KF, and Mourier C, Gut microbiota and metabolic health: The potential beneficial effects of a medium chain triglyceride diet in obese individuals, *Nutrients*, 8, 281, 2016.
10. Million M, Lagier YC, Yahav D, and Paul M. Gut bacterial microbiota and obesity. *Clin Microbiol Infect.*, 19, 305–13, 2013.
11. Kasai C, Sugimoto K, Moritani I, et al., Comparison of the gut microbiota composition between obese and non-obese individuals in a Japanese population, as analyzed by terminal restriction fragment length polymorphism and next-generation sequencing, *BMC Gastroenterol.*, 15, 100, 2015.
12. Davis-Richardson AG, Ardissone AN, Dias R, et al., Bacteroides dorei dominates gut microbiome prior to autoimmunity in Finnish children at high risk for type 1 diabetes, *Front Microbio.*, 5, 678, 2014.
13. Mullaney J, Stephens JE, Costello ME, et al., Type 1 diabetes susceptibility alleles are associated with distinct alterations in the gut microbiota, *Microbiome*, 6, 35, 2018.
14. Yamanouchi J, Rainbow D, Serra P, et al., Interleukin-2 gene variation impairs regulatory T cell function and causes autoimmunity, *Nat Genet.*, 39, 329, 2007.
15. Hunter K, Rainbow D, Plagnol V, et al., Interactions between Idd5.1/Ctla4 and other type 1 diabetes genes, *J Immunol.*,179, 8341, 2007.
16. Boulange CL, Nieves AL, Chilloux J, et al., Impact of the gut microbiota on inflammation, obesity, and metabolic disease, *Genome Med.*, 8, 42, 2016.
17. Pociot F and Lernmark A, Genetic risk factors for type 1 diabetes*, Lancet*, 387, 2331, 2016.
18. Million M, Angelakis E, Paul M, et al., Comparative meta-analysis of the effect of *Lactobacillus* species on weight gain in humans and animals, *Microb Pathog.*, 53, 100, 2012.
19. Rabiei S, Shakkerhosseini R, and Saadat N. The effects of symbiotic therapy on anthropometric measures, body composition and blood pressure in patient with metabolic syndrome: A triple blind RCT, *Med J Islam Repub Iran*, 29, 213, 2015.

20. Tajabadi-Ebrahimi M, Sharifi N, Farrokihan A, et al., A randomized controlled clinical trial investigating the effect of synbiotic administration on markers of insulin metabolism and lipid profiles in overweight type 2 diabetic patients with coronary heart disease, *Exp Clin Endocrinol Diabetes*, 125, 21, 2017.
21. Shin NR, Lee JC, Lee HY, et al., An increase in the *Akkermansia* spp. population induced by metformin treatment improves glucose homeostasis in diet-induced obese mice, *Gut Microbiota*, 2, 167, 2013.
22. Tremaroli V, Karlsson F, Werling M, et al., Rou-en-Y Gastric bypass and vertical banded gastroplasty induce long term changes on the human gut microbiome contributing to fat mass regulation, *Cell Metabol.*, 22, 228, 2015.
23. Cohen RV, Pinheiro JC, Schiavon CA, et al., Effects of gastric bypass surgery in patients with type 2 diabetes and only mild obesity, *Diabetes Care*, 35, 1420, 2012.
24. Kikuchi R, Irie J, Yamada-Goto, N, et al., The impact of laparoscopic sleeve gastrectomy with duodeno-jejunal bypass on intestinal microbiota differs from that of laparoscopic sleeve gastrectomy in Japanese patients with obesity, *Clin Drug Investig.*, 38, 545, 2018.
25. McGrice M and Don PM, Interventions to improve long-term weight loss in patients following bariatric surgery: Challenges and solutions, *Diabetes Metab Syndr Obes.*, 8, 263, 2015.
26. Jackson FW, Foods containing prebiotics, *Prebiotin Prebiotic*, 2015. https://www.prebiotin.com/foods-containing-prebiotics/.

17 Achieving a Healthy Body Weight in Later Life
Interventions to Reduce Type 2 Diabetes Risk

Kathryn N. Porter Starr, Kenlyn R. Young, and Connie W. Bales

CONTENTS

17.1 THE CONVERGENCE OF GLOBAL GRAYING WITH THE OBESITY EPIDEMIC

Type 2 diabetes has long been a major health concern for older adults, as it is strongly associated with age-related declines in insulin sensitivity. However, recent demographic trends have precipitated an unprecedented increase in the occurrence of diabetes and its associated health complications in older individuals. The convergence of the epidemic of obesity with worldwide population shifts toward a higher proportion of older adults has created a serious public health challenge in the form of obesity- and age-related diabetes [1].

17.1.1 MAJOR DEMOGRAPHIC TRENDS AFFECTING LATE-LIFE DIABETES PREVALENCE

17.1.1.1 Global Graying

Due to tremendous strides in prevention and treatment of infectious diseases and remarkable increases in life expectancy, the reality of global aging is now being fully realized. By the year 2050, the number of adults in the United States who are age 65 and older will nearly double to almost 83 million, up from approximately 43 million in 2012 [2]. This will include a sharp escalation of the number of those 85 and older, which is expected to grow to 19 million by 2050 [3]. The same trends are anticipated on a global level. Today, 8.5% of people worldwide (617 million) are aged 65 and older, and this percentage is projected to increase to nearly 17% by 2050 (1.6 billion) [4], when there will be twice as many adults aged 65 years and older as children 5 and under [5].

17.1.1.2 Pandemic of Obesity

Concerns about the health impact of the obesity epidemic for the general population are well known. A trend toward steadily increasing body weights began to be recognized decades ago, although there has been little success to date in reversing the trend [6]. Overweight (body mass index [BMI] of 25–29.9 kg/m^2) and obesity (BMI $\geq$ 30 kg/m^2) have also become a major health concern on a global scale. Worldwide obesity has more than doubled since 1980, with more than 1.9 billion adults (39%) 18 years and older being overweight. Of these, over 600 million are obese. These trends are bringing a major shift in causes of mortality; most of the world's population now live in countries where overweight/obesity is responsible for more deaths than underweight [1].

17.1.2 LATE-LIFE OBESITY AMPLIFIES DIABETES RISK

The convergence of global graying with the obesity epidemic has increased the prevalence of geriatric obesity so that it is now very common. Almost 40% of older ($\geq$ 60 years of age) adults in the United States have a BMI exceeding 30 kg/m^2 [7], and similar trends are being recorded globally in both the developed and developing world [8]. Obesity levels of class II (BMI 35.0–39.9 kg/m^2) and higher are becoming increasingly common even at advanced ages. This creates a major health concern because both aging and obesity increase the risk of chronic conditions, including type 2 diabetes. This double threat hastens progression of the disease and accelerates the development of related complications and disabilities [9].

Considering the influence of these dramatic population trends, it is not surprising that older adults have the highest rates of diabetes of any population age group. More than 25% of all adults in the U.S. aged 65 years and older have diabetes; this represents 20.8% who have been diagnosed, along with 4.4% who are undiagnosed. An additional 48.3% of older adults have prediabetes, although only 14.1% are aware of their diagnosis [10]. In addition to threatening overall mortality, diabetes in later life compromises health-related quality of life by increasing the number of years lived with disability. In the Western world, diabetes ranks as the eighth leading cause of disability-adjusted life-years [11].

17.2 IMPACT OF LATE-LIFE OBESITY ON INSULIN SENSITIVITY AND PHYSICAL FUNCTION

The relationship between obesity and diabetes is exceedingly strong, with the prevalence of type 2 diabetes increasing along with obesity in a dose-dependent manner [12–14]. The need to optimize body mass and composition is well-recognized for all segments of the adult population, but it is particularly critical for the older individuals with type 2 diabetes. Insulin sensitivity declines with age; however, in the obese older adult, glucose tolerance is worsened due to increased release of pro-inflammatory cytokines from adipose stores, leading to insulin resistance, and impaired glucose handling [15]. Furthermore, higher BMI, age, and comorbidity are being identified as significant co-risk factors for functional decline [16]. As illustrated in Figure 17.1, and discussed subsequently, the combination of aging, obesity, and insulin resistance detrimentally affect muscle quality and muscle function.

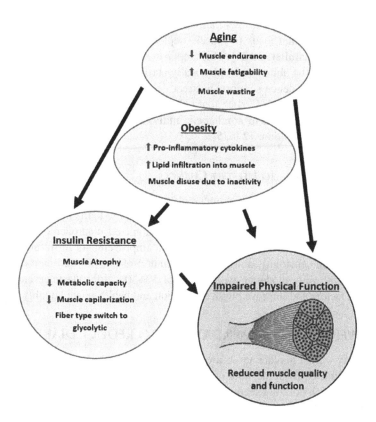

FIGURE 17.1   Impact of aging, obesity, and insulin resistance on muscle function and quality.

17.2.1   DETRIMENTAL HEALTH OUTCOMES

The risk to mortality posed by obesity is greatly enhanced by the coexistence of diabetes; moreover, the risk of microvascular and cardiovascular disease—major causes of mortality and morbidity in individuals with diabetes—is heightened due to obesity-linked hypertension and dyslipidemia [17]. Furthermore, cardiovascular disease (CVD) (ischemic heart disease, stroke, and congestive heart failure) and microvascular disease in the presence of both obesity and type 2 diabetes negatively impact function, independence, and ultimately quality of life. In addition to CVD, hypoglycemia is one of the most frequent nonfatal events to occur in older adults with type 2 diabetes [17]. Individuals with poor glycemic control, dementia, and renal impairment are most at risk [11]. In a large cohort study of 72,310 older adults with diabetes, Huang and colleagues found that age and duration of diabetes had significant impact on health outcomes. Specifically, older adults with diabetes for 10 or more years have significantly higher incidence rates of complications compared to those of the same age with diabetes less than 10 years [18]. The highest complications included acute hypoglycemic event, eye disease, coronary artery disease, congestive heart failure, and mortality [18]. It is important to note that not only is life expectancy shortened for older adults with diabetes, but the number of good-quality years and functional independence is also dramatically reduced. It was estimated that older adults with type 2 diabetes have reduced number of years of good quality of life by 11.1 in men and 13.8 in women [19].

Lean muscle mass is also greatly impacted by the co-occurrence of obesity and type 2 diabetes, leading to impaired physical function. As shown in Figure 17.1, aging is accompanied by loss of lean muscle mass, decline in muscle strength, and increase in fat mass. Furthermore, greater adiposity favors the accumulation of lipid between and within muscles (reduced muscle quality). In most obese individuals, there is persistent, low-grade inflammation resulting from chronic activation of the innate immune system that leads to muscle depletion by enhancing protein breakdown and impairing myogenesis in parallel [20,21]. This impairment is further exacerbated by the fact that obesity markedly reduces the ability to be physically active, leading to progressive muscle atrophy due to disuse. Increasing evidence supports a direct detrimental effect of obesity and diabetes on muscle quality and performance [22], such that older persons with diabetes have reduced walking speed and impaired gait compared to nondiabetic individuals of similar age, and up to 70% have lower-extremity mobility limitations [23–25].

17.2.2 BENEFICIAL RESPONSES TO LIFESTYLE CHANGES

Recognizing the need for prompt effective interventions to disrupt the cycle of obesity and diabetes is essential in the rapidly growing older adult population. In response to the impact of obesity and type 2 diabetes on age-associated physiological changes, recent randomized, controlled weight loss and physical activity intervention trials have documented significant improvements in intrahepatic fat content, insulin secretion, insulin sensitivity, and greater likelihood of partial remission of type 2 diabetes [26,27]. Moreover, with only moderate weight loss of 5%–10%, lifestyle interventions also reduce cardiovascular risk factors and improve physical function and health-related quality of life [28–30].

17.3 BODY WEIGHT RECOMMENDATIONS TO REDUCE DIABETES RISK

Concerns about body weight in older adults are mainly focused on those having a BMI of 30 kg/m^2 or more. This is distinguished from the state of being mildly to moderately overweight (BMI >25 but less than 30 kg/m^2), which does not seem to be strongly linked with detrimental effects on morbidity and mortality in older adults [31,32]. In contrast, frank obesity contributes to an array of negative health outcomes in the older population, leading to significant morbidity, disability, decreased quality of life and, in some cases, even increased rates of mortality [33–35]. Based on this evidence, the general recommendation has been that overweight older adults should not be encouraged to reduce their weight, in part because of concerns about potential detrimental side effects of weight loss [36]. However, in the case of diabetes or even prediabetes, there may be some benefit in modest weight reduction, especially if the BMI is approaching 30 kg/m^2 [37]. To be sure, there are exceptional situations when weight reduction may not be recommended even in the face of obesity; examples include life-threatening illnesses such as later-stage cancer and in the case of advanced dementia [38].

In setting body-weight goals for this population, the limitations of using BMI as an indicator of excessive adiposity should be considered. The BMI does not fully capture the extent of adiposity in this population because, as adults age, they accumulate a greater proportion of body weight as fat compared to lean tissue [39]; also, the change in distribution to more intra-abdominal than subcutaneous fat is not reflected in the BMI. Moreover, the commonly observed loss of height with aging due to vertebral body compression and spinal kyphosis can distort the BMI measurement. Because visceral adiposity is strongly linked with metabolic derangements, assessing it by measuring waist circumference has been suggested (> 102 cm in men and > 88 cm in women), although there are no age-specific recommendations. The indication of ethnic differences in BMI cutoffs for detrimental health changes has also been noted, although this has not been well-described in older adults [40,41].

17.4 INTERVENTIONS TO ACHIEVE A HEALTH BODY WEIGHT

For all obese individuals who have type 2 diabetes or prediabetes, weight reduction is recommended. Likewise, for overweight persons with prediabetes or type 2 diabetes, especially those at the upper end of the BMI range for overweight, weight reduction can be beneficial. While the metabolic benefits will be driven by the amount of weight lost, it is important for older adults to have a realistic weight loss goal that is likely to be achievable and sustainable, as well as moderate and gradual. Regardless of the starting weight, a weight loss as small as 5%–10% of baseline can lead to significant positive effects on health [33,42]. Weight reduction provides a number of indirect benefits (improved function, self-esteem, sense of control), in addition to wide-ranging improvements in health and mortality. Even if pharmacologic agents are needed to achieve adequate glycemic control, lifestyle interventions can help minimize necessary doses and maximize health benefits.

17.4.1 WEIGHT REDUCTION

Weight reduction is difficult to achieve in adults of all ages [43,44] and it is especially challenging in older adults, who have lower basal metabolic rates, calorie requirements, and rates of physical activity [45–47]. Moreover, efforts to reduce body weight in obese older adults raise concerns about the loss of lean body mass [48]. Lowering of muscle mass is a concern not only for function, but it is also linked with impaired glucose uptake and tolerance [49]. When weight reduction is recommended, it should be approached in a medically supervised program that includes a hypocaloric diet and an individualized exercise program aiming to preserve muscle tissue [20]. Unfortunately, the nature of diabetes and its treatment can hinder weight loss and even promote weight gain. This is because the progressive dysfunction of pancreatic B cells and increasing insulin resistance necessitate increasingly higher insulin dosages. This, in turn, promotes weight gain and, in a negative vicious cycle, makes weight loss even more difficult to achieve than for nondiabetic overweight/obese individuals [50].

A negative energy (calorie) balance must be achieved for meaningful weight loss to occur. Energy intake (amount of calories consumed) must be brought moderately below energy expenditure over time so as to achieve a safe but consistent negative balance. Especially in older adults, it is important for the rate of weight loss to be gradual. Published equations, such as the Harris Benedict equation [51], are used to determine the total energy expenditure (TEE) as a means of estimating the energy requirement for an individual. Table 17.1 shows the steps required for calculating TEE using the Harris Benedict equation.

The TEE can also be calculated using the predictive equations derived from studies with doubly labeled water and published by the Food and Nutrition Board of the Institute of Medicine (IOM) [52]. The equations in Table 17.2 published by the IOM were developed for use in overweight and obese individuals aged 19 years and older.

Once the TEE is determined, an individualized calorie prescription of 250–500 kcal per day below TEE will typically lead to a moderate but steady weight loss of approximately 0.5–1.0 lbs per week. To avoid nutrient shortfalls (see also the section on Nutritional Adequacy), the calorie prescription should be a minimum of 1,200 kcal per day for women and 1,800 kcal per day for men [52].

TABLE 17.1

Calculation of Total Energy Expenditure Using the Harris Benedict Equation

Males: BMR = $[66.5 + (13.75 \times \text{wt [kg]}) + (5.003 \times \text{ht [cm]}) - (6.775 \times \text{age [yr]})]$

Females: BMR = $[655.1 + (9.563 \times \text{wt [kg]}) + (1.850 \times \text{ht [cm]}) - (4.676 \times \text{age [yr]})]$

To determine the TEE, make the following activity level adjustments:

Sedentary (little or no exercise)	BMR × 1.2
Lightly active (light ex/sports 1–3 days/wk)	BMR × 1.375
Moderately active (moderate ex/sports 3–5 days/wk)	BMR × 1.55
Very active (hard exercise/sports 6–7 days/wk)	BMR × 1.725
Extra active (very hard daily exercise/sports and physical job or twice-daily training)	BMR × 1.9

BMR, basal metabolic rate; ht, height; TEE, total energy expenditure; wt, weight.

TABLE 17.2

Calculation of Total Energy Expenditure Using the Institute of Medicine Equations

Overweight/obese males: TEE = 864 − 9.72 × age [yr] + PA × 14.2 × wt [kg] + 503 × ht [m]

Overweight/obese females: TEE = 387 − 7.31 × age [yr] + PA × (10.9 × wt [kg] + 660.7 × ht [m]

Where PA is the physical activity coefficient:

Sedentary	PA = 1.00 if PAL is estimated to be ≥ 1.0 < 1.4
Low active	PA = 1.11 if PAL is estimated to be ≥ 1.4 < 1.6
Active	PA = 1.25 if PAL is estimated to be ≥ 1.6 < 1.9
Very active	PA = 1.48 if PAL is estimated to be ≥ 1.9 < 2.5

PAL, physical activity level.

17.4.2 PHYSICAL ACTIVITY RECOMMENDATIONS FOR OLDER ADULTS

The Physical Activity Guidelines for Americans recommend that adults 65 years of age and older should get 150 minutes of moderate physical activity every week and muscle strength activities, targeting all of the major muscle groups, on 2 or more days a week [53]. The prevalence of older adults meeting these recommendations ranges from 27.3% to 44.3% [54]. It is important to note that older adults unable to meet the current physical activity recommendations can still benefit from smaller amounts of physical activity [55]. For example, when prolonged sitting is interrupted by brief bouts of walking or simple resistance activities, persons with diabetes have improvements in postprandial glucose, insulin, C-peptide, and triglycerides [56]. Furthermore, in the English Longitudinal Study of Ageing, older adults who exercised but did not meet the 150-minute, moderate-intensity exercise recommendations still had reduced risk of all-cause mortality, cardiovascular mortality, and death by other causes. These findings illustrate that meaningful benefits can still be gained, even at lower intensity and smaller amounts than the physical activity guidelines [57].

17.4.3 WEIGHT MAINTENANCE

Once the weight reduction target is met, the calorie restriction can be eased to the point of weight maintenance. Exercise has been shown to be particularly helpful in helping to sustain a recent weight reduction [58] and should be recommended as a part of the weight maintenance regimen [59]. However, some level of calorie restriction may continue to be required for long-term calorie maintenance of a healthy body mass in this target population. As an additional challenge, obese individuals with type 2 diabetes may be more resistant to the maintenance of weight loss, because some antidiabetic drugs promote weight gain [60].

17.4.4 NUTRITIONAL ADEQUACY

Calorie requirements decrease with age, so the prescribed calorie deficit to produce the target rate of weight loss may represent a challenge to nutritional adequacy in older adults needing a weight loss intervention. It is important that the weight loss diet plan provides a wide variety of food choices to enhance long-term compliance and that it does not limit the intakes of essential nutrients (e.g., protein, vitamins, minerals). A diet history or typical diet record or recall may be collected to provide a profile of the usual intake and food preferences so that these can be considered in the diet plan to the fullest possible extent. Given that the prescribed hypocaloric intakes could limit food choices, the advice of a registered dietitian/nutritionist should be sought for the design and personalization of the dietary plan for older individuals beginning a weight loss regimen. Any need for nutritional supplements (e.g., vitamins or minerals at risk for inadequate

TABLE 17.3

Selected Dietary Reference Intakes for Adults Aged 51 Years and Older

Macronutrients

	Female 51 yrs+	Male 51 yrs+
Calorie level	1,600	2,000
Protein, g	46	56
Protein, % kcal	10–35	10–35
Carbohydrate, g	130	130
Carbohydrate, % kcal	45–65	45–65
Dietary fiber, g	22.4	28
Added sugar, % kcal	< 10%	< 10%
Total fat, % kcal	20–35	20–35
Saturated fat, % kcal	< 10%	< 10%

Vitamins

	Female 51 yrs+	Male 51 yrs+
Calorie level	1,600	2,000
Vitamin A, mg	700	900
Vitamin E, mg	15	15
Vitamin D, IU	600	600
Vitamin C, mg	75	75
Thiamin, mg	1.1	1.2
Riboflavin, mg	1.1	1.3
Niacin, mg	14	16
Vitamin B_6, mg	1.5	1.7
Vitamin B_{12}, mcg	2.4	2.4
Choline, mg	425	450
Vitamin K, mg	90	120
Folate, mcg	400	400

Minerals

	Female 51 yrs+	Male 51 yrs+
Calorie level	1,600	2,000
Calcium, mg	1,200	1,000
Iron, mg	8	8
Magnesium, mg	320	420
Phosphorous, mg	700	700
Potassium, mg	4,700	4,700
Sodium, mg	2,300	2,300
Zinc, mg	8	11
Copper, mcg	900	900
Manganese, mg	1.8	2.3
Selenium, mcg	55	55

Source: Institute of Medicine, *Dietary Reference Intakes for Energy, Carbohydrate, Fiber, Fat, Fatty Acids, Cholesterol, Protein, and Amino Acids*, The National Academies Press, Washington, DC, 2005.

consumption) should also be identified and addressed. Table 17.3 presents the Dietary Reference Intakes for key essential micronutrients for women and men aged 51 years or more [52].

General guidelines for healthy eating patterns can also be helpful for developing a long-term diet plan. According to the 2015–2020 US Department of Agriculture Dietary Recommendations [61], a healthy eating pattern limits intakes of the following:

- Saturated fat: Limit to less than 10% of total kcal per day.
- Sugar: Limit to less than 10% of total kcal per day.

- Sodium: If not hypertensive, aim for 2,400 mg per day or less.
- Alcohol: Men limit to two drinks per day; women limit to one drink per day, consumed with food.

These are general guidelines for the population but can be especially beneficial in the case of diabetes risk.

17.5   DIABETES MANAGEMENT IN OLDER ADULTS

While the role of diet in diabetes management is addressed elsewhere in this volume, it is important to note some unique points concerning diet management in older persons. In the case of marked obesity, weight reduction is an important therapeutic requirement [17,18]. Reductions in fasting glucose levels correspond directly to the amount of weight reduction [62]. As in all obese adults with glucose intolerance, weight reduction will bring improvements in insulin action and blood glucose concentrations, and required doses of diabetes medications may be reduced. Blood glucose regulation may need to be approached more carefully in older adults with diabetes. Important findings from the ACCORD and ADVANCE studies showed that tight glucose control may not be warranted in elderly diabetic patients. In fact, near-normal glucose control was linked with significantly increased risks of death from any cause and death from cardiovascular causes [63]. In the case of serious comorbidities, there may be more harm than benefit from intensive glucose-lowering therapy [64]. Thus, relaxing blood glucose and hemoglobin A1c (HgbA1c) targets is often recommended in the management of diabetes in older adults. This underscores and increases focus on the importance of maintaining a healthy body weight and optimizing essential nutrient intakes for older adults at diabetes risk.

17.6   CONCLUDING COMMENTS AND RECOMMENDATIONS

Achieving and maintaining a healthy body weight and a generous intake of key nutrients is a low risk, high gain component of health management for older adults with type 2 diabetes or at risk of developing it. Apart from more invasive and expensive treatments and medications, lifestyle changes aimed at optimizing body weight also promote a variety of other advantageous health outcomes. A healthy BMI plays a vital role in preserving the cardiometabolic profile, slowing the course of the disease, and extending the life expectancy [60]. The lifestyle recommendations offered in this chapter to achieve a healthy BMI and diet composition are summarized in Table 17.4.

TABLE 17.4
Lifestyle Recommendations for a Healthy Body Weight

1. In most cases, weight loss is recommended for obese older adults, whether they have prediabetes or type 2 diabetes.
2. Older adults with a body mass index (BMI) in the upper range of the overweight BMI category may also benefit from modest weight loss.
3. The weight loss strategy should include a reduced calorie intake (250–500 kcal below the total energy expenditure) in the context of a nutritionally adequate and palatable diet.
4. The diet should apply recommendations from the Dietary Guidelines to moderate intakes of sugar, saturated fat, sodium, and alcohol.
5. Moderate physical activity (150 min/wk plus muscle strength activities on 2 or more days per week) is strongly encouraged, although lesser amounts of physical activity will also convey important benefits.
6. Relaxation of blood glucose and HgbA1c targets is often recommended in the management of diabetes in older adults, thus these lifestyle measures are particularly useful as a safe and effective way to manage diabetes risk in later life.

REFERENCES

1. World Health Organization. *Obesity and Overweight Fact Sheet 2016.* http://www.who.int/mediacentre/factsheets/fs311/en/. Accessed online October 25, 2017.
2. He W, Goodkind D, Kowal P. International Population Reports, *P95/16-1, An Aging World: 2015.* In: Bureau USC, ed. Washington, DC: U.S. Government Publishing Office, 2016.
3. Federal Interagency Forum on Aging-Related Statistics. *Older Americans 2016: Key Indicators of Well-Being.* Federal Interagency Forum on Aging-Related Statistics. Washington, DC: U.S. Government Printing Office, August 2016.
4. Kowal P, Goodkind D, He W. U.S. *Census Bureau, International Population Reports, P95/16-1, An Aging World: 2015.* Washington, DC: U.S. Government Publishing Office, 2016.
5. United Nations, Department of Economic and Social Affairs, Population Division (2011). *World Population Prospects: The 2010 Revision, Volume I: Comprehensive Tables.* ST/ESA/SER.A/313.
6. Flegal KM, Carroll MD, Kit BK, Ogden CL. Prevalence of obesity and trends in the distribution of body mass index among us adults, 1999–2010. *JAMA.* 2012;307(5):491–7.
7. Flegal KM, Kruszon-Moran D, Carroll MD, Fryar CD, Ogden CL. Trends in obesity among adults in the United States, 2005 to 2014. *JAMA.* 2016;315(21):2284–91.
8. Ng M, Fleming T, Robinson M, Thomson B, Graetz N, Margono C, et al. Global, regional, and national prevalence of overweight and obesity in children and adults during 1980–2013: A systematic analysis for the Global Burden of Disease Study 2013. *Lancet.* 2014;384(9945):766–81.
9. Ahima RS. Connecting obesity, aging and diabetes. *Nat Med.* 2009;15(9):996–7.
10. Centers for Disease Control and Prevention. *National Diabetes Statistics Report A.* Washington, DC: US Department of Health and Human Services, 2017.
11. Sinclair A, Dunning T, Rodriguez-Mañas L. Diabetes in older people: New insights and remaining challenges. *Lancet Diabetes Endocrinol.* 2015;3(4):275–85.
12. Esser N, Legrand-Poels S, Piette J, Scheen AJ, Paquot N. Inflammation as a link between obesity, metabolic syndrome and type 2 diabetes. *Diabetes Res Clin Pract.* 2014;105(2):141–50.
13. Must A, Spadano J, Coakley EH, Field AE, Colditz G, Dietz WH. The disease burden associated with overweight and obesity. *JAMA.* 1999;282(16):1523–9.
14. Narayan KMV, Boyle JP, Thompson TJ, Gregg EW, Williamson DF. Effect of BMI on lifetime risk for diabetes in the U.S. *Diabetes Care.* 2007;30(6):1562–6.
15. Batsis JA, Silvio B. Sarcopenia, sarcopenic obesity and insulin resistance. In: C Croniger, ed. *Medical Complications of Type 2 Diabetes:* InTech, 2011. Doi: 10.5772/22008. Available from: https://www.intechopen.com/books/medical-complications-of-type-2-diabetes/sarcopenia-sarcopenic-obesity-and-insulin-resistance
16. Cheng FW, Gao X, Bao L, Mitchell DC, Wood C, Sliwinski MJ, et al. Obesity as a risk factor for developing functional limitation among older adults: A conditional inference tree analysis. *Obesity (Silver Spring).* 2017;25(7):1263–9.
17. Halter JB, Musi N, McFarland Horne F, Crandall JP, Goldberg A, Harkless L, et al. *Diabetes and cardiovascular disease in older adults: Current status and future directions. Diabetes.* 2014;63(8):2578–89.
18. Huang ES, Laiteerapong N, Liu JY, John PM, Moffet HH, Karter AJ. Rates of complications and mortality in older patients with diabetes mellitus: The diabetes and aging study. *JAMA Intern Med.* 2014;174(2):251–8.
19. Narayan KM, Boyle JP, Thompson TJ, Sorensen SW, Williamson DF. Lifetime risk for diabetes mellitus in the United States. *JAMA.* 2003;290(14):1884–90.
20. Costamagna D, Costelli P, Sampaolesi M, Penna F. Role of inflammation in muscle homeostasis and myogenesis. *Mediat Inflamm.* 2015;2015:805172.
21. Porter Starr KN, McDonald SR, Bales CW. Obesity and physical frailty in older adults: A scoping review of lifestyle intervention trials. *J Am Med Dir Assoc.* 2014;15(4):240–50.
22. Volpato S, Bianchi L, Lauretani F, Lauretani F, Bandinelli S, Guralnik JM, et al. Role of muscle mass and muscle quality in the association between diabetes and gait speed. *Diabetes Care.* 2012;35(8):1672–9.
23. Šimundić A-M. Measures of diagnostic accuracy: Basic definitions. *Med Biol Sci.* 2008;22(4):61–5.
24. Kalyani RR, Corriere M, Ferrucci L. Age-related and disease-related muscle loss: The effect of diabetes, obesity, and other diseases. *Lancet Diabetes Endocrinol.* 2014;2(10):819–29.
25. Kalyani RR, Saudek CD, Brancati FL, Selvin E. Association of diabetes, comorbidities, and A1C with functional disability in older adults: Results from the National Health and Nutrition Examination Survey (NHANES), 1999–2006. *Diabetes Care.* 2010;33(5):1055–60.

26. Bouchonville M, Armamento-Villareal R, Shah K, Napoli N, Sinacore DR, Qualls C, et al. Weight loss, exercise or both and cardiometabolic risk factors in obese older adults: Results of a randomized controlled trial. *Int J Obes (Lond).* 2014;38(3):423–31.

27. Gregg EW, Chen H, Wagenknecht LE, et al. Association of an intensive lifestyle intervention with remission of type 2 diabetes. *JAMA.* 2012;308(23):2489–96.

28. Purnell JQ, Kahn SE, Albers JJ, Nevin DN, Brunzell JD, Schwartz RS. Effect of weight loss with reduction of intra-abdominal fat on lipid metabolism in older men. *J Clin Endocrinol Metab.* 2000;85(3):977–82.

29. Villareal DT, Banks M, Sinacore DR, Siener C, Klein S. Effect of weight loss and exercise on frailty in obese older adults. *Arch Intern Med.* 2006;166(8):860–6.

30. Mazzali G, Di Francesco V, Zoico E, Fantin F, Zamboni G, Benati C, et al. Interrelations between fat distribution, muscle lipid content, adipocytokines, and insulin resistance: Effect of moderate weight loss in older women. *Am J Clin Nutr.* 2006;84(5):1193–9.

31. Chapman IM. Obesity paradox during aging. *Interdiscip Top Gerontol.* 2010;37:20–36.

32. van Uffelen JG, Berecki-Gisolf J, Brown WJ, Dobson AJ. What is a healthy body mass index for women in their seventies? Results from the Australian longitudinal study on women's health. *J Gerontol A Biol Sci Med Sci.* 2010;65(8):847–53.

33. Mathus-Vliegen EM. Prevalence, pathophysiology, health consequences and treatment options of obesity in the elderly: A guideline. *Obes Facts.* 2012;5(3):460–83.

34. Whitmer RA, Gunderson EP, Barrett-Connor E, Quesenberry CP, Jr., Yaffe K. Obesity in middle age and future risk of dementia: A 27 year longitudinal population based study. *BMJ.* 2005;330(7504):1360.

35. Valdes AM, Andrew T, Gardner JP, Kimura M, Oelsner E, Cherkas LF, et al. Obesity, cigarette smoking, and telomere length in women. *Lancet.* 2005; 366(9486):662–4.

36. Brown RE, Kuk JL. Consequences of obesity and weight loss: A devil's advocate position. *Obes Rev.* 2015;16(1):77–87.

37. Kirkman MS, Briscoe VJ, Clark N, Florez H, Haas LB, Halter JB, et al. Diabetes in older adults. *Diabetes Care.* 2012;35(12):2650–64.

38. Porter Starr K, McDonald S, Weidner J, Bales C. Challenges in the management of geriatric obesity in high risk populations. *Nutrients.* 2016;8(5):262.

39. Newman AB, Lee JS, Visser M, Goodpaster BH, Kritchevsky SB, Tylavsky FA, et al. Weight change and the conservation of lean mass in old age: The Health, Aging and Body Composition Study. *Am J Clin Nutr.* 2005;82(4):872–8; quiz 915–6.

40. Chan RSM, Woo J. Prevention of overweight and obesity: How effective is the current public health approach. *Int J Environ Res Public Health.* 2010;7(3):765–83.

41. Hunma S, Ramuth H, Miles-Chan JL, Schutz Y, Montani JP, Joonas N, et al. Body composition-derived BMI cut-offs for overweight and obesity in Indians and Creoles of Mauritius: Comparison with Caucasians. *Int J Obes (2005).* 2016;40(12):1906–14.

42. Han E, Sohn HS, Lee JY, Jang S. Health behaviors and medication adherence in elderly patients. *Am J Health Promot.* 2017;31(4):278–86.

43. Cannon CP, Kumar A. Treatment of overweight and obesity: Lifestyle, pharmacologic, and surgical options. *Clin Cornerstone.* 2009;9(4):55–68; discussion 9-71.

44. Ross R. The challenge of obesity treatment: Avoiding weight regain. *CMAJ.* 2009;180(10):997–8.

45. Tzankoff SP, Norris AH. Effect of muscle mass decrease on age-related BMR changes. *J Appl Physiol Respir Environ Exerc Physiol.* 1977;43(6):1001–6.

46. Elia M, Ritz P, Stubbs RJ. Total energy expenditure in the elderly. *Eur J Clin Nutr.* 2000;54 Suppl 3:S92–103.

47. Villareal DT, Apovian CM, Kushner RF, Klein S. Obesity in older adults: Technical review and position statement of the American Society for Nutrition and NAASO, The Obesity Society. *Am J Clin Nutr.* 2005;82(5):923–34.

48. Weinheimer EM, Sands LP, Campbell WW. A systematic review of the separate and combined effects of energy restriction and exercise on fat-free mass in middle-aged and older adults: Implications for sarcopenic obesity. *Nutr Rev.* 2010;68(7):375–88.

49. Kalyani RR, Metter EJ, Ramachandran R, Chia CW, Saudek CD, Ferrucci L. Glucose and insulin measurements from the oral glucose tolerance test and relationship to muscle mass. *J Gerontol A Biol Sci Med Sci.* 2012;67(1):74–81.

50. Al-Goblan AS, Al-Alfi MA, Khan MZ. Mechanism linking diabetes mellitus and obesity. *Diabetes Metab Syndr Obes.* 2014;7:587–91.

51. Harris JA, Benedict FG. A biometric study of basal metabolism in man. *Proc Natl Acad Sci U S A.* 1918;4(12):370–3.

52. Institute of Medicine. *Dietary Reference Intakes for Energy, Carbohydrate, Fiber, Fat, Fatty Acids, Cholesterol, Protein, and Amino Acids.* Washington, DC: The National Academies Press, 2005.

53. Physical Activity Guidelines Advisory Committee. *Physical Activity Guidelines Advisory Committee Report, 2008.* Washington, DC: U.S. Department of Health and Human Services, 2008.

54. Keadle SK, McKinnon R, Graubard BI, Troiano RP. Prevalence and trends in physical activity among older adults in the United States: A comparison across three national surveys. *Prev Med.* 2016;89(Supplement C):37–43.

55. Garber CE, Blissmer B, Deschenes MR, Franklin BA, Lamonte MJ, Lee IM, et al. American College of Sports Medicine position stand. Quantity and quality of exercise for developing and maintaining cardiorespiratory, musculoskeletal, and neuromotor fitness in apparently healthy adults: Guidance for prescribing exercise. *Med Sci Sports Exerc.* 2011;43(7):1334–59.

56. Dempsey PC, Larsen RN, Sethi P, Sacre JW, Straznicky NE, Cohen ND, et al. Benefits for type 2 diabetes of interrupting prolonged sitting with brief bouts of light walking or simple resistance activities. *Diabetes Care.* 2016;39(6):964–72.

57. Hamer M, de Oliveira C, Demakakos P. Non-exercise physical activity and survival: English longitudinal study of ageing. *Am J Prev Med.* 2014;47(4):452–60.

58. Catenacci VA, Grunwald GK, Ingebrigtsen JP, Jakicic JM, McDermott MD, Phelan S, et al. Physical activity patterns using accelerometry in the National Weight Control Registry. *Obesity (Silver Spring).* 2011;19(6):1163–70.

59. Dietz WH, Baur LA, Hall K, Puhl RM, Taveras EM, Uauy R, et al. Management of obesity: Improvement of health-care training and systems for prevention and care. *Lancet.* 2015;385(9986):2521–33.

60. Schwartz S, Herman M. Revisiting weight reduction and management in the diabetic patient: Novel therapies provide new strategies. *Postgrad Med.* 2015;127(5):480–93.

61. U.S. Department of Health and Human Services and U.S. Department of Agriculture. 2015 – 2020 Dietary Guidelines for Americans. 8th Edition. December 2015. https://health.gov/dietaryguidelines/2015/guidelines/. Accessed online October 25, 2017.

62. Klein S, Sheard NF, Pi-Sunyer X, Daly A, Wylie-Rosett J, Kulkarni K, et al. Weight management through lifestyle modification for the prevention and management of type 2 diabetes: Rationale and strategies: A statement of the American Diabetes Association, the North American Association for the Study of Obesity, and the American Society for Clinical Nutrition. *Diabetes Care.* 2004;27(8):2067–73.

63. Dluhy RG, McMahon GT. Intensive glycemic control in the ACCORD and ADVANCE trials. *N Engl J Med.* 2008;358(24):2630–3.

64. Muller N, Khunti K, Kuss O, Lindblad U, Nolan JJ, Rutten GE, et al. Is there evidence of potential overtreatment of glycaemia in elderly people with type 2 diabetes? Data from the GUIDANCE study. *Acta Diabetol.* 2017;54(2):209–14.

18 Primary Prevention of Type 2 Diabetes
From Research to Community

Natascha Thompson and Sam Dagogo-Jack

CONTENTS

18.1 INTRODUCTION

Type 2 diabetes (T2DM), a global epidemic, now ranks among the leading noncommunicable public health challenges of the present era [1–3]. In 2015, The International Diabetes Federation (IDF) estimated that 415 million adults had diabetes worldwide, with T2DM accounting for 90%–95% of all diabetes cases [1]. The public health burden imposed by diabetes is underscored by the fact that diabetes now is the leading cause of blindness, end-stage renal failure, and nontraumatic limb amputations, and a major contributor to heart disease, stroke, and peripheral vascular disease [4–7]. There is now abundant evidence from clinical trials that T2DM is preventable in adults through implementation of lifestyle interventions and/or medications. However, the achievement of sustained glycemic control to the level necessary for prevention of complications often proves elusive, even in countries in the developed economies [8,9]. Optimal glycemic control requires a highly motivated patient and regular contact points of that patient with the diabetic care team. The care process for an individual with diabetes includes many challenges: the use of multiple medications; frequent clinic visits; adherence to challenging lifestyle prescriptions; performance of demanding self-management tasks; paying for cumulative costs of home blood glucose monitoring equipment; sustained engagement by a team of physicians, nurses, dietitians, diabetes educators, ophthalmologists, podiatrists, behaviorists, and other specialized professionals; and the implementation of sundry other recommendations [10,11]. Translation of the results of clinical trials on diabetes prevention to the community at large presents additional challenges and involves focus on health and nutrition literacy, identification of persons at risk for T2DM, promotion of lifestyle intervention efforts, provision of community resources, and pertinent legislative action that rewards preventive behavior.

18.1.1 PATHOPHYSIOLOGY

Current understanding indicates that multiple pathophysiological defects underlie T2DM (Figure 18.1). Generally, at least eight unique pathophysiological defects are currently recognized in T2DM: insulin resistance, impaired insulin secretion, impaired glucagon suppression, increased lipolysis, exaggerated hepatic glucose production, incretin deficiency/resistance, maladaptive renal glucose reabsorption, and central nervous system defects (including impaired dopaminergic tone and dysregulation of satiety) [12–14]. Insulin resistance can be inherited or acquired. Obesity, aging, physical inactivity, overeating, increased lipolysis, and accumulation of excessive amounts of nonesterified (free) fatty acids are known causes of insulin resistance. Normally, cytoplasmic long-chain fatty acids are transported into mitochondria as long-chain fatty acyl coenzyme A (LCFA-CoA) for beta-oxidation, a process that is gated by carnitine palmitoyl transferase (CPT)-1 and 2 (the shuttle enzymes located in the outer and inner mitochondrial membrane). This shuttle process ensures that fatty acids do not accumulate excessively in the cytoplasm. Inhibition of that process leads to intracellular accumulation of long-chain fatty acids, which can induce lipotoxicity, cellular dysfunction, and cell death [13,14]. Further, intracellular accumulation of long-chain fatty acids along with diacylglycerol (DAG) can activate certain isoforms of protein kinase C (PKC), leading to aberrant phosphorylation of the insulin receptor and consequent insulin resistance.

Acetyl-CoA, a product of glycolysis for the Krebs cycle, can be converted to malonyl CoA by the enzyme acetyl-CoA carboxylase (ACC). Malonyl-CoA is the activated two-carbon donor required for fatty acid synthesis. Malonyl-CoA also is a potent inhibitor of CPT-1, thereby blocking the delivery and oxidation of fatty acids in mitochondria. The result is accumulation of long-chain fatty acids in the cytosol and eventual lipotoxicity [14,15]. Glucose abundance also increases the formation of intracellular DAG. Thus, multiple metabolic pathways link intracellular glucose abundance (usually derived from carbohydrate consumption) to impaired fat oxidation, fatty acid synthesis, accumulation of long-chain fatty acids, risk of lipotoxicity, and insulin resistance. Among the potent interventions that have been demonstrated to ameliorate the pathological cellular and molecular processes leading to insulin resistance are caloric restriction (reduction of carbohydrate and fat intake), physical activity, and weight loss [16–24].

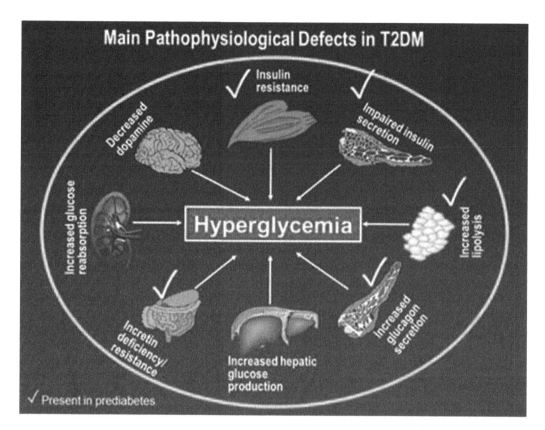

FIGURE 18.1 Recognized pathophysiological defects in type 2 diabetes mellitus and prediabetes. (Adapted from Dagogo-Jack, S., *Diabetes Risks from Prescription and Nonprescription Drugs*, ADA Press, Alexandria, VA, 2016.)

18.1.2 Risk Factors for Type 2 Diabetes

Both genetic and environmental factors underlie the development of T2DM [25,26]. To date, more than 60 gene variants associated with T2DM have been identified; however, the effect size of these individual gene variants is rather modest [27–31]. The environmental risk factors strongly associated with T2DM risk include obesity, physical inactivity, history of gestational diabetes, hypertension, and dyslipidemia, among others [10,25,26]. These risk factors interact with genetic predisposition (indicated by a family history of diabetes and/or high-risk ethnic heritage) to promote the development of diabetes. Such a phenomenon was clearly demonstrated in the studies that showed a threefold increase in the rate of T2DM in recent Japanese immigrants to the United States compared with native Japanese [32]. Since a dramatic increase in disease prevalence over a relatively short time frame in humans is unlikely to be due to sudden new genetic mutations, environmental factors (notably changes in diet, physical activity, and perhaps microbial flora) probably trigger the surging diabetes rates among genetically predisposed populations. The exact mechanisms whereby these environmental triggers induce diabetes in genetically predisposed persons remain to be fully elucidated.

18.1.3 Prediabetes

The term *prediabetes* refers to impaired glucose tolerance (IGT) and impaired fasting glucose (IFG), two intermediate metabolic states between normal glucose tolerance and diabetes. IGT is defined by a plasma glucose level of 140 mg/dl to 199 mg/dl (7.8–11.1 mmol/l), 2 hours following ingestion of a 75-gram oral solution. IFG is defined by a fasting plasma glucose level of 100 mg/dl to 125 mg/dl (5.6–6.9 mmol/l) [10]. There is considerable overlap in the risk factors and pathophysiological defects that underlie T2DM and prediabetes. Although the exact sequence of evolution of individual pathophysiological defects has not been determined precisely, many of the defects co-evolve during the pathogenesis of T2DM and are demonstrable even at the stage of prediabetes [33–43]. Estimates by the US Centers for Disease Control and Prevention (CDC) indicated that there were approximately 29 million adults with diabetes and 86 million with prediabetes in 2014 [44]. Worldwide, there are more than 400 million people with prediabetes [1]. Individuals with prediabetes progress to T2DM at an annual rate of approximately 10% [36,37].

18.1.4 PREDICTORS OF PROGRESSION FROM PREDIABETES TO TYPE 2 DIABETES

An analysis of six prospective studies [45] on progression from IGT to diabetes revealed the following features: (1) baseline fasting plasma glucose (FPG) and 2-hour oral glucose tolerance test (OGTT) glucose values are positively associated with diabetes risk; (2) the rate of progression from IGT to T2DM was exponential among subjects in the top quartile of baseline FPG, but increased linearly with increasing 2-hour OGTT glucose levels; (3) incident diabetes occurred at higher rates in Hispanic, Mexican American, Pima, and Nauruan populations than among Caucasians; (4) the degree of obesity, as measured by the body mass index (BMI), predicted T2DM risk in three studies with the lowest incidence rates of diabetes, but not in the studies that recorded the highest incidence of T2DM; and (5) a family history of diabetes did not predict the risk of progression from IGT to diabetes in these studies, suggesting that genetic effects probably are fully established by stage of IGT [45]. Thus, the magnitude of fasting and postchallenge dysglycemia (a reflection of insulin action and insulin secretion), ethnicity, and weight gain are major predictors of progression to T2DM.

Longitudinal studies in subjects from a high-risk population (Pima Indians) [46] with baseline normal glucose tolerance (NGT) indicated that weight gain, insulin resistance, and progressive loss of insulin secretory response to glucose predicted the development of T2DM [47]. Weight gain predicted progression from NGT to IGT and progression from IGT to T2DM during a 6-year follow-up period, with a twofold increase noted when comparing progressors to nonprogressors [47]. The greater weight gain in the progressors was accompanied by approximately 30% worsening of insulin resistance and a significant decline in acute insulin secretory response to intravenous glucose [47]. Weight gain also predicted incident T2DM in African Americans in the Atherosclerosis Risk in Communities study [48]. It follows that interventions that induce weight loss (e.g., diet, exercise, medications) could prevent progression from prediabetes to T2DM. In the prospective study of Pima Indians [47], progressive impairment of first-phase insulin secretion proved to be a critical determinant of progression from NGT to IGT and from IGT to T2DM. Progression from IGT to diabetes was associated with an approximately 75% decline in acute insulin secretory response to intravenous glucose [47]. A high concordance rate for impaired insulin secretion has also been reported among elderly identical twins discordant for T2DM [12], which suggests a genetic basis for pancreatic beta-cell dysfunction. The role of beta-cell dysfunction in predicting progression to T2DM indicates that interventions that prevent or replenish the progressive decline in insulin secretion can be expected to prevent the development of diabetes.

18.1.5 PREDICTORS OF INITIAL TRANSITION TO PREDIABETES

In contrast to the numerous studies on the transition from prediabetes to T2DM [45–48], information on the incidence of prediabetes among initially normoglycemic persons is scant. In a study of 254 Pima Indians with normoglycemia, 79 subjects (31%) progressed to prediabetes (IGT) during a mean follow-up period of 4 years [49]. Based on those results, the incidence of prediabetes among

Pima Indians can be estimated at approximately 8% per year [49]. Study of the Pima Indians also highlights that defects in insulin secretion and action occur early in the transition from NGT to IGT, and that increase in basal endogenous glucose output is a relatively late event during transition from IGT to DM [47]. Of the 468 subjects with NGT at enrollment in the Baltimore Longitudinal Study on Aging (BLSA), more than half were followed for at least 10 years [50]. By 10 years, 62% of the initially NGT participants had progressed to prediabetes, yielding an incidence rate of prediabetes of 6.2% in the BLSA cohort (96% of whom were European American) [50]. Dagogo-Jack et al. followed 343 healthy African American and European American offspring of parents with T2DM in the Pathobiology of Prediabetes in a Biracial Cohort (POP-ABC) study and observed that 100 had developed incident prediabetes (IGT and/or IFG) during a mean follow-up period of approximately 3 years, without evidence of ethnic disparities [51]. Thus, among black and white subjects with a parental history of T2DM, the incidence of prediabetes was approximately 10% per year. These data indicate that the risk of incident prediabetes among offspring of parents with T2DM in the general United States population is similar to or higher than the risk observed among Pima Indians, a group with the world's highest rate of T2DM [46]. The POP-ABC data underscore the importance of heredity, familial, and genetic T2DM. Taken together, these studies found that normoglycemic individuals develop prediabetes at an annual rate of 6%–10%, the higher rate being more likely among those with a strong family history of T2DM. Based on findings in the Pima Indian [46] and the POP-ABC [51] studies, the predictors of incident prediabetes include older age, male gender, overweight/obesity, lower insulin sensitivity, and impaired acute insulin secretory response to glucose [51]. Other predictors of incident prediabetes included food habits, physical inactivity, higher C-reactive protein, and lower adiponectin levels [51–53]. Obesity is a likely unifying factor that links the various pathophysiological mechanisms leading to dysglycemia. Comparison of several measures of adiposity indicates higher values in people who progress from normoglycemia to prediabetes compared with those who maintain normal glucose metabolism.

18.2 APPROACH TO PREVENTION OF TYPE 2 DIABETES

18.2.1 LIFESTYLE MODIFICATION

The view that T2DM is a preventable disease has been demonstrated to be accurate based on the results from a few landmark, randomized trials [54–57]. All studies focused on interventions in individuals identified as high risk, primarily defined as individuals with impaired glucose tolerance and including impaired fasting glucose in one of the studies (Table 18.1). The lifestyle interventions consisted of diet and exercise prescriptions, with the addition of weight loss or BMI goals. Dietary strategies included adoption of healthy eating patterns, calorie reduction (by approximately 500–1,000 kcal/day), dietary fat intake limitation (to 30% or less of calorie intake) and increase in fiber intake (in one of the studies). Physical activity strategies varied from goals of 150 minutes of physical activity per week (similar in intensity to brisk walking) to moderate intensity physical activity for at least 30 minutes per day (with a recommendation for endurance exercise) to increasing exercise by one to two defined units per day. Weight loss goals generally attempted to achieve weight reduction of 5%–7% of initial body weight or BMI reduction to less than 23 kg/m². All studies demonstrated reductions in the rate of progression from prediabetes to T2DM when compared to the control population at rates of 29%–58% over study periods that ranged from approximately 3 to 6 years [54–57].

18.2.1.1 Da Qing Study

The Da Qing Study [54] identified 577 individuals with IGT following a screening process of 110,660 men and women from 33 healthcare clinics in the city of Da Qing, China and subsequently randomized the subjects to either a control group or to one of three active treatment groups: diet only, exercise only, or diet plus exercise. The mean age of participants in this study was 45 years,

TABLE 18.1

Randomized, Controlled Trials of Lifestyle Intervention for Diabetes Prevention

Study [Reference]	Duration	Strategies	Weight Goals	Diet Goals	Physical Activity Goals	Diabetes Risk Reduction
DaQing [54]	6 years	Individualized counseling by physician; small-group counseling sessions weekly for 1 month, monthly for 3 months, then once every 3 months thereafter	Reduction of 0.5–1.0 kg/mo for BMI ≥ 25 kg/m² until goal of 23 kg/m² reached	BMI < 25 kg/m²: 25–30 kcal/kg, 55%–65% carbohydrate, 10%–15% protein, 25%–30% fat BMI ≥ 25 kg/m²: Reduce intake for weight loss of 0.5–1.0 kg/mo until BMI of 23 kg/m² reached	Increase leisure physical exercise by 1 U/day and by 2 U/day if < 50 yrs with no cardiovascular disease or arthritis	31% in diet group 46% in exercise group 42% in diet-plus-exercise group
DPS [55]	3 years	7 face-to-face, individualized consultation sessions during the first year and every 3 months thereafter	Reduction ≥ 5%; not more than 0.5–1.0 kg/wk	Dietary fat < 30 E% (proportion of total energy); saturated fat <10 E%; fiber ≥15 gm/1,000 kcal; very-low-calorie diet allowed after 6 months	Moderate-intensity physical activity ≥ 30 min/day; resistance training sessions offered; exercise competition between study centers; voluntary group walking and hiking available	58%
DPP [56]	2.8 years	16-session core curriculum; face-to-face (usually one-on-one) meeting every 2 months for the duration of the trial; self-monitoring of intake for 1 week every month during maintenance	Reduction of 7% of initial body weight in the first 6 months; weight loss rate of 1–2 lbs/wk	Calorie reduction of 500–1,000 calories/day; 25% calories from fat	≥ 700 kcal/wk = 150 min of moderate physical activities (similar in intensity to brisk walking); minimum frequency of 3×/wk, with ≥ 10 min/ session	58%
IDDP-1 [57]	3 years	Monthly telephone contact; personal sessions every 6 months	No defined weight loss goals	Reduction in total calories, refined carbohydrates, and fats, avoidance of sugar and inclusion of fiber-rich foods	>30 min/day exercise to include physical labor, brisk walking, and cycling	28.5%

and the mean BMI was 26 kg/m^2. Dietary advice varied based on BMI classification as lean or overweight, and the exercise prescription was focused on increase in exercise by one to two units per day, defined by time and intensity of exercise. Counseling sessions (either individual or group) were a key component in this study and occurred at a frequency of weekly for 1 month, monthly for 3 months, and then once every 3 months for the remainder of the study.

The primary endpoint, the cumulative incidence of diabetes at 6 years, was 67.7% in the control group, 43.8% in the diet-only group, 41.1% in the exercise-only group, and 46% in the diet-plus-exercise group. As the dietary advice differed based on BMI stratification, the study investigators also looked at incidence rate of diabetes in those with a BMI baseline less than 25 kg/m^2 compared to those with BMI of 25 kg/m^2 or greater. Findings showed similar relative decreases in diabetes incidence rates (when compared to the control group), regardless of BMI stratification of lean versus overweight. After adjustments for baseline differences in BMI and fasting glucose, the diet, exercise, and diet-plus-exercise interventions were associated with reductions in risk of developing diabetes by 31%, 46%, and 42%, respectively [54]. Interestingly, the diet-plus-exercise group did not show additive benefit when compared to the diet-only and exercise-only groups.

18.2.1.2 Finnish Diabetes Prevention Study

The Finnish Diabetes Prevention Study (DPS) [55] randomized 522 middle-aged, overweight subjects (mean age of 55 years and mean BMI of 31 kg/m^2) with IGT to either a usual-care control group or to an intensive lifestyle intervention group. The control group was provided general information, either individually or in one group session, and included some printed information, with the overall message of weight reduction, increased physical activity, and healthy diet changes. The intervention group received individual counseling sessions with the study nutritionist, focused on specific diet and exercise goals, for a total of seven visits over the course of the first year of the study and then every 3 months for the remainder of the study. The primary goals for lifestyle intervention included weight reduction of 5% or more (not to exceed 0.5–1.0 kg per week), moderate physical activity of 30 minutes or more per day (endurance exercise recommended), total fat and saturated fat reduction, and increased fiber intake (15 g/1,000 kcal or more). A very-low-calorie diet was acceptable (after 6 months of onset of the study) if preferred by the subject to enhance weight loss.

Results of the DPS study showed a decrease in the proportion of sedentary individuals, a decrease in fat intake, and an increase in fiber intake in the intervention group compared to the control group at 1 and 3 years, with weight reductions of 3.5–4.5 kg (higher weight reduction at year 1 compared to year 3) compared to 0.9–1.0 kg in the control group. This translated to a risk reduction for diabetes development of 58% in the lifestyle intervention group compared to the control group [55]. It is worth noting that use of a very-low-calorie diet did not affect diabetes risk. The study investigators believed that the type of intensive lifestyle intervention used in the study (individualized and by skilled professionals) was a practice feasible to implement in the primary healthcare setting.

18.2.1.3 Diabetes Prevention Program

The Diabetes Prevention Program (DPP) randomized 3,234 subjects 25 years or older (mean age, 51 years) with fasting glucose values of 95–125 mg/dl and IGT to placebo, metformin, or a lifestyle intervention program [56]. The mean BMI was around 34 in all study groups, and participants in the study allowed for a diverse representation of ethnic and racial groups in the US population (American Indians, Hispanics, African Americans, Asians, and Pacific Islanders), with 45% of the study cohort constituting individuals of non-European ancestry. Individuals assigned to the intensive lifestyle intervention group were provided an individualized, flexible and culturally sensitive 16-lesson curriculum, administered by case managers and designed to help these participants achieve the following goals: at least 7% weight reduction, consumption of a low-calorie/low-fat diet, and at least 150 minutes per week of moderate physical activity (similar in intensity to brisk walking).

Results of the DPP, after an average follow-up period of 2.8 years, showed a 58% reduction in diabetes incidence in the intensive lifestyle intervention group and a 31% reduction in diabetes incidence in the metformin group when compared to the control group [56]. The treatment effect of intensive lifestyle intervention was significant in all subgroups and was greater in individuals with lower baseline glucose concentrations 2 hours after a glucose load when compared to those with higher baseline glucose concentrations. Lifestyle intervention was also noted to be more effective in older persons and those with a lower BMI. Restoration of normal glucose tolerance was noted in nearly 40% of individuals in the intensive lifestyle intervention group, a greater effect than seen with metformin or placebo [56].

The reduction in diabetes incidence in the DPP study was the same as the Finnish DPS but was higher than the reductions associated with interventions in the Da Qing study. The reversion to normal glucose tolerance in the DPP lifestyle intervention group is significant in that these individuals were 50% less likely to develop diabetes during long-term follow-up when compared to those who had persistent IGT status [58]. Additionally, post-study follow-up periods of 10–20 years demonstrated continued benefit of lifestyle intervention in decreasing diabetes incidence [59–61].

18.2.1.4   Indian Diabetes Prevention Program

The Indian Diabetes Prevention Program (IDPP) randomized South Asians with IGT to four arms: control (with standard advice, N = 136), lifestyle modification (N = 133), low-dose metformin (N = 133), and lifestyle modification plus low-dose metformin (N = 136) [57]. Participants in lifestyle modification groups received counseling sessions aimed at promoting healthy eating habits (decreased intake of refined carbohydrates and fats and increased intake of dietary fiber) and boosting physical activity (at least 30 minutes daily). After a median follow-up of 30 months, the relative reductions in diabetes incidence were 28.5% with lifestyle modification, 26.4% with metformin, and 28.2% with lifestyle modification and metformin [62]. Remarkably, these benefits of lifestyle modification occurred despite the lack of significant weight change in the two groups that focused on lifestyle change.

18.2.2   Medications for Diabetes Prevention

Even in the most successful of the randomized controlled trials, the risk reduction for incident diabetes following lifestyle intervention was approximately 60% [54–57]. This figure raises the question as to whether additive benefit in terms of diabetes risk reduction would be noted with medication use and whether medications could be offered to high-risk persons who are unable or unwilling to implement lifestyle changes, or in whom lifestyle modifications have failed to halt glycemic progression. Several of the landmark diabetes prevention trials also included pharmacological arms, and additional studies have specifically tested medications for diabetes prevention. Given the linear relationship between diabetes risk reduction and the amount of weight loss (approximately 10% for every 1 kg weight loss) [56,63], a medication that enhances or maintains weight loss would be a rational adjunct to lifestyle. What follows is a summary of medications that have been studied for the prevention of T2DM (Table 18.2).

Medications that have been studied for diabetes prevention include sulfonylureas, metformin, acarbose, orlistat, rosiglitazone, and pioglitazone. The DPP demonstrated that utilization of metformin, at 850-mg twice-daily dosing, decreased the development of diabetes in adults with IGT by 31% [56]. The diabetes prevention efficacy of metformin was observed primarily in younger, obese (BMI > 35 kg/m^2) individuals; among older or leaner participants, the effect of metformin in diabetes risk reduction was no better than that of placebo. In addition, restoration of normal fasting glucose values in the DPP study was achieved with similar efficacy in the metformin and lifestyle intervention arms, but metformin was less effective than lifestyle intervention in restoring normal post-load glucose levels. Mean weight loss in the metformin group was 2.1 kg, and rates of gastrointestinal side effects were highest in the metformin group [56].

TABLE 18.2

Randomized, Controlled Trials of Medications for Diabetes Prevention

Study	Intervention	Duration	Weight Effect (Mean Loss or Gain)	Risk of Progression to Diabetes Mellitus	Significant Side Effects of Medication	Reference
DPP	Metformin (850 mg BID) vs. lifestyle modification vs placebo	2.8 years	Loss of 2.1 kg	Reduction by 31%	GI symptoms	56
IDPP-1	Metformin (250–500 mg BID) vs. lifestyle modification + metformin vs lifestyle modification	3 years	No significant change	Reduction by 26%–28% but no additive benefit of metformin to lifestyle	Symptoms of hypoglycemia with higher metformin dosing regimen	57
STOP-NIDDM	Acarbose (100 mg TID) vs placebo	3.3 years	Loss of 2.8 kg	Reduction by 25%	Mild-moderate GI symptoms	64
XENDOS	Orlistat (120 mg TID) vs placebo	4 years	Loss of 5.8 kg	Reduction by 37%	Mild-moderate GI symptoms	65
IDDP-2	Pioglitazone (30 mg daily) + lifestyle modification vs placebo + lifestyle modification	3 years	Gain in pioglitazone group	No additive benefit of pioglitazone to lifestyle	No significant difference	73
DREAM	Rosiglitazone (8 mg daily) vs placebo	3 years	Gain of 2.2 kg	Reduction by 60%	Peripheral edema, weight gain, and heart failure	66
ACT NOW	Pioglitazone (30–45 mg daily) vs placebo	2.4 years	Gain of 3.6 kg	Reduction by 72%	Edema and weight gain	67
CANOE	Rosiglitazone (2 mg BID) + metformin (500 mg BID) vs placebo	3.9 years	No significant change	Reduction by 66%	Diarrhea	68

BID, twice daily; GI, gastrointestinal; TID, three times per day.

The STOP-NIDDM (Study to Prevent Non-Insulin-Dependent Diabetes Mellitus) utilized acarbose as the intervention drug and demonstrated a 25% decrease in the rate of progression to diabetes when compared to placebo [64]. Acarbose also increased the probability that IGT will revert to normal glucose tolerance over time. Mean weight loss was 2.8 kg with acarbose use, and mild to moderate gastrointestinal symptoms were the most significant side effect with acarbose use [64].

In the XENDOS (XENical in the Prevention of Diabetes in Obese Subjects) study, the pancreatic lipase inhibitor orlistat (when prescribed in combination with lifestyle modification) resulted in a 37% risk reduction in incident diabetes among subjects with impaired glucose tolerance, compared with lifestyle intervention alone [65]. In comparison to other medications used in diabetes prevention trials, orlistat demonstrated one of the greatest weight loss benefits, with a mean weight loss of 5.8 kg over a 4-year period. The weight loss benefit was noted in both the IGT and the NGT subgroups, although the reduction in diabetes incidence was only noted in the IGT subgroup. Mild to moderate gastrointestinal side effects were listed as the most common side effects with orlistat [65].

Thiazolidinedione drugs were tested in the DREAM (Diabetes Reduction Assessment with Ramipril and Rosiglitazone Medication) [66], ACT NOW (ACTos NOW for the Prevention of Diabetes) [67], and CANOE (CAnadian Normoglycemia Outcomes Evaluation) [68] studies. A risk reduction in diabetes of 60% was demonstrated in the DREAM study, which utilized rosiglitazone (8 mg daily) in conjunction with basic lifestyle recommendations. Rosiglitazone additionally increased the likelihood of regression to normoglycemia by 70%–80% when compared to placebo. Peripheral edema, weight gain, and heart failure were reported as side effects of rosiglitazone use [66]. The ACT NOW trial demonstrated a 72% diabetes risk reduction with pioglitazone use and a 48% conversion to normal glucose tolerance, with edema and weight gain as reported adverse effects of the medication [67]. A follow-up study examining effects of pioglitazone approximately 12 months after discontinuation of the medication demonstrated that a greater number of individuals achieved normoglycemia with pioglitazone in comparison to placebo, but the rate of conversion from IGT to T2DM was similar in the medication-treated group and the placebo group [69]. The CANOE trial showed that low-dose combination therapy with metformin (500 mg twice daily) and rosiglitazone (2 mg twice daily) decreased incident type 2 diabetes by 66% compared with placebo in IGT subjects. Regression to normal glucose tolerance was noted in almost 80% of the treatment group. Of note, the low doses were well-tolerated, with minimal effect on clinically relevant adverse events of the individual drugs [68].

In the NAVIGATOR trial, the use of valsartan for 5 years, along with lifestyle modification, led to a relative reduction of 14% in the incidence of diabetes among subjects with IGT, but the effect of nateglinide was not better than placebo [70].

18.2.2.1 Limitations of Medications

The drugs that have been tested for diabetes prevention are associated with a range of adverse effects, the need for continuous therapy to maintain their effects, and consequent adherence barriers. In the studies that tested the effect of interruption of metformin, rosiglitazone, and pioglitazone therapy for diabetes prevention, no sustained effect off medication was observed, which indicates that those medications did not fundamentally improve the underlying pathophysiology of prediabetes [69,71,72]. Moreover, in the IDPP-1 and IDPP-2, neither low-dose metformin nor pioglitazone, when tested in combination with lifestyle modification, achieved additive reduction of diabetes risk, compared to the effects of lifestyle modification alone [57,73]. Clearly, the cumulative costs of long-term (probably lifelong) therapy with medications (even where generic versions are available and no adverse effects occur) can be prohibitive, particularly for low-resource areas.

For reasons that have already been argued, the use of drugs for diabetes prevention cannot be recommended as a first-line approach in the general population. The latter conclusion is not to eschew societal expectation of safe, effective, and durable medications for diabetes prevention. Indeed, the poor human record of long-term adherence to behavioral recommendations and the known physiological adaptations that limit weight loss and trigger counterveiling mechanisms that promote weight regain [74] create a need for such adjunctive pharmacological agents. The ideal drug for diabetes prevention (Figure 18.2) should be nontoxic, well-tolerated, and at least as efficacious as lifestyle modification [33,75]. Additionally, such a drug should repair or improve the pathophysiological defects that underlie prediabetes, so that a durable effect that outlasts the period of medication can be expected. The latter attribute would permit withdrawal of the medication after a defined period of intervention, without the risk of prediabetes relapse. Finally, the cost of such a drug must not be prohibitive, bearing in mind the large number of people with prediabetes (86 million in the United States and more than 400 million worldwide).

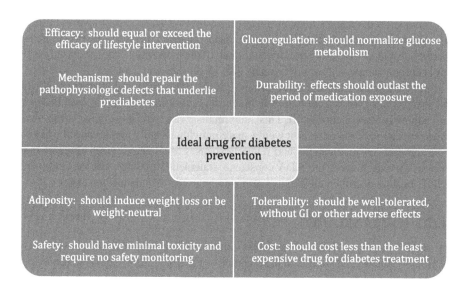

FIGURE 18.2 Desirable characteristics of an ideal drug for diabetes prevention.

18.2.2.2 Current Guidelines for Use of Medication for Diabetes Prevention

The American Diabetes Association (ADA) consensus statement [76] recommends lifestyle modification with a weight loss goal of 5%–10%, along with moderate physical activity of approximately 30 minutes daily for patients with IFG or IGT. Although no drug has been approved by the US Food and Drug Administration (FDA) for diabetes prevention, the ADA has suggested that treatment with metformin be considered as an adjunct to diet and exercise for the prevention of T2DM in selected high-risk persons [10,76]. Based on the subgroup analysis of the efficacy of metformin in the DPP, metformin was most effective in preventing diabetes in high-risk, very obese (BMI > 35 kg/m^2) prediabetic subjects younger than 60 years of age [56]. Additional selection criteria when considering metformin use in prediabetic subjects include a family history of diabetes in first-degree relatives, prior gestational diabetes mellitus, hypertriglyceridemia, subnormal high-density lipoprotein (HDL)-cholesterol levels, hypertension, and hemoglobin A1c (HbA1c) 5.7%–6.4% [10,76].

Even in persons who harbor all or most of these risk factors, active lifestyle modification is the preferred initial intervention; metformin can then be considered for individuals who fail to make significant progress. Currently, there are no clear guidelines for determining the optimal timing of metformin therapy, but failure of lifestyle intervention can be determined fairly empirically. The DPP participants assigned to lifestyle intervention lost approximately 7% of their baseline body weight during the first 6 months (i.e., approximately 1% per month). Thus, candidates for diabetes prevention who are unable to meet the lifestyle response target of losing approximately 1% per month of body weight during the initial 3–6 months of behavioral intervention may be considered for adjunctive metformin therapy.

The guidelines on the management of prediabetes, issued by the Indian Health Services (IHS) and the Australian Diabetes Society/Australian Diabetes Educators Association, emphasize lifestyle intervention prior to consideration of medications. The Australian guidelines recommend trying lifestyle intervention for a minimum of 6 months before considering drugs for diabetes prevention [77]. The IHS guidelines recommend addition of either metformin or pioglitazone if initial lifestyle intervention fails to improve dysglycemia in people with prediabetes [78]. The IHS guidelines state that the decision to use medication for diabetes prevention must be made on an individual basis and with the patient's full understanding [78].

Prediabetes is diagnosed based on the presence of either IFG alone, IGT alone (determined during oral glucose tolerance test), or both IFG and IGT. Individuals who have both IFG and IGT (so-called "double prediabetes") show more severe insulin resistance and impairment of beta-cell function compared to persons with a single prediabetes marker [76,79,80]. Nearly all persons with double prediabetes (approximately 96%) would qualify for metformin therapy, based on the ADA consensus criteria, whereas only approximately 30% of persons with isolated IFG would be eligible for metformin treatment using the same criteria [76,81]. This means that the use of OGTT can refine and sharply tailor the selection of individuals at greatest risk (i.e., those with IFG + IGT) for metformin adjunctive treatment [76,81]. This "maximalist" risk and "minimalist" drug intervention approach has much to commend it, as it would spare individuals and governments the huge expense of covering the costs of medications and related expenses for a much wider range of individuals from lower-risk pools. Indeed, the ADA consensus statement stipulates that the presence of both IFG and IGT must be documented if metformin is to be used for diabetes prevention [76].

18.3   KEYS TO TRANSLATION

In general, the keys to the translation of any new concept or discovery related to health consist of (1) adequate comprehension, evaluation, and acceptance of the new information within a specialized professional community; (2) processing and conversion of the new information into the professional knowledge base and dissemination to a wider circle of professionals and students; (3) diffusion of the conceptual information to the general public, through demonstrative education by convinced professionals; and (4) adoption of evidenced-based changes in practices and behaviors, triggered by the new knowledge. The preceding construct of translational cascade is somewhat akin to the sequential steps in Prochaska's transtheoretical model of behavior modification: *Pre-Contemplative, Contemplative, Preparation, Action, and Change* [82,83].

18.3.1   DISSEMINATION OF DIABETES PREVENTION KNOWLEDGE

The preponderance of evidence from randomized, clinical trials on the efficacy of lifestyle intervention in preventing T2DM has established the rationale for diabetes prevention as self-evident among health professionals. However, the screening for prediabetes and institution of prompt lifestyle counseling has not become routine practice, even in economically advanced countries. Bridging the hiatus between philosophical acceptance of the idea of diabetes prevention among health professionals and the adoption of pragmatic steps to detect and act upon high-risk persons requires a methodical approach.

The information and knowledge base of healthcare professionals must be steered toward a more pragmatic approach to primary prevention of diabetes through a number of established approaches. First, curriculum development in primary and high schools should begin to introduce seminal data from the behavioral components of the landmark diabetes prevention studies within a wider context of instruction in wellness and health promotion. Second, students in schools of medicine, nursing, pharmacy, and allied medical fields should receive exposure to formal instruction in the design and key findings of the major diabetes prevention studies—again, within the wider context of wellness and health promotion. Third, mastery of the principles and methods of primary prevention of T2DM ought to be a priority item in the core curriculum of residency training programs for physicians. The latter can be implemented through lectures and workshops by intramural experts and invited speakers. Finally, practicing physicians in all disciplines (including internists, family physicians, endocrinologists, cardiologists, nephrologists, and general and specialist surgeons), podiatrists, nurse practitioners, and other primary care providers must have their knowledge base updated to include the tenets of primary prevention of diabetes.

Operationally, the increased awareness about diabetes prevention at the primary care level should lead to increased zeal for screening and detection of individuals with prediabetes (often relatives of patients with established T2DM). Once individuals have been diagnosed with prediabetes, appropriate referral for lifestyle counseling can follow, as recommended by the ADA [10].

Convinced healthcare workers and their families become conduits for the dissemination and diffusion of diabetes prevention ideas in targeted segments of the public (hospital communities, established patients and their relatives, schools, neighborhoods, social media and outlets, religious forums, etc.). Most human societies have encountered diabetes and are probably preconditioned for receptive attention to diabetes campaigns, having been primed by awareness of the more obvious complications, such as blindness, amputation, and end-stage kidney disease. Such a preconditioning of societal awareness of diabetes and its complications bodes well for the dissemination of ideas regarding the rationale and feasibility of diabetes prevention. Yet, the fact that T2DM can be prevented by modest caloric restriction and physical activity is yet to enter folklore. That gap in the popular consciousness (despite the raging global epidemic of diabetes) presents an enormous opportunity for leadership by healthcare professionals and civic leaders. To convince and motivate large segments of society for preventive action against diabetes requires coordinated efforts at the local, regional, state, national, and international leadership levels. Creative programs anchored by ministries and departments of health, information, education, and other agencies would also be important catalysts for public education, awareness, and action. The expertise and contributions from philanthropic organizations and other nongovernmental bodies, especially local, national, and international diabetes associations, can be invaluable during the process of program building and facilitation.

18.3.2 Strategies for Diabetes Prevention in the Community

Five key elements can be distilled from the lifestyle intervention protocols utilized by the DPP and other major diabetes prevention trials. Most or all of these strategies can readily be adapted for widespread application in the community.

18.3.2.1 Selection of Persons at Risk

All diabetes prevention trials targeted, screened, and enrolled a defined group of at-risk persons, using well-known risk factors for T2DM. The merit of that approach is underscored by the finding that the participants randomized to placebo did in fact develop diabetes at an alarming rate (approximately 12% per year in DPP, approximately 18% per year in IDPP) [56]. Thus, the published criteria used for selecting at-risk persons for diabetes prevention appear to be of high fidelity and can be adopted for translation of diabetes prevention in the general populace. Specifically, a positive family history of T2DM in first-degree relatives, overweight or obesity (using ethnic-specific BMI cut-offs), and an FPG in the range of 96–125 mg/dl predict a high yield of eligible individuals for community diabetes prevention efforts. The appropriate BMI cutoff for identifying overweight subjects appears to be 22 kg/m^2 or more for Asians, compared with 25 kg/m^2 or more for most other ethnicities [84,85]. The inclusive age range for the published diabetes prevention studies was at least 25 years for DPP and Da Qing studies, 40–65 years for FDPS, and 30–55 years for IDPP [54–57]. None of the published diabetes prevention studies enrolled individuals younger than age 25 years, which is a major limitation, given the increasing prevalence of T2DM in children and adolescents [86,87]. Obesity and physical inactivity are major risk factors for T2DM in children, as in adults. Other risk factors include female gender, ethnicity, family history of T2DM, peripubertal age, and intrauterine exposure to diabetes [88–90]. Because the long-term complications of diabetes become established over a more than 10-year period, the epidemic of T2DM in children and adolescents predicts dire consequences for patients at the prime of their youth [91]. Primary prevention of childhood T2DM, therefore, is of utmost public health importance. For the aforementioned reasons, it is desirable for community diabetes prevention initiatives to lower the inclusive age for screening at-risk persons well into the childhood and adolescent years. A school-based pilot study sponsored by the US National Institutes of Health showed that obesity and diabetes risk factors can be decreased by lifestyle intervention in sixth-grade pupils [92].

18.3.2.2 Delivery of Physical Activity Intervention

The physical activity component of lifestyle intervention in the reported diabetes prevention studies was of moderate intensity (approximately 55% VO_2 max) and duration (approximately 30 minutes daily in the DPP). Out of an abundance of caution, participants in the DPP lifestyle intervention arm underwent submaximal cardiac stress testing prior to commencement of the physical activity program [93]; however, that was not a routine requirement for physical activity in the majority of diabetes prevention trials [54,55,57]. It must be stressed that physical activity was well-tolerated in the DPP, and no untoward cardiovascular events or musculoskeletal injuries were reported. A routine requirement for prescreening with cardiac stress would be a serious logistical and economic hindrance to the widespread translation of diabetes prevention, and may not be necessary for the majority of free-living individuals who are candidates for diabetes prevention in the community. The DPP exercise goal of 150 minutes per week was similar to that prescribed in the Malmo [94] and Da Qing [54] studies but lower than the 210 minutes per week prescribed in the Finnish study [55]. The DPP and all other landmark studies have demonstrated the efficacy, tolerability, and safety of moderate-intensity physical activity (150–210 minutes per week) as used for the prevention of T2DM [54–57,94]. Walking was the preferred activity for the vast majority of participants in these studies.

Given the generally low rates of voluntary physical activity in urbanized communities (58,95), innovative motivational strategies [95,96] will be required to build physical activity into daily routine, especially in high-risk populations. In clinical trials, the physical activity intervention component often required exercise physiologists or other skilled staff to implement. For large-scale community translation, these specialists may not be essential, as lay persons can be trained to deliver physical activity intervention. However, the infrastructure required for effective large-scale implementation of physical activity intervention—well-lit and safe walkways, public parks, biking trail, health and fitness clubs, et cetera—may not be readily available in many developing countries, especially at overcrowded urban centers. One innovative approach to the problem of space for physical activity is to establish partnerships with schools and houses of religious worship, so that their large real estate can be utilized for diabetes prevention activity after school hours and during nonworship days.

A tropical environment (especially high temperature, humidity, and torrential rain) constitutes an additional barrier to regular outdoor exercise. Cultural barriers to exercise may also exist in some communities, where obesity may be venerated as a sign of well-being and evidence of freedom from wasting diseases (such as malnutrition, HIV/AIDS, and tuberculosis). A less-obvious obstacle is a cultural mindset among blue collar workers that associates exercise with the privileged elite. These (mis)-perceptions must be confronted using education and public awareness campaigns. Such grassroots educational campaigns should emphasize the risks of obesity and the health benefits of modest increases in physical activity, thereby shifting the focus from exercise as indulgent leisure of the bourgeoisie to exercise as an engine of health promotion among the proletariat. Civic and local government leadership should collaborate to create community resources for participatory health promotion and wellness. The lowest reported dose of exercise that was effective in preventing diabetes was approximately 150 minutes per week (or approximately 30 minutes/day) [56]; however, significant metabolic benefits can be derived from shorter bouts of activity (10–15 minutes spread across two or three periods during the day) [97]. This specific point is worth emphasizing when counseling time-pressed subjects. Additionally, whenever appropriate, participatory physical activity and health promotion should be built into scheduled cultural festivals and other activities. The latter could include student-teacher and parent-child low-to-moderate intensity sporting events, parades, pageants, mini-carnivals, and other civic celebrations.

18.3.2.3 Frequent Contacts

The frequency of contacts between participants in diabetes prevention programs and lifestyle interventionists was weekly, monthly, bi-monthly, or quarterly, depending on the specific study protocols and phase of study. In the DPP, the greatest weight loss occurred during the initial

24 weeks of intensive individual weekly sessions with lifestyle coaches [56]. When the visit frequency was relaxed to monthly sessions, some weight regain was noted. Other studies, notably FDPS and Da Qing, used lower overall contact frequency (every 2 months to quarterly) and achieved comparable results to those achieved by the DPP [54,55]. Clearly, regular contact at some frequency between interventionists and participants is desirable for successful diabetes prevention. Such contacts could create favorable dynamics and "bonding" between lifestyle coach and participant. Moreover, the repeated objective recording of weight, waist circumference, and other metabolic measures could have important motivational effects. However, the optimal frequency of physical contacts necessary for successful diabetes prevention in the community is unclear and could well differ by cultural and regional peculiarities. Thus, such data would need to be determined through pilot studies in different communities. Fewer face-to-face counseling sessions in group format, supplemented by virtual contacts (via SMS text messaging, e-mail, or web-based platforms) could be a less-expensive approach to harnessing the power of contact in diabetes prevention efforts. Along these lines, web-based lifestyle programs have been reported to have modest but variable effects on weight loss in studies reported from Australia, the United States, Europe, and Asia [98–102]; however, extrapolation to populations with lower literacy and uncertain digital access is questionable.

18.3.2.4 Delivery of Dietary Intervention

The participants in the landmark diabetes prevention studies [54–57] were asked to reduce their daily intake of fat calories and total calories. Consumption of meals high in dietary fiber was also promoted. To help participants maintain a healthy eating pattern, additional training regarding reading and understanding food labels was provided. The nutritional counseling was delivered in person during the regular visits. As already discussed, there appeared to be a relationship between frequency of counseling visits and the magnitude of weight loss in the DPP. However, other programs that used less-frequent visits achieved comparable efficacy in diabetes prevention. Thus, following initial run-in and initiation of the dietary intervention, maintenance visits at approximately 3-month intervals may be sufficient to yield desirable results in a community setting.

Pragmatically, implementing dietary intervention for diabetes prevention in local communities in sub-Saharan Africa and other developing regions would be fraught with challenges. First, of course, is the shortage of trained and culturally adapted dietitians and medical nutritionists. Second, mandatory food labeling, the result of legislation passed some decades ago in the West, is not yet a routine practice in many developing countries. In fact, nutritional information may be lacking for many staple foods. Third, even where food labeling exists, low literacy rates mitigate against their comprehension. Furthermore, the popularity of informal retail markets (especially for grains, flour, corn, cereal, rice, beans, cassava powder [garri], and other tuber-derived staples) that do not offer standardized packaging calls for creative approaches to the implementation of caloric control. Thus, effective dietary intervention strategies for diabetes prevention in developing countries must anticipate and creatively overcome or circumvent these apparent translational obstacles. In that regard, the value of local pilot and feasibility studies cannot be overemphasized. In low-literacy regions, a visual (pictorial) approach to dietary modification could be an effective alternative to text-based formats. The Dietary Guidelines for Americans, issued by the USDA, advocates a simple plate method: Half of the plate contains fruits and vegetables; the other half is divided roughly equally into grains and protein [103]. The plate method [103,104] is an attractive model that can be evaluated as the basis for teaching portion control and optimal dietary habits in developing countries. The visual approach uses a graphic display of a typical plate, divided into segments that contain desirable food classes in optimal proportions [104].

18.3.2.5 Self-monitoring

Extensive self-monitoring of nutrient intake and minutes spent each day in physical activity (and type of activity) was an integral part of the lifestyle intervention in the DPP [56,93]. In other studies, the frequent self-monitoring of weight and anthropometrics has been reported to be associated with long-term maintenance of weight loss [105]. The exact mechanism whereby self-monitoring of eating and exercise behavior predicts good metabolic outcome is unclear. It is plausible that such a level of involvement in one's health could have a beneficial heuristic effect by guiding food choices and lifestyle decisions. For most persons in psychic equilibrium, the potential adverse psychological impact of frequent self-monitoring of nutrient intake and physical activity is probably negligible. For these reasons, it seems prudent to incorporate some element of self-monitoring component into a community-based diabetes prevention campaign. The focus of such monitoring could be type and amount (serving size) of food intake, daily physical activity minutes, and other lifestyle endpoints, as appropriate. In low-literacy situations, the use of domestic surrogates (spouses, relatives, school age children, neighbors, family friends, etc.) to capture these endpoints could be considered. Where feasible, self-monitored data can be transmitted via SMS text to the community diabetes prevention centers (CDPCs) for tracking and real-time interventional feedback purposes.

18.3.3 COMMUNITY DIABETES PREVENTION CENTERS

The sheer magnitude of the current and projected escalation of the diabetes epidemic in developing countries mandates the broadest possible response at the community level. One practical, efficient approach is the establishment of CDPCs at several locations on the African continent and in the Caribbean region, India and South Asia, the Pacific Rim, South and Central America, Australia, and New Zealand, as well as in communities inhabited by high-risk populations in Europe and North America. Such a groundswell of CDPCs can serve as essential focal points for the dissemination of diabetes prevention practices. Operationally, the CDPCs can be administered and staffed by the noncommunicable diseases branch of ministries and departments of health, or through partnership with nongovernmental organizations. The primary purpose of CDPCs would be to test and implement culturally and regionally appropriate models for the delivery of physical activity and dietary interventions. Referral to CDPCs can be based on a risk factor approach that focuses on genetic (e.g., family history of diabetes) and other risk markers. Individuals with diagnosed T2DM can be the conduits for referral of family members to CDPCs for prediabetes screening and intervention.

18.3.4 UNIQUE VULNERABILITIES IN DEVELOPING COUNTRIES AND TRANSLATING DIABETES PREVENTION TO COMMUNITIES IN DEVELOPING COUNTRIES

People with diabetes in developing countries, assuming current trends remain unabated, will account for over 70% of the global diabetes burden by the year 2035. Additional data from surveys in developing countries indicate that diabetes predominantly affects younger age groups: The majority of people with diabetes fall within the age range of 40–59 years, as compared to 60 years or older in developed countries [75]. It has also been predicted that future increases in diabetes numbers would affect all age groups in developing countries, whereas in developed countries, an increase is expected predominantly among persons older than 60 years, with a slight decrease in the younger age groups [75]. This younger age predilection means that individuals in developing countries in their prime productivity years are the ones burdened with diabetes and its complications, with dire consequences on national economics. Besides the enormous direct medical costs, the additional lost productivity from absenteeism and presenteeism inflict compounding negative effects on current and future economic performance in the developing world. Furthermore, the preponderance of diabetes in young women of childbearing age perpetuates a vicious cycle through the effects of intrauterine fetal programming for increased susceptibility to cardiometabolic disorders in postnatal life [62,106]. A more recent vulnerability is the unexpected association of successful antiretroviral therapy in HIV patients with treatment-emergent metabolic perturbations, including diabetes, dyslipidemia, and lipodystrophy [95,107].

Clearly, lifestyle modification is a remarkably and consistently effective intervention for preventing the development of T2DM in high-risk populations in China, India, Europe, and the United States. Some pilot projects have reported promising results among indigenous (Maori) New Zealanders [108]. However, the efficacy of lifestyle intervention needs to be confirmed in large randomized, controlled trials (RCTs) or pragmatic studies in other regions of the world (including Africa, Latin America, Australia, New Zealand, Middle-East, and Caribbean regions). There is overwhelming evidence that lifestyle modification is a more compelling approach to diabetes prevention than medications. However, the landmark lifestyle intervention programs that achieved remarkable success in preventing diabetes were designed as RCTs and conducted predominantly at academic medical centers. The protocols of many of the RCTs entailed frequent clinic visits, utilized specialized multidisciplinary teams (including physicians, nurses, dietitians, psychologists, exercise physiologists, and others), and consumed substantial resources and support from institutions and funding agencies. Notably, all protocol-mandated services and interventions were provided at no cost to participants in the diabetes prevention RCTs, many of whom also received incentives and stipends. Thus, the odds were stacked heavily toward success in these RCTs, and it is crucial to determine whether the sterling results obtained in the landmark RCTs could be reproduced in the community, without all the inbuilt advantages, specialized professionals, and resources. Some community initiatives are currently underway to determine the feasibility of community programs for diabetes prevention [109,110]. The CDC has been training and certifying community diabetes prevention personnel under the aegis of the National DPP [111]. Programs using trained laypersons to deliver adaptations of the DPP lifestyle intervention to groups (rather than one-on-one sessions) in the community have been shown to produce promising results [109,110,112].

18.3.5 Costs of Preventing Type 2 Diabetes

Analysis of costs associated with the DPP indicates that the overall expense to society of preventing diabetes was cost-effective [113–116]. Over 3 years, the direct medical costs of the DPP interventions were $79 per participant in the placebo group, $2,542 in the metformin group, and $2,780 in the lifestyle group [113,114]. Further, longer-term analysis indicated that lifestyle modification remained cost-effective, and metformin was potentially cost-saving when used for preventing diabetes [116]. Cost analysis in the IDPP showed that the T2DM prevention strategies in India, especially lifestyle intervention, were cost-effective [117]. The total cost of identifying one person with IGT was $117. The direct medical costs were $61 per person in the control group and $225 in the lifestyle intervention group [117]. The cost of preventing one case of T2DM through lifestyle modification in India was $1,052 [117]. The DPP, IDPP, and other trials were, by the nature of their design, quite resource-intensive.

Clearly, the adaptation of diabetes prevention programs to developing countries would require extensive cost-containment and cost-shifting strategies. Reduction in contact frequency, optimization of the size of the intervention personnel, and the use of group (rather than one-on-one) counseling format should decrease costs significantly. Furthermore, the use of trained lay (nonmedical) workers to implement lifestyle modification protocols in group sessions at CDPCs and prorated cost-sharing could be additional approaches to the implementation of affordable diabetes prevention programs in developing countries [109,118]. Even with a markedly scaled-down cost schedule, the low gross domestic product (approximately $500 per capita) in many developing countries suggests that these nations cannot afford to underwrite the costs of even a limited national diabetes prevention program. Given the immense future benefits to society from prevention of T2DM, novel funding sources (private, industry, international, philanthropic, and other agencies) would need to be explored and mobilized for successful implementation of diabetes prevention initiatives in most low- and middle-income countries.

18.4 CONCLUSION

Nearly 90 million adults in the United States and more than 400 million people around the world have prediabetes. Perhaps one of the most significant public health advances of the present era is the demonstration that progression from prediabetes to T2DM can be interrupted by effective interventions. Among the different interventions that have been demonstrated to prevent diabetes, lifestyle modification is the most appealing because of its superior efficacy, nontoxicity, and generalizable effects in persons from various ethnic backgrounds [54–57]. Based on data from the DPP, US ethnic minority groups showed similar sensitivity to the effects of lifestyle intervention, as did Caucasians in the DPP [56]. In contrast to well-known data demonstrating higher risk for diabetes development in certain ethnic minority groups, the DPP demonstrated relatively similar incidence of T2DM (around 12%) among African Americans, Asian Americans and Pacific Islanders, Caucasian Americans, Hispanic Americans, and Native Americans [56]. The finding of similar incident diabetes rates among individuals from different US racial and ethnic groups suggests that once individuals have progressed from normal glucose tolerance to IGT, the risk of further progression to diabetes may be less dependent on ethnic/racial factors. Further research is needed to identify the mechanisms and mediators of early glycemic progression. Additional support for lifestyle modifications as the primary intervention strategy is the durability of sustained benefits of diabetes prevention for up to 20 years following cessation of formal intervention [59–61]. The durability of medication effect in diabetes prevention has not clearly been demonstrated to date.

The effective translation of diabetes prevention across communities requires engagement and coordination at multiple levels within the healthcare establishment, civic society, and government agencies (Figure 18.3). Environmental and policy changes are needed to stimulate broad societal participation in wellness and diabetes prevention activities. Pilot and feasibility projects are needed to customize

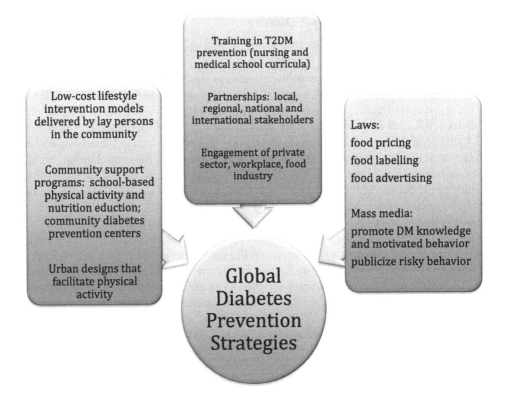

FIGURE 18.3 Global diabetes prevention strategies.

generally proven methodologies to local specificities and realities in developing countries and under-served communities. Ecological improvements that result in improved access to safe walking trails, well-lit and well-kept public parks, subsidized or affordable neighborhood fitness centers, and other appurtenances for health promotion would all augur well for the practice of community diabetes prevention. The establishment of CDPCs to serve as a hub for harmonizing the planning, delivery, and evaluation of lifestyle intervention activities would be an efficient approach to community diabetes prevention. Appropriate legislation that promotes food labeling, rewards healthful behavior, and redistributes revenue from "sin" taxes on tobacco and alcohol to fund community diabetes prevention initiatives would be well-directed. Clearly, great opportunities exist for innovative partnerships among governmental, civic, philanthropic, and other nongovernmental organizations toward a common purpose of stemming the global diabetes epidemic by focusing on primary prevention.

ACKNOWLEDGMENTS

SD-J is supported, in part, by grants (R01 DK067269, DK62203, DK48411) from the National Institutes of Health.

Disclosures: The authors have no conflicts of interest regarding the content of this chapter.

REFERENCES

1. International Diabetes Federation. *IDF Diabetes Atlas 2015; Seventh Edition.* Brussels, Belgium: International Diabetes Federation 2015.
2. World Health Organization. *Global Status Report on Noncommunicable Diseases 2014.* Geneva, Switzerland: WHO Press 2014.
3. Shaw JE, Sicree RA, Zimmet PZ. Global estimates of the prevalence of diabetes for 2010 and 2030. *Diabetes Res Clin Pract.* 2010;87:4–14.
4. Beran D, Yudkin, JS. Diabetes care in sub-Saharan Africa. *Lancet.* 2006;368:1689–95.
5. Dagogo-Jack S. Pattern of foot ulcer in diabetic Nigerians. *Pract Diabetes Dig.* 1991;2:75–8.
6. Dagogo-Jack S. Diabetic in-patient mortality in Nigeria. *Pract Diabetes Dig.* 1991;2:117–9.
7. Dagogo-Jack S. Primary prevention of cardiovascular disease in diabetic patients. *Cardiol Q.* 2006;12:20–5.
8. Banegas JR, Lopez-Garcia E, Dallongeville J, Guallar E, Halcox JP, Borghi C, et al. Achievement of treatment goals for primary prevention of cardiovascular disease in clinical practice across Europe: The EURIKA study. *Eur Heart J.* 2011;32:2143–53.
9. Ali MK, Bullard KM, Saaddine JB, Cowie CC, Imperatore G, Gregg EW. Achievement of goals in U.S. diabetes care, 1999–2010. *New Engl J Med.* 2013;368:1613–24.
10. American Diabetes Association. Standards of medical care in diabetes—2018. *Diabetes Care.* 2018;41:S1–S156.
11. Dagogo-Jack S. Preventing diabetes-related morbidity and mortality in the primary care setting. *J Natl Med Assoc.* 2002;94:549–60.
12. Dagogo-Jack S, Santiago JV. Pathophysiology of type 2 diabetes and modes of action of therapeutic interventions. *Arch Intern Med.* 1997;157:1802–17.
13. Defronzo RA. Banting Lecture. From the triumvirate to the ominous octet: A new paradigm for the treatment of type 2 diabetes mellitus. *Diabetes.* 2009;58:773–95.
14. DeFronzo RA. Insulin resistance, lipotoxicity, type 2 diabetes and atherosclerosis: The missing links. The Claude Bernard Lecture 2009. *Diabetologia.* 2010;53:1270–87.
15. Rasmussen BB, Holmbäck UC, Volpi E, Morio-Liondore B, Paddon-Jones D, Wolfe RR. Malonyl coenzyme A and the regulation of functional carnitine palmitoyltransferase-1 activity and fat oxidation in human skeletal muscle. *J Clin Invest.* 2002;110:1687–93.
16. Kitabchi AE, Temprosa M, Knowler WC, Kahn SE, Fowler SE, Haffner SM, et al. Role of insulin secretion and sensitivity in the evolution of type 2 diabetes in the diabetes prevention program: Effects of lifestyle intervention and metformin. *Diabetes.* 2005;54:2404–14.
17. Larson-Meyer DE, Heilbronn LK, Redman LM, Newcomer BR, Frisard MI, Anton S, et al. Effect of calorie restriction with or without exercise on insulin sensitivity, β-cell function, fat cell size, and ectopic lipid in overweight subjects. *Diabetes Care.* 2006;29:1337–44.

18. Kelley DE. Effects of weight loss on glucose homeostasis in NIDDM. *Diabetes Rev.* 1995;3:366–77.

19. Schneider SH, Morgado A. Effects of fitness and physical training on carbohydrate metabolism and associated cardiovascular risk factors in patients with diabetes. *Diabetes Rev.* 1995;3:378–407.

20. Rogers MA, Yamamoto C, King DS, Harberg JM, Ensani AA, Holloszy JO. Improvement in glucose tolerance after one week of exercise in patients with mild NIDDM. *Diabetes Care.* 1988;11:613–8.

21. Eriksson KF, Lindgarde F. Prevention of type 2 diabetes mellitus by diet and physical exercise. *Diabetologia.* 1991;34:891–8.

22. Mikines KJ, Sonne B, Farrell PA, Tronier B, Galbo H. Effect of physical exercise on sensitivity and responsiveness to insulin in humans. *Am J Physiol.* 1988;254:E248–59.

23. Goodyear LJ, Kahn BB. Exercise, glucose transport, and insulin sensitivity. *Annu Rev Med.* 1998;49:235–61.

24. Steven S, Hollingsworth KG, Al-Mrabeh A, Avery L, Aribisala B, Caslake M, et al. Very-low-calorie diet and 6 months of weight stability in type 2 diabetes: Pathophysiologic changes in responders and nonresponders. *Diabetes Care.* 2016. pii: dc151942. [Epub ahead of print].

25. Hu F. Globalization of diabetes: The role of diet, lifestyle, and genes. *Diabetes Care.* 2011;34:1249–57.

26. Egede LE, Dagogo-Jack S. Epidemiology of type 2 diabetes: Focus on ethnic minorities. *Med Clin N Am.* 2005;89:949–75.

27. Tanizawa Y, Riggs AC, Dagogo-Jack S, Vaxillaire M, Froguel P, Liu L, et al. Isolation of the human LIM/homeodomain gene islet-1 and identification of a simple sequence repeat polymorphism. *Diabetes.* 2004;43:935–41.

28. Ehm MG, Karnoub MC, Sakul H, Gottschalk K, Holt DC, Weber JL, et al; American Diabetes Association GENNID Study Group. Genetics of NIDDM. Genome wide search for type 2 diabetes susceptibility genes in four American populations. *Am J Hum Genet.* 2000;66:1871–81.

29. McCarthy M, Zeggini E. Genome-wide association studies in type 2 diabetes. *Curr Diab Rep.* 2009; 9:164–71.

30. Hivert MF, Jablonski KA, Perreault L, Saxena R, McAteer JB, Franks PW, et al. Updated genetic score based on 34 confirmed type 2 diabetes Loci is associated with diabetes incidence and regression to normoglycemia in the diabetes prevention program. *Diabetes.* 2011;60:1340–8.

31. Dagogo-Jack S. Predicting Diabetes: Our relentless quest for genomic nuggets. *Diabetes Care.* 2012; 35:193–5.

32. Fujimoto WY, Leonetti DL, Kinyoun JL, Newell-Morris L, Shuman WP, Stolov WC, et al. Prevalence of diabetes mellitus and impaired glucose tolerance among second-generation Japanese-American men. *Diabetes.* 1987;36:721–9.

33. Dagogo-Jack S, Edeoga C. Understanding and identifying pre-diabetes – Can we halt the diabetes epidemic? *Eur Endocrinol.* 2008;4:16–8.

34. Pour OR, Dagogo-Jack S. Prediabetes as a therapeutic target. *Clin Chem.* 2011;57:215–20.

35. Maschirow L, Khalaf K, Al-Aubaidy HA, Jelinek HF. Inflammation, coagulation, endothelial dysfunction and oxidative stress in prediabetes—Biomarkers as a possible tool for early disease detection for rural screening. *Clin Biochem.* 2015;48:581–5.

36. Nyenwe EA, Dagogo-Jack S. Metabolic syndrome, prediabetes and the science of primary prevention. *Minerva Endocrinol.* 2011;36:129–45.

37. Tabák A, Herder C, Rathmann W, Brunner E, Kivimäki M. Prediabetes: A high-risk state for diabetes development. *Lancet.* 2012;379:2279–90.

38. Weir G, Bonner-Weir S. Five stages of evolving progression to diabetes. *Diabetes.* 2004;53:S16–21.

39. Weyer C, Bogardus C, Mott DM, Pratley R. The natural history of insulin secretory dysfunction and insulin resistance in the pathogenesis of type 2 diabetes mellitus. *J Clin Invest.* 1999;104:787–94.

40. Toft-Nielsen MB, Damholt MB, Madsbad S, Hilsted LM, Hughes TE, Michelsen BK, et al. Determinants of the impaired secretion of glucagon-like peptide-1 in type 2 diabetic patients. *J Clin Endocrinol Metab.* 2001;86:3717–23.

41. Papaetis G. Incretin-based therapies in prediabetes: Current evidence and future perspectives. *World J Diabetes.* 2014;5:817–34.

42. Lopategi A, López-Vicario C, Alcaraz-Quiles J, García-Alonso V, Titos E, Clària J, et al. Role of bioactive lipid mediators in obese adipose tissue inflammation and endocrine dysfunction. *Mol Cell Endocrinol.* 2016;419:44–59.

43. Cerasi E, Luft R. The prediabetic state, its nature and consequences—A look toward the future. *Diabetes.* 1972;21 (Suppl. 2):685–94.

44. Centers for Disease Control and Prevention. National Diabetes Statistics Report: Estimates of Diabetes and Its Burden in the United States, 2014. Atlanta, GA: US Department of Health and Human Services; 2014.

45. Edelstein SL, Knowler WC, Bain RP, et al. Predictors of progression from impaired glucose tolerance to NIDDM: An analysis of six prospective studies. *Diabetes*. 46:701–10, 1997.

46. Knowler WC, Bennett PH, Hamman RF, Miller M. Diabetes incidence and prevalence in Pima Indians: A 19-fold greater incidence than in Rochester, Minnesota. *Am J Epidemiol*. 1978;108:497–505.

47. Weyer C, Bogardus C, Mott DM, Pratley R. The natural history of insulin secretory dysfunction and insulin resistance in the pathogenesis of type 2 diabetes mellitus. *J Clin Invest*. 1999;104:787–94.

48. Brancati FL, Kao WH, Folsom AR, Watson RL, Szklo M. Incident type 2 diabetes mellitus in African American and white adults: The Atherosclerosis Risk in Communities Study. *JAMA*. 2000;283:2253–9.

49. Weyer C, Tataranni PA, Bogardus C, Pratley R. Insulin resistance and insulin secretory dysfunction are independent predictors of worsening glucose tolerance during each stage of type 2 diabetes development. *Diabetes Care*. 2001;24:89–94.

50. Meigs JB, Muller DC, Nathan DM, Blake DR, Andres R. The natural history of progression from normal glucose tolerance to type 2 diabetes in the Baltimore longitudinal study of aging. *Diabetes*. 2003;52:1475–84.

51. Dagogo-Jack S, Edeoga C, Ebenibo S, Nyenwe E, Wan J. Lack of racial disparity in incident prediabetes and glycemic progression among black and white offspring of parents with type 2 diabetes: The pathobiology of prediabetes in a biracial cohort (POP-ABC) study. *J Clin Endocrinol Metab*. 2014;99:E1078–87.

52. Boucher AB, Adesanya EAO, Owei I, Gilles AK, Ebenibo S, Wan J, Edeoga C, Dagogo-Jack S. Dietary habits and leisure-time physical activity in relation to adiposity, dyslipidemia, and incident dysglycemia in the Pathobiology of Prediabetes in A Biracial Cohort Study. *Metabolism*. 2015;64:1060–7.

53. Jiang Y, Owei I, Wan J, Ebenibo S, Dagogo-Jack S. Adiponectin levels predict prediabetes risk: The Pathobiology of Prediabetes in A Biracial Cohort (POP-ABC) Study. *BMJ Open Diabetes Res Care*. 2016;4:e000194. doi:10.1136/bmjdrc-2016.

54. Pan XR, Li GW, Hu YH, Wang JX, Yang WY, An ZX, et al. Effects of diet and exercise in preventing NIDDM in people with impaired glucose tolerance: The Da Qing IGT and Diabetes Study. *Diabetes Care*. 1997;20:537–44.

55. Tuomilehto J, Lindstrom J, Eriksson J, Valle T, Hamalainen H. Prevention of type 2 diabetes mellitus by changes in lifestyle among subjects with impaired glucose tolerance. *N Engl J Med*. 2001;344:1343–50.

56. DPP Research Group. Reduction in the incidence of type 2 diabetes with lifestyle intervention or metformin. *N Engl J Med*. 2002;346:393–403.

57. Ramachandran A, Snehalatha C, Mary S, Mukesh B, Bhaskar AD, Vijay V; Indian Diabetes Prevention Programme (IDPP). The Indian Diabetes Prevention Programme shows that lifestyle modification and metformin prevent type 2 diabetes in Asian Indian subjects with impaired glucose tolerance (IDPP-1). *Diabetologia*. 2006;49:289–97.

58. Perreault L, Pan Q, Mather KJ, Watson KE, Hamman RF, Kahn SE; Diabetes Prevention Program Research Group. Effect of regression from prediabetes to normal glucose regulation on long-term reduction in diabetes risk: Results from the Diabetes Prevention Program Outcomes Study. *Lancet*. 2012;379:2243–51.

59. Diabetes Prevention Program Research Group. 10-year follow-up of diabetes incidence and weight loss in the Diabetes Prevention Program Outcomes Study. *Lancet*. 2009;374:1677–86.

60. Lindström J, Ilanne-Parikka P, Peltonen M, Aunola S, Eriksson JG, Hemiö K, Sustained reduction in the incidence of type 2 diabetes by lifestyle intervention: Follow-up of the Finnish Diabetes Prevention Study. *Lancet*. 2006;368:1673–79.

61. Li G, Zhang P, Wang J, An Y, Gong Q, Gregg EW, et al. Cardiovascular mortality, all-cause mortality, and diabetes incidence after lifestyle intervention for people with impaired glucose tolerance in the Da Qing Diabetes Prevention Study: A 23-year follow-up study. *Lancet Diabetes Endocrinol*. 2014;2:474–80.

62. Francis-Emmanuel PM, Thompson DS, Barnett AT, Osmond C, Byrne CD, Hanson MA, et al. Glucose metabolism in adult survivors of severe acute malnutrition. *J Clin Endocrinol Metab*. 2014;99:2233–40.

63. Hamman RF, Wing RR, Edelstein SL, Lachin JM, Bray GA, Delahanty L, et al. Effect of weight loss with lifestyle intervention on risk of diabetes. *Diabetes Care*. 2006;29:2102–7.

64. Chiasson JL, Josse RG, Gomis R, Hanefeld M, Karasik A, Laakso M. STOP-NIDDM Trial Research Group. Acarbose for prevention of type 2 diabetes mellitus: The STOP-NIDDM randomised trial. *Lancet*. 2002;359:2072–7.

65. Orgerson JS, Hauptman J, Boldrin MN, Sjöström L. XENical in the prevention of Diabetes in Obese Subjects (XENDOS) study: A randomized study of orlistat as an adjunct to lifestyle changes for the prevention of type 2 diabetes in obese patients. *Diabetes Care*. 2004;27:155–61.

66. DREAM (Diabetes REduction Assessment with ramipril and rosiglitazone Medication) Trial Investigators. Effect of rosiglitazone on the frequency of diabetes in patients with impaired glucose tolerance or impaired fasting glucose: A randomised controlled trial. *Lancet.* 2006;368:1096–105.

67. DeFronzo RA, Tripathy D, Schwenke DC, Banerji M, Bray GA, Buchanan TA, et al. ACT NOW Study. Pioglitazone for diabetes prevention in impaired glucose tolerance. *N Engl J Med.* 2011;364:1104–15.

68. Zinman B, Harris SB, Neuman J, Gerstein HC, Retnakaran RR, Raboud J, et al. Low-dose combination therapy with rosiglitazone and metformin to prevent type 2 diabetes mellitus (CANOE trial): A double-blind randomised controlled study. *Lancet.* 2010;376:103–11.

69. Tripathy D, Schwenke DC, Banerji M, Bray GA, Buchanan TA, Clement SC, et al. Diabetes incidence and glucose tolerance after termination of pioglitazone therapy: Results from ACT NOW. *J Clin Endocrinol Metab.* 2016;101(5):2056–2062.

70. NAVIGATOR Study Group. Effect of valsartan on the incidence of diabetes and cardiovascular events. *N Engl J Med.* 2010;362:1477–90.

71. DPP Research Group. Effects of withdrawal from metformin on the development of diabetes in the diabetes prevention program. *Diabetes Care.* 2003;26:977–80.

72. DREAM Trial Investigators. Incidence of diabetes following ramipril or rosiglitazone withdrawal. *Diabetes Care.* 2011;34:1265–9.

73. Ramachandran A, Snehalatha C, Mary S, Selvam S, Kumar CK, Seeli AC, Shetty AS. Pioglitazone does not enhance the effectiveness of lifestyle modification in preventing conversion of impaired glucose tolerance to diabetes in Asian Indians: Results of the Indian Diabetes Prevention Programme-2 (IDPP-2). *Diabetologia.* 2009;52:1019–26.

74. Greenway FL. Physiological adaptations to weight loss and factors favouring weight regain. *Int J Obes (Lond)* 2015. doi:10.1038/ijo.2015.59.

75. Echouffo-Tcheugui JB, Dagogo-Jack S. Preventing diabetes mellitus in developing countries. *Nat Rev Endocrinol.* 2012;8:557–62.

76. Nathan DM, Davidson MB, DeFronzo RA, Heine RJ, Henry RR, Pratley R, Zinman B. Impaired fasting glucose and impaired glucose tolerance. *Diabetes Care.* 2007;30:753–9.

77. Twigg SM, Kamp MC, Davis TM, Neylon EK, Flack JR; Australian Diabetes Society and Australian Diabetes Educators Association. Prediabetes: A position statement from the Australian Diabetes Society and Australian Diabetes Educators Association. *Med J Aust.* 2007;186:461–5.

78. Indian Health Services. *2008 IHS Guidelines for Care of Adults With Prediabetes and/or the Metabolic Syndrome in Clinical Settings*; 2005. http://www.unitefordiabetessjc.org/Portals/0/2005 NDPPPreDMMetsynGuidelines042605%20(1).pdf (Accessed April 3, 2016).

79. Dagogo-Jack S, Askari H, Tykodi G. Glucoregulatory physiology in subjects with low-normal, high-normal, or impaired fasting glucose. *J Clin Endocrinol Metab.* 2009;94:2031–6.

80. Kanat M, Mari A, Norton L, Winnier D, DeFronzo RA, Jenkinson C, Abdul-Ghani MA. Distinct β-cell defects in impaired fasting glucose and impaired glucose tolerance. *Diabetes.* 2012;61:447–53.

81. Rhee MK, Herrick K, Ziemer DC, Vaccarino V, Weintraub WS, Narayan KM, et al. Many Americans have pre-diabetes and should be considered for metformin therapy. *Diabetes Care.* 2010;33:49–54.

82. Velicer WF, Brick LA, Fava JL, Prochaska JO. Testing 40 predictions from the transtheoretical model again, with confidence. *Multivariate Behav Res.* 2013;48:220–40.

83. Norcross JC, Krebs PM, Prochaska JO. Stages of change. *J Clin Psychol.* 2011;67:143–54.

84. Pan WH, Flegal KM, Chang HY, Yeh WT, Yeh CJ, Lee WC. Body mass index and obesity-related metabolic disorders in Taiwanese and US whites and blacks: Implications for definitions of overweight and obesity for Asians. *Am J Clin Nutr.* 2004;79:31–39.

85. Yang W, Lu J, Weng J, Jia W, Ji L, Xiao J, Prevalence of diabetes among men and women in China. *N Engl J Med.* 2010;362:1090–101.

86. Pohl JH, Greer JA, Hasan KS. Type 2 diabetes mellitus in children. *Endocr Pract.* 1998;4:413–6.

87. Kaufman FR. Type 2 diabetes mellitus in children and youth: A new epidemic. *J Pediatr Endocrinol Metab.* 2002;15 (Suppl 2):737–44.

88. Alberti G, Zimmet P, Shaw J, Bloomgarden Z, Kaufman F, Silink M; Consensus Workshop Group. Type 2 diabetes in the young: The evolving epidemic: The international diabetes federation consensus workshop. *Diabetes Care.* 2004;27:1798–811.

89. Wiegand S, Maikowski U, Blankenstein O, Biebermann H, Tarnow P, Gruters A. Type 2 diabetes and impaired glucose tolerance in European children and adolescents with obesity – A problem that is no longer restricted to minority groups. *Eur J Endocrinol.* 2004;151:199–206.

90. Caprio S. Development of type 2 diabetes mellitus in the obese adolescent: A growing challenge. *Endocr Pract.* 2012;18:791–5.

91. TODAY Study Group. Rapid rise in hypertension and nephropathy in youth with type 2 diabetes: The TODAY clinical trial. *Diabetes Care.* 2013;36:1735–41.

92. HEALTHY Study Group. A school-based intervention for diabetes risk reduction. *N Engl J Med.* 2010; 363:443–45.

93. The Diabetes Prevention Program Research Group. The Diabetes Prevention Program (DPP): Description of lifestyle intervention. *Diabetes Care.* 2002;25:2165–71.

94. Eriksson KF, Lindgarde F. Prevention of type 2 (noninsulin-dependent) diabetes mellitus by diet and physical exercise: The 6-year Malmo feasibility study. *Diabetologia.* 1991;4:891–8.

95. Pate RR, Pratt M, Blair SN, Haskell WL, Macera CA, Bouchard C, et al. Physical activity and public health: Recommendation from the Centers for Disease Control and Prevention and the American College of Sports Medicine. *JAMA.* 1995;273:402–7.

96. Kimm SY, Glynn NW, Kriska AM, Barton BA, Kronsberg SS, Daniels SR, et. al. Decline in physical activity in black and white girls during adolescence. *N Engl J Med.* 2002;347:709–15.

97. Hood MS, Little JP, Tarnopolsky MA, Myslik F, Gibala MJ. Low-volume interval training improves muscle oxidative capacity in sedentary adults. *Med Sci Sports Exerc.* 2011;43:1849–56.

98. Tate DF, Wing RR, Winett RA. Using Internet technology to deliver a behavioral weight loss program. *JAMA.* 2001;285:1172–7.

99. Neve M, Morgan PJ, Jones PR, Collins CE. Effectiveness of web-based interventions in achieving weight loss and weight loss maintenance in overweight and obese adults: A systematic review with meta-analysis. *Obes Rev.* 2010;11:306–21.

100. Kodama S, Saito K, Tanaka S, Horikawa C, Fujiwara K, Hirasawa R, et al. Effect of Web-based lifestyle modification on weight control: A meta-analysis. *Int J Obes (Lond).* 2012;36:675–85.

101. Kohl LF, Crutzen R, de Vries NK. Online prevention aimed at lifestyle behaviors: A systematic review of reviews. *J Med Internet Res.* 2013;15:e146. doi: 10.2196/jmir.2665.

102. Watson S, Woodside JV, Ware LJ, Hunter SJ, McGrath A, Cardwell CR, et al. Effect of a web-based behavior change program on weight loss and cardiovascular risk factors in overweight and obese adults at high risk of developing cardiovascular disease: Randomized controlled trial. *J Med Internet Res.* 2015;17(7):e177. doi: 10.2196/jmir.3828.

103. US Department of Agriculture Center for Nutrition Policy and Promotion. Dietary Guidelines for Americans; 2015. http://www.cnpp.usda.gov/dietaryguidelines.htm (Accessed April 5, 2016).

104. Camelon KM, Hådell K, Jämsén PT, Ketonen KJ, Kohtamäki HM, Mäkimatilla S, et al. The Plate Model: A visual method of teaching meal planning. DAIS Project Group. Diabetes Atherosclerosis Intervention Study. *J Am Diet Assoc.* 1998;98:1155–8.

105. Wing RR, Phelan S. Long-term weight loss maintenance. *Am J Clin Nutr.* 2005;82 (Suppl.):222S–5S.

106. Dabelea D, Knowler WC, Pettitt DJ. Effect of diabetes in pregnancy on offspring: Follow-up research in the Pima Indians. *J Matern Fetal Med.* 2000;9:83–8.

107. Dagogo-Jack S. HIV therapy and diabetes risk (Editorial). *Diabetes Care.* 2008;31:1267–68.

108. Simmons, D, Rush E, Crook, N. Development and piloting of a community health worker-based intervention for the prevention of diabetes among New Zealand Maori in Te Wai o Rona: Diabetes Prevention Strategy. *Public Health Nutr.* 2008;11:1318–25.

109. Ackermann RT, Marrero DG. Adapting the Diabetes Prevention Program lifestyle intervention for delivery in the community: The YMCA model. *Diabetes Educ.* 2007;33:69, 74–5, 77–8.

110. Albright AL, Gregg EW. Preventing type 2 diabetes in communities across the U.S.: The National Diabetes Prevention Program. *Am J Prev Med.* 2013;44(4 Suppl 4):S346–51.

111. Albright A. The national diabetes prevention program: From research to reality. *Diabetes Care Educ Newsl.* 2012 Summer;33(4):4–7.

112. Hays LM, Finch EA, Saha C, Marrero DG, Ackermann RT. Effect of self-efficacy on weight loss: A psychosocial analysis of a community-based adaptation of the diabetes prevention program lifestyle intervention. *Diabetes Spectr.* 2014;27:270–5.

113. Diabetes Prevention Program (DPP) Research Group. Cost associated with the primary prevention of type 2 diabetes mellitus in the diabetes prevention program. *Diabetes Care.* 2003;26:36–47.

114. Diabetes Prevention Program Research Group. Within-trial cost-effectiveness of lifestyle intervention or metformin for the primary prevention of type 2 diabetes. *Diabetes Care.* 2003;26:2518–23.

115. Herman WH, Hoerger TJ, Brandle M, Hicks K, Sorensen S, Zhang P, et al. Diabetes Prevention Program Research Group. The cost-effectiveness of lifestyle modification or metformin in preventing type 2 diabetes in adults with impaired glucose tolerance. *Ann Intern Med.* 2005;142:323–32.

116. Diabetes Prevention Program Research Group. The 10-year cost-effectiveness of lifestyle intervention or metformin for diabetes prevention: An intent-to-treat analysis of the DPP/DPPOS. *Diabetes Care.* 2012;35:723–30.

117. Ramachandran A, Snehalatha C, Yamuna A, Mary S., Ping Z. Cost-effectiveness of the interventions in the primary prevention of diabetes among Asian Indians: Within-trial results of the Indian Diabetes Prevention Programme (IDPP). *Diabetes Care.* 2007;30:2548–52.

118. Ackermann RT, Marrero DG, Hicks KA, Hoerger TJ, Sorensen S, Zhang P, et al. An evaluation of cost sharing to finance a diet and physical activity intervention to prevent diabetes. *Diabetes Care.* 2006;29:1237–41.

19 Management of Diabetes Mellitus in Sub-Saharan Africa
Focus on Nigeria

Olufemi A. Fasanmade, Amie A. Ogunsakin, and Sam Dagogo-Jack

CONTENTS

19.1   INTRODUCTION

Management of any medical condition starts with obtaining a good history, performing careful physical examination, generating differential diagnoses, and confirming a definitive diagnosis through appropriate clinical and laboratory investigations. Management of diabetes mellitus (DM), a common noncommunicable disease (NCD), follows this same pattern. However, the management of diabetes in sub-Saharan Africa and other developing countries has some peculiarities that will be highlighted in this chapter, using Nigeria and other countries as reference points.

19.1.1   PRESENTATION OF DIABETES MELLITUS IN DEVELOPING COUNTRIES

Developing countries are often low income and low-medium income countries with varying levels of literacy and access to social amenities and infrastructure. The gross domestic product (GDP) of Nigeria is low at $5,900. The literacy rate of Nigeria is up to 51%–80% in urban cities among the youth but as low as 20%–30% in rural areas. Literacy in women is much lower than for males. Tragically, life expectancy at birth in Nigeria and several developing countries is approximately 50 years for men and approximately 55 years for women.[1-4] These stark realities have substantial impact on the clinical presentation and quality of care of DM.[5-7] Low scientific literacy (especially health illiteracy) permits the flourishing of substituted (typically unscientific) traditional beliefs and perceptions about etiology, pathophysiology, and management of diverse medical conditions.[7] Consequently, many patients delay in presenting to orthodox medical clinics, thereby exposing themselves to the deleterious effects of the unorthodox care and the risk of harboring advanced disease.[7] In many sub-Saharan African countries, 50%–75% of patients with diabetes are undiagnosed, one of the highest undiagnosed rates amongst the various regions[8] (Table 19.1). The reasons adduced for the high rate of undiagnosed diabetes center mostly around poor literacy, belief in local traditional explanations of illness, and misguided search for "cures"

TABLE 19.1

Prevalence Estimates of Diagnosed Diabetes Mellitus in Selected Regions and Countries of Sub-Saharan Africa

African Region	Country	Diagnosed DM Cases	Prevalence (%)
West	Nigeria	1,731,811	1.8
East	Kenya	463,903	1.8
Central	DRC	151,729	6.1
South	South Africa	1,865,021	5.1

Source: International Diabetes Federation Diabetes Atlas, 8th edition, www.diabetesatlas.org, 2017.

Note: Estimates for undiagnosed DM are unreliable but believed to be 50%–75% of all diabetes patients in the region.[8]

DM, diabetes mellitus; DRC, Democratic Republic of Congo.

from traditional healers. Polyuria and polydipsia often do not lead to prompt presentation until the patients become very ill. Weight loss, blurred vision, and malaise are often self-diagnosed as "malaria" or attributed to stressful work and sometimes to evil forces.[9,10] Even among persons with diagnosed diabetes, symptoms of the diabetic complications tend to be attributed to strange or unseen forces. These beliefs and practices markedly delay presentation to modern health care facilities, and usually occur after trial of herbal concoctions dispensed by traditional healers. These traditional remedies further complicate the presentation of the disease.[9–11] Paresthesia is often treated by scarification marks or application of hot or sometimes corrosive topical agents, all worsening the already-complicated diabetes.

In the urban areas of these developing countries, earlier presentation may occur, and less use of herbal or traditional medications is observed, but the patients still present late, symptoms often being attributed to other factors or diseases. Almost every case is treated first for malaria, then typhoid fever, sometimes once or twice, with little evidence to support either of these wrong diagnoses.[12]

19.1.2 CHALLENGES OF DIAGNOSIS AND TREATMENT

The diagnosis of DM is often made after the first or second visit to the primary or secondary care center because of a dearth of point-of-care testing or bedside urine or blood testing facilities. Due to these diagnostic deficiencies and treatment delays, many patients lose confidence in the health-care system and bypass primary/secondary levels of health care to present directly at tertiary centers. The latter contributes to the characteristic overcrowding of the tertiary centers in developing countries, which leads to long clinic hours, exhausted and time-pressed health care providers, and suboptimal patient engagement during the delivery of care. Many patients do not get an hemoglobin A1c (HbA1c) test done for years due to poverty, ignorance, or lack of equipment or reagents/cartridges, or a combination of these factors. Getting an HbA1c done can cost up to N7000 ($19), which is approximately one-third of the Nigerian monthly minimum wage, thus disenfranchising 75% of the populace.[13,14] Thus, most treatment regimens are based on only the fasting blood glucose (FBG) result, random/postprandial glucose tests, or urine glucose testing in rural or suburban centers. The resultant imprecision of urine and blood glucose measurements as estimates of chronic glycemic burden leads to suboptimal treatment to target. In many instances, there are no targets set by the attending medical personnel, and little else apart from the blood sugars and blood pressures are monitored. Lipid profile measurements are beyond the reach of many patients at primary and secondary care levels, which hampers documentation of comorbid cardiovascular risks.[15] Overall, the management of DM in most sub-Saharan African countries is generally suboptimal, with consequent poor health outcomes (Table 19.2).

TABLE 19.2

Challenges to Effective Diabetes Care in Sub-Saharan Africa

Screening/Prevention	Policy and Guidelines	Healthcare System	Access
Prompt and early intervention not readily available	No operational policy/action plan to avoid obesity and overweight	Scarcity of widely available comprehensive diabetes care centers	Limited availability and affordability of medicines
Suboptimal routine surveillance and management of complications	Lack of integrated management of diabetes and other chronic health conditions	Near absence of standard diabetes multidisciplinary team	Limited access to diabetes technologies
Low awareness of diabetes as a chronic condition	Lack of local research data to guide policies and improve care	Poor communication infrastructure	Low socioeconomic status and health literacy

19.2 ORGANIZATION OF DIABETES IN SUB-SAHARAN AFRICA: EXAMPLE FROM NIGERIA

Most of the people with DM are seen in secondary institutions (general hospitals, specialist hospitals, private hospitals). More complicated cases are seen in the few tertiary centers (less than 60 of such centers exist) in Nigeria, a country of 182 million people spread over 36 states and the Federal Capital Territory (Abuja).[16] There are approximately 2–5 million people with DM in Nigeria, the most populous black country (accurate prevalence studies are scarce). More than half of these people living with DM remain undiagnosed.[8,17] Approximately one-third of these are found in the rural areas, and the rest are in the urban areas.[18,19] Frequently, DM cases are only suspected when the patient has polyuria, polydipsia, and weight loss, the classic symptoms of DM, or when presenting to the emergency room or outpatient clinics with diabetic complications. The diagnosis of DM is often missed because routine or mandatory blood glucose testing on all admitted patients is only done in few centers. The common complications patients present with include acute metabolic complications, such as hyperglycemic emergencies, or symptoms pointing to chronic complications, such as paresthesia of the lower limbs, blurred vision, poor obstetric history, erectile dysfunction, carbuncles, or poorly healing foot ulcers.[20,21] A small number of DM cases are discovered during public health screening programs, routine community medical screening programs, pre-employment medical checks, and for investigation of other conditions, such as infertility, hypertension, stroke, and others.[22,23] Four to five percent of people with HIV/AIDS or tuberculosis (TB) have DM diagnosed during their evaluation.[24,25]

19.2.1 PRIMARY CARE CENTERS

There are 33,303 general hospitals, 20,278 primary health centers, and 59 teaching hospitals and federal medical centers in Nigeria. Approximately 70% of health care is provided by private vendors, and only 30% by government (federal and state).[26] There is a poor referral system, with only unidirectional flow from primary to secondary and tertiary. This leads to congestion of patients at the higher levels of care and paucity of patients at the lower tiers of health care.[27]

The primary care centers typically are small medical centers, usually a bungalow or a block in the community or ward, and are often not able to manage or follow up the DM patients who often have co-morbidities or complications, as they are often staffed by nurses, junior medical officers, and equipped with little diagnostic and monitoring equipment. Most primary care centers have only urine testing for monitoring DM control, and very few have functioning blood glucose meters. The dispensaries of such primary centers also rarely have more than metformin and sulfonylureas as antidiabetic medications.

Few primary care centers have insulin stocked in their dispensaries or pharmacies, and when available, storage is often suboptimal. Healthcare practitioners like dietitians, nutritionists, diabetes educators, and chiropodists are hardly ever present at this tier of care, due to financial limitations, poor infrastructure, and lack of incentives needed to attract and retain such professionals in these primary care centers—most of which are found in the rural or suburban villages and towns. The few patients diagnosed at the scantily staffed and poorly equipped primary care centers are therefore mostly referred to the secondary care centers, where most of them are better staffed and equipped to treat such patients.

19.2.2 SECONDARY CARE CENTERS

The secondary care centers (general hospitals and comprehensive health centers) are bigger medical centers, often comprised of a few buildings or blocks; they often have family physicians, internists, general nurses, dietitians, and physical therapists (physiotherapists). Some have a wide range of surgical consultants and ophthalmologists, to whom the patients can be referred if the need arises.

Other patients who cannot be managed at the secondary health centers are referred to tertiary health institutions (state specialist hospitals, federal medical centers, or teaching hospitals) by the care providers at the secondary care center or at the behest of the patient being treated or their relatives. In countries like Nigeria, with understaffed secondary care providers, the tertiary centers are sometimes forced to play the role of both secondary and tertiary care centers, leading to overcrowding and overstretching of these centers, with the consequent delays in service or provision of consultation in a hurried, perfunctory fashion. Details such as foot examination and fundoscopy are often thus omitted by the overwhelmed medical practitioners to "save time" and cover all patients scheduled for that clinic.

Secondary care centers in developing countries almost always have a good number of nurses, pharmacists, dietitians, and internists but rarely have any diabetologists/endocrinologists or podiatrists. The patients at this level of care are treated by internists, family physicians, or experienced medical officers with basic medical degrees and limited formal or informal post-graduate training. Diabetes educators, registered dietitians, exercise physiologists, and foot care specialists (podiatrists/chiropodists) are scarce, and the medical officers must increase their knowledge to be able to serve in multiple roles; nurses also frequently take on the role of diabetes educator. However, these substitute functionaries of the standard diabetes care team lack the specific training for the roles they discharge. Some secondary care centers have functioning glucose meters, point-of-care HbA1c equipment, and full laboratory and other diagnostic services. However, they generally lack capability for managing most patients with diabetic complications.

19.2.3 TERTIARY CARE CENTERS

Tertiary centers are the highest tier of medical services, often made of several buildings, medical centers, with several departments. These centers also often have affiliated medical schools and other training programs for a diverse cadre of paramedical or allied medical professions. They are better equipped, with availability of specialized units for some advanced procedures, including retinal surgery, laser eye treatment, and echocardiography. However, cardiac catheterization and other advanced cardiac procedures are usually lacking. Few tertiary centers have vascular surgery facilities, and the number of bypass surgeries for peripheral or coronary artery disease is minimal, even in the best of these centers, in many sub-Saharan countries. Some tertiary care centers have a full diabetes team, comprised of endocrinologists/diabetologists, dietitians, nutritionists, physiotherapists, and diabetes nurse specialists. It is uncommon to find a tertiary center hospital that has readily available chiropodists/podiatrists or certified diabetes educators. In addition to the usual services available in the secondary centers, a few tertiary care centers have renal dialysis and renal transplant units for management of patients with end-stage renal disease (few of whom can afford the heavily subsidized procedure). The few government-run centers on average have volumes of approximately 10 renal transplants. In the private sector, St. Nicholas Hospital in Lagos, Nigeria is a leading center, with volumes of 100–150 kidney transplants over the last decade.[28] At the time of writing, no medical center performs whole pancreatic or islet cell transplants. Some of the centers also have access to high-end devices/investigations like MRI, high performance liquid chromatography for HbA1c, and reagents for fructosamine levels.[29]

Most tertiary centers have point-of-care HbA1c measurement capability. Given the high prevalence of nutritional anemia, sickle cell disease, and sickle trait in the region that often leads to false HbA1c results, fructosamine assays ought to be more widely available to inform local experience, research, and practice. Despite these limitations, adherence of patients to the medications and glucose monitoring is considerable, with 60% being adherent to hypoglycemic medications and knowing their latest blood glucose readings.[30] Very few patients carry out self-monitoring of blood glucose (SMBG). Insulin pump therapy, continuous glucose monitoring, and more recent or emerging diabetes technologies, such as closed-loop systems, are conspicuously absent.

Most sub-Saharan patients needing specialized procedures, such as bariatric surgery, renal transplants, pancreas/islet cell transplants, lower-extremity and cardiac vascular bypass surgeries, or angioplasty, travel abroad (typically to Europe, India, and the United Arab Emirates) for such services.[31] South Africa has well-developed infrastructure for these services and attracts an increasing number of referrals. Renal replacement care (including transplantation) is available in a few centers in Nigeria, but the scale is vastly inadequate for the population. Notably, these expensive healthcare procedures usually are out-of-pocket expenses for most patients, except government officials, who are usually sponsored. The development of local capabilities in advanced care for diabetes and its complications should stem the tide of expensive medical tourism abroad and reverse the economic drain.[31]

19.3 HUMAN RESOURCES/PERSONNEL FOR DIABETES CARE

The categories of personnel who care for DM patients in sub-Saharan Africa include nurses, physicians, and other cadres of healthcare professionals.

19.3.1 NURSES

There is no regional tradition of the nurse-specialist for diabetes care. Instead, all nurses are trained to provide basic care for the patients with and other diseases. Nurses perform urinalysis and point-of-care blood glucose tests, provide basic nutritional advice, and teach patients self-injection techniques, among other tasks. Some of these nurses have been exposed to informal or ad hoc DM training sponsored by nongovernmental organizations or multinational pharmaceutical companies.[32] In general, nurses do not have drug prescribing authority, except in some rural areas that lack physician presence. However, prescribing authority is a moot point, as patent medicine stores and pharmacies in several countries in the region can sell medications directly to patients without prescriptions. Indeed, self-medication based on hearsay from neighbors and friends is rife in sub-Saharan Africa.

19.3.2 DOCTORS

The doctor-to-patient ratio is typically inadequate across the region: In both secondary and tertiary centers, diabetes clinics are often overloaded with patients. The ratio declines precipitously when specialist physicians are considered. In Nigeria, a relatively upward country in the region, there are fewer than 150 endocrinologists in Nigeria to cater for the approximately 5 million patients with diabetes. That number, though, is more than the combined number of all endocrinologists in other west African countries. There are insufficient diabetes clinics and grossly inadequate diabetes specialists. The chaotic, oversubscribed nature of the few clinics means doctors typically spend less than 15 minutes per patient, allowing little time for foot examination, funduscopy, or review of self–glucose monitoring charts. Many such clinics are run by internists or family physicians, and few are run by specialist endocrinologists. The number of endocrinologists and diabetologists has, however, increased significantly in the last three decades. In the 1980s, there were fewer than 10 endocrinologists/diabetologists in Nigeria, which has recently increased to approximately 150 (including pediatric endocrinologists).[33]

19.3.3 OTHER ALLIED HEALTH PERSONNEL

Routine availability of the full-spectrum diabetes care team (comprising nutritionist, certified diabetes educator, podiatrist, dietitian, exercise physiologists/physical therapist, etc.) is a general rarity in healthcare facilities in the region. Even in Nigeria, few secondary or tertiary centers have all these categories of staff. In fact, there are less than five certified diabetes educators and podiatrists in Nigeria.[33] This contrasts sharply with South Africa, where a robust diabetes educator presence exists, along with other cadres of the diabetes care team.

19.4 PROFILE OF DIABETIC PATIENTS

The typical DM patients seen in Nigeria are diagnosed in the fifth to sixth decade of life. Over 95% are type 2 DM, while type 1 and other forms of DM account for 5%.[33] In most hospital-based studies in Nigeria, type 2 DM patients are overweight or normal weight (<15% being obese; BMI > 30 kg/m^2). The mean HbA1c is usually between 8% and 9% in tertiary centers, with scant data from the secondary and primary centers.[34,35] Less than a third of patients attain glycemic targets specified by International Diabetes Federation (IDF) or the American Diabetes Association (ADA). Fewer than 10% of people with diabetes in Nigeria are covered by National Health Insurance Service (NHIS) or any third-party insurance. Thus, the cost of care is borne directly by the patients and their relatives.

19.4.1 DIABETES COMORBIDITIES

Based on limited surveys and anecdotal experience, approximately 60% of patients with diabetes in Nigeria are hypertensive, and a substantial proportion have some form of dyslipidemia. Some 30%–60% of the patients with hypertension in Nigerian clinics have prediabetes or diabetes. There is also an increased number of diabetes patients amongst the psychiatric clinic population. The relationship between diabetes and psychiatric disorders is rather complex. Although the two conditions can arise independently, mental illness and antipsychotic drugs are independent risk factors for diabetes, and diabetes appears to increase the risk for depression.[36]

19.4.2 DIABETES AND INFECTIOUS DISEASE

Approximately 12% of patients with pulmonary tuberculosis screened positive for DM, compared with 5.6% of the population without tuberculosis in Lagos, Nigeria.[33,37] Diabetes is also common in patients being treated for HIV/AIDS. Antiretroviral agents commonly used for HIV treatment have been associated with increased risk of dysglycemia.[38]

19.5 EXPERIENCE OF THE NIGERIAN PATIENT WITH DIABETES

19.5.1 FEAR AND DESPAIR

The level of care received by DM patients is often perceived by them as poor, as the patients find themselves in unfamiliar terrain of living with incurable disease that differs from what they are used to: infectious diseases for which the treatment or cure only takes a few days or weeks. The patients rate care as low, due to prolonged waiting times before appointments can be made and long waiting hours in the outpatient clinics and in the long queues waiting for medications. This has led to a greater reliance on unorthodox medicine, complimentary or alternative medicine, and faith healers, which appear less cumbersome and are appealing to the patients but are fraught with disastrous consequences.[39,40]

19.5.2 REDUCED QUALITY OF LIFE

DM as a chronic disease leads to a reduction in the quality of life, because the people living with it spend several days off work per year due to ill health, high cost of care, need for regular clinic appointments, and several comorbidities and complications, all of which weigh down the strongest people.

19.5.3 ABANDONMENT

Patients with DM also feel abandoned, as there is no support, nor is cost of their treatment or investigations borne by government agencies; neither employers nor families can provide the needed supplies and medications. This feeling of abandonment is heightened when the patients compare their care with those with TB or HIV/AIDS in the same clinic space or medical center, who have free (sponsored or subsidized) treatment. Many patients with DM find it hard to come to terms with the concept of the disease being a lifelong, chronic disease and thus seek cures and treatment in the strangest quarters and through the most unusual means, including consulting herbalists, spiritualists, and faith healers. Many of the patients also express distrust for their physicians and go shopping for new ones every now and then, with several disruptions in their care. This is even more heightened by what the patients feel are conflicting instructions from one care provider to another.

19.6 PROGNOSTIC INDICES OF DIABETES MELLITUS IN NIGERIA

Several previous studies have reported on diabetes-related morbidity and mortality in various parts of Nigeria. Earlier Nigerian reports demonstrated the large role of infections and metabolic complications in DM mortality, with many patients having sepsis as one of the factors leading to their admission and demise. Reports of cardiovascular morbidity in this period was mainly from stroke, with very few people reporting myocardial infarction or heart failure.[41]

19.6.1 EMERGENCE OF CARDIOVASCULAR MORBIDITY IN NIGERIA

The evolving pattern of cardiovascular morbidity over the years has seen more patients being diagnosed. The younger patients are usually congenital heart disease patients, while the elderly and middle aged are usually hypertensive or diabetic, or both, and require valve replacement, angioplasty, et cetera, especially among obese subjects with diabetes. Coronary artery disease cases are gradually increasing to the extent that open-heart-surgery programs and angioplasty programs have commenced in several states across Nigeria as cases seen over the past two decades have steadily risen.[42,43]

19.6.2 DIABETES MELLITUS FOOT SYNDROME

DM foot syndrome (DMFS; previously called *diabetic foot gangrene*) is a leading complication and cause of diabetes-related morbidity and mortality. Lower-extremity amputation from DMFS is the leading cause of major limb amputation in Nigeria.[44,45] Unfortunately, many lives are lost while patients procrastinate about whether to allow the amputation to be carried out, and some who are willing can't afford the fees required for such life-saving measures. Not uncommonly, medical wards are occupied by many patients with varying stages of DMFS, and in a few cases autoamputation of digits or a whole leg may supervene. Severe sepsis leading to septic shock and death is the eventual outcome in the unfortunate patient with DMFS.[46]

19.6.3 HOSPITAL MORBIDITY AND MORTALITY ATTRIBUTABLE TO DIABETES MELLITUS

Overall morbidity and mortality rates attributable to DM vary across different hospitals in different parts of the country. The rates range from single- to double-digit percentage points. Studies in the South South Zone of Nigeria revealed that 5%–20% of all admissions were diabetes related, and that the case fatality of diabetes was one of the highest of all conditions. Hyperglycemic emergencies, DMFS, and stroke accounted for most of the causes of mortality in patients with diabetes.[33,46–48] This has resulted in the need to ramp up acute and chronic care for patients in most secondary and tertiary centers in Nigeria. Tertiary care centers, including many university teaching hospitals, in Nigeria are beginning to set up specialized units to manage stroke and other complications.

In a retrospective study of the admission pattern in a tertiary center in Lagos, Nigeria, a total of 1,703 patients were admitted through the adult emergency wards during the period March 2011 to February 2012. Diabetes-related admissions comprised 166 (9.74%) of total medical admissions, with a case fatality rate of 21.6%.[49] The leading causes of death were hyperglycemic emergencies (diabetic ketoacidosis, hyperosmolar hyperglycemic states, and other mixed hyperglycemic emergencies), hypoglycemia, and DMFS. In a similar study in Port Harcourt, Nigeria, the case fatality of diabetes-related admissions was 17%, and the leading causes of mortality were acute metabolic complications (hyperglycemic and hypoglycemic emergencies) seen in 39.8% of the subjects.[46] In yet another retrospective study, 8.8% of inpatients admitted with diabetes died (70% of deaths occurring within the first week of admission).[50] These dismal data have been replicated at other locations.[33,46–48,51–53] In neighboring Ghana, in a study conducted between 1983 and 2014, the most common reasons for diabetes-related hospital admissions were hyperglycemic emergencies (accounting for 80%) and cardiovascular-related causes. Case fatality in that study ranged from 15% to 21%.[54]

19.7   DIABETES SUPPORT GROUPS

19.7.1   Diabetes Association of Nigeria

There is no pan-African diabetes-focused association like the European Association for the Study of Diabetes (EASD). However, there are a few scattered national diabetes support groups across the region. Examples include the Diabetes Association of Nigeria (DAN), a nonprofit, nongovernment, patient-centered organization devoted to patient support. Historically, promotion or funding of diabetes research has not been within the ambit of DAN's activities. Having a large membership spanning almost all the states of the country, DAN has collaborated with the IDF and other associations to increase awareness of diabetes in the region and pursue a common goal of providing support for persons with the diabetes.[19,33,55]

19.7.2   Community Initiatives

The Structured Health Initiative (STRUHI) is a not-for-profit organization dedicated to the advancement of health care in Nigeria, with diabetes as a key area of focus.[33,56] STRUHI operates mainly out of Lagos, Nigeria and is partnering with international agencies to study diabetes, tuberculosis, and other noncommunicable diseases, as well as communicable diseases that coexist with diabetes. Through this initiative, several healthcare providers, including doctors and nurses, have been trained. Additionally, STRUHI has sponsored screening programs for DM and the development of guidelines for diabetes management. Talabi Centre for Diabetes Studies, established more than 10 years ago in Ogun state, is another charitable community initiative that focuses on screening, prevention, and monitoring of DM, and training of personnel involved in diabetes care and education.

19.7.3   Strategies for Improving Diabetes Care in Nigeria Study Group (SIDCAIN)

The Strategies for Improving Diabetes Care in Nigeria Study Group (SIDCAIN) was formed approximately 8 years ago by physicians from three tertiary hospitals in southwestern Nigeria with the aim of optimizing care for patients with diabetes and hypertension. The SIDCAIN group operates several primary and secondary centers for screening, diagnosis, and management of noncommunicable diseases. Other notable activities include training of health workers involved in diabetes and hypertension care, production of treatment guidelines and educational material, and patient support programs.[57]

19.7.4   Podiatry Initiative in Nigeria

Two podiatry initiatives in Nigeria aimed at limb preservation are described here. The World Diabetes Foundation (WDF)13-830 program's goal was to strengthen 11 clinics, train 301 healthcare providers, and screen 10,000 people with DM for foot complications in Lagos, Nigeria within 3 years.[58] These targets were met and in some areas exceeded. Similarly, the WDF 13-806 project established 20 foot clinics, trained more than 400 healthcare providers, and provided audiovisual and printed training material for DMFS prevention and treatment.[59] These WDF projects serve to create model systems that can be replicated nationally and regionally, to confront and ameliorate one of the most costly diabetic complications in low-income countries.[11] DMFS afflicts 10% of all DM patients in Nigeria and accounts for 12% of DM admissions.[21,33]

19.8   HEALTHCARE SYSTEM

The healthcare system in sub-Saharan Africa varies across and within countries in the region.

19.8.1   Healthcare Financing

Approximately 80% of patients in Nigeria finance their medical bills from their personal income or funds contributed by members of their immediate or extended family.[5,60] Such resources barely cover the cost of tests and medications in a stable, uncomplicated patient, and often are inadequate for the care of patients with expensive complications (e.g., DMFS, end-stage renal disease, eye disease, stroke, or heart disease). Fewer than 10% of Nigerian patients with diabetes have third-party health insurance coverage.[61] In fact, a survey found that 65% of the population in Ghana was enrolled in the National Health Insurance program, as compared to a mere 3.5% in Nigeria.[62] The much larger overall population of Nigeria compared to Ghana is an obvious challenge in the organization of healthcare delivery and financing.

19.8.2   Monitoring of Diabetes Mellitus Control

With the pervasive poverty and low health literacy, only an estimated 20%–40% of Nigerian patients with DM perform SMBG regularly.[60,63] Many patients have blood glucose meters donated by various entities but fail to use them due to illiteracy and/or lack of test strips. There may also be a role of trypanophobia (extreme fear of medical procedures involving injections or needles). The lack of SMBG is compounded by a general lack of patients' familiarity with the medications they are taking for diabetes.[61] Where affordability of glucose test strips is an issue, the frequency of SMBG can be negotiated on an individual basis. Patients treated with short- or intermediate-acting insulin and sulfonylureas need to self-monitor more frequently than those treated with basal insulin alone or oral agents that are not associated with increased risk of hypoglycemia.

There are anecdotes of patients successfully extending the days of SMBG coverage by splitting test strips in half. However, it is unknown whether blood glucose measurements using half of the standard test strip would be consistently accurate. Even less known is whether the exposure of reagent in the split test strip in a tropical environment would inactivate glucose oxidase, hexokinase, or other embedded enzymatic catalysts required for accurate SBMG readings. There is evidence that split test strips might be reliable for visual reading of blood glucose in a temperate environment[64]; however, local research is needed to determine whether this form of "stretching" of resources would be reliable for meter-read glucose values in sub-Saharan Africa.

19.8.3   Complementary and Alternative Medicine

Healthcare management of most diabetic patients is pluralistic, with many patients using spiritual, traditional, complementary, and alternative medicine options.[5,9,40] The large use of these unorthodox (and often unproven) remedies is due to the general culture and belief system prevalent in most parts of sub-Saharan Africa, which lays a lot of emphasis on the spiritual basis of any disease, especially chronic illnesses like diabetes. Patients seldom agree or understand that disease is a disease without a cure and are thus prone to false promises of cure from unconventional sources. Thus, it not surprising that many patients seen in the orthodox (Western-style) clinics still consult spiritualists, faith healers, herbalists, and other traditional medicine practitioners.

The quest for cure that results in patronage of multiple unconventional alternative medical sources comes at a steep price for many patients. The loss of personal and family funds siphoned off by these alternative practitioners depletes resources for funding approved diabetes medications and self-management items. The high dependence on complementary/alternative medicine is corroborated by a study in Lagos (arguably the most enlightened and cosmopolitan Nigeria city), which demonstrated that 46% of DM patients use complementary and alternative medicine.[40] The extent of patronage and dependence must be even higher among patients in semirural and rural areas.

19.9 IMPROVING HEALTH OUTCOMES

Improving health outcomes in people with DM and reducing the high morbidity and mortality from diabetes require several measures.

19.9.1 COPING WITH INCREASING NONCOMMUNICABLE DISEASES

Developing countries such as Nigeria will require devising innovative and locally adapted approaches to combating the surging numbers of people with NCDs like hypertension and DM.[65] These NCDs are all closely related, and simple lifestyle changes can decrease: Among the lifestyle targets are optimal nutrition, physical activity, smoking cessation, moderation of alcohol intake, and stress reduction. This is more important with the dwindling resources of the national budget to health (in Nigeria, the budget for health has been 2%–7% of the total annual budget) in the last decade or two, and the low coverage of the population by the NHIS. Nigeria, which champions universal health coverage in regional health summits and congresses, has very low enrollment rates (insured people in Nigeria are less than 5%) than other countries like Ghana and South Africa, which have insurance coverage of up to 40%–50%.[66,67]

19.9.2 HOME-GROWN SOLUTIONS TO IMPROVE OUTCOMES

It is desirable to develop ingenious, home-grown solutions to tackle the problems in NCD care.[33,68] Building partnerships with well-funded communicable disease programs (e.g., HIV/AIDS) could elevate NCDs like diabetes and hypertension to greater prominence and awareness. Indeed, several HIV/AIDS treatment centers now serve as centers for screening for and treating diabetes, hypertension, and other conditions, with great cost savings.[69] Increasingly, government agencies are involved in promoting health through lifestyle changes and promotion of screening programs in vulnerable groups, thereby encouraging early detection and timely intervention. Attention to antenatal and obstetric care, as well as maternal and child health, likely would break the chain of fetal programming of adult cardiometabolic diseases. Social programs aimed at poverty alleviation, improved literacy, health education, better healthcare funding, and wider access to health insurance coverage will all improve overall outcomes in diabetes and other NCDs (Table 19.3).

TABLE 19.3

Strategies for Improving Diabetes Care in Sub-Saharan Africa

- Investment in local and regional diabetes focused research
- Expansion of the pool of trained specialists in the standard diabetes care team (educators, nutritionists, podiatrists, endocrinologists, etc.)
- Development of local capabilities in the manufacture and distribution of medicines and devices in diabetes
- Culture of patient-centered and outcomes-focused diabetes care delivery
- Optimization of standardized surveillance system for diabetes mellitus complications
- Community involvement and improvement in health literacy

19.9.3 Diabetes Prevention Programs

Type 2 DM is a preventable condition. The earliest prevention opportunity presents before birth ("primordial" prevention), when improved management during pregnancy can be beneficial in reducing the risk of diabetes in later life for the offspring.[70] Children and youth can be taught healthy lifestyles and adequate space provided for play, leisure, sports, and any form of physical activity.

Community screening programs can help discover the large number of asymptomatic people with differing degrees of dysglycemia.[71] The World Diabetes Day celebrated on November 14 provides opportunity for nationwide community screening and awareness campaigns. Persons with prediabetes benefit from lifestyle intervention to prevent future diabetes. The US Diabetes Prevention Program (DPP) clearly demonstrated the ability of lifestyle or medication to halt progression of prediabetes to diabetes.[72] Patients in the DPP were randomized into three groups, which were placed on healthy lifestyle (diet and exercise), metformin, or placebo. The results demonstrated that a healthy, active lifestyle, as compared with placebo, reduced the occurrence of type 2 DM by 58%. In the same study, those treated with metformin experienced 31% diabetes risk reduction (Figure 19.1). The DPP results of lifestyle intervention have been replicated in Finland, China, and India and can be readily adapted to populations in sub-Saharan African countries.[73,74]

19.9.4 Optimizing Diabetes Mellitus Control

It has been estimated that more than half of the persons with diabetes in sub-Saharan Africa are not diagnosed and, of those diagnosed, only one-half are usually on any treatment. Of those receiving treatment, fewer than 50% achieve glycemic targets, most likely due to poor adherence or socioeconomic factors.[75,76] This ominous "rule of halves" is associated with high morbidity and mortality from diabetes, and other NCDs have a high mortality. Efforts directed at improving health literacy, adherence, and access to proper care would be essential for improving patient outcomes.[27] The well-established oral antidiabetes medications, such as sulfonylureas and metformin, are generally available and mostly affordable as generics. The cost of the newer branded agents exceeds minimum wage for many low-income patients. Similarly, older insulin formulations (neutral protamine Hagedorn [NPH], regular insulin) are more affordable than the expensive analogues (Table 19.4). For patients who are adherent to lifestyle and medications, little evidence supports superiority of more expensive oral agents or analogue insulin formulations over the generic, older alternatives. Therefore, it is prudent for physicians to use sound judgment

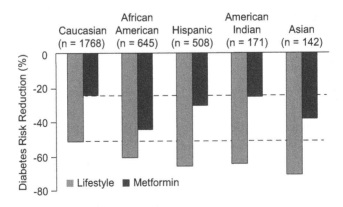

FIGURE 19.1 Primary results of the US Diabetes Prevention Program (DPP) showing efficacy of lifestyle intervention versus placebo in preventing progression from prediabetes to type 2 diabetes mellitus by race-ethnicity. (Adapted from Diabetes Prevention Program Research Group, *N. Engl. J. Med.*, 346, 393–403, 2002.)

TABLE 19.4

Drugs Used for Diabetes Mellitus in Sub-Saharan Africa

More Commonly Available	Newer Agents Not Widely Available or Affordable
Oral Agents	
Metformin	DPP4 inhibitors
Sulfonylureas	SGLT2 inhibitors
Thiazolidinediones	GLP1-agonists
Insulin Formulations	
Regular insulin	Insulin analogues
NPH	• Analogue basal
Premixed 70/30	• Analogue short acting
	• Inhaled insulin

Source: 2017 Diabetes Program managing hyperglycemia in low resource settings, www.who.int/diabetes/en.

DPP4, dipeptidyl peptidase 4; GLP glucagonlike peptide 1; NPH, neutral protamine Hagedorn; SGLT2, sodium glucose transporter 2.

when selecting antidiabetes agents for patients in sub-Saharan Africa. Even in resource-poor communities, much more can be done to improve diabetes outcomes (Figure 19.2). Simple measures like healthy lifestyle changes, minimizing fried foods, taking more walks, avoiding cheap motorbike rides for short commutes, and reinforcing patient education could go a long way in improving the metabolic profile (Figure 19.1).

The problems of poverty and limited access and affordability of care loom large in the region. As advocates for their patients, physicians should seize every opportunity for obtaining gratuitous samples, discount vouchers, and assistance programs from pharmaceutical companies for the benefit of their diabetes patients.

Along with appropriate medications, medical nutrition therapy, regular SMBG, and regular clinic attendance and follow-up are practices that improve health outcomes in people with diabetes.[76] As discussed, the frequency of SMBG can be negotiated with patients unable to afford

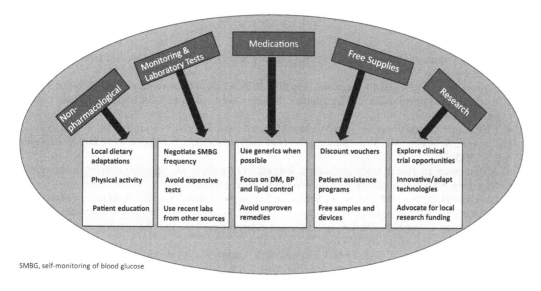

SMBG, self-monitoring of blood glucose

FIGURE 19.2 Approach to management of diabetes in sub-Saharan Africa: doing more with less.

test strips. basis. Patients treated with short- or intermediate-acting insulin and sulfonylureas need to self-monitor more frequently than those treated with basal insulin alone or oral agents that are not associated with increased risk of hypoglycemia. If multiple daily SMBG is not feasible, SMBG performed at staggered time periods (before breakfast, approximately 2 hours post-lunch, before dinner, or bedtime) on 3 days each week could still provide reasonable data to inform adjustments to diabetes regimen.[77] Regular foot examination, eradication of barefoot walking, and use of appropriate footwear would decrease the risk of foot injuries and DMFS. Educating patients with apparently minor foot conditions like tinea pedis or small bullae to seek early medical attention is critical to preventing limb loss.

Beyond these measures, the seminal role of locally generated research in informing best practices in the region cannot be overemphasized. Local research on optimal nutrition, glycemic index of traditional foods, efficacy of "stretching" strategies like splitting glucose test strips, and viability of recently expired insulin and other medications would be invaluable in advancing evidence-based practices (Figure 19.2).

19.10 SUMMARY

This chapter describes the peculiarities of DM in sub-Saharan Africa. Using Nigeria (the most populous country in the region) as a focal point, we highlight the roles of socioeconomic constraints, low literacy, late presentation, harmful cultural practices, lack of health insurance coverage, limited human and technical resources, and an overstretched healthcare delivery system. These factors militate against optimal control of DM, with often disastrous consequences. Investment in education, leading to improvement in health literacy and trained health personnel, would be a critical step toward better DM care in the region. The development and implementation of local guidelines for optimal DM care is desirable. Such guidelines must emphasize efficient practices, avoidance of unproven remedies, "doing more with less," and a holistic approach. Expanding the rudimentary health insurance programs in some countries in the region also would improve access to care. Importantly, entrepreneurial initiatives in local production of pharmaceutical products, reagents, and devices used for DM management would break the precarious dependency on imported drugs and appurtenances for DM care. Efforts aimed at building patient support groups across the region would help translate DM self-management practices to local communities.

REFERENCES

1. National Bureau of Statistics 2014. National Literacy Survey, quarter four. Accessed from www.nigerianstat.gov.ng on 16/3/18.
2. Nigeria Country Profile, GDP – per capita (PPP). 2017;16(2). Accessed from www.indexmundi.com on 20/3/18.
3. World Health Organization. 2017. Countries: Nigeria. Accessed from www.who.int/countries/nigeria. on 16/3/18.
4. UNESCO; Countries/Nigeria. 2018. Accessed from en.unesco.org/Nigeria on 16/3/18.
5. Chinenye S, Ogbera AO. Sociocultural aspects of diabetes mellitus in Nigeria. *J Soc Health Diabetes.* 2013:1;15–21.
6. Abdulraheem IS. Health needs assessment and determinants of health seeking behavior among elderly Nigerians: A household survey. *Ann Afr Med.* 2007;6(2):58–63.
7. Onyeonoro UU, Ogah OS, Moses AO. Urban rural differences in health care seeking pattern of residents of Abia State, Nigeria and the implications of control of NCDs. *Healthserv Insight.* 2016;9:29–36.
8. International Diabetes Federation. IDF Diabetes Atlas: 8th edition 2017. Accessed from www.idf.org/diabeteseatlas.org/Africa on 19/3/18.
9. Adejumo H, Odusan O, Sogbein O, Laiteerapong N, Dauda M, Ahmed O. The impact of religion and culture in diabetes care in Nigeria. *Afr J Diab Med.* 2015;23(2):1–3.
10. Awak PK. An ethnographic study of diabetes: Implications for the application of patient centered care in Cameroon. *J Anthropology* 2014: Article ID 937898:1–12.

11. Ogbera A, Fasanmade O, Ohwovoriole A. High costs, low awareness and a lack of care – The diabetic foot in Nigeria. *Diabetes Voice* 2016;51(3):30–32.
12. Igbeneghu C, Olisekodiaka MJ, Onuegbu JA, Malaria and typhoid fever among adult patients presenting with fever in Ibadan, Southwest Nigeria. *Int J Trop Med* 2009;4(3):112–116.
13. Adesina OF, Oduniyi AO, Olutunde AO, Ogunlana MO, Ogunkoya JO, Alalade BA. Is HBA1c testing in Nigeria only for the rich? *Afr J Diab Med.* 2012;20(2):47.
14. Adebayo JK. Monitoring diabetes mellitus with HBA1c: The Abakaliki Nigeria experience. *J Health Med Nurs.* 2015:12;118–124.
15. Oguomba VM, Nwose EU, Skinner TC, Digban KA, Onyia IC. Prevalence of cardiovascular diseases risk factors among a Nigerian population: Relationship with income level and accessibility to CVD risk screening. *BMC Public Health.* 2015;15:397.
16. National Bureau of Statistics 2014. Nigerian Gross Domestic Product Report, quarter 4. Accessed from www.nigerianstat.gov.ng on 16/3/18.
17. Sabir A, Ohwovoriole A, Isezuo S, Fasanmade O, Abubakar S, Iwuala S. Type 2 diabetes mellitus and its risk factors among the rural Fulanis of Northern Nigeria. *Ann Afr Med.* 2013;12(4):217–222. doi:10.4103/1596-3519.122689.
18. Enang OE, Otu AA, Essien OE, Okpara H, Fasanmade OA, Ohwovoriole AE, Searle J. Prevalence of dysglycemia in Calabar: A cross-sectional observational study among residents of Calabar, Nigeria. *BMJ Open Diabetes Res Care.* 2014;20;2(1):e000032. doi:10.1136/bmjdrc-2014-000032.
19. Ogbera AO, Ekpebegh C. Diabetes mellitus in Nigeria: The past, present and future. *World J Diabetes.* 2014;5(6):905–911.
20. Ogbera AO, Awobusuyi J, Unachukwu C, Fasanmade O. Clinical features, predictive factors and outcome of hyperglycaemic emergencies in a developing country. *BMC Endocr Disord.* 2009;9:9. doi:10.1186/1472-6823-9-9.
21. Ogbera AO, Fasanmade O, Ohwovoriole AE, Adediran O. An assessment of the disease burden of foot ulcers in patients with diabetes mellitus attending a teaching hospital in Lagos, Nigeria. *Int J Low Extrem Wounds.* 2006;5(4);244–249.
22. Nyenwe EA, Odia OJ, Ihekwaba AE, Ojule A, Babatunde S. Type diabetes in adult Nigerians: A study of its prevalence and risk factors in Port Harcourt Nigeria. *Diab Res Clin Pract* 2003:62(3);177–185.
23. Oluwayemi IO, Brink SJ, Oyenusi EE, Oduwole OA, Oluwayemi MA. Fasting blood glucose profile among secondary school adolescents in Ado Ekiti, Nigeria. *J Nutr Metab.* 2015:2015:417859. doi:10.1155/2015/417859.
24. Ogbera AO, Kapur A, Odeyemi K, Longe-Peters K, Adeyeye OO, Odeniyi I, Ogunnowo BE. Screening for diabetes mellitus and human immune deficiency virus infection in persons with tuberculosis. *J Prev Med Hyg.* 2014;55(2):42–45.
25. Ogbera AO, Kapur A, Chinenye S, Fasanmade O, Uloko A, Odeyemi K. Undiagnosed diabetes mellitus in tuberculosis: A Lagos report. *Indian J Endocrinol Metab.* 2014;18(4):475–479.
26. Welcome MO. The Nigeria health care system: Need for integrating and surveillance system. *J Pharm Bioallied Sci.* 2011;3(4): 470–478.
27. Oguejiofor O, Odenigbo C, Onwukwe C. Diabetes in Nigeria: Impact, challenges, future directions. *Endocrinol Metab Syndr.* 2014;3(2):1–9.
28. Arogundade FA. Kidney transplantation in a low-resource setting: Nigeria. *Kidney Int Suppl.* 2013;3(2):241–245.
29. Rehlenbeck SI. Monitoring diabetic control in developing countries: A review of glycated haemoglobin and fructosamine assays. *Trop Doct* 1998;28:9–15.
30. Adisa R, Alutundu MB, Fakeye TO. Factors contributing to non-adherence to oral hypoglycemic medications among ambulatory type 2 diabetes patients in Southwestern Nigeria. *Pharm Pract.* 2009;7:163–169.
31. Medical tourism costs Nigeria over N400bn annually–Minister. 2017. Accessed from www.tribuneonlineng.com on 18/3/18.
32. Case study: Lilly diabetes/ Healthy interactions. 2018. Accessed from www.healthyinteractions.com on 19/3/18.
33. Fasanmade OA, Dagogo-Jack S. Diabetes care in Nigeria. *Ann Glob Health.* 2015;81(6):821–829.
34. Uloko AE, Ofoegbu EM, Chinenye S, Fasanmade OA, Fasanmade AA, Ogbera AO, Ogbu OO, Oli JM, Girei BA, Adamu A. Profile of Nigerians with diabetes mellitus—Diabetes Nigeria Study Group (2008): Results of a multi-centre Study. *Indian J Endocrinol Metab.* 2012;16:558–564.
35. Ogbera AO, Chinenye S, Onyekwere A, Fasanmade O. Prognostic indices of diabetes mortality. *Ethn Dis.* 2007;17:721–725.

36. Dagogo-Jack S. The role of antipsychotic agents in the development of diabetes. *Nat Clin Pract Endocrinol Metab*. 2009;5:22–23.

37. Ogbera AO, Kapur A, Chinenye S, Fasanmade O, Uloko A, Odeyemi K. Undiagnosed diabetes mellitus in tuberculosis: A Lagos report. *Indian J Endocrinol Metab*. 2014;18(4):475–479.

38. Dagogo-Jack S. HIV therapy and diabetes risk (Editorial). *Diabetes Care*. 2008;31:1267–1268.

39. Chinenye S, Young E. State of diabetes care in Nigeria; a review. *Nigerian Health J*. 2011;11(4);101–106.

40. Ogbera AO, Dada O, Adeyeye F, Jewo PI. Complementary and alternative medicine use in diabetes mellitus. *W Afr J Med*. 2010:29;158–162.

41. Dagogo-Jack S, Odia OJ. Myocardial infarction in Nigerian Africans. *Orient J Med*. 1990;2:129–132.

42. Eze JC, Ezemba N. Open heart surgery in Nigeria. *Texas Health Inst J*. 2007;34(1):8–10.

43. Falase B, Sanusi M, Majekodunmi A, Animashaun B, Ajose I, Idowu A, Oke A. *J Cardiothorac Surg*. 2013;8:6. doi:10.1186/1749-8090-8-6.

44. Dagogo-Jack S. Pattern of foot ulcer in diabetic Nigerians. *Pract Diabetes Digest*. 1991;2:75–78.

45. Ndukwu CU, Muoneme CA. Prevalence and pattern of major extremity amputation in a tertiary Hospital in Nnewi, south eastern Nigeria. *Trop J Med Res*. 2015;18:104–108.

46. Dagogo-Jack S. Diabetic in-patient mortality in Nigeria. *Pract Diabetes Dig*. 1991;2:117–119.

47. Unachukwu CN, Uchenna DI, Young E. Mortality among diabetes in patients in Port-Harcourt, Nigeria. *Afr J Endocrinol Metab*. 2008;7:1–5.

48. Aguocha BU, Ukpabi JO, Onyeonoro UU, Njoku P, Ukegbu AU Pattern of diabetic mortality in a tertiary health facility in south eastern Nigeria. *Afr J Diab Med*. 2013;21;1–3.

49. Anyanwu AC, Odeniyi IA, Fasanmade OA, Adewunmi AJ, Adegoke O, Mojeed AC, Olofin KE, Ohwovoriole AE. Endocrine related diseases in the emergency unit of a tertiary health center in Lagos: A study of the admission and mortality patterns. *Niger Med J*. 2013;54(4):254–257.

50. Adekanle O, Ayodeji OO, Olatunde LO, Folorunso TR. A 7-year retrospective study of diabetes related deaths in a Nigerian tertiary hospital. *Diabetes Int*. 2008;16(2):15–17.

51. Unadike BC, Essien I, Essien O, Akpan NA, Peters EJ, Ekott JU. Indications for and outcome of diabetic admissions at the University of Uyo Teaching hospital, Uyo. *Ibom Med J*. 2013;6(2):16–22.

52. Ezeala-Adikaibe B, Aneke E, Orjioke C, Ezeala-Adikaibe N, Mbadiwe N, Chime P, Okafor U. Pattern of medical admissions at Enugu State University of Science and Technology Hospital: A 5-year review. *Ann Med Health Sci Res*. 2014;4(3):426–431.

53. Chijioke A, Adamu AM, Makusidi AM. Mortality patterns among type 2 diabetes mellitus patients in Ilorin, Nigeria. *JEMDSA*. 2010;15(2):79–82.

54. Sarfo-Kantanka O, Sarfo FS, Ansah EO, Eghan BA, Ayisi-Boateng NK, Acheamfour-Akowuah. Secular trends in admissions and mortality rates from diabetes mellitus in the central belt of Ghana: A 31-year review. *PLoS One*. 2016. doi:10.1371/journal.pone.0169505.

55. Dagogo-Jack S. Experience with the organization of a local diabetic association in Port Harcourt, Nigeria. *Pract Diabetes Dig*. 1990;1:145–147.

56. Ogbera AO, Kapur A, Abdur-Razzaq H, Harries AD, Ramaiya K, Adeleye O, et al. Clinical profile of diabetes mellitus in tuberculosis. *BMJ Open Res Care*. 2015;3(1):e000112.

57. Raimi TH, Alebiosu OC, Adeleye JO, Balogun WO, Kolawole BA, Familoni OB et al. Diabetes education: Strategy for improving diabetes care in Nigeria. *Afr J Diab Med*. 2014:22;9–11.

58. Diabetes Podiatry Initiative in Nigeria WDF 13-830. 2014. Accessed from www.worlddiabetesfoundation.org on 20/3/18.

59. Improving Diabetes Foot Care in Lagos, WDF 13-806. 2014. Accessed from www.worlddiabetesfoundation.org on 20/3/18.

60. Nwankwo CH, Nandy B, Nwankwo BO. Factors influencing diabetes management outcome among patients attending government health facilities in South east Nigeria. *Int J Trop Med*. 2010;5:28–36.

61. Awodele O, Osuolale JA. Medication adherence in type 2 diabetes patients: Study of patients in Alimosho General Hospital, Igando, Lagos, Nigeria. *Afr Health Sci*. 2015;15(2):513–22.

62. Odeyemi IAO, Nixon J. Assessing equity in health care through the national health insurance schemes of Nigeria and Ghana: A review based comparative analysis. *Int J Equity Health*. 2013;12:9.

63. Iwuala SO, Olamoyegun MA, Sabir AA, Fasanmade OA. The relationship between self-monitoring of blood glucose and glycaemia control among patients attending an urban diabetes clinic in Nigeria. *Ann Afr Med*. 2015;14(4);182–187.

64. Spraul M, Sonnenberg GE, Berger M. Less expensive, reliable blood glucose self-monitoring. *Diabetes Care*. 1987;10(3):357–359.

65. Maiyaki MB, Garbati MA. The burden of non-communicable diseases in Nigeria; in the context of globalization. *Ann Afr Med*. 2014;13:1–10.

66. Wang H, Otoo N, Dsane-Selby L. 2017. World Bank Group. Ghana National Health Insurance Scheme. Improving financial sustainability based on expenditure review. Accessed from openknowledge.worldbank.org on 3/5/18, pages 1–71.

67. Valrie J. 2010. South Africa in International Health systems: Snapshots of health in 16 countries. Physicians for a National Health Programme. Accessed from http://www.euro.who int/document/e85400.pdf.

68. Welcome MO. The Nigerian health care system: Need for integrating and surveillance system. *J Pharm Bio Allied Sci.* 2011:3(4):470–478.

69. Oputa RN, Chinenye S. Diabetes in Nigeria: A translational approach. *Afr J Diabetes Med.* 2015;23(1):7–10.

70. Olagbuji BN, Atiba AS, Olofinbiyi BA, Akintayo AA, Awoleke JO, Ade-Ojo IP, Fasubaa OB; Gestational Diabetes Study Group-Nigeria. Prevalence of and risk factors for gestational diabetes using 1999, 2013 WHO and IADPSG criteria upon implementation of a universal one step screening and diagnostic strategy in a sub- Saharan Africa population. *Eur J Obstet Gynecol Reprod Biol.* 2015. doi:101016/jejogrb.2015.02.030.

71. Pascal IG, Ofoedu JN, Uchenna NP, Uchamma G-UE. Blood glucose control and medication adherence among adult type 2 diabetic Nigerians attending a primary care clinic in under-resourced environment of eastern Nigeria. *N Am J Med Sci.* 2012;4(7):310–315.

72. Diabetes Prevention Program Research Group. Reduction in the incidence of type 2 diabetes with lifestyle intervention or metformin. *N Engl J Med.* 2002;346:393–403.

73. Dagogo-Jack S. Primary prevention of type 2 diabetes in developing countries. *J Natl Med Assoc.* 2006;98:415–419.

74. Echouffo-Tcheugui JB, Dagogo-Jack S. Preventing diabetes mellitus in developing countries. *Nat Rev Endocrinol.* 2012;8:557–562.

75. Hart J. Rule of halves: Implications of increasing diagnosis and reducing drop out for future workload and prescribing costs in primary care. *Br J Gen Pract.* 1992;42:116–119.

76. Oghagbon EK. Commentary: Improving persistently elevated HBA1c in diabetes mellitus patients in Nigeria. *Ethn Dis.* 2014;24(4):502–507.

77. Dagogo-Jack S. Preventing diabetes-related morbidity and mortality in the primary care setting. *J Natl Med Assoc.* 2002;94:549–560.

78. Prevention and Control of Noncommunicable Diseases: Guidelines for primary health care in low-resource settings. 2012. Accessed from www.apps.who.int on 10/10/18.

20 Gestational Diabetes
Focus on Pregestational, Gestational, and Postnatal Weight Management

Jacques E. Samson

CONTENTS

20.1 INTRODUCTION

The prevalence of obesity is increasing worldwide and is associated with increased rates of gestational diabetes. This greatly impacts the developing fetus and has the potential for detrimental influences not only in utero, but also long-term, throughout the offspring's lifespan. Various metabolic changes occur in pregnancy, which leads to hyperinsulinemia, insulin resistance, and a relative fasting hypoglycemia. The placenta is a complex endocrine organ that is capable of synthesizing various hormones, growth factors, and cytokines whose function is to provide the necessary nutrients to the developing and growing fetus.

20.1.1 EPIDEMIOLOGY

Diabetes is a common medical complication of pregnancy that poses a threat both to the mother and her fetus. It is estimated that up to 6%–9% of pregnancies are complicated by diabetes mellitus, and approximately 90% of these cases represents women with gestational diabetes (GDM) (1). More than 8 million women in the United States have pre-GDM (2). The increase in obesity parallels the risk of developing diabetes (3). Complications of uncontrolled diabetes in pregnancy include spontaneous abortion, fetal anomalies, macrosomia, fetal demise, preterm delivery, preeclampsia, neonatal hypoglycemia, neonatal hyperbilirubinemia, increased risk of obesity, and type 2 diabetes in the offspring later in life (4,5). Pregnancy is a motivating time and presents a window of opportunity for lifestyle modification and optimization of diabetes control. A multidisciplinary approach in an intensified manner may assist the diabetic patient in optimizing her care, which may lead to excellent perinatal outcomes.

20.1.2 CLASSIFICATION OF DIABETES IN PREGNANCY

20.1.2.1 Historical Perspective

In 1949, Dr. Priscilla White developed a classification system for diabetes in pregnancy (6):

Class A: Diagnosis made on glucose tolerance test, which deviates slightly from the normal
Class B: Duration of less than 10 years and onset age of at least 20 years with no vascular disease
Class C: Duration 10–19 years or onset 10–19 years of age; minimal vascular disease
Class D: Duration ≥20 years or onset <10 years of age or evidence of vascular disease
Class E: Calcified pelvic arteries on X-ray
Class F: Nephritis
Class T: Transplantation

The White classification was revised in 1965, 1972, and 1980. In 1994, the American College of Obstetrician and Gynecologists (ACOG) Technical Bulletin noted "improvements in fetal assessment and neonatal care, and metabolic management of the pregnant woman have rendered the White classification system less helpful" (7,8). The most recent ACOG practice bulletin makes no mention of White's classification (8,9). The above classification is of historical importance, as many authors use various revisions in their publications.

20.1.2.2 Diabetes Classification (American Diabetes Association)

The American Diabetes Association (ADA) has classified diabetes into the following categories (10):

1. Type 1 diabetes: Caused by β-cell destruction leading to absolute insulin deficiency.
2. Type 2 diabetes: Progressive loss of β-cell insulin secretion frequently on the background of insulin resistance.
3. GDM: Diabetes diagnosed in the second or third trimester of pregnancy that was not clearly overt diabetes prior to gestation.
4. Specific type of diabetes due to other causes: Monogenic diabetes syndromes (neonatal diabetes and maturity-onset diabetes of the young), diseases of the exocrine pancreas (cystic fibrosis), and drug- or chemical-induced diabetes (glucocorticoids, treatment of HIV/ AIDS, or organ transplantation).

20.1.3 DEFINITION OF GESTATIONAL DIABETES

GDM has been defined as any degree of carbohydrate intolerance first recognized during pregnancy, regardless of whether the condition may have predated pregnancy or persisted after the pregnancy (11). The prevailing maternal adaptation in pregnancy is the shift in glucose metabolism from insulin sensitivity to insulin resistance, exemplified by higher circulating lipids, heightened postprandial glucose, and increased β-cell demand/response (12,13).

When women cannot adapt to the glycemic demands of pregnancy, hyperglycemia and glucose intolerance manifest by the late second trimester, and this is recognized as GDM (1).

20.2 IMPACT OF GESTATIONAL DIABETES ON PREGNANCY AND BEYOND

20.2.1 NEONATAL RISKS

The offspring of women with GDM are at increased risk of macrosomia, neonatal hypoglycemia, hyperbilirubinemia, shoulder dystocia, birth trauma, and stillbirth (14). Maternal diabetes also impacts the offspring's metabolism and contributes to childhood and adult-onset obesity and diabetes (5,15). Anomalies have also been associated with diabetes in pregnancy; however, they seem to be more common in pre-GDM first diagnosed during pregnancy (Figures 20.1 and 20.2). Observational studies show an increased risk of anencephaly, microcephaly, congenital heart disease, and caudal regression (3).

20.2.2 MATERNAL RISKS

Women with GDM are at greater risk of developing preeclampsia, undergoing a cesarean delivery, and, in up to 70% of women, developing diabetes mellitus later in life (14).

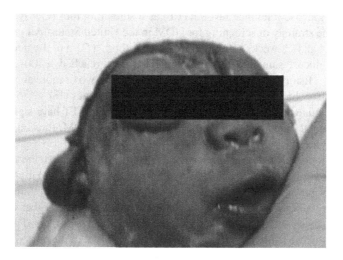

FIGURE 20.1 Neonate with anencephaly of a diabetic mother. (Courtesy of Jacques E. Samson's.)

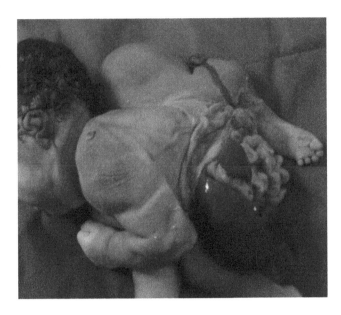

FIGURE 20.2   Neonate with body stalk anomaly born of a diabetic patient with an HbA1c of 12.4%. (Courtesy of Jacques E. Samson's.)

20.3   DIAGNOSIS OF GESTATIONAL DIABETES MELLITUS

Debate continues regarding the diagnosis and treatment of GDM, despite several large studies. In the United States, screening for GDM historically consisted of obtaining the patient's medical history, focused on past obstetric outcomes and a family history of type 2 diabetes (14). This strategy failed to identify half of women with GDM (16). In 1973, O'Sullivan proposed the use of a 50-g, 1-hour oral glucose tolerance test (OGTT) as a screening tool (17). A two-step screening tool has remained the strategy of screening for GDM in the United States. All pregnant patients are screened between 24 and 28 weeks using the two-step method: a 50-g oral glucose screen followed by a 1-hour venous glucose sample. Once a threshold has been reached, a 100-g, 3-hour diagnostic OGTT is performed. Historically, the diagnosis was made with two or more abnormal values; however, a recent study has challenged the need for two abnormal values (18).

Women with even one abnormal value on the 100-g, 3-hour OGTT have significantly increased risk of adverse perinatal outcomes compared with women with GDM, thus one elevated value, as opposed to two, may be used for the diagnosis of GDM (14,19).

There are no randomized trials that have evaluated the threshold value of the 1-hour glucose challenge that should be used. It varies from 130 to 140 mg/dL. A value of 140 mg/dL has lower false-positives and greater positive predictive values across various racial and ethnic groups. Although sensitivities are marginally improved using lower thresholds, there are higher false-positives (20). An elevated 1-hour screen should prompt a confirmatory test with a 100-g oral glucose solution followed by a 3-hour glucose sampling. The diagnosis of gestational diabetes is made when a 1-hour screen is higher than 190 or at least one value of plasma or serum glucose levels is elevated after a 3-hour OGTT (14). The Carpenter Coustan criteria for diagnosis of GDM uses a lower threshold than the National Diabetes Data Group and may result in higher rates of diagnosis (14,21):

Fasting: at least 95 mg/dL (5.3 mmol/L)
1 hour: at least 180 mg/dL (10.0 mmol/L)
2 hours: at least 155 mg/dL (8.6 mmol/L)
3 hours: at least 140 mg/dL (7.8 mmol/L)

In an attempt to identify pregnant women with glucose intolerance who are at increased risk for adverse perinatal outcomes, the Hyperglycemia and Adverse Pregnancy Outcomes (HAPO) Study Cooperative Research Group conducted a study to clarify the risks of adverse outcomes associated with various degrees of maternal glucose tolerance lower than those in overt diabetes mellitus (22). A one-step, 75-g OGTT was used followed by 2-hour plasma glucose to identify thresholds for preselected primary and secondary outcomes. In order to standardize the diagnosis of GDM, The International Association of Diabetes and Pregnancy Study Group (IADPSG) in 2010 recommended that a universal 75-g, 2-hour OGTT be performed during pregnancy and that the diagnosis of GDM be made when any single threshold value was met or exceeded (19).

Fasting: at least 92 mg/dL (5.1 mmol/L)
1 hour: at least 180 mg/dL (10.0 mmol/L)
2 hour: at least 153 mg/dL (8.5 mmol/L)

The adoption of the IADPSG would identify approximately 18% of pregnant women in the United States as having GDM. The Eunice Kennedy Shriver National Institute of Child Health and Human Development Consensus Development Conference on Diagnosing Gestational Diabetes recommended the use of a two-step method to screen and diagnose GDM, as there is lack of evidence that the one-step, 75-g OGTT leads to clinically significant improvements in maternal or newborn outcomes. In addition, implementation of this one-step method would significantly increase healthcare costs (23).

The ACOG supports the two-step process. The ADA continues to recognize that there is no clear evidence that supports the IADPSG-recommended diagnostic approach (10).

Early screening is recommended in order to diagnose early GDM or pre-GDM. Women with the following risk factors should be screened at their first prenatal visit: overweight, obese, polycystic ovarian syndrome, previous history of GDM, previous child weighing at least 4,000 g, first-degree relative with diabetes and hypertension (10).

20.4 MANAGEMENT OF GESTATIONAL DIABETES MELLITUS

20.4.1 BENEFITS OF TREATING GESTATIONAL DIABETES

The Australian Carbohydrate Intolerance Study in Pregnant Women trial was the first large-scale, randomized treatment trial for GDM. In 2005, they found that treatment was associated with significant reduction in the rate of a composite of serious newborn complications: perinatal death, shoulder dystocia, birth trauma including fracture, and nerve palsy. Other comorbidities, such as large-for-gestational-age infants, reduced neonatal fat, preeclampsia, and rates of cesarean delivery have been reported to be reduced (24–26).

Treatment of diabetes in pregnancy begins with lifestyle modification, which includes medical nutrition therapy, physical activity, and weight management depending on pregestational weight gain (3). It is suggested that 70%–85% of women diagnosed with GDM can have optimal glycemic control with lifestyle modification alone.

Two large clinical trials have shown the effectiveness of intensive lifestyle interventions in high-risk patients with a relative risk reduction of 58% in the diagnosis of diabetes (27). A recent meta-analysis that included 15 trials (4,501 women and 3,768 infants) concluded that lifestyle interventions are the primary therapeutic strategy for women with GDM. The lifetime interventions included a variety of components, such as education, diet, exercise, and self-monitoring of blood glucose. Women who adopted lifestyle modification were less likely to have postnatal depression and were more likely to achieve postpartum weight goals. There was also a decrease in large-for-gestational-age neonates and decreased neonatal adiposity (28). The goal of lifestyle modification in

GDM is to achieve normal blood glucose, provide adequate weight gain, and contribute to appropriate fetal growth and development (14). The ADA recommends nutritional counseling by a registered dietician and development of a personalized nutrition plan based on the individual's BMI for all patients with GDM (3).

20.4.2 DIETARY MODIFICATIONS

The conventional approach to nutrition therapy in GDM has focused on carbohydrate restriction. Although effective, this approach is the most challenging component to treatment adherence in GDM. Furthermore, there is little evidence supporting carbohydrate restriction or any diet prescription in GDM (29). Although there is no consensus on the optimal diet for women with GDM, a recent meta-analysis of 19 trials attempted to determine which dietary advice for women with GDM was the best for reducing perinatal complications. Ten different diets, ranging from low-moderate glycemic index (GI) diets to ethnic-specific diet with standard healthy diet, were analyzed. The review found no clear difference between the different types of diets in reducing poor perinatal outcomes, except for a possible reduction in cesarean section rates (30). More evidence is needed to assess the effects of different types of diets for women with GDM.

The goal of medical nutrition therapy in women with GDM is to achieve normal blood glucose levels, prevent ketosis, provide adequate weight gain, and contribute to appropriate fetal growth and development (14). The ADA recommends nutritional counseling by a registered dietician and development of a personalized nutrition plan based on the patient's BMI (3). Nutritional counseling should include recommendations about caloric allotment, carbohydrate intake, and caloric distribution. Although the dietary composition that optimizes perinatal outcomes is unknown, it is suggested that carbohydrate intake be from complex carbohydrates and be limited to 33%–40% of calories. The remaining calories should be from proteins comprising of 20% protein and 40% fat (31). Three meals and two to three snacks are recommended to distribute carbohydrate intake and reduce postprandial glucose fluctuations (14).

20.4.3 PHYSICAL ACTIVITY

There is a paucity of published trials addressing physical activity in patients with GDM. Most studies are small in sample size and have not shown improvements in glucose levels. Benefits of exercise in managing diabetes are extrapolated from the nonpregnant literature. Weight training exercise tends to have the most impact as it increases lean muscle mass and improves tissue sensitivity to insulin. Women with GDM should aim for 30 minutes of moderate-intensity aerobic exercise at least five times per week or a minimum of 150 minutes per week. Furthermore, simple regimens, such as walking for 10–15 minutes after each meal, can lead to improved glycemic control and are recommended (32,33).

Appropriate weight gain based on BMI is another cornerstone in optimizing outcomes in pregnancy. The Institute of Medicine guidelines recommend a total weight gain of 6.8–11.3 kg (15–25 lbs) for overweight pregnant women (BMI of 25.0–29.9). It is recommended that all obese women (BMI ≥ 30) gain 5.0–9.1 kg (11–20 lbs). Excessive gestational weight gain is associated with short-term and long-term postpartum weight retention and large-for-gestational-age neonates (34). Weight loss, however, is not recommended during pregnancy. Several studies have consistently identified increased risk of small-for-gestational-age (less than tenth percentile) neonates (34).

20.4.4 MEDICATION MANAGEMENT

Oral medications such as metformin and glyburide have been used to treat gestational diabetes, however, the US Food and Drug Administration (FDA) has not approved them for this indication.

20.4.4.1 Metformin

Metformin, a biguanide that inhibits hepatic gluconeogenesis and glucose absorption and stimulates glucose uptake by the peripheral tissue, gained acceptance to be used in pregnancy after several studies demonstrated its safety. A large, randomized controlled trial (RCT) assigned 751 women with GDM to receive insulin or metformin. The composite outcome of perinatal morbidity, which included neonatal hypoglycemia, respiratory distress, phototherapy, birth trauma, prematurity and low APGAR scores, was noted to be similar in both groups; however, 46% of women who took metformin eventually required insulin (35). Another RCT of 47 women per arm evaluated glycemic control in women receiving metformin or insulin in GDM to identify factors predicting the need for supplemental insulin in those treated with metformin. Metformin was noted to provide adequate glycemic control with lower mean glucose levels, less weight gain, and lower frequency of neonatal hypoglycemia; however, 26% of women receiving metformin required supplemental insulin (36). A meta-analysis of six randomized clinical trials that included 1,420 patients suggested that metformin use in pregnancy did not significantly increase adverse maternal outcomes and neonatal outcomes. There was less weight gain and less rates of neonatal hypoglycemia; however, there was a higher incidence of premature births (37). Another meta-analysis including 2,509 patients found no difference when comparing metformin and insulin; however, metformin had a higher rate of preterm birth, with a risk ratio of 1.5 (38).

Metformin crosses the placenta with levels that can be as high as maternal concentration. Long-term metabolic effects on the fetus are unknown (39). These concerns along, with an increased risk of preterm birth, are reasons the ADA continues to recommend insulin as the first line treatment when pharmacologic agents are indicated to treat GDM (3).

Some women may decline insulin use; therefore, metformin may be used as a second-line drug for the treatment of GDM (14). Metformin can be given at 500 mg nightly for 1 week at initiation, then increased to 500 mg twice daily (9).

20.4.4.2 Glyburide

Glyburide is a sulfonylurea that binds to pancreatic β-cell adenosine triphosphate calcium channel receptors to increase insulin secretion and insulin sensitivity of peripheral tissues.

Several studies have described the efficacy of glyburide as a treatment option for GDM. A secondary analysis of an RCT of 404 women sought to evaluate glyburide versus insulin and severity level of GDM and pregnancy outcome. It was concluded that glyburide and insulin were equally effective for treatment of GDM at all levels of severity (40). A recent meta-analysis of 18 randomized, clinical trials to evaluate the efficacy and safety of oral antidiabetic drugs for treatment of gestational diabetes concluded that both metformin and glyburide might be suitable for use in pregnancy. Glyburide, however, was associated with increased risk of neonatal hypoglycemia, high maternal weight gain, high neonatal birth weight, and macrosomia (41). Another meta-analysis concluded that significant differences in the primary outcomes in glyburide versus insulin were obtained in birthweight (mean difference of 109 g), macrosomia (risk ratio, 2.62), and neonatal hypoglycemia (risk ratio, 2.04). The study also concluded that glyburide is clearly inferior to insulin and should not be used for treatment of women with GDM (38). The ACOG have stated that, although glyburide use has increased in the treatment of GDM, it should not be recommended as a first-line pharmacologic treatment because, in most studies, it does not yield equivalent outcomes to insulin (14).

20.4.4.3 Insulin

Insulin does not cross the placenta and is the only pharmacologic treatment approved by the FDA for the treatment of GDM in the United States. The ADA continues to recommend insulin as the drug of choice for treatment of GDM. Oral medications have not been approved by the FDA for use in pregnancy.

The mainstay of insulin management in pregnancy includes a combination of short-acting insulin, such as lispro and aspart, and intermediate-acting insulin, such as neutral protamine Hagedorn (NPH). The typical starting dose is 0.7–1.0 U/kg daily in divided doses. Dosage adjustments should

TABLE 20.1
Action Profiles of Various Insulin Regimens

Type	Onset of Action	Peak of Action (h)	Duration of Action (h)
Insulin lispro	1–15 min	1–2	4–5
Insulin aspart	1–15 min	1–2	4–5
Regular insulin	30–60 min	2–4	6–8
Isophane insulin (NPH)	1–3 h	5–7	13–18
Insulin glargine	1–2 h	No peak	24
Insulin detemir	1–3 h	Minimal peak 8–10	18–26

Source: Gabbe, S.G. and Graves, C.R., *Obstet. Gynecol.*, 102, 857–868, 2003; Committee on Practice Bulletins-Obstetrics, *Obstet. Gynecol.*, 130, e17–e37, 2017.

be based on blood glucose levels (1). Long-acting insulins, such as glargine and detemir, have been evaluated in pregnancy and have been to be as effective as the combination of short and intermediate insulin (42,43). Action profiles for various insulin regimens are delineated in Table 20.1. Further high-quality RCTs are needed to determine the best treatment options for diabetes in pregnancy.

20.4.4.4 Glucose Monitoring

Surveillance of blood glucose values is required to determine glycemic control. Unfortunately, there is insufficient data to delineate the optimal frequency of blood glucose testing in women with GDM. The general recommendation is for daily glucose monitoring four times a day—fasting and after each meal (14). Tight metabolic control occurs when fasting blood glucose levels are less than or equal to 95 mg/dL; 1-hour levels are less than or equal to 140 mg/dL; or 2-hour levels are less than or equal to 120 mg/dL.

Real-time continuous glucose monitoring (CGM) measures interstitial glucose in an ongoing fashion. Studies in nonpregnant patients indicate that real-time CGM lowers hemoglobin A1c (HbA1c) and may reduce the tendency for biochemical hypoglycemia (44). Secher et al. randomized pregnant women with pre-GDM, both type 1 and type 2, to intermittent CGM or routine care in order to determine whether CGM improves maternal glycemic control and pregnancy outcomes. They concluded that intermittent, real-time CGM did not improve glycemic control or pregnancy outcomes (45). A recent multicenter RCT by Feig et al. randomized 325 women with type 1 diabetes for 12 months (46). Patients who were planning on becoming pregnant or were already pregnant were selected and randomized to CGM in addition to capillary glucose monitoring or capillary glucose monitoring alone with the aim to evaluate maternal glucose control, obstetric outcomes, and neonatal health outcomes. Women randomized to CGM had a greater reduction in HbA1c, reduced hyperglycemia, less glycemic variability, reduction in large-for-gestational-age fetuses, and reduction in neonatal hypoglycemia and admission to the neonatal ICU. This trial has been evaluated in nonpregnant patients and pregnancy in women with type 1 diabetes. CGM should therefore be considered in pregnant patients with type 1 diabetes using intensive insulin therapy (46).

20.5 INTERVENTIONS FOR PREVENTION OF GESTATIONAL DIABETES

20.5.1 LIFESTYLE MODIFICATIONS (DIET AND PHYSICAL ACTIVITY)

There is a direct link between obesity and the risk of developing GDM. In women with pre-GDM, optimal control should occur prior to pregnancy. Observational studies show an increased risk of diabetic embryopathy with poor glycemic control. In patients with pre-GDM, associations between elevated periconceptional HbA1c and embryopathy are convincing; therefore, it is recommended to optimize glycemic control prior to conception with an HbA1c below 6.5% (48 mmol/mol) in order to minimize this risk (47,48).

Although there is no robust evidence to provide guidance on the primary prevention of GDM, lifestyle modification including dietary changes and exercise has been effective in the management of obesity and appears to be a promising strategy. In addition, lifestyle modification has been found to reduce the incidence of developing diabetes in high-risk patients (49). It has been established that obese women who have even small weight reductions prior to pregnancy may have improved pregnancy outcomes (34). Although achieving a normal BMI is ideal, a weight loss of 5%–7% can significantly improve metabolic health (50). Motivational interviewing, a directive, patient-centered counseling approach focused on exploring and resolving ambivalence, has emerged as an effective adjunctive therapeutic approach in lifestyle modification. A systemic review and meta-analysis of 29 RCTs demonstrated that lifestyle modification with diet or physical activity prior to 15 weeks' gestation resulted in an 18% reduction in the risk of GDM (51). The US Preventive Task Force recommends that all adults 18 years and older with a BMI of 30 or higher be offered and referred to intensive, multicomponent behavior interventions (52).

Nutritional supplements that incorporate bioactive agents with positive effect on insulin sensitivity, such as myo-inositol (2 g twice daily) and probiotics, have shown promising results in reducing the incidence of GDM (53). Limited evidence conducted in women at risk of developing GDM from one study using probiotics and three small trials using myo-inositol have shown a 60%–70% reduction in the risk of developing GDM. Various dietary interventions including diet counseling, low-GI diet, energy restriction diet (33% reduction in caloric intake), and low-carbohydrate diet have demonstrated a reduction in the risk of GDM and lower gestational weight gain (54). In addition, the ADA recommends dietary strategies to prevent development of diabetes including reduced calories and reduced intake of dietary fat, dietary fiber of 14 g/1,000 kcal and foods containing whole grains (55).

Women with preexisting diabetes may benefit from a very low-carbohydrate ketogenic diet prior to pregnancy. A recent randomized trial demonstrated a greater reduction in HbA1c, greater weight loss, and reduced medication requirement when compared to patients with a moderate-carbohydrate, calorie-restricted, low-fat diet (56).

Exercise, defined as purposeful physical activity carried out to sustain or improve health or fitness, is effective in improving metabolic health. The ADA recommends regular physical activity of 150 minutes per week (55). High-intensity interval training, which involves alternating periods of relatively intense exercise with periods of rest or low intensity for 60 minutes, 5 days per week, have been described by RCTs and meta-analysis to improve fasting blood glucose, HbA1c, and body composition (57–59).

20.5.2 Weight Loss

Long-term maintenance of glycemic control ideally should involve a multidisciplinary approach, including nutrition counseling and visits with a diabetes nurse and certified diabetes educator. Postpartum weight loss, involving behavioral modification, nutritional counseling, diet, and physical activity is recommended for all overweight and obese women. A systematic review and meta-analysis of 12 RCTs concluded that motivational interviewing appears to enhance weight loss in overweight and obese patients when used alongside behavioral weight-management programs (50). The optimal macronutrient distribution of weight loss diets has not been established. The recommended minimum dietary allowance for digestible carbohydrate is 130 g/day. Fats should be limited to below 7% of total calories (< 200 mg/day). Two or more servings of fish per week are recommended. Protein intake should account for 15%–20% of ingested energy (55).

Surgical interventions such as gastric bypass have also been shown to improve medical comorbidities and may be considered prior to pregnancy. Long-term observational studies have shown considerable improvements in glycemic control and associated comorbidities among patients who have undergone bariatric surgery.

20.6   FETAL MONITORING AND TIMING OF DELIVERY

Assignment of gestational age is performed with the patient's known last menstrual period, in addition to an early dating ultrasound. This should ideally be performed during the first trimester. An anatomy ultrasound or fetal survey is usually performed between 18 and 20 weeks' gestations. Since macrosomia, defined as an estimated fetal weight of 4,000 g or greater, may occur as a result of gestational diabetes, it is also reasonable to assess fetal growth in the third trimester. Although there is no consensus regarding antepartum fetal testing in well-controlled patients with GDM who are not medically treated, patients with GDM who require medications or patients with pre-GDM are recommended to have twice-weekly antenatal surveillance starting around 32 weeks (14). Timing of delivery depends on glycemic control. In well-controlled GDM not requiring medications, expectant management may be considered until 40 weeks 6 days. In GDM requiring medications, delivery is recommended between 39 weeks 0 days to 39 weeks and 6 days. Experts have supported earlier delivery for women with poorly controlled GDM (60,61).

Screening between 4 and 12 weeks postpartum is recommended for all women who had GDM. The Fifth International Workshop on Gestational Diabetes Mellitus recommends that women with GDM undergo a 75-g, 2-hour OGTT in the postpartum period. This should include a fasting and 2-hour value. Testing should occur every 1–3 years thereafter (62).

20.7   CONCLUSION

GDM management should focus on lifestyle modification. Education, dietary modifications, exercise, and glucose monitoring are the hallmarks of nonpharmacologic management. When pharmacologic treatment of GDM is indicated, insulin is considered first line. Screening 4–12 weeks postpartum is recommended for all women with a diagnosis of GDM. This should be repeated every 1–3 years thereafter. Postpartum weight loss and maintenance, involving behavioral modification, nutritional counseling, diet, and physical activity, are recommended for all overweight and obese women and may be the strategy to delay and even prevent progression to diabetes.

REFERENCES

1. Committee on Practice Bulletins-Obstetrics. Practice bulletin no. 137: Gestational diabetes mellitus. *Obstet Gynecol*. 2013;122(2 Pt 1):406–416.
2. ACOG Committee on Practice Bulletins. ACOG practice bulletin no. 58. Ultrasonography in pregnancy. *Obstet Gynecol*. 2004;104(6):1449–1458.
3. American Diabetes Association. 13. Management of diabetes in pregnancy. *Diabetes Care*. 2017;40(Suppl 1):S114–S119.
4. Holmes VA, Young IS, Patterson CC, Pearson DW, Walker JD, Maresh MJ et al. Optimal glycemic control, pre-eclampsia, and gestational hypertension in women with type 1 diabetes in the diabetes and pre-eclampsia intervention trial. *Diabetes Care*. 2011;34(8):1683–1688.
5. Dabelea D, Hanson RL, Lindsay RS, Pettitt DJ, Imperatore G, Gabir MM et al. Intrauterine exposure to diabetes conveys risks for type 2 diabetes and obesity: A study of discordant sibships. *Diabetes*. 2000;49(12):2208–2211.
6. White P. Pregnancy complicating diabetes. *Am J Med*. 1949;7(5):609–616.
7. ACOG technical bulletin. Diabetes and pregnancy. Number 200–December 1994 (replaces No. 92, May 1986). Committee on Technical Bulletins of the American College of Obstetricians and Gynecologists. *Int J Gynaecol Obstet*. 1995;48(3):331–339.
8. Sacks DA, Metzger BE. Classification of diabetes in pregnancy: Time to reassess the alphabet. *Obstet Gynecol*. 2013;121(2 Pt 1):345–348.
9. American College of Obstetricians and Gynecologists Committee on Practice Bulletins-Obstetrics. ACOG practice bulletin. Clinical management guidelines for obstetrician-gynecologists. Number 30, September 2001 (replaces Technical Bulletin Number 200, December 1994). Gestational diabetes. *Obstet Gynecol*. 2001;98(3):525–538.

10. American Diabetes Association. 2. Classification and diagnosis of diabetes. *Diabetes Care.* 2017;40(Suppl 1):S11–S24.

11. Report of the Expert Committee on the diagnosis and classification of diabetes mellitus. *Diabetes Care.* 1997;20(7):1183–1197.

12. Di Cianni G, Miccoli R, Volpe L, Lencioni C, Del Prato S. Intermediate metabolism in normal pregnancy and in gestational diabetes. *Diabetes Metab Res Rev.* 2003;19(4):259–270.

13. Butte NF. Carbohydrate and lipid metabolism in pregnancy: Normal compared with gestational diabetes mellitus. *Am J Clin Nutr.* 2000;71(5 Suppl):1256S–1261S.

14. Committee on Practice Bulletins-Obstetrics. Practice bulletin no. 180: Gestational diabetes mellitus. *Obstet Gynecol.* 2017;130(1):e17–e37.

15. Clausen TD, Mathiesen ER, Hansen T, Pedersen O, Jensen DM, Lauenborg J et al. Overweight and the metabolic syndrome in adult offspring of women with diet-treated gestational diabetes mellitus or type 1 diabetes. *J Clin Endocrinol Metab.* 2009;94(7):2464–2470.

16. Coustan DR, Nelson C, Carpenter MW, Carr SR, Rotondo L, Widness JA. Maternal age and screening for gestational diabetes: A population-based study. *Obstet Gynecol.* 1989;73(4):557–561.

17. O'Sullivan JB, Mahan CM, Charles D, Dandrow RV. Screening criteria for high-risk gestational diabetic patients. *Am J Obstet Gynecol.* 1973;116(7):895–900.

18. Roeckner JT, Sanchez-Ramos L, Jijon-Knupp R, Kaunitz AM. Single abnormal value on 3-hour oral glucose tolerance test during pregnancy is associated with adverse maternal and neonatal outcomes: A systematic review and metaanalysis. *Am J Obstet Gynecol.* 2016;215(3):287–297.

19. International Association of Diabetes and Pregnancy Study Groups Consensus Panel, Metzger BE, Gabbe SG, Persson B, Buchanan TA et al. International association of diabetes and pregnancy study groups recommendations on the diagnosis and classification of hyperglycemia in pregnancy. *Diabetes Care.* 2010;33(3):676–682.

20. Esakoff TF, Cheng YW, Caughey AB. Screening for gestational diabetes: Different cut-offs for different ethnicities? *Am J Obstet Gynecol.* 2005;193(3 Pt 2):1040–1044.

21. Carpenter MW, Coustan DR. Criteria for screening tests for gestational diabetes. *Am J Obstet Gynecol.* 1982;144(7):768–773.

22. HAPO Study Cooperative Research Group, Metzger BE, Lowe LP, Dyer AR, Trimble ER, Chaovarindr U et al. Hyperglycemia and adverse pregnancy outcomes. *N Engl J Med.* 2008;358(19):1991–2002.

23. Vandorsten JP, Dodson WC, Espeland MA, Grobman WA, Guise JM, Mercer BM et al. NIH consensus development conference: Diagnosing gestational diabetes mellitus. *NIH Consens State Sci Statements.* 2013;29(1):1–31.

24. Crowther CA, Hiller JE, Moss JR, McPhee AJ, Jeffries WS, Robinson JS et al. Effect of treatment of gestational diabetes mellitus on pregnancy outcomes. *N Engl J Med.* 2005;352(24):2477–2486.

25. Landon MB, Spong CY, Thom E, Carpenter MW, Ramin SM, Casey B et al. A multicenter, randomized trial of treatment for mild gestational diabetes. *N Engl J Med.* 2009;361(14):1339–1348.

26. Hartling L, Dryden DM, Guthrie A, Muise M, Vandermeer B, Donovan L. Benefits and harms of treating gestational diabetes mellitus: A systematic review and meta-analysis for the U.S. Preventive Services Task Force and the National Institutes of Health Office of Medical Applications of Research. *Ann Intern Med.* 2013;159(2):123–129.

27. Inzucchi SE. Diagnosis of diabetes. *N Engl J Med.* 2013;368(2):193.

28. Brown J, Alwan NA, West J, Brown S, McKinlay CJ, Farrar D et al. Lifestyle interventions for the treatment of women with gestational diabetes. *Cochrane Database Syst Rev.* 2017;5:CD011970.

29. Hernandez TL. Carbohydrate content in the GDM diet: Two views: View 1: Nutrition therapy in gestational diabetes: The case for complex carbohydrates. *Diabetes Spectr.* 2016;29(2):82–88.

30. Han S, Middleton P, Shepherd E, Van Ryswyk E, Crowther CA. Different types of dietary advice for women with gestational diabetes mellitus. *Cochrane Database Syst Rev.* 2017;2:CD009275.

31. Mulford MI, Jovanovic-Peterson L, Peterson CM. Alternative therapies for the management of gestational diabetes. *Clin Perinatol.* 1993;20(3):619–634.

32. Basevi V, Di Mario S, Morciano C, Nonino F, Magrini N. Comment on: American Diabetes Association. Standards of medical care in diabetes–2011. *Diabetes Care.* 2011;34(Suppl. 1):S11–S61. *Diabetes Care.* 2011;34(5):e53; author reply e4.

33. Davenport MH, Mottola MF, McManus R, Gratton R. A walking intervention improves capillary glucose control in women with gestational diabetes mellitus: A pilot study. *Appl Physiol Nutr Metab.* 2008;33(3):511–517.

34. Practice bulletin no. 156: Obesity in pregnancy: Correction. *Obstet Gynecol.* 2016;128(6):1450.

35. Rowan JA, Hague WM, Gao W, Battin MR, Moore MP, Mi GTI. Metformin versus insulin for the treatment of gestational diabetes. *N Engl J Med*. 2008;358(19):2003–2015.

36. Spaulonci CP, Bernardes LS, Trindade TC, Zugaib M, Francisco RP. Randomized trial of metformin vs insulin in the management of gestational diabetes. *Am J Obstet Gynecol*. 2013;209(1):34e1-7.

37. Su DF, Wang XY. Metformin vs insulin in the management of gestational diabetes: A systematic review and meta-analysis. *Diabetes Res Clin Pract*. 2014;104(3):353–357.

38. Balsells M, Garcia-Patterson A, Sola I, Roque M, Gich I, Corcoy R. Glibenclamide, metformin, and insulin for the treatment of gestational diabetes: a systematic review and meta-analysis. *BMJ*. 2015;350:h102.

39. Eyal S, Easterling TR, Carr D, Umans JG, Miodovnik M, Hankins GD et al. Pharmacokinetics of metformin during pregnancy. *Drug Metab Dispos*. 2010;38(5):833–840.

40. Langer O, Yogev Y, Xenakis EM, Rosenn B. Insulin and glyburide therapy: Dosage, severity level of gestational diabetes, and pregnancy outcome. *Am J Obstet Gynecol*. 2005;192(1):134–139.

41. Jiang YF, Chen XY, Ding T, Wang XF, Zhu ZN, Su SW. Comparative efficacy and safety of OADs in management of GDM: Network meta-analysis of randomized controlled trials. *J Clin Endocrinol Metab*. 2015;100(5):2071–2080.

42. Herrera KM, Rosenn BM, Foroutan J, Bimson BE, Al Ibraheemi Z, Moshier EL et al. Randomized controlled trial of insulin detemir versus NPH for the treatment of pregnant women with diabetes. *Am J Obstet Gynecol*. 2015;213(3):426e1-7.

43. Lv S, Wang J, Xu Y. Safety of insulin analogs during pregnancy: A meta-analysis. *Arch Gynecol Obstet*. 2015;292(4):749–756.

44. Juvenile Diabetes Research Foundation Continuous Glucose Monitoring Study Group, Beck RW, Hirsch IB, Laffel L, Tamborlane WV, Bode BW et al. The effect of continuous glucose monitoring in well-controlled type 1 diabetes. *Diabetes Care*. 2009;32(8):1378–1383.

45. Secher AL, Ringholm L, Andersen HU, Damm P, Mathiesen ER. The effect of real-time continuous glucose monitoring in pregnant women with diabetes: A randomized controlled trial. *Diabetes Care*. 2013;36(7):1877–1883.

46. Feig DS, Donovan LE, Corcoy R, Murphy KE, Amiel SA, Hunt KF et al. Continuous glucose monitoring in pregnant women with type 1 diabetes (CONCEPTT): A multicentre international randomised controlled trial. *Lancet*. 2017;390(10110):2347–2359.

47. Guerin A, Nisenbaum R, Ray JG. Use of maternal GHb concentration to estimate the risk of congenital anomalies in the offspring of women with prepregnancy diabetes. *Diabetes Care*. 2007;30(7):1920–1925.

48. Jensen DM, Korsholm L, Ovesen P, Beck-Nielsen H, Moelsted-Pedersen L, Westergaard JG et al. Periconceptional A1C and risk of serious adverse pregnancy outcome in 933 women with type 1 diabetes. *Diabetes Care*. 2009;32(6):1046–1048.

49. Knowler WC, Barrett-Connor E, Fowler SE, Hamman RF, Lachin JM, Walker EA et al. Reduction in the incidence of type 2 diabetes with lifestyle intervention or metformin. *N Engl J Med*. 2002;346(6):393–403.

50. Armstrong MJ, Mottershead TA, Ronksley PE, Sigal RJ, Campbell TS, Hemmelgarn BR. Motivational interviewing to improve weight loss in overweight and/or obese patients: A systematic review and meta-analysis of randomized controlled trials. *Obes Rev*. 2011;12(9):709–723.

51. Song C, Li J, Leng J, Ma RC, Yang X. Lifestyle intervention can reduce the risk of gestational diabetes: A meta-analysis of randomized controlled trials. *Obes Rev*. 2016;17(10):960–969.

52. Moyer VA, U.S. Preventive Services Task Force. Screening for and management of obesity in adults: U.S. Preventive Services Task Force recommendation statement. *Ann Intern Med*. 2012;157(5):373–378.

53. Rogozinska E, Chamillard M, Hitman GA, Khan KS, Thangaratinam S. Nutritional manipulation for the primary prevention of gestational diabetes mellitus: A meta-analysis of randomised studies. *PLoS One*. 2015;10(2):e0115526.

54. Silva-Zolezzi I, Samuel TM, Spieldenner J. Maternal nutrition: Opportunities in the prevention of gestational diabetes. *Nutr Rev*. 2017;75(suppl 1):32–50.

55. American Diabetes Association, Bantle JP, Wylie-Rosett J, Albright AL, Apovian CM, Clark NG et al. Nutrition recommendations and interventions for diabetes: A position statement of the American Diabetes Association. *Diabetes Care*. 2008;31 Suppl 1:S61–S78.

56. Saslow LR, Daubenmier JJ, Moskowitz JT, Kim S, Murphy EJ, Phinney SD et al. Twelve-month outcomes of a randomized trial of a moderate-carbohydrate versus very low-carbohydrate diet in overweight adults with type 2 diabetes mellitus or prediabetes. *Nutr Diabetes*. 2017;7(12):304.

57. Karstoft K, Winding K, Knudsen SH, Nielsen JS, Thomsen C, Pedersen BK et al. The effects of free-living interval-walking training on glycemic control, body composition, and physical fitness in type 2 diabetic patients: A randomized, controlled trial. *Diabetes Care*. 2013;36(2):228–236.

58. Karstoft K, Winding K, Knudsen SH, James NG, Scheel MM, Olesen J et al. Mechanisms behind the superior effects of interval vs continuous training on glycaemic control in individuals with type 2 diabetes: A randomised controlled trial. *Diabetologia.* 2014;57(10):2081–2093.

59. Jelleyman C, Yates T, O'Donovan G, Gray LJ, King JA, Khunti K et al. The effects of high-intensity interval training on glucose regulation and insulin resistance: A meta-analysis. *Obes Rev.* 2015;16(11):942–961.

60. Spong CY, Mercer BM, D'Alton M, Kilpatrick S, Blackwell S, Saade G. Timing of indicated late-preterm and early-term birth. *Obstet Gynecol.* 2011;118(2 Pt 1):323–333.

61. American College of Obstetricians and Gynecologists. ACOG committee opinion no. 560: Medically indicated late-preterm and early-term deliveries. *Obstet Gynecol.* 2013;121(4):908–910.

62. Metzger BE, Buchanan TA, Coustan DR, de Leiva A, Dunger DB, Hadden DR et al. Summary and recommendations of the Fifth International Workshop-Conference on Gestational Diabetes Mellitus. *Diabetes Care.* 2007;30 Suppl 2:S251–S260.

63. Gabbe SG, Graves CR. Management of diabetes mellitus complicating pregnancy. *Obstet Gynecol.* 2003;102(4):857–868.

21 Pathophysiology and Management of Type 1 Diabetes
Rational Design of Insulin Therapy

Schafer Boeder and Steven Edelman

CONTENTS

21.1 INTRODUCTION

In this chapter, we will review the basic epidemiology and pathophysiology of type 1 diabetes (T1D) before discussing the role of nutrition and exercise therapy. The evidence for use of home glucose monitoring via blood glucose meters and continuous glucose monitors will be presented. We will then examine the medical therapies available for treatment of T1D, including insulin and insulin analogues, synthetic amylin (pramlintide), and off-label medications. An approach to designing and optimizing the insulin therapy regimen will be discussed.

21.2 EPIDEMIOLOGY AND PATHOPHYSIOLOGY OF TYPE 1 DIABETES

T1D is a chronic disease characterized by destruction of the insulin-producing β cells of the pancreas and the subsequent need for exogenous insulin therapy. Roughly 5%–10% of all diabetes cases worldwide are due to T1D (1). It remains the most common form of diabetes among children and adolescents, though the onset may occur at any age (2). Multiple large, population-based registry studies have helped elucidate the incidence and prevalence of T1D among children and adolescence across the globe and over time.

In 1990, the World Health Organization (WHO) initiated the Multinational Project for Childhood Diabetes (DIAMOND) project to study T1D in children 14 years of age and younger living in 50 countries around the world. The project reported an incidence of T1D in this population of roughly 4.5% between the years of 1990–1994 (3). However, the incidence varied greatly country to country, and even within different regions of the same country. Populations from China and South America had the lowest incidence (< 1/100,000 per year), whereas populations from Sardinia, Portugal, Canada, the United Kingdom, New Zealand, and the Scandinavian Peninsula had the highest incidence (> 20/100,000) (Figure 21.1). In general, the incidence increased with age and was greatest among those who were 10–14 years old. A follow-up of the DIAMOND project, describing data from 57 countries during 1990–1999, reported an average annual increase in incidence of 2.8% (95% confidence interval [CI], 2.4%–3.2%) (4). The authors suggest that such a rapid increase in incidence cannot be explained by changes in population genetics, and that environmental triggers or gene-environment interactions may be playing a role.

The SEARCH for Diabetes in Youth study, funded by the US Centers for Disease Control (CDC) and the National Institute of Digestive Health and Kidney Disease, examined the incidence and prevalence of diabetes among individuals younger than 20 years in the United States in 2002–2003 (5). The incidence of T1D was greatest among age groups 5–9 years (22.1/100,000 person-years) and 10–14 years (25.9/100,000 person-years), and non-Hispanic white youth had the highest rates when compared to other ethnicities. Data from the SEARCH study and the Colorado insulin-dependent diabetes mellitus (IDDM) study registry were used to compare the incidence of T1D over a 26-year period in the state of Colorado (6). The incidence went from 14.8/100,000 per year (95% CI, 14.0–15.6) in 1978–1988 to 23.9/100,000 per year (95% CI, 22.2–25.6) in 2002–2004, increasing by an average of 2.3% (95% CI, 1.6–3.1) per year.

The EURODIAB ACE study group examined the incidence of T1D throughout Europe and Israel from 1989 to 1994 (7), reporting a wide variation between regions ranging from 3.2/100,000 person-years in Macedonia to 40.2/100,000 person-years in parts of Finland. The incidence rate of T1D increased by 3.4% (95% CI, 2.5%–4.4%) annually during the years studied, with the highest rates of increase occurring in the youngest age group (0–4 years). Taken together, data from the registry studies demonstrate striking differences in T1D rates around the globe, illustrated by a 400-fold variation in incidence among studied countries (8). Unfortunately, there is a relative paucity of data

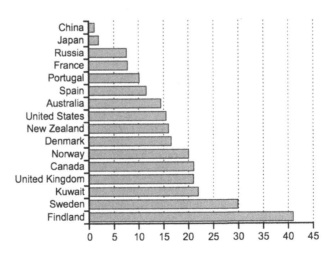

FIGURE 21.1 Age-standardized incidence of type 1 diabetes in children younger than 14 years. (From Edelman, S. et al., *Practical Management of Type 1 Diabetes*, 2nd ed., Professional Communications, West Islip, NY, 399 p, 2014.)

on the incidence and prevalence of T1D in adults, although an estimated 85% of people living with the disease, and 25%–50% of those who are newly diagnosed, are adults (9).

The pathophysiology of T1D involves the autoimmune-mediated destruction of pancreatic β cells. While the precise cause remains unclear, there are various hypotheses. Chief among them is that exposure to infectious or environmental triggers leads to autoimmunity against β cells in the setting of underlying genetic risk (10). Researchers have identified a number of risk factors associated with the development of T1D, as well as a significant genetic component, including the association with certain human leukocyte antigen (HLA) class II alleles (11).

A longstanding theory of T1D pathophysiology is that exposure to viral infections triggers autoimmune destruction of β cells. Unfortunately, there have not been conclusive findings correlating specific infections with the development of T1D (12). There are, however, data showing seasonal patterns of diabetes onset (seasonality of onset) with increased incidence during late autumn through early spring, correlating to times with higher rates of viral infections (13). There are also patterns for seasonality of birth among youth with T1D, with increased rates among those born during the spring and decreased rates among those born during the fall (14). It has been hypothesized that seasonal variability in the levels of maternal vitamin D, which may have effects on β-cell autoimmunity, can explain seasonality of birth observations. Increased maternal vitamin D intake during pregnancy has been associated with a lower risk of islet autoimmunity in children (15), and increased vitamin D supplementation during the first year of life has been associated with a reduced risk of T1D in infants (16). Studies have investigated the role of other nutritional factors, including breastfeeding, vitamin E, and exposures to cow's milk and gluten, though results have been mixed and no clear association with T1D risk has been established (17).

Genetic risk factors play a significant role in the development of T1D. While most individuals with T1D have no family history, first-degree relatives of a person with T1D have a roughly 15-fold increased lifetime risk of developing the disease (1 in 20) compared with the general population (1 in 300) in the United States (18). The lifetime concordance rate is 6%–10% for dizygotic twins, and more than 60% for monozygotic twins (19). Risk for offspring of fathers with T1D (7%) is greater than that of offspring of affected mothers (2%–3%) (20). The timing of disease onset may be related to the relative contribution of genetic risk, with earlier onset of diabetes in children correlating with a higher genetic susceptibility. Siblings of individuals diagnosed before 5 years of age have a higher risk of developing T1D during childhood or adolescence compared to siblings of individuals diagnosed later (between age 5 and 15 years) (21).

Multiple genes have been described to correlate with increased (or decreased) risk for the development of T1D. However, the principal markers of increased risk are two susceptibility haplotypes, DR3 and DR4, in the HLA class II region on chromosome 6 (22). The HLA class II molecule plays a central role in immune recognition of foreign and self-antigens. Misrecognition of antigens by specific HLA class II haplotypes may lead to autoimmune destruction of β cells. Over 90% of children with T1D carry the DR3 or DR4 susceptibility haplotypes (23), compared to only 20% of the general population. It is estimated that HLA region variation accounts for 40%–50% of T1D genetic risk (24), with numerous other genes affecting susceptibility to a lesser degree.

21.3 NUTRITION THERAPY AND EXERCISE

Appropriate nutrition is an essential component in the management of T1D. Medical providers must be well-versed in diabetes-specific nutrition and proficient in sharing this knowledge with patients. Ideally, individuals with T1D should have access to a multidisciplinary team including a certified diabetes educator and a registered dietitian specializing in diabetes-related nutrition. Understanding the effects of carbohydrates and other macronutrients on blood glucose levels and insulin requirements can empower people with T1D to make informed dietary and treatment decisions.

Diabetes-specific medical nutrition therapy (MNT) delivered by a registered dietician is associated with a 0.3%–1.0% reduction in A1c for patients with T1D (25–27). The American Diabetes Association (ADA) Standards of Medical Care in Diabetes recommend that every patient with diabetes receive education on nutrition therapy and assistance in designing an individualized eating plan (28). The ADA guidelines emphasize healthful eating: the intake of high-quality, nutrient-dense foods. They do not endorse specific dietary interventions, but they do provide examples of healthful eating patterns, such as the Mediterranean diet and the Dietary Approaches to Stop Hypertension (DASH) diet. Body weight management should also be considered as an important component of nutrition therapy, as data from the T1D exchange has demonstrated that two-thirds of patients aged 31–64 years are either overweight or obese (29).

There remains no agreed-upon ideal "diabetic diet" or specific macronutrient breakdown. Nutritional recommendations should focus on designing a well-balanced diet that is congruent with individual culinary and cultural preferences. The Institute of Medicine has published general dietary reference intakes that suggest the total daily energy intake be comprised of 45%–65% carbohydrates, 20%–35% fat, and 10%–35% protein (30). In T1D, the nutritional focus has long been on carbohydrate intake and its relationship to insulin dosing and timing. Compared to other macronutrients, carbohydrates—which are rapidly metabolized and absorbed as molecules of glucose and other sugars—have a more striking effect on blood glucose levels. For this reason, most individuals with T1D attempt to match their insulin dose with their carbohydrate intake in order to maximize mealtime glucose control.

The various approaches to mealtime insulin dosing include utilizing carbohydrate counting, eating a consistent carbohydrate diet, and using carbohydrate estimation. In choosing which method to employ, the provider must assess each patient's literacy, cognitive ability, and desire to engage in diabetes management. All patients, however, should be referred for T1D-specific education that includes characterizing what a carbohydrate is and the relative carbohydrate content of common foods (in particular those eaten by the patient) (Figure 21.2). A more intensive training was studied in the Dose Adjusted for Normal Eating (DAFNE) trial, in which individuals with T1D were randomized to a 5-day educational course on matching insulin to carbohydrate intake versus usual care (31). Compared to controls, the treatment group demonstrated a 1% decrease in A1c without increased hypoglycemia, as well as increased treatment satisfaction and overall wellbeing. A meta-analysis reported that, among five studies with parallel design, a 0.64% A1c reduction was seen in carbohydrate-counting groups compared to controls (32).

The motivated patient should be taught how to calculate the number of carbohydrates in meals. Free smartphone apps or handbooks can be used to look up the carbohydrate content of specific foods and can help calculate the total carbohydrate content of a meal based on portion size. The patient can then determine a mealtime insulin dose based on the insulin-to-carbohydrate ratio (e.g., 1 unit for every 10 g of carbs) assigned by their provider. Counting carbohydrates is difficult, and errors are common. In one study, adults with T1D miscounted the carbohydrate content of meals by an average of approximately 20% (or 15 g), usually underestimating the carbohydrate intake (33). Higher degrees of error in carbohydrate counting were associated with increased glycemic variability. Patients should return for periodic assessment and ongoing education relating to carbohydrate counting to maintain or improve their skills.

An alternative to using an insulin-to-carbohydrate ratio can be considered in patients who do not have the ability or desire to count carbohydrates. A less-flexible but somewhat simpler approach is to use a fixed insulin dose with a consistent carbohydrate diet. As an example, a patient with an insulin-to-carbohydrate ratio of 1:10 (1 unit for every 10 g of carbs) may be instructed to take 6 units of insulin and eat 60 g of carbohydrates with each meal. Designing set meals, including content and portion size, that match the desired carbohydrate content can provide a framework for the patient's home meal plan. This approach works best for individuals who have fairly static dietary preferences and uniform food intake.

(a)

- All breads (even whole-wheat and 9-grain breads)
- Rolls, crackers, bagels, baguettes, breadsticks
- All cereals (cold and hot cereals, including "healthy" oatmeal)
- All beans (healthy beans such as kidney beans, chick peas, black-eyed peas, etc)
- All starchy vegetables (white and sweet potatoes, green peas, and corn)
- All fruits (even fruits that are not sweet, such as grapefruit; and fruits in every form: juice, canned, frozen, and dried)
- All grains (from the exotic to the traditional: amaranth, barley, buckwheat, corn, emmer, granola, kammut, millet, oats, quinoa, rice, rye, sorghum, spelt, teff, triticale, wheat, wild rice) and foods made with these grains, such as pasta, tortillas, couscous, etc
- Milk and yogurt (whole milk, low-fat milk, and fat-free milk)
- Candy, baked goods, regular sodas, and beverages
- Seasonings and sauces: barbeque sauce, marinades, mayonnaise, ketchup, etc

(b)

Each of these foods contain 15 grams of carbohydrate:
- 1 slice of bread
- ½ cup cooked cereal
- ¾ cup cold cereal
- ½ cup starchy vegetable (corn, peas)
- ½ plantain – ½ cup cooked taro, cassava, or tannier
- ⅓ cup cooked rice, pasta
- ½ cup beans
- 1 small potato
- 1 small fruit
- 4 oz (½ small glass) juice
- 1 glass milk
- 6 oz plain yogurt

Carbohydrate bargains are ½ cup of cooked vegetable or 1 cup of raw vegetable. These have only 5 grams of carbohydrates.

FIGURE 21.2 (a) Foods with carbohydrates and (b) carbohydrate content of common foods (From Edelman, S. et al., *Practical Management of Type 1 Diabetes*, 2nd ed., Professional Communications, West Islip, NY, 399 p, 2014.)

An even more simplified approach, for those who cannot count carbohydrates or maintain a consistent carbohydrate diet, is to dose insulin based on estimated carbohydrate content or meal size. For example, a patient may be instructed to take 3 units for a small or low-carbohydrate meal, 5 units for an average meal, and 7 units for a large or high-carbohydrate meal. While this approach provides some guidance for adjusting insulin based on nutritional intake, it is relatively imprecise and is likely to lead to increased glycemic variability. When appropriate, patients should be encouraged to adopt more sophisticated methods of carbohydrate counting and insulin dosing. Ongoing interaction with certified diabetes educators and registered dieticians is important for all individuals with diabetes in order to achieve or maintain treatment goals.

Given the focus on dietary carbohydrates during nutrition and insulin training for T1D, the importance of other primary macronutrients (namely fat and protein) is often overlooked. These macronutrients play a major role not only in general nutrition, but also in blood glucose management. For example, there is evidence from the Diabetes Control and Complications Trial (DCCT) that diets lower in carbohydrates and higher in fats may be associated with increased glycosylated hemoglobin (A1c) values, possibly due to effects on insulin signaling and insulin resistance (34). High-fat and high-protein foods will raise blood glucose levels, and it appears their effects are additive. One study compared consistent carbohydrate meals containing low-fat/low-protein, low-fat/high-protein, high-fat/low-protein, and high-fat/high-protein contents in adolescents with

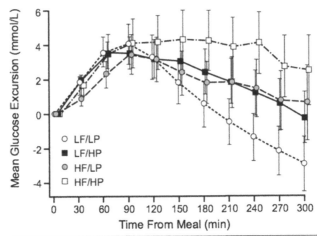

Mean postprandial glucose excursions from 0 to 300 min for 33 subjects after test meals of LF/LP, LF/HP, HF/LP, and HF/HP content. Carbohydrate amount was the same in all meals. There were significant differences in glucose excursions between meal types from 150 to 300 min (P <0.03). Error bars represent 95% CIs.

Smart CEM, et al. *Diabetes Care*. 2013;36:3897-3902.

FIGURE 21.3 Mean postprandial glucose excursions after test meals. (From Edelman, S. et al. *Practical Management of Type 1 Diabetes*, 2nd ed. West Islip, NY: Professional Communications, 2014; page 399.)

T1D using individualized premeal insulin dosing (35). The high-fat/high-protein meal led to a mean glucose excursion that was 97 mg/dL higher at 300 minutes compared to the low-fat/low-protein meal (Figure 21.3). This pattern of increased and prolonged hyperglycemic excursion after meals that are high in fat or protein can be addressed in some patients by giving an additional insulin dose 1–2 hours after the meal, or—for individuals using an insulin pump—by using a dual-wave bolus.

Physical activity and exercise are also important considerations for individuals with T1D. The ADA Standards of Medical Care recommend that all adults with diabetes get 150 minutes or more per week of moderate-to-vigorous activity (spread over at least 3 days, and including 2–3 weekly session of resistance exercise), and that they reduce time spent in sedentary behaviors such as prolonged sitting (28). Regular exercise has been shown to have many benefits for people with T1D, including increased insulin sensitivity, reduced insulin requirements, improved cardiovascular and respiratory fitness, greater muscle strength, and increased sense of well-being (36), as well as curtailing the decline in mobility experienced by some overweight patients (37).

Although there are many benefits of exercise, potential risks exist. Most adults with diabetes—especially those who have additional cardiovascular risk factors, such as heart disease, a prior stroke, hypertension, dyslipidemia, a history of smoking, or age over 45 years for males or 55 years for females—should consult with their healthcare provider before engaging in increased physical activity or initiating an exercise routine. Diabetes-related complications such as retinopathy, neuropathy, and foot ulcers or Charcot foot can limit exercise options and predispose to injury. In general, patients should start slowly with frequent, low-intensity physical activity and then increase the duration and intensity of exercise as tolerated.

A common and justified concern among people with T1D is exercise-induced hypoglycemia, which can occur during and up to 11 hours after exercise, sometimes continuing into the nocturnal period (36,38). This phenomenon is due in part to the increase in glucose uptake by skeletal muscles, which is required to support a heightened workload during physical activity. In people without diabetes, the response to falling blood glucose levels during exercise includes a reduction in insulin production and an increase in glucagon secretion. The net effect is to stimulate the production and release of glucose by the liver. Individuals with T1D lack the ability to autoregulate insulin levels and fully counteract this exercise-mediated glucose uptake. Exercise-induced hypoglycemia is most commonly associated with moderate-intensity aerobic activity of longer duration, such as distance running, swimming, and cycling. Further exacerbating the situation is the increase in insulin sensitivity that occurs during and for hours after exercise.

An active approach to mitigating exercise-induced hypoglycemia via preventive measures and preparedness is essential. The basic principles are blood glucose monitoring, increasing carbohydrate intake, and decreasing prandial insulin. Prior to, during (if prolonged), and after exercise, patients should follow blood glucose levels using self-monitoring of blood glucose (SMBG) or continuous glucose monitoring (CGM). Prior to physical activity, rapid-acting insulin doses can be reduced by 25%–75%, depending on the intensity and duration of exercise. Another strategy is to ingest carbohydrates—for example, 10–20 g of glucose prior to exercise. If hypoglycemia is experienced during activity, another 15–20 g of simple carbohydrates (such as glucose tablets or juice) should be taken with a repeat blood glucose check 15 minutes later. After exercise, a complex carbohydrate with an appropriate (possibly decreased) bolus of insulin can be considered to replete glycogen stores (36). Each individual responds differently to exercise, insulin, and carbohydrate intake, as well as to other factors including duration and intensity of exercise. Thus, patients should be advised to observe and record how they respond to such variables and to make appropriate adjustments to minimize hypoglycemia.

Exercise-related hyperglycemia can also occur, especially during high-intensity or anaerobic exercise such as weightlifting, sprinting, gymnastics, wrestling, and many team or competitive sports. During such activities, there is a surge in epinephrine and other counter-regulatory stress hormones that act to oppose the action of insulin by stimulating hepatic glucose production and release. Glucose from the liver can exceed the uptake by muscle and other tissues, leading to hyperglycemia and even predisposing some individuals with T1D to ketosis (36,38). In patients who experience hyperglycemia during or after intense exercise, careful treatment with a dose of rapid-acting insulin at the time of the activity (or shortly after) can be considered. Adequate fluid intake is essential to prevent dehydration, especially in the setting of hyperglycemia. As with all exercise, frequent SMBG or the use of CGM is recommended. If blood glucose is above 250 mg/dL and ketosis is present, exercise should be deferred. If blood glucose is above 300 (without ketosis), caution is recommended (36).

21.4   HOME AND CONTINUOUS GLUCOSE MONITORING

A primary goal in the management of T1D is to maintain blood glucose near euglycemia while avoiding large hyper- and hypoglycemic excursions. It is well established that improved glycemic control is associated with reduced rates of microvascular and neuropathic complications (39), and there is evidence that intensive glycemic control improves cardiovascular outcomes when initiated early in the course of disease (40,41). The traditional measures of glucose control are the serum blood glucose, including fasting plasma glucose (FPG) and postprandial glucose (PPG), and the A1c. In clinical practice, SMBG is often utilized in place of the serum glucose to measure FPG and PPG values.

Home SMBG has long been an important tool for individuals living with T1D. Patients should be educated regarding the appropriate technique for using a blood glucose meter, and how to make use of the information obtained from glucose checks. SMBG can inform decisions related to insulin dosing, exercise, nutrition intake, and the prevention and treatment of both hypo- and hyperglycemia. In their Standards of Medical Care, the ADA recommends that patients on intensive insulin regimens perform SMBG before each meal and snack (and occasionally in the postprandial setting), at bedtime, during suspected hypoglycemia, after treatment for hypoglycemia until euglycemia is achieved, and before activities such as exercise or driving (42). Data from the T1D Exchange clinic registry demonstrates an association between increased frequency of SMBG and lower A1c, as well as a decrease in acute complications (43).

While A1c and SMBG are useful for both patients and providers, these tests have limitations. The A1c is a measure of average glucose control over a period of several months. It cannot be used to assess for blood glucose excursion or hypoglycemia (44), and its accuracy can be adversely affected by conditions that influence the turnover of red blood cells (45). SMBG represents blood glucose levels at specific time points but provides no information about the glucose trend or the frequency or duration of hyper- or hypoglycemia between glucose checks. Neither A1c or SMBG can be used to accurately characterize blood glucose variability, which is an important predictor of poor outcomes. Acute glucose fluctuations, which lead to endothelial dysfunction via increased oxidative stress, likely play a major role in the development of vascular disease, leading to long-term diabetic complications (46,47). High glucose variability with frequent acute hyperglycemic episodes may be even more damaging to blood vessels than uninterrupted hyperglycemia (48).

Real-time continuous glucose monitoring (RT-CGM) provides patients with estimates of their blood glucose measurement at frequent, regular intervals (e.g., every 5 minutes). Technological advances during recent decades have made RT-CGM more accurate, more portable, and increasingly relevant to clinical diabetes care. A RT-CGM system is made of up three components. The first is a small sensor that is inserted into the subcutaneous tissue to measure glucose within the interstitial fluid, usually by enzymatic detection via glucose oxidase (49). Attached to the sensor is an external transmitter that sends data to a device, such as a smartphone or dedicated receiver, that can store, process, and display information including real-time glucose values and glucose trends. The RT-CGM allows the user to set alerts for low and high glucose, as well as for rapidly changing glucose levels. Blinded CGM, in which real-time measurements are not shown to the patient but are stored for later review, is used frequently in research and sometimes in the clinical setting as a diagnostic tool.

A limitation inherent to currently available RT-CGM systems is the time lag between changes in the blood glucose and corresponding changes in the interstitial fluid, which can be up to 20 minutes (50). The difference between blood and interstitial glucose is greatest when the blood level is changing rapidly. Additionally, some of these systems require multiple daily calibrations using values obtained from capillary blood glucose.

Studies in patients with T1D have consistently demonstrated that the use of RT-CGM leads to improved glycemic control and/or reduced hypoglycemia. In one such study, 81 children and 81 adults with poorly controlled T1D (A1c $\geq$ 8.1%) were randomized to SMGB, intermittent RT-CGM, and continuous RT-CGM (51). Patients in the continuous RT-CGM group had an average reduction in A1c of 1%, compared to a reduction of 0.4% in the SMBG group. Another study evaluated 62 patients with T1D randomized to RT-CGM-guided insulin pump therapy or standard insulin pump therapy without CGM and found the RT-CGM group had an average A1c 0.43% lower than controls at 3 months, without increased hypoglycemia (52). Within the CGM group, those who wore the glucose sensor for more than 70% of the time had A1c improvements 0.5% greater than those who wore the device for less than 70% of the time, suggesting a "dose-dependent" effect. The Juvenile Diabetes Research Foundation (JDRF) conducted a trial of 322 patients with T1D and showed that RT-CGM, when compared to SMBG, improved A1c among adult patients over the age of 25 years by 0.5% (53). A study of 129 adults and children with well-controlled T1D (A1c < 7.0%) using either RT-CGM or SMBG for 26 weeks demonstrated significant differences between the groups in A1c, time spent with glucose at or below 60 mg/dL, and time out of range ($\leq$ 70 or > 180 mg/dL), favoring the RT-CGM group (54). Another trial showed significantly reduced time spent in hypoglycemia (< 63 mg/dL), lower A1c, and increased time at goal glycemia when using RT-CGM compared to SMBG in 120 children and adults with T1D and A1c below 7.5% (55).

Given the strength of evidence for the benefits of RT-CGM in lowering A1c and reducing hypoglycemia, both the Endocrine Society (56) and the ADA (42) recommend the use of RT-CGM in children, adolescents, and adults with T1D who can adhere to regular use of the device. The American Association of Clinical Endocrinologists consensus statement on glucose monitoring recommends CGM for all patients with T1D (57). Prior to initiating CGM, patient readiness should be assessed and training on the use of the device should be provided. Assessment of the frequency of CGM use, as well as further device training, should be a part of each patient's ongoing diabetes education.

21.5 DESIGNING A MEDICAL THERAPY REGIMEN

21.5.1 INSULIN AND INSULIN ANALOGUES

The standard of care in the treatment of T1D is to use insulin and insulin analogues to attempt to mimic, as closely as possible, the release of insulin by the functioning pancreas. This can be done using either multiple daily injection (MDI) therapy or continuous subcutaneous insulin infusion (CSII) therapy, both described in further detail below. The clinical utility of the various insulin products is related in part to their pharmacodynamic and pharmacokinetic properties (Figure 21.4), which must be considered when designing a regimen to approximate physiologic insulin replacement. This includes providing a relatively flat "basal" component (meant to suppress glucose production by the liver while in the fasting state), and a prandial "bolus" component (to promote glucose disposal during meals or other hyperglycemic states).

The insulin products best suited for mealtime bolus dosing are the genetically engineered "rapid-acting" insulin analogues, including insulin lispro, aspart, and glulisine. When injected

Insulin Preparation	Onset of Action	Peak Action	Duration of Action
Mealtime Insulins			
Rapid-Acting :			
Regular	30-60 minutes	1.5-5 hours	6-8 hours
Fast-Acting :			
Subcutaneous			
Aspart (Novolog)[b]	10-20 minutes	40-50 minutes	3-5 hours
Glulisine (Apidra)[b]	25 minutes	40-50 minutes	4-5 hours
Lispro (Humalog)[b]	15-30 minutes	0.5-2.5 hours	3-6.5 hours
Inhaled:			
Afrezza	1-5 minutes	12-15 minutes	3-4 hours
Basal Insulins			
Intermediate-Acting:			
Isophane (NPH)	1-2 hours	4-12 hours	14-24 hours

	Onset of Action	Peak Action	Duration of Action
Long-Acting:			
Detemir (Levemir)[b]	1-2 hours	3-9 hours	6-23 hours
Glargine (Lantus)[b]	1-1.5 hours	No peak	11 to >24 hours
Ultralong-Acting:			
Glargine (Toujeo)[b]	Develops over 6 hours	12-18 hours[c]	28 hours[c]
Degludec (Tresiba)	1 hour	9-12 hours	At least 48 hours

FIGURE 21.4 (a) This table summarizes the typical time course of action (pharmacokinetics) of various insulin preparations. Values are highly variable among individuals, depending on the site and depth of injection, local tissue blood flow, skin temperature, and exercise. (b) Reproducibility of time course of action and efficacy may be improved with insulin analogues. (c) For a single 0.6 U/kg doses of Toujeo. Duration of action and time to peak action differ for 0.4, 0.9 U/kg doses. See prescribing information for more details. (From Edelman, S. and Henry, R., *Diagnosis and Management of Type 2 Diabetes*, 13th ed., Professional Communications, West Islip, NY, 2017.)

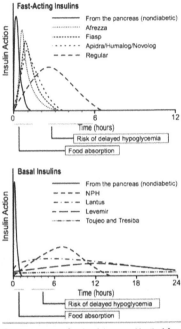

Fast-Acting Insulins

Insulin Action

- From the pancreas (nondiabetic)
- Afrezza
- Fiasp
- Apidra/Humalog/Novolog
- Regular

Time (hours)   0 ... 6 ... 12

Risk of delayed hypoglycemia

Food absorption

Basal Insulins

Insulin Action

- From the pancreas (nondiabetic)
- NPH
- Lantus
- Levemir
- Toujeo and Tresiba

Time (hours)   0 ... 6 ... 12 ... 18 ... 24

Risk of delayed hypoglycemia

Food absorption

The time course of action (pharmacokinetics) for the rapid-acting insulin analogues (Apidra [glulisine], Humalog [lispro], Novolog [aspart]) is not as fast as insulin from the pancreas of an individual that does not have diabetes, but it is much more physiologic than the older Regular insulin preparation. Afrezza, the inhalable action is faster-acting than Apidra/Humalog/Novolog/Admelog, but is still not as fast as the human pancreas. Also shown is the time course of action of the intermediate-acting insulin NPH (isophane) and long-acting insulins Lantus (glargine), Levemir (detemir), and Basaglar (glargine). The newer basal insulins discussed (Toujeo and Tresiba) also have long, flat durations of action.

FIGURE 21.5 Time course of action of currently available insulins. (From Edelman, S. *Taking Control of Your Diabetes*, 5th ed. West Islip, NY: Professional Communications, 2018.)

subcutaneously, these preparations begin to work in 15–30 minutes, reach peak effect in 30–90 minutes, and have a duration of action of 4–6 hours (Figure 21.5). A new, faster-acting aspart starts to work in 15–20 minutes, peaks in 40–50 minutes, and is active for 2–4 hours. In comparison, the "short-acting" human (regular) insulin—which self-aggregates in solution after subcutaneous injection—has a delayed onset of 30–60 minutes, peaks at 2–3 hours, and is active for 8–10 hours. The faster onset and shorter duration of action of "rapid-acting" insulin analogues allow for more flexible mealtime dosing and less post-meal hypoglycemia. Thus, with a few exceptions, including insurance/cost factors or the presence of delayed food absorption due to moderate to severe gastroparesis, regular insulin is rarely appropriate for use in T1D.

Basal insulin preparations that are effective in T1D include the "long-acting" insulin analogues (detemir and glargine), as well as the "ultra-long-acting" products (glargine U-300 and degludec). As with the "rapid-acting" analogues, these insulin formulations contain altered amino acid sequences that give them their distinct absorption and clearance profiles. Detemir has an onset of action of 2–4 hours, and a duration of action lasting 14–24 hours. Therefore, some patients with T1D can use detemir as a once-daily injection, though the majority will require two injections per day to maintain a stable basal action. Insulin glargine also starts to work within 2–4 hours, but has a slightly longer duration, lasting for 20–24 hours. A split (twice-daily) dose can be considered for those patients in whom the therapeutic effect wears off in less than 24 hours. Two newer products, insulin degludec and insulin glargine U-300 (concentrated glargine), are considered "ultra-long-acting" insulin analogues. Glargine U-300 has a slow onset over 6 hours and a prolonged action of around 28 hours. Degludec begins to work after 1 hour and remains active for over 48 hours. The "ultra-long-acting" basal insulins offer modest advantages over their predecessors, including a more consistent profile throughout the day, reduced hypoglycemia, and more flexible dosing.

Neutral protamine Hagedorn (NPH), the sole "intermediate-acting" insulin, was previously used in T1D as a twice-daily basal insulin with some prandial effect. However, unpredictable peak times (4–10 hours) can lead to increased glucose variability and hypoglycemia, making NPH inappropriate for most T1D patients. Likewise, available premixed insulin preparations—for example, insulin lispro protamine suspension with insulin lispro, and insulin aspart protamine suspension with insulin aspart—provide inflexible dosing and are not standard of care in T1D.

21.5.2 Multiple Daily Injection Therapy

To design a basal-bolus MDI regimen, the provider must work with the patient to establish a total daily dose (TDD) of insulin, an insulin-to-carbohydrate ratio, and an insulin sensitivity factor. Most patients have a daily insulin requirement of 0.3–1.5 units of insulin for each kilogram of body weight. As a starting point, the TDD of insulin for a newly diagnosed patient can be estimated to be 0.5 units/kg/day. For example, an estimated TDD for a patient weighing 72 kg would be 36 units. The basal component should equal roughly 50% of the TDD, or approximately 18 units per day in this example. Note that some individuals—such as those who eat a high-carbohydrate diet or who continue to make some endogenous insulin—may require a lower percentage of their TDD as basal insulin. Once a starting basal dose is decided, the prandial insulin component should be calculated. For a patient planning to use a fixed insulin dose with a consistent carbohydrate diet at three meals per day, the mealtime dose can be estimated as the TDD minus the basal dose, divided by three. In our example, the insulin calculation would be as follows: (36 units TDD – 18 units basal)/3 meals per day = 6 units per meal.

However, most patients should develop a personalized premeal dosing regimen consisting of an insulin-to-carbohydrate ratio and an insulin sensitivity factor (ISF). A typical insulin-to-carbohydrate ratio would be 1 unit of insulin for every 10–15 g of carbohydrates consumed. The ISF, also known as *correctional factor*, is used to correct glucose values that are above goal (for example, > 100 mg/dL). A common ISF would be 1 unit of insulin to lower the blood glucose by 50 mg/dL. Consider a patient with a premeal blood glucose of 200 mg/dL who is planning to eat a meal containing 60 g of carbohydrates. If their insulin-to-carbohydrate ratio is 1:10, and their ISF is 1 unit/50 mg/dL (goal, 100 mg/dL), they would need 6 units to cover the carbohydrates plus 2 units to correct for the hyperglycemia, for a total premeal dose of 8 units of rapid-acting insulin.

21.5.3 Continuous Subcutaneous Insulin Infusion Therapy

Another approach to imitating physiologic insulin delivery is to use an insulin pump to administer CSII. Currently available pumps infuse a rapid-acting insulin analogue to provide both basal and bolus insulin components. While not appropriate for all individuals with T1D, CSII has a number of advantages over MDI regimens. The basal insulin is given as a constant infusion at a programmed rate that can be fine-tuned to match diurnal variations in insulin sensitivity. This may be useful for patients who experience early-morning insulin resistance (the dawn phenomenon). Also, insulin delivery can be completely suspended if necessary (e.g., during exercise) to avoid or mitigate hypoglycemia.

Patients also use the pump to give bolus insulin to cover nutritional intake and correct for elevated blood glucose. Individualized insulin-to-carbohydrate ratios and insulin sensitivity factors can be programmed into the device to assist in calculating appropriate bolus doses based on carbohydrate intake and blood glucose values. Advanced features such as "square-wave" and "dual-wave" boluses allow for prandial insulin to be delivered over an extended period of time. This can be useful for meals high in protein and fat, or for patients with delayed absorption (e.g., gastroparesis). Pumps can also infuse very small insulin doses with high accuracy, which can be difficult to do via subcutaneous injection.

21.5.4 Optimizing Insulin Therapy Using Blood Glucose Data

The effectiveness of the insulin regimen—be it MDI or CSII—should be frequently evaluated, and adjustments should be made to optimize glucose control. Careful review of blood glucose data collected by the patient using SMBG can reveal patterns of hyper- or hypoglycemia that require attention. Even more information can be obtained by downloading and reviewing CGM data, which may help identify inappropriate basal dosing, postprandial hyperglycemia, asymptomatic hypoglycemia, or other previously unidentified patterns. In general, the first step in reviewing blood glucose data should always be to assess for hypoglycemia, followed by looking for recurrent hyperglycemia, episodes of glucose variability, and other patterns such as dawn phenomenon. The average blood glucose, variation from the mean, and percent time spent below, within, and above goal glycemic targets should also be reviewed if possible.

When assessing the insulin regimen, the basal insulin dose should be interrogated and adjusted first. This can be accomplished using blood glucose values collected during a period of fasting when the patient does not require any rapid-acting insulin (i.e., overnight for most individuals). To do a basal test, patients can be instructed to eat an early dinner with a normal dose of prandial insulin. After dinner, they should fast (except for water) for the rest of the evening, overnight, and into the morning for as long as they feel comfortable (until breakfast, or even lunchtime, the following day). During the fast, they should check their blood glucose every 3–4 hours, or at a minimum at bedtime and again first thing in the morning. If the fasting blood glucose values remain within 20% of the glucose at bedtime, then the basal insulin dose is appropriate. If there is a significant rise or fall in blood glucose, the basal dose should be adjusted accordingly.

Once the basal dose is established, the appropriateness of the bolus component should be examined. The insulin-to-carbohydrate ratio and the insulin sensitivity factor should each be considered separately. A pattern of fasting or premeal euglycemia with postprandial hyperglycemia suggests an insulin-to-carbohydrate mismatch, possibly due to an insufficient insulin-to-carbohydrate ratio. A pattern of consistent hyperglycemia that fails to correct despite the patient giving the recommended correctional dose would suggest an insufficient insulin sensitivity factor. Dysglycemia after meals can be related to many others factors as well, including poor insulin timing, unreliable carbohydrate counting, delayed absorption of nutrients, and improper insulin injection technique. These issues must be considered and reviewed with the patient during ongoing education provided by the multidisciplinary care team.

21.5.5 Inhaled Insulin, Pramlintide Therapy, and Off-Label Medications

When compared to type 2 diabetes, there remains a dearth of treatment options for people living with T1D. Insulin is not only the mainstay of therapy, but is in fact the only medication used to treat T1D by the majority of patients. Aside from the insulin products previously discussed, which are administered by the patient via subcutaneous injection or infusion, there is a single available insulin human inhalation powder (Afrezza). Approved in 2014, Afrezza is packaged in single-dose cartridges of 4 and 8 units. It is inhaled using a thumb-sized inhaler and then rapidly absorbed into the systemic circulation via the lung. Its biologic activity is similar to that of the rapid-acting insulin analogues, but with a faster onset of action, peak effect, and elimination time, giving it a profile that better mimics physiologic insulin activity. Inhaled insulin may have effects on pulmonary function and is contraindicated in patients with chronic lung or reactive airway disease. Caution should be taken in patients with a history of, or risk factors for, lung cancer.

The only noninsulin medication that is FDA approved for use in adults with T1D is the synthetic amylin analogue pramlintide. Like amylin, pramlintide slows gastric emptying, increases satiety, and reduces hepatic glucose production by suppressing the release of glucagon. Pramlintide has been shown to reduce insulin requirements, lower A1c, and lead to weight reduction. However, drawbacks include nausea in some patients, hypoglycemia (if prandial insulin doses are not decreased sufficiently), and the need for an additional injection before each meal. These issues have hindered the widespread adoption of pramlintide.

There are several therapies approved for type 2 diabetes—including GLP-1 agonists, sodium-glucose cotransporter 2 (SGLT2) inhibitors, and metformin—that are sometimes used off-label in the treatment of T1D. Like pramlintide, the glucagon-like peptide 1 (GLP-1) agonists can delay gastric emptying, increase satiety, suppress glucagon release, lower insulin needs, and promote weight loss. They are being studied for use in T1D but are not yet FDA approved for this indication. The SGLT2 inhibitors block reabsorption of glucose in the proximal nephron, leading to glucosuria and reduced blood glucose levels. These medications, which may increase the risk of diabetic ketoacidosis, are also being investigated further. Metformin decreases hepatic glucose production and may help to reduce insulin doses and weight in T1D, though it is not approved for this use.

21.6 IATROGENIC HYPOGLYCEMIA

Insulin therapy is associated with a risk of hypoglycemia, which can represent a significant barrier to optimizing blood glucose control for individuals with T1D. Patients can experience a wide array of symptoms related to hypoglycemia, which are categorized as either neurogenic (adrenergic or cholinergic) or neuroglycopenic (58). Neurogenic symptoms—manifestations of the physiologic response to hypoglycemia—can include tremors, diaphoresis, tachycardia, palpitations, anxiety, and hunger. Neuroglycopenic symptoms—representing the direct effect of hypoglycemia in the brain—can include confusion, cognitive delay, slurred speech, behavioral changes, blurry vision, fatigue, loss of consciousness, seizure, and even death.

Because the signs and symptoms of low blood glucose can be highly variable between individuals, it is difficult to define hypoglycemia using specific glucose concentration cutoffs. However, the ADA and the International Hypoglycaemia Study Group recommend classifying hypoglycemia in three levels: glucose alert value (level 1), clinically significant hypoglycemia (level 2), and severe hypoglycemia (level 3) (42). A glucose alert value is any measured glucose 70 mg/dL or lower, which may elicit symptoms and should be treated. Single or multiple glucose alert values may prompt adjustments to the diabetes treatment plan. Clinically significant hypoglycemia occurs with any measured glucose 54 mg/dL or lower and represents increased risk to the patient (e.g., falls/injuries, arrhythmias, neurologic injury) and to others (e.g., motor vehicle accidents). Severe hypoglycemia is characterized by cognitive impairment requiring assistance from another individual for treatment and recovery.

Many factors can contribute to the development of hypoglycemia in insulin-treated individuals. These include changes in insulin sensitivity (e.g., weight loss, exercise), mismatches between insulin dosing and carbohydrate/caloric intake (e.g., excessive insulin, poor insulin timing, skipped or delayed meals, gastroparesis, errors in carbohydrate counting or estimation), and comorbid medical conditions (e.g., liver disease, renal failure, adrenal insufficiency, and critical illness) (59). Other risk factors include lower A1c, elderly age, longer duration of diabetes, and prior history of severe hypoglycemia (60). Patients who have experienced recurrent hypoglycemia may develop impaired counterregulatory hormone activity and a reduced autonomic response to low blood glucose, known as *hypoglycemia-associated autonomic failure*. This leads to hypoglycemia unawareness (the attenuation or absence of adrenergic symptoms during hypoglycemia) and increases the risk for subsequent hypoglycemia (58).

People living with T1D, as well as their loved ones and caregivers, should be educated on the proper treatment for hypoglycemia. A patient who is conscious and able to eat during an episode of hypoglycemia should ingest 15–20 g of oral glucose (or other fast-acting carbohydrate) with the goal of normalizing blood glucose as quickly as possible. Examples of appropriate treatments include 2–4 glucose tablets (5 g each), 4–6 oz of fruit juice or regular soda, or a single-serving package of candies (such as Skittles or fruit snacks). Foods with a mixed macronutrient profile (e.g., candy bars) should be avoided, as the fat and protein content will lead to delayed recovery and contribute an unnecessary caloric load (8). The blood glucose should be rechecked via SMBG 15 minutes after treatment, and if glycemia has not normalized, the treatment should be repeated. Once euglycemia is achieved, a meal or snack should be considered in order to prevent hypoglycemia recurrence (60). The treatment for severe hypoglycemia is injection of glucagon by a trained family member or caregiver.

Patient education and blood glucose monitoring are key components of hypoglycemia prevention (58). Individuals with T1D should be aware of behaviors that can predispose them to low blood glucose, including fasting for tests or procedures, skipping meals, and exercising. By anticipating such events, patients can proactively decrease their insulin dose or increase carbohydrate intake to prevent hypoglycemia. Regular blood glucose checks via SMBG or CGM are essential for reducing the rate and severity of hypoglycemic events, and for early detection and treatment when hypoglycemia does occur. At each clinic visit, the provider should review the home blood glucose data, evaluate for symptomatic and asymptomatic hypoglycemic episodes, and adjust the insulin regimen accordingly. For patients with hypoglycemia unawareness, relaxation of glycemic targets should be considered (60). Strict avoidance of hypoglycemia can help reestablish the counterregulatory hormone response and restore hypoglycemia awareness (61).

21.7   CONCLUSION

T1D is a disease of impaired insulin production with a pathogenesis that remains incompletely characterized. Evidence suggests that the incidence of T1D is increasing among children, adolescence, and adults around the world. Thankfully, there are an increasing number of insulin products and devices—such as continuous glucose monitors and insulin pumps—available for use in the management of T1D. Further advances in diabetes-related treatment and technologies, including noninsulin medications, wearable sensors, and automated closed-loop insulin delivery systems, promise a brighter future. Still, the lifestyle interventions of nutrition therapy and exercise remain fundamental to a well-rounded, multidisciplinary approach to diabetes care.

REFERENCES

1. Diagnosis and classification of diabetes mellitus. *Diabetes Care*. 2009;32 Suppl 1:S62–S67. doi:10.2337/dc09-S062.
2. Stanescu DE, Lord K, Lipman TH. The epidemiology of type 1 diabetes in children. *Endocrinol Metab Clin North Am*. 2012;41(4):679–694. doi:10.1016/j.ecl.2012.08.001.
3. Karvonen M, Viik-Kajander M, Moltchanova E, Libman I, LaPorte R, Tuomilehto J. Incidence of childhood type 1 diabetes worldwide. Diabetes Mondiale (DiaMond) Project Group. *Diabetes Care*. 2000;23(10):1516–1526.
4. Incidence and trends of childhood type 1 diabetes worldwide 1990-1999. *Diabet Med*. 2006;23(8):857–866. doi:10.1111/j.1464-5491.2006.01925.x.
5. Dabelea D, Bell RA, D'Agostino RB, Jr., Imperatore G, Johansen JM, Linder B et al. Incidence of diabetes in youth in the United States. *JAMA*. 2007;297(24):2716–2724. doi:10.1001/jama.297.24.2716.
6. Vehik K, Hamman RF, Lezotte D, Norris JM, Klingensmith G, Bloch C et al. Increasing incidence of type 1 diabetes in 0- to 17-year-old Colorado youth. *Diabetes Care*. 2007;30(3):503–509. doi:10.2337/dc06-1837.
7. Variation and trends in incidence of childhood diabetes in Europe. EURODIAB ACE Study Group. *Lancet*. 2000;355(9207):873–876.
8. Edelman S, Hirsch I, Pettus J. *Practical Management of Type 1 Diabetes*. 2nd ed. West Islip, NY: Professional Communications; 2014. 399 p.

9. Haller MJ. Type 1 diabetes in the 21st century: A review of the landscape. In: Peters A, Laffel L, editors. *Type 1 Diabetes Sourcebook*. Alexandria, VA: American Diabetes Association; 2013.

10. Eisenbarth GS. Type I diabetes mellitus. A chronic autoimmune disease. *N Engl J Med*. 1986;314(21):1360–1368. doi:10.1056/nejm198605223142106.

11. Atkinson MA, Eisenbarth GS, Michels AW. Type 1 diabetes. *Lancet*. 2014;383(9911):69–82. doi:10.1016/s0140-6736(13)60591-7.

12. Goldberg E, Krause I. Infection and type 1 diabetes mellitus - A two edged sword? *Autoimmun Rev*. 2009;8(8):682–686. doi:10.1016/j.autrev.2009.02.017.

13. Ostman J, Lonnberg G, Arnqvist HJ, Blohme G, Bolinder J, Ekbom Schnell A et al. Gender differences and temporal variation in the incidence of type 1 diabetes: Results of 8012 cases in the nationwide Diabetes Incidence Study in Sweden 1983-2002. *J Intern Med*. 2008;263(4):386–394. doi:10.1111/j.1365-2796.2007.01896.x.

14. Maahs DM, West NA, Lawrence JM, Mayer-Davis EJ. Chapter 1: Epidemiology of type 1 diabetes. *Endocrinol Metab Clin North Am*. 2010;39(3):481–497. doi:10.1016/j.ecl.2010.05.011.

15. Fronczak CM, Baron AE, Chase HP, Ross C, Brady HL, Hoffman M et al. In utero dietary exposures and risk of islet autoimmunity in children. *Diabetes Care*. 2003;26(12):3237–3242.

16. Hypponen E, Laara E, Reunanen A, Jarvelin MR, Virtanen SM. Intake of vitamin D and risk of type 1 diabetes: A birth-cohort study. *Lancet*. 2001;358(9292):1500–1503. doi:10.1016/s0140-6736(01)06580-1.

17. Virtanen SM, Knip M. Nutritional risk predictors of beta cell autoimmunity and type 1 diabetes at a young age. *Am J Clin Nutr*. 2003;78(6):1053–1067.

18. Redondo MJ, Fain PR, Eisenbarth GS. Genetics of type 1A diabetes. *Recent Prog Horm Res*. 2001;56:69–89.

19. Redondo MJ, Jeffrey J, Fain PR, Eisenbarth GS, Orban T. Concordance for islet autoimmunity among monozygotic twins. *N Engl J Med*. 2008;359:2849–2850.

20. Hamalainen AM, Knip M. Autoimmunity and familial risk of type 1 diabetes. *Curr Diab Rep*. 2002;2(4):347–353.

21. Gillespie KM, Gale EA, Bingley PJ. High familial risk and genetic susceptibility in early onset childhood diabetes. *Diabetes*. 2002;51(1):210–214.

22. Mehers KL, Gillespie KM. The genetic basis for type 1 diabetes. *Br Med Bull*. 2008;88(1):115–129. doi:10.1093/bmb/ldn045.

23. Noble JA, Valdes AM. Genetics of the HLA region in the prediction of type 1 diabetes. *Curr Diab Rep*. 2011;11(6):533–542. doi:10.1007/s11892-011-0223-x.

24. Concannon P, Erlich HA, Julier C, Morahan G, Nerup J, Pociot F et al. Type 1 diabetes: Evidence for susceptibility loci from four genome-wide linkage scans in 1,435 multiplex families. *Diabetes*. 2005;54(10):2995–3001.

25. Kulkarni K, Castle G, Gregory R, Holmes A, Leontos C, Powers M et al. Nutrition practice guidelines for type 1 diabetes mellitus positively affect dietitian practices and patient outcomes. The Diabetes Care and Education Dietetic Practice Group. *J Am Diet Assoc*. 1998;98(1):62–70; quiz 1–2.

26. Rossi MC, Nicolucci A, Di Bartolo P, Bruttomesso D, Girelli A, Ampudia FJ et al. Diabetes interactive diary: A new telemedicine system enabling flexible diet and insulin therapy while improving quality of life: An open-label, international, multicenter, randomized study. *Diabetes Care*. 2010;33(1):109–115. doi:10.2337/dc09-1327.

27. Scavone G, Manto A, Pitocco D, Gagliardi L, Caputo S, Mancini L et al. Effect of carbohydrate counting and medical nutritional therapy on glycaemic control in type 1 diabetic subjects: A pilot study. *Diabet Med*. 2010;27(4):477–479. doi:10.1111/j.1464-5491.2010.02963.x.

28. 4. Lifestyle management. *Diabetes Care*. 2017;40(Suppl 1):S33–S43. doi:10.2337/dc17-S007.

29. Weinstock RS, DuBose SN, Aleppo GM et al. Characteristics of older adults with type 1 diabetes: Data from the T1D Exchange. *Paper presented at: American Diabetes Association 72nd Scientific Sessions*; June 8–12, 2012; Philadelphia, PA.

30. Trumbo P, Schlicker S, Yates AA, Poos M. Dietary reference intakes for energy, carbohydrate, fiber, fat, fatty acids, cholesterol, protein and amino acids. *J Am Diet Assoc*. 2002;102(11):1621–1630.

31. Training in flexible, intensive insulin management to enable dietary freedom in people with type 1 diabetes: Dose adjustment for normal eating (DAFNE) randomised controlled trial. *BMJ*. 2002;325(7367):746.

32. Bell KJ, Barclay AW, Petocz P, Colagiuri S, Brand-Miller JC. Efficacy of carbohydrate counting in type 1 diabetes: A systematic review and meta-analysis. *Lancet Diabetes Endocrinol*. 2014;2(2):133–140. doi:10.1016/s2213-8587(13)70144-x.

33. Brazeau AS, Mircescu H, Desjardins K, Leroux C, Strychar I, Ekoe JM et al. Carbohydrate count-
    ing accuracy and blood glucose variability in adults with type 1 diabetes. *Diabetes Res Clin Pract.*
    2013;99(1):19–23. doi:10.1016/j.diabres.2012.10.024.

34. Savage DB, Petersen KF, Shulman GI. Disordered lipid metabolism and the pathogenesis of insulin
    resistance. *Physiol Rev.* 2007;87(2):507–520. doi:10.1152/physrev.00024.2006.

35. Smart CE, Evans M, O'Connell SM, McElduff P, Lopez PE, Jones TW et al. Both dietary protein and
    fat increase postprandial glucose excursions in children with type 1 diabetes, and the effect is additive.
    Diabetes Care. 2013;36(12):3897–3902. doi:10.2337/dc13-1195.

36. Colberg SR, Riddell MC. Physical activity: Regulation of glucose metabolism, clinicial management
    strategies, and weight control. In: Peters A, Laffel L, editors. *American Diabetes Association/JDRF
    Type 1 Diabetes Sourcebook.* Alexandria, VA: American Diabetes Association; 2013.

37. Rejeski WJ, Ip EH, Bertoni AG, Bray GA, Evans G, Gregg EW et al. Lifestyle change and mobility in
    obese adults with type 2 diabetes. *N Engl J Med.* 2012;366(13):1209–1217. doi:10.1056/NEJMoa1110294.

38. Yardley J, Mollard R, MacIntosh A, MacMillan F, Wicklow B, Berard L et al. Vigorous intensity
    exercise for glycemic control in patients with type 1 diabetes. *Can J Diabetes.* 2013;37(6):427–432.
    doi:10.1016/j.jcjd.2013.08.269.

39. The effect of intensive treatment of diabetes on the development and progression of long-term complica-
    tions in insulin-dependent diabetes mellitus. The Diabetes Control and Complications Trial Research
    Group. *N Engl J Med.* 1993;329(14):977–986. doi:10.1056/NEJM199309303291401.

40. Nathan DM, Cleary PA, Backlund JY, Genuth SM, Lachin JM, Orchard TJ et al. Intensive diabetes treat-
    ment and cardiovascular disease in patients with type 1 diabetes. *N Engl J Med.* 2005;353(25):2643–
    2653. doi:10.1056/NEJMoa052187.

41. Nathan DM, Zinman B, Cleary PA, Backlund JY, Genuth S, Miller R et al. Modern-day clinical
    course of type 1 diabetes mellitus after 30 years' duration: The diabetes control and complications
    trial/epidemiology of diabetes interventions and complications and Pittsburgh epidemiology of dia-
    betes complications experience (1983–2005). *Arch Intern Med.* 2009;169(14):1307–1316. doi:10.1001/
    archinternmed.2009.193.

42. 6. Glycemic targets. *Diabetes Care.* 2017;40(Suppl 1):S48–S56. doi:10.2337/dc17-S009.

43. Miller KM, Beck RW, Bergenstal RM, Goland RS, Haller MJ, McGill JB et al. Evidence of a strong
    association between frequency of self-monitoring of blood glucose and hemoglobin A1c levels in T1D
    exchange clinic registry participants. *Diabetes Care.* 2013;36(7):2009–2014. doi:10.2337/dc12-1770.

44. Brownlee M, Hirsch IB. Glycemic variability: A hemoglobin A1c–independent risk factor for diabetic
    complications. *JAMA.* 2006;295(14):1707–1708. doi:10.1001/jama.295.14.1707.

45. American Diabetes Association. 5. Glycemic targets. *Diabetes Care.* 2016;39 Suppl 1:S39–S46.
    doi:10.2337/dc16-S008.

46. Chang CM, Hsieh CJ, Huang JC, Huang IC. Acute and chronic fluctuations in blood glucose levels
    can increase oxidative stress in type 2 diabetes mellitus. *Acta Diabetol.* 2012;49 Suppl 1:S171–S177.
    doi:10.1007/s00592-012-0398-x.

47. Monnier L, Mas E, Ginet C, Michel F, Villon L, Cristol JP et al. Activation of oxidative stress by acute
    glucose fluctuations compared with sustained chronic hyperglycemia in patients with type 2 diabetes.
    JAMA. 2006;295(14):1681–1687. doi:10.1001/jama.295.14.1681.

48. Ceriello A, Esposito K, Piconi L, Ihnat MA, Thorpe JE, Testa R et al. Oscillating glucose is more del-
    eterious to endothelial function and oxidative stress than mean glucose in normal and type 2 diabetic
    patients. *Diabetes.* 2008;57(5):1349–1354. doi:10.2337/db08-0063.

49. Vaddiraju S, Burgess DJ, Tomazos I, Jain FC, Papadimitrakopoulos F. Technologies for continuous
    glucose monitoring: Current problems and future promises. *J Diabetes Sci Technol.* 2010;4:1540–1562.

50. Maurizi AR, Pozzilli P. Do we need continuous glucose monitoring in type 2 diabetes? *Diabetes/Metab
    Res Rev.* 2016. doi:10.1002/dmrr.2450.

51. Deiss D, Bolinder J, Riveline JP, Battelino T, Bosi E, Tubiana-Rufi N et al. Improved glycemic control in
    poorly controlled patients with type 1 diabetes using real-time continuous glucose monitoring. *Diabetes
    Care.* 2006;29(12):2730–2732. doi:10.2337/dc06-1134.

52. O'Connell MA, Donath S, O'Neal DN, Colman PG, Ambler GR, Jones TW et al. Glycaemic impact
    of patient-led use of sensor-guided pump therapy in type 1 diabetes: A randomised controlled trial.
    Diabetologia. 2009;52(7):1250–1257. doi:10.1007/s00125-009-1365-0.

53. Tamborlane WV, Beck RW, Bode BW, Buckingham B, Chase HP, Clemons R et al. Continuous glu-
    cose monitoring and intensive treatment of type 1 diabetes. *N Engl J Med.* 2008;359(14):1464–1476.
    doi:10.1056/NEJMoa0805017.

54. Beck RW, Hirsch IB, Laffel L, Tamborlane WV, Bode BW, Buckingham B et al. The effect of continuous glucose monitoring in well-controlled type 1 diabetes. *Diabetes Care*. 2009;32(8):1378–1383. doi:10.2337/dc09-0108.

55. Battelino T, Phillip M, Bratina N, Nimri R, Oskarsson P, Bolinder J. Effect of continuous glucose monitoring on hypoglycemia in type 1 diabetes. *Diabetes Care*. 2011;34(4):795–800. doi:10.2337/dc10-1989.

56. Klonoff DC, Buckingham B, Christiansen JS, Montori VM, Tamborlane WV, Vigersky RA et al. Continuous glucose monitoring: An endocrine society clinical practice guideline. *J Clin Endocrinol Metab*. 2011;96(10):2968–2979. doi:10.1210/jc.2010-2756.

57. Bailey TS, Grunberger G, Bode BW, Handelsman Y, Hirsch IB, Jovanovič L et al. American Association of Clinical Endocrinologists and American College of Endocrinology 2016 outpatient glucose monitoring consensus statement. *Endocr Pract*. 2016;22(2):231–261. doi:10.4158/EP151124.CS.

58. Awoniyi O, Rehman R, Dagogo-Jack S. Hypoglycemia in patients with type 1 diabetes: Epidemiology, pathogenesis, and prevention. *Curr Diab Rep*. 2013;13(5):669–678. doi:10.1007/s11892-013-0411-y.

59. Cryer PE. The barrier of hypoglycemia in diabetes. *Diabetes*. 2008;57(12):3169–3176. doi:10.2337/db08-1084.

60. Chiang JL, Kirkman MS, Laffel LM, Peters AL. Type 1 diabetes through the life span: A position statement of the American Diabetes Association. *Diabetes Care*. 2014;37(7):2034–2054. doi:10.2337/dc14-1140.

61. Cryer PE. Diverse causes of hypoglycemia-associated autonomic failure in diabetes. *N Engl J Med*. 2004;350(22):2272–2279. doi:10.1056/NEJMra031354.

62. Edelman S, Henry, R. *Diagnosis and Management of Type 2 Diabetes*. 13th ed. West Islip, NY: Professional Communications,; 2017.

63. Edelman S. *Taking Control of Your Diabetes*. 5th ed. West Islip, NY: Professional Communications; 2018.

22 Meal Detection Module in an Artificial Pancreas System for People with Type 1 Diabetes

S. Samadi, K. Turksoy, I. Hajizadeh, J. Feng,
M. Sevil, C. Lazaro, N. Hobbs, R. Brandt,
J. Kilkus, E. Littlejohn, and A. Cinar

CONTENTS

22.1 INTRODUCTION

Artificial pancreas (AP) control systems aim to achieve automated regulation of blood glucose concentration in people with type 1 diabetes (T1D). While in open-loop insulin administration, the individual, with physician supervision, makes all the decisions regarding the insulin adjustments. AP is a closed-loop system that automatically manipulates the insulin doses and infusion [1–6]. An AP system consists of a minimum of four components: (1) a person with T1D, (2) a continuous glucose monitor (CGM) that measures and reports the interstitial glucose concentration, (3) a control algorithm that makes decisions regarding the insulin infusion rate, and (4) an insulin pump that administers the insulin to the patient. The AP may utilize additional measuring devices in order to feed more comprehensive information to the controller about the subject's physiological condition [7]. The physiological conditions, such as physical activity or exercise, stress, and sleep, are assessed by the interpretation of physiological variables reported by wearable devices, such as heart rate, energy expenditure, etc. [8–10]. Using the measured physiological variables in addition to CGM data enables a multivariable AP with a controller to manage the effect of otherwise unknown (unannounced) disturbances [11]. In a fully automated AP (no manual entries), while the measured physiological variables relieve the need for manual entries about the physiological conditions, integration of meal detection and meal size estimation components into AP systems is needed to compensate for meal announcements.

Control of postprandial glucose is one of the most important challenges in diabetes therapy. Several factors influence glycemic response to food, including food form (e.g., solid, liquid), degree of cooking and processing (degree of hydration, degree of starch gelatinization, particle size), ripeness, macronutrient composition, fiber, antinutrients (e.g., amylase inhibitors), amount of food consumed at one time, meal frequency, rate of ingestion, and physiological effects [12–14]. Absorption of nutrients is related to the inherent qualities of the nutrients themselves and their interactions with each other and with nonabsorbable food components (i.e., fiber) [13]. Any of these factors, alone or in combination, will impact the overall rate of digestion and absorption and subsequent glycemic response that must be predicted by AP systems.

Carbohydrates belong to one of four groups: mono- and disaccharides (sugars), oligosaccharides (chains of 3–10 glucose or fructose polymers), and polysaccharides (fiber and starch) [15,16]. During digestion, the body breaks down all sugars into monosaccharides for absorption, but not all carbohydrates are metabolized fully into glucose. Although fiber itself is resistant to digestion by dietary enzymes, it does play an important role in the rate of nutrient absorption. Soluble fiber, in particular, delays gastric emptying and slows nutrient absorption; however, there is inconclusive evidence that increasing dietary fiber will influence glycemic outcomes in diabetic individuals [16–20]. Because a multitude of factors influence glycemic response, it is not possible to predict the physiological effect of food based on chemical composition alone. An index of the physiological effects of food, also known as the *glycemic index*, is available to supplement data on chemical composition of foods [20]. Glycemic index (appearance rate at which various carbs are absorbed in to the bloodstream) thus can aid in variable insulin dosing predictions for AP systems.

Currently, people with T1D who use insulin pumps manually enter the estimates of the carbohydrate content of a meal into the pump to compute the meal insulin bolus. In addition to the drive to eliminate human errors, such as forgetting to enter meal information and unreliable carbohydrate estimation, the desire to reduce the burden of manual entries inspired the development of meal detection methods over the last decade.

This chapter reviews meal detection methods developed to date and used in the closed-loop control of glucose concentration and focuses on two meal detection algorithms that are integrated into a multivariable AP system.

22.2   DIFFERENT TECHNIQUES FOR MEAL DETECTION

Automation of meal information requires a meal module that first detects the meals automatically and then plans a meal insulin bolus strategy for detected meals. Some methods addressed only detect the meals, while the others either estimate the meal carbohydrate size or define rules for insulin meal boluses based on detected meal impulses.

Meal detection algorithms can be categorized into five techniques:

1. The techniques based on calculation or estimation of glucose rate of change (ROC): Meal detection methods that use real-time glucose ROC or first or second derivatives of glucose level variation in a brief period of time based on successive CGM readings [21–25]. These change metrics are used in some threshold rules to detect the occurrence of the meal [21,22,26] or estimate the meal impulses [26,25].
2. The techniques that use estimation theory: Some detection methods consider an insulin-glucose dynamics model and use a Kalman filter estimation to estimate the unmeasured meal-related glucose rise parameters or variables (state variables of the insulin-glucose model). The estimation error is corrected at every sampling time based on the deviation of measured output and estimated output of the model (in this case, the difference in interstitial glucose concentration measured by CGM and estimated by the insulin-glucose model). The estimated meal-related parameters or variables are then processed by threshold rules

to differentiate between meal or nonmeal situations. The insulin-glucose models used to detect the meal based on the Kalman filter approach belong to one of two categories:

    a. A linear data-driven model consisting of three differential equations describing glucose (G), first (G'), and second (G'') derivatives of glucose [21,26]. Some threshold rules on the estimated values of first and second derivatives will detect the occurrence of a meal.

    b. A first-principles minimal metabolic model that describes the glucose-insulin dynamics [27].

3. The techniques that use a meal library: A simple insulin-glucose model predicts the glucose trajectory without meal, and with meals with different magnitude and different start times. The probability of matching computed ROC of measured glucose by CGM and of models with various meals decides about the shape, time, and magnitude of the meal [28].

4. The techniques based on signal processing and statistics literature:

    a. Variable state dimension (VSD) approach: The method identifies two data-driven state-space glucose concentration models (the number of states are different in the two models), with and without meal as the input. Based on the value of defined detection statistics computed at every sample time, a Kalman filter switches its operation (estimation) between two models, and the meal size is estimated [29].

    b. Parameter invariant (PAIN) detector. Using measured glucose (output), the method builds two statistics tests invariant to the parameters of the model. The algorithm defines a score based on the statistics equivalent to the confidence level in the occurrence of a meal [30].

5. Knowledge-based detector without any glucose models: The method transforms the derivatives computed based on CGM data to different qualitative variables. Qualitative variables are distinct from each other, representing different patterns of glucose variation. Using qualitative variables, a detection feature is defined. The detection feature is processed with some threshold-type criteria to detect the meal. The carbohydrate content of the meal is estimated by a knowledge-based (fuzzy logic-based) system at every sampling time. The estimator uses CGM and subcutaneous insulin delivery data [24,31].

ROC-based methods have quick detections but the risk of false-positives (erroneous indication of a meal) is high. They may detect the glucose rise caused by other factors such as psychological stress as consumption of meals. The risk of hypoglycemia is high, especially if the estimation of the size of the meal is not included in the algorithm and any detection is treated with the same insulin dosing.

For Kalman filter-based methods, relying only on a fixed glucose model that applies for all people with T1D and using a constant threshold for detection feature disregards inter- and intrapatient variability.

Considering 5 minutes as the sampling time of measured glucose, using meal library and PAIN techniques imposes high detection delay if the confidence level is high enough.

False-positive detections may increase if physiological information is not incorporated in the knowledge-based approach. But the estimation of carbohydrate is incremental and conservative, which reduces hypoglycemia risk in case of false-positive detection.

22.3 TWO MEAL DETECTION METHODS USED IN THE MULTIVARIABLE ARTIFICIAL PANCREAS SYSTEM

We have discussed the importance of the presence of a meal detection module in an automated AP system. The module has the task of determining the time and amount of carbohydrates consumed and suggesting the insulin bolus to control postprandial glucose. Based on the aforementioned strengths and weakness of different techniques, we consider two different algorithms developed based on entirely different approaches [24,27].

22.3.1 ALGORITHM A: DETECTION BASED ON AN INSULIN-GLUCOSE MODEL AND ESTIMATION THEORY

The first algorithm (algorithm A) considered an extended Bergman glucose-insulin compartmental model and applied an unscented Kalman filter algorithm on the discretized model to estimate the states and parameters of the model. The detection of the meal depends on the value of the estimated rate of appearance of glucose $R_a(t)$. The meal flag raises if the estimated $R_a(t)$ is above 2 mg/dL/min and a meal bolus is given [27,32].

22.3.2 ALGORITHM B: DETECTION BASED ON QUALITATIVE VALUES AND ESTIMATION BASED ON FUZZY LOGIC-BASED SYSTEM

Modeling in fuzzy logic is inspired by the knowledge stemming from the human interpretation of changes expressed as some general qualitative rules. The output of a fuzzy logic-based model is built on the use of descriptive rules. Rules involve the combination of qualitative values (e.g., low, medium, large) of all model inputs. While rules are originated from physiological principles or human findings based on the experience or observation of large data sets, building proper inputs using measured variables that can fit in rules to describe the input-output relation is an important task for mathematics.

The algorithm (algorithm B) does not use any physiology-based model. The variation of real-time measured glucose by CGM is modeled by qualitative variables. Qualitive variables have a different combination of first and second glucose derivatives. In Figure 22.1, $G'(k)$ and $G''(k)$ are the first and

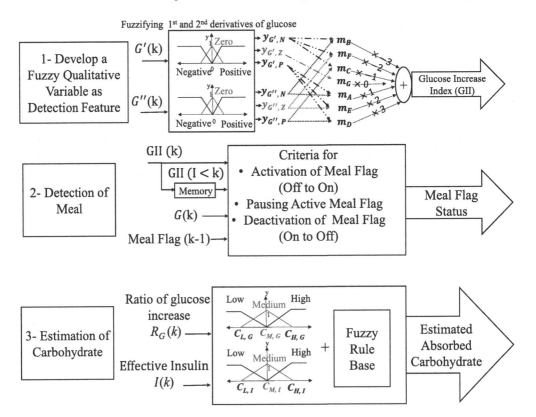

FIGURE 22.1 Algorithm B flowchart: Step1: A detection feature is computed based on the first and second derivatives of glucose concentration changes. Step 2: Based on rules used for meal detection, detect the presence of a meal. Step 3: The carbohydrate content is estimated for detected meals.

second derivatives of glucose at current time step. [$y_{G',N}$ $y_{G',Z}$ $y_{G',P}$] are the set of membership degrees assigned to input G' (similarly for G''), where subscripts N, Z, and P denote negative, zero, and positive ranges. Membership degree is a concept in fuzzy logic-based math (vs crisp math) expressing how much an input (in this case $G'(k)$) belongs to qualitative values (in this case positive, zero, and negative). As shown in Figure 22.1 (see first row), if $G'(k)$ is centered around zero, the membership degree of $G'(k)$ to the zero qualitative value (middle triangular section) is higher compared to the negative and positive qualitative values (yG', $Z > yG'$, P and yG', $Z > yG'$, N). As input $G'(k)$ movies away from $G'(k) = 0$, yG', Z linearly reduces from 1 to 0. The variable m_i, $i = A$, B, ..., F (Figure 22.1) denotes the membership degree of glucose concentration derivatives at time step k ($G'(k)$, $G''(k)$) to qualitative variable i. Qualitative variables (A-F) each represent accelerating, linear, or decelerating increase or decrease of glucose concentration variations. Glucose increase index (GII) is a defined detection feature. The threshold criteria on the detection feature and current glucose concentration determine the status of meal flag (second row in Figure 22.1). A fuzzy logic-based system estimates the carbohydrate content of the detected meal once a meal is detected (third row in Figure 22.1).

22.4   ASSESSMENT OF ALGORITHMS A AND B WITH CLINICAL EXPERIMENTS

Clinical experiments for real-time evaluation of the multivariable AP control system are conducted at the University of Chicago Clinical Research Center. Subjects with T1D use their own insulin type and pump during the experiments. Each subject undergoes a 60-hour closed-loop experiment without any manual meal and exercise announcements. The time and amount of all infused insulin doses are computed by the AP system. Based on the study protocol, breakfast, lunch, dinner, and one or two snacks per day were provided. In addition, the hypoglycemia module of the AP system suggests occasionally the consumption of rescue carbohydrates as needed to prevent potential hypoglycemia [10]. The decisions of the AP system are made every 5 minutes, when the AP receives new glucose concentration data from the CGM. All modules, including the meal detection module, update their outputs with the same sampling rate. The frequency of physiological signal collection from wearable devices is higher, and the timing of the information is synchronized with the CGM sampling rate.

The meal detection module of the AP system includes both algorithms. During clinical experiments, both algorithms are executed simultaneously. They use measured glucose concentration (CGM) and insulin pump data to detect the meals and estimate the meal insulin or carbohydrate based on their own approaches. In the current stage, the AP system uses only the algorithm A to determine the insulin meal bolus, and the detection and estimation of the second algorithm is used for confirmation. Running both algorithms in parallel in real time for the same clinical data allows us to assess the strengths and limitations of each and find a strategy to reconcile their decisions. The conclusions reached by both algorithms will be reconciled in the future to improve the meal detection goals, which are (1) high sensitivity for detection of the true meals before a remarkable rise in glucose concentration takes place, and (2) low occurrence of false-positive detections.

Figure 22.2 shows the glucose regulation for one of the clinical experiments with subject 1 within the postprandial period (2 hours after the start of meals), where meal detection algorithm A decides the infused insulin meal boluses. All meals are detected by the algorithm (one snack is not detected [Figure 22.2d] because the glucose trend is decreasing within all 24 time steps). The meal is considered detected when the first insulin bolus after the start of the meal is given. The bars in the figure correspond to insulin boluses given for breakfast, lunch, dinner, and evening snack, and the actual carbohydrate (CHO) content of meals/snacks is written at the top of each column. The same food contents are repeated over the 3 days of the experiment (lasting for 60 hours). The experiment ends on the third day in the afternoon. The right y-axis indicates the change of glucose with respect to base glucose concentration (G_b) at the start of the meal. In x-axis, sampling time = 0 corresponds to start of the meal. Detection time varies from 5 to 18 sampling times (5 minutes). Except for cases c and e, the infused insulin was able to bring back the glucose concentration close to G_b or to an acceptable decreasing trend.

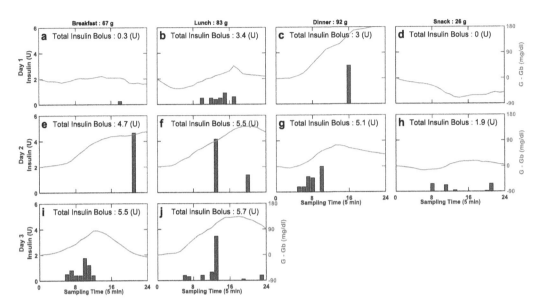

FIGURE 22.2 Variations in the measured glucose concentration (G) from the glucose concentration at the start of meal (*Gb*) within the first 2 hours after start of meals/ snacks when algorithm A computes the insulin meal boluses (right y-axis). *The bars show* the suggested insulin meal boluses (left y-axis) by algorithm A. Data of subject 1 during a 3-day clinical experiment.

Figure 22.3 shows the estimation of carbohydrate by algorithm B for the same clinical experiment displayed in Figure 22.2 by algorithm A. The change of glucose is entirely controlled by algorithm A. The outcome of algorithm B is recorded only for later assessment. A meal is considered as detected by algorithm B when the first estimation (bars in Figure 22.3) stands out. The total estimated carbohydrate within a period of 24 sampling times after a meal (within 2 hours) is noted

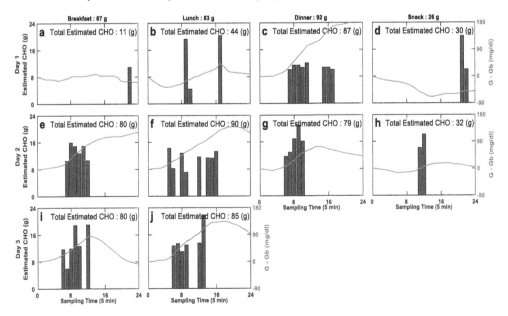

FIGURE 22.3 Estimation of carbohydrate (CHO) content (bars) of meals/snacks by algorithm B (left y-axis). The curves indicate the variations in the glucose concentration (G) from the glucose concentration at the start of meal (*Gb*) within the first 2 hours after start of meals/snacks when algorithm A computes the insulin meal boluses (right y-axis). Data of subject 1 during a 3-day clinical experiment.

in each subfigure as the meal size estimation for the corresponding actual meal. For example, subfigure *i* shows that algorithm B has detected a meal at the sixth sampling time (30 minutes after the start of the meal) and estimated 80 g of carbohydrate for the breakfast on the third day, where the actual carbohydrate amount was 67 g. The amount of meal bolus is proportional to the estimated carbohydrate based on patient-specific carbohydrate-to-insulin ratio.

Figures 22.4 through 22.7 present the experimental results for each algorithm with subjects 2 and 3.

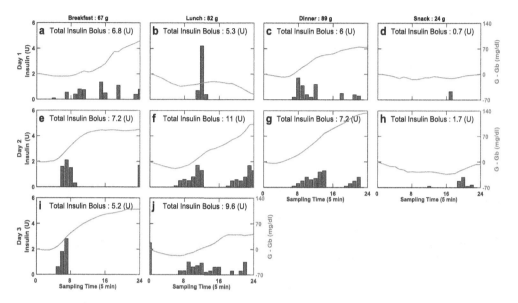

FIGURE 22.4   The change in glucose concentration (G) from the glucose concentration at the start of meal (*Gb*) within the first 2 hours after start of meals/snacks when algorithm A computes the insulin meal boluses (right y-axis). *The bars show* the suggested insulin meal boluses (left y-axis) by algorithm A. Data of subject 2 during a 3-day clinical experiment.

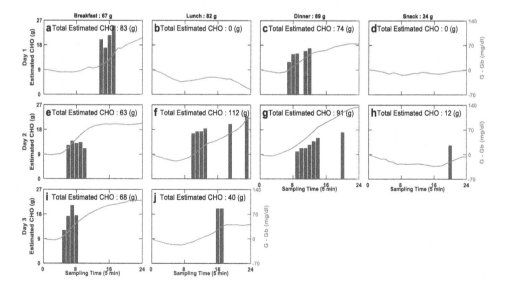

FIGURE 22.5   Estimation of carbohydrate (CHO) content (bars) of meals/snacks by algorithm B (left y-axis). The curves indicate the variations in the glucose concentration (G) from the glucose concentration at the start of meal (*Gb*) within the first 2 hours after start of meals/ snacks when algorithm A computes the insulin meal boluses (right y-axis). Data of subject 2 during a 3-day clinical experiment.

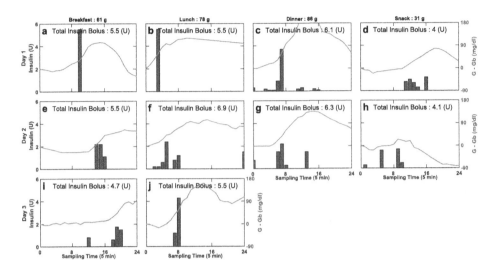

FIGURE 22.6 The change in glucose concentration (G) from the glucose concentration at the start of meal (*Gb*) within the first 2 hours after start of meals/snacks when algorithm A computes the insulin meal boluses (right y-axis). *The bars show* the suggested insulin meal boluses (left y-axis) by algorithm A. Data of subject 3 during a 3-day clinical experiment.

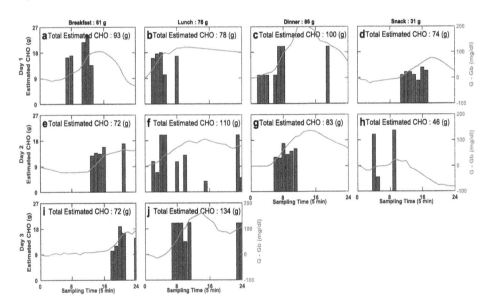

FIGURE 22.7 Estimation of carbohydrate (CHO) content (bars) of meals/snacks by algorithm B (left y-axis). The curves indicate the variations in the glucose concentration (G) from the glucose concentration at the start of meal (*Gb*) within the first 2 hours after start of meals/snacks when algorithm A computes the insulin meal boluses (right y-axis). Data of subject 3 during a 3-day clinical experiment.

The detection rate is 85% and 92% for algorithm A and B, respectively. For detected meals, Figure 22.8 displays the detection delay for both algorithms (for the nondetected meals, detection delay is not defined). Based on Figure 22.8, the mediums of detection delay for algorithms are comparable (35 minutes for algorithm A and 30 minutes for algorithm B). However, the cases with high detection delay (> 50 min) are rare for algorithm B. For algorithm B, false detection is 1.2 occurrences per day. Figures 22.9 and 22.10 show statistical results for detected meals by algorithm B for 13 clinical experiments, in which the algorithm is assessed retrospectively for 10 experiments and for three experiments

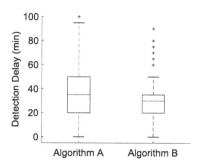

FIGURE 22.8   Distribution of detection delay, defined as the time between the start of meal and the time meal is detected by algorithm.

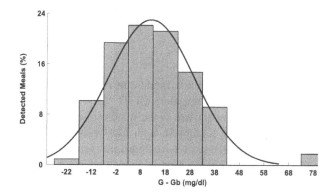

FIGURE 22.9   Distribution of the change of measured glucose concentration at the detection time (G) based on glucose concentration at the start of meal (Gb) (for algorithm B).

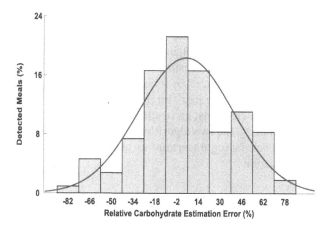

FIGURE 22.10   Distribution of relative carbohydrate estimation error (for algorithm B) defined as the absolute estimation error divided by the magnitude of the actual value of consumed carbohydrate.

in real time (the results are presented in Figures 22.3, 22.5, and 22.7 in detail). Figure 22.9 indicates that 98% of detected meals were identified early enough when the measured glucose (CGM) increased less than 43 mg/dL. The estimation error (Figure 22.10) depends on the appearance of the effect of the meal on glucose levels that might be lower (than usual appearance) because of high insulin on board before a meal or physical activity. Also, the appearance of glucose rise may be higher due to some digested rescue carbohydrates or other (unmeasured) reasons, such as stress.

22.5 DISCUSSION

A high rate of true-positive detection, low rate of false-positive detection, and reliable amount of meal bolus for detected meals are essential goals for a meal module as a component of an unannounced meal AP control system. We discussed the performance of two meal detection algorithms built on different approaches. The dependency on the glucose dynamic model is the hallmark of distinction of two algorithms. A model-dependent approach has better tolerance to sudden change of measured glucose and potentially takes less risk of false detection. However, assuming a fixed-model structure is a deficiency of this approach that may reduce the detection rate and extend detection delay. Algorithm A is a model-dependent approach and updates the model parameters to manage the inter- and intrapatient variability to some extent. This approach also has a higher computation load. The model-free meal detection approach, such as algorithm B, has higher detection rates (both true and false). The computation load and detection delay are low (compared to model-dependent approach). The estimation of carbohydrate included in algorithm B is also a benefit to determine a reliable amount of meal bolus.

22.6 CONCLUSIONS

Integration of a reliable and fast meal detection module in AP systems is a big step toward fully automated regulation of blood glucose concentration in T1D. Missed or late detection leads to hyperglycemia, while false detections may induce extra insulin administration and cause hypoglycemia. Hence, the meal detector must be able to achieve high true-positive and low false-positive meal detections. Reconciling the decisions made by two algorithms representative of model-dependent and model-free meal detection approaches is a promising method to achieve a fast and reliable meal detector.

22.7 FUTURE WORK: RECONCILING ALGORITHMS A AND B TO ENHANCE RELIABILITY OF DETECTION

Comparing both algorithms, algorithm B detects the meal faster, while the probability of false-detection rate is also higher. To increase the reliability of detection without a long waiting time, algorithm A checks the validity. If Algorithm B detects a meal and starts carbohydrate estimation (and proportionally a bolus infusion) while algorithm A has not detected a meal, the estimated carbohydrate can be reduced by a confidence factor until the meal is confirmed or denied by algorithm A. The same strategy might be followed if a meal is detected only by algorithm A. In case of double detections, an insulin dose might be administered based on the highest suggested insulin value by the two algorithms. The decision made by a combined meal detector is more accurate when facing uncertainties of daily life, such as exercise and stress affecting blood glucose variation.

REFERENCES

1. B. P. Kovatchev, E. Renard, C. Cobelli, H. C. Zisser, P. Keith-Hynes, S. M. Anderson, S. A. Brown. et al., "Safety of outpatient closed-loop control: First randomized crossover trials of a wearable artificial pancreas," *Diabetes Care*, vol. 37, no. 7, pp. 1789–1796, 2014.
2. K. Turksoy and A. Cinar, "Adaptive control of artificial pancreas systems-A review," *J. Healthc. Eng.*, vol. 5, no. 1, pp. 1–22, 2013.
3. S. Trevitt, S. Simpson, and A. Wood, "Artificial pancreas device systems for the closed-Loop control of type 1 diabetes what systems are in development?," *J. Diabetes Sci. Technol.*, p. 1932296815617968, 2015.
4. F. Chee, T. Fernando, and P. V. van Heerden, "Closed-loop control of blood glucose levels in critically ill patients," *Anaesth Intensive Care*, vol. 30, no. 3, pp. 295–307, 2002.
5. A. Haidar, "The artificial pancreas: How closed-Loop control is revolutionizing diabetes," *IEEE Control Syst.*, vol. 36, no. 5, pp. 28–47, 2016.

6. K. Turksoy, N. Frantz, L. Quinn, M. Dumin, J. Kilkus, B. Hibner, A. Cinar, and E. Littlejohn, "Automated insulin delivery—The light at the end of the tunnel," *J. Pediatr.*, vol. 186, pp. 17–28.e9, 2017.

7. A. Cinar, "Multivariable adaptive artificial pancreas system in Type 1 diabetes," *Curr Diab Rep.*, vol. 17, no. 10. 2017.

8. K. Turksoy, T. M. L. Paulino, D. P. Zaharieva, L. Yavelberg, V. Jamnik, M. C. Riddell, and A. Cinar, "Classification of physical activity: Information to artificial pancreas control systems in real time.," *J. Diabetes Sci. Technol.*, vol. 9, no. 6, pp. 1200–1207, 2015.

9. K. Turksoy, C. Monforti, M. Park, G. Griffith, L. Quinn, and A. Cinar, "Use of wearable sensors and biometric variables in an artificial pancreas system," *Sensors (Switzerland)*, vol. 17, no. 3, 2017.

10. K. Turksoy, J. Kilkus, I. Hajizadeh, S. Samadi, J. Feng, M. Sevil, C. Lazaro, N. Frantz, E. Littlejohn, and A. Cinar, "Hypoglycemia detection and carbohydrate suggestion in an artificial pancreas," *J. Diabetes Sci. Technol.*, vol. 10, no. 6, pp. 1236–1244, 2016.

11. K. Turksoy, L. Quinn, E. Littlejohn, and A. Cinar, "Multivariable adaptive identification and control for artificial pancreas systems," *IEEE Trans. Biomed. Eng.*, vol. 61, no. 3, pp. 883–891, 2014.

12. J. M. W. Wong and D. J. A. Jenkins, "Carbohydrate digestibility and metabolic effects," *J. Nutr.*, vol. 137, no. 11 Suppl, pp. 2539S–2546S, 2007.

13. M. E. Shils, J. A. Olson, M. Shike, and A. C. Ross. "Fiber and other dietary factors affecting nutrient absorption and metabolism," in *Modern Nutrition in Health and Disease*. 9th ed. Baltimore, MD, 1998, pp. 679–698.

14. "Nutrition recommendations and interventions for diabetes: A position statement of the American diabetes association," *Diabetes Care*, vol. 31, no. Suppl. 1. 2008.

15. M. J. Franz, J. P. Bantle, C. A. Beebe, J. D. Brunzell, J. L. Chiasson, A. Garg, L. A. Holzmeister et al., "Evidence-based nutrition principles and recommendations for the treatment and prevention of diabetes and related complications," *Diabetes Care*, vol. 25, no. Suppl. 1. 2002.

16. M. L. Wheeler and F. X. Pi-Sunyer, "Carbohydrate issues: Type and amount," *J. Am. Diet. Assoc.*, vol. 108, no. 4 Suppl., 2008.

17. D. J. Jenkins, T. M. Wolever, A. R. Leeds, M. A. Gassull, P. Haisman, J. Dilawari, D. V. Goff, G. L. Metz, and K. G. Alberti, "Dietary fibres, fibre analogues, and glucose tolerance: Importance of viscosity," *BMJ.*, vol. 1, no. 6124, pp. 1392–1394, 1978.

18. S. Holt, D. Carter, P. Tothill, R. Heading, and L. Prescott, "Effect of gel fibre on gastric emptying and absorption of glucose and paracetamol," *Lancet*, vol. 313, no. 8117, pp. 636–639, 1979.

19. M. J. Franz, M. A. Powers, C. Leontos, L. A. Holzmeister, K. Kulkarni, A. Monk, N. Wedel, and E. Gradwell, "The evidence for medical nutrition therapy for type 1 and type 2 diabetes in adults," *J Am Diet Assoc.*, vol. 110, no. 12. pp. 1852–1889, 2010.

20. D. J. A. Jenkins, T. M. S. Wolever, and R. H. Taylor, "Glycemic index of foods: A physiological basis for carbohydrate exchange," *Am. J. Clin. Nutr.*, vol. 34, no. 3, pp. 362–366, 1981.

21. E. Dassau, B. W. Bequette, B. A. Buckingham, and F. J. Doyle 3rd, "Detection of a meal using continuous glucose monitoring: Implications for an artificial beta-cell," *Diabetes Care*, vol. 31, no. 2, pp. 295–300, 2008.

22. R. A. Harvey, E. Dassau, H. Zisser, D. E. Seborg, and F. J. Doyle, "Design of the glucose rate increase detector a meal detection module for the health monitoring system," *J. Diabetes Sci. Technol.*, p. 1932296814523881, 2014.

23. H. Lee, B. A. Buckingham, D. M. Wilson, and B. W. Bequette, "A closed-loop artificial pancreas using model predictive control and a sliding meal size estimator," *J. Diabetes Sci. Technol.*, vol. 3, no. 5, pp. 1082–1090, 2009.

24. S. Samadi, K. Turksoy, I. Hajizadeh, J. Feng, M. Sevil, and A. Cinar, "Meal detection and carbohydrate estimation using continuous glucose sensor data," *IEEE J. Biomed. Health Inform.*, vol. 21, no. 3, pp. 619–627, 2017.

25. H. Lee, B. A. Buckingham, D. M. Wilson, and B. W. Bequette, "A closed-loop artificial pancreas using model predictive control and a sliding meal size estimator," *J Diabetes Sci Technol.*, vol. 3, no. 5, pp. 1082–1090, 2009.

26. H. Lee and B. W. Bequette, "A closed-loop artificial pancreas based on model predictive control: Human-friendly identification and automatic meal disturbance rejection," *Biomed. Signal Process. Control*, vol. 4, no. 4, pp. 347–354, 2009.

27. K. Turksoy, S. Samadi, J. Feng, E. Littlejohn, L. Quinn, and A. Cinar, "Meal detection in patients with type 1 diabetes: A new module for the multivariable adaptive artificial pancreas control system," *IEEE J. Biomed. Health Informatics*, vol. 20, no. 1, pp. 47–54, 2016.

28. F. Cameron, G. Niemeyer, and B. A. Buckingham, "Probabilistic evolving meal detection and estimation of meal total glucose appearance," *J. Diabetes Sci. Technol.*, vol. 3, pp. 1022–1030, 2009.

29. J. Xie and Q. Wang, "A variable state dimension approach to meal detection and meal size estimation: In silico evaluation through basal-bolus insulin therapy for type 1 diabetes," *IEEE Trans Biomed Eng.*, vol. 64, no. 6, pp. 1249–1260, 2017.

30. J. Weimer, S. Chen, A. Peleckis, M. R. Rickels, and I. Lee, "Physiology-invariant meal detection for type 1 diabetes," *Diabetes Technol. Ther.*, vol. 18, no. 10, pp. 616–624, 2016.

31. S. Sediqeh, M. Rashid, K. Turksoy, J. Feng, I. Hajizadeh, N. Hobbs, C. Lazaro, M. Sevil, E. Littlejohn, and A. Cinar, "Automatic detection and estimation of unannounced meals for multivariable artificial pancreas system," *Diabetes Technol. Ther.*, vol. 20, no. 3, pp. 235–246, 2018.

32. K. Turksoy, I. Hajizadeh, S. Samadi, J. Feng, M. Sevil, M. Park, L. Quinn, E. Littlejohn, and A. Cinar, "Real-time estimation of glucose concentration and insulin bolusing for unannounced meals with artificial pancreas," *Control Eng. Pract.*, vol. 59, pp. 159–164, 2017. Doi:10.1016/j.conengprac.2016.08.001.

23 Oxidative Stress and the Effects of Dietary Supplements on Glycemic Control in Type 2 Diabetes

Emmanuel C. Opara

CONTENTS

23.1 INTRODUCTION

Oxidative stress can be defined as a situation of imbalance in which the levels of pro-oxidants, referred to as *reactive oxygen species* (ROS) present in tissues, by far outweigh the amounts of neutralizing substances, otherwise known as *antioxidants*, as previously discussed [1]. There is overwhelming evidence in the literature to show that this phenomenon is associated with both type 1 and type 2 diabetes [1–7]. Many experimental approaches have been used to demonstrate the association of oxidative stress with diabetes. Some investigators have examined levels of ROS or their degradation products, while others have assessed tissue and blood levels of micronutrient antioxidants and/or the levels and activities of antioxidant enzymes in experimental animals and in individuals afflicted with diabetes. While it has been fairly accepted that oxidative stress may play a role in the etiology of type 1 diabetes [4,8,9], it is presently not clear that it plays any role in the pathogenesis of type 2 diabetes. Previous studies had suggested that oxidative stress is a consequence of type 2 diabetes and may be primarily involved in the development of secondary complications of the disease [10–15]. However, there is a growing body of evidence to show that it may actually play a role, even if secondary, in the pathogenesis of the disease [1–3,6,7,16–20]. In this chapter, we will review the literature to determine the relationship between oxidative stress and type 2 diabetes, with particular attention to the role played by oxidative stress in the pathogenesis of the disease. We will then determine if there is a valid scientific basis for a beneficial role of antioxidant supplementation in the prevention and as adjunct therapy for glycemic control in human subjects afflicted with type 2 diabetes, as reported in some studies.

23.2   ASSOCIATION BETWEEN OXIDATIVE STRESS AND TYPE 2 DIABETES

As indicated earlier, it has been shown in numerous studies that oxidative stress is present in type 2 diabetes. The strong association between oxidative stress and type 2 diabetes can be illustrated by a study that we reported several years ago [21]. In that study, we distinguished between two groups of type 2 diabetic patients on the basis of the absence or presence of microalbuminuria. We showed that those patients who had diabetes for longer duration presented with microalbuminuria and had higher incidence of diabetic complications. The diabetic patients typically presented with hyperglycemia, hyperinsulinemia, and hyperlipidemia. We assessed oxidative stress in these patients by measurements of plasma lipid peroxide levels and total antioxidant capacity. We found that the diabetic patients had increased plasma levels of lipid peroxides and decreased levels of plasma total antioxidant capacity compared to control nondiabetic subjects. The degree of oxidative stress was more pronounced in the group of diabetic patients with microalbuminuria and a higher incidence of diabetic complications [21]. Using total antioxidant capacity assay as an index of oxidative stress, other investigators have also found that patients with type 2 diabetes have reduced antioxidant status [13–15,22–24]. However, using the total peroxyl radical-trapping potential (TRAP) assay to assess antioxidant status, it has also been reported that there is no major defect in the antioxidant potential in the plasma of patients suffering from type 2 diabetes [25]. The reason for this discrepancy is unclear, since other investigators have used the same assay to report a deficiency of antioxidant status in type 2 diabetes [13,22–24].

Many studies have found deficiencies in the levels of individual antioxidant substances in type 2 diabetes. Thus, reduced blood levels of α-tocopherol (vitamin E), ascorbic acid (vitamin C), carotenoids, zinc, chromium, and reduced glutathione (GSH) have been reported in individuals afflicted with type 2 diabetes [3,26–32]. Since patients with the metabolic syndrome and type 2 diabetes present with hyperinsulinemia, it is of interest that it has been observed that insulin infusion acutely depletes circulating vitamin E levels in humans [33]. Complementary to these reports, are also data showing that high blood levels of certain antioxidant substances, including α-tocopherol, β-carotene, and lycopene, are associated with decreased risk of type 2 diabetes [34,35].

Another approach used by some investigators to demonstrate the presence of oxidative stress in type 2 diabetes is the measurement of lipid peroxide levels and their degradation products. Using a validated technique for measuring authentic plasma lipid peroxide levels, it has been shown that individuals with type 2 diabetes have higher levels of thiobarbituric acid–reactive substances (TBARS) compared to nondiabetic subjects [21,29,30,36–41]. In one study, lipid peroxides, expressed as malondialdehyde (MDA), were measured along with certain hemostatic variables: fibrinogen, von Willebrand factor (vWf), plasminogen activator inhibitor (PAI-1), tissue plasminogen activator (t-PA), and plasmin activity in patients with type 2 diabetes. It was found that MDA was elevated in the patients with microalbuminuria compared with patients without microalbuminuria and control nondiabetic patients. All the hemostatic parameters were also increased in the diabetic patients compared to the control subjects [42]. Isoprostanes are widely recognized products of lipid peroxidation, whose measurement provides a reliable index of oxidant injury [43]. Hence, it has also been used to assess the presence of oxidative stress in diabetes. In one study, plasma F2 isoprostane levels were measured at baseline and 90 minutes after a glucose load in diabetic patients. It was found that the isoprostane levels increased during acute hyperglycemia in type 2 diabetes, thus providing direct evidence of free radical–mediated oxidative damage in the disease [44].

In other studies, investigators have also measured antioxidant enzyme levels and activities in the assessment of oxidative stress in type 2 diabetes. In two reports from the same group of investigators, Cu-Zn superoxide dismutase (SOD) and glutathione peroxidase (GPX) activities in red blood cells were measured and found to be normal in diabetic patients [30,36]. In another study, serum SOD levels and the activities of serum SOD and GPX were reported to be lower in diabetic patients compared to control nondiabetic individuals [37]. However, it has also been reported that diabetic patients have increased serum SOD activity when compared to healthy subjects [29,45]. The reason for the discrepancies in these reports is unclear. However, in an *in vitro* study designed to link hyperglycemia to oxidative stress, it has been shown that high glucose levels induced an overexpression of the antioxidant enzymes, SOD, catalase, and GPX, in human endothelial cells in culture [46]. This observation is consistent with the findings in the reports by Seghrouchni et al. [29] and Sozmen et al. [45].

23.3   ROLE OF OXIDATIVE STRESS IN THE PATHOGENESIS OF TYPE 2 DIABETES

It is clear that oxidative stress is strongly associated with type 2 diabetes, as shown by various studies using different approaches, as outlined in the preceding section. The crucial question from these studies showing association between oxidative stress and type 2 diabetes is the role, if any, that oxidative stress may play in the pathogenesis of type 2 diabetes. To address this question, it is pertinent to review the metabolic pathways of glucose disposal. The primary pathway of glucose metabolism is glycolysis, through which pyruvate is generated and enters the second pathway, known as the *Krebs cycle,* for complete oxidation [47]. The complete oxidation of glucose to yield ATP is achieved by oxidative phosphorylation that is coupled to an electron transport chain. In the glycolytic pathway, glyceraldehyde-3-phosphate dehydrogenase enzyme catalyzes the degradation of glyceraldehyde-3-phosphate to 1,3-bisphosphoglycerate. This enzyme is a heme-containing protein that can be inhibited when oxidized severely by a burden of oxidants [48,49]. Also, the cytochrome enzymes of the electron transport chain contain the transition metal copper (Cu^{++}), which can also be inhibited when oxidized by the abundance of ROS. The consequence of these blockages to glucose metabolism by oxidative stress would contribute to an elevation of blood glucose or hyperglycemia.

There are several mechanisms by which oxidative stress may be involved in the pathogenesis of type 2 diabetes. First, it could impair glucose metabolism at the level of the major tissues responsible for glucose disposal. The site of major glucose utilization in the body is the skeletal muscle. It is therefore not surprising that it has been reported that the pathogenesis of type 2 diabetes involves perturbations to the antioxidant defense systems within the skeletal muscle [17]. In the study, muscle samples were obtained from seven patients with type 2 diabetes and five age-matched, as well as nine young, nondiabetic subjects, before and after a euglycemic-hyperinsulinemic clamp for 120 minutes. The samples were analyzed for heat shock protein (HSP)-72 and heme oxygenase(HO)-1 mRNA, intramuscular triglyceride content, and the maximal activities of β-hydroxyacyl-CoA dehydrogenase (β-HAD) and citrate synthase (CS). Basal expression of both HSP72 and HO-1 mRNA were lower by 33% and 55%, respectively, when comparing diabetic patients with age-matched and young control subjects, with no differences between the latter groups. Both basal HSP72 and HO-1 mRNA correlated with glucose infusion rate during the clamp. Significant correlations were also observed between HSP72 mRNA, and both β-HAD and CS. HSP72 mRNA was induced by the clamp in all groups. The data thus provided evidence that the genes involved in providing cellular protection against oxidative stress are defective in individuals afflicted with type 2 diabetes [17]. In an experimental model of diabetes, it has also been reported that oxidative stress may impair muscle repair [16], which probably would diminish the capacity of skeletal muscle to dispose of glucose.

Secondly, oxidative stress activates certain signaling pathways, such as nuclear factor-κB, p38 MAPK, and NH_2-terminal Jun kinases, which underlie the development of diabetic complications. It has recently been proposed that the activation of these same stress pathways by glucose and fatty acids may lead to both insulin resistance and impaired insulin secretion [6]. Thirdly, the progressive decline in β-cell function frequently seen in patients with type 2 diabetes has been attributed to glucose toxicity and lipotoxicity, which are associated with oxidative stress [2]. Of interest, it has also been shown that oxidative stress causes depolarization and Ca^{2+} uptake in a β-cell line [50], a phenomenon that stimulates insulin secretion and may contribute to the hyperinsulinemia seen in type 2 diabetes.

Also, as illustrated in our study [21] described earlier, type 2 diabetes generally presents with a triangular relationship of hyperlipidemia, hyperglycemia, and hyperinsulinemia, and it is a matter of debate which of these factors is a cause or consequence of the other. The scenario this author would propose is that the problem starts with hyperlipidemia, in which increased fatty acid oxidation would stimulate insulin secretion [51], resulting in increased plasma levels of insulin or hyperinsulinemia. Hyperinsulinemia would down-regulate insulin receptor numbers and insulin action [52,53], leading to diminished insulin sensitivity and an increase in blood glucose levels. Simultaneously, the products of the fatty oxidation would cause inhibition of glucose metabolism while enhancing hepatic glucose synthesis [54,55], thereby exacerbating the hyperglycemia. Among the products of fatty acid metabolism are increased levels of ROS that would inhibit glucose metabolism and further enhance the elevation of glucose in the blood, as outlined earlier. Blood glucose overload in the face of impediments to its oxidation would activate minor pathways of glucose metabolism, such as glucose auto-oxidation, which generate more ROS and exacerbate oxidative stress, and type 2 diabetes, as previously illustrated [1]. Finally, it is well established that type 2 diabetes is a multifactorial disease with a strong genetic component [56]. It is therefore of significant interest that oxidative stress has been reported to be associated with gene polymorphisms in patients with type 2 diabetes and diabetic nephropathy [57].

23.4 STUDIES OF ANTIOXIDANT SUPPLEMENTATION FOR GLYCEMIC CONTROL IN TYPE 2 DIABETES

The abundance of evidence in support of the association between oxidative stress and type 2 diabetes has led to numerous studies that have examined the effects of various antioxidant supplements as adjunct therapy in type 2 diabetic patients [1,19,27]. Also, it is fairly established that the incidence of type 2 diabetes increases with age, which has been associated with increased oxidative stress in many studies [5,19,31]. It is therefore necessary to explore the potential of antioxidant supplementation as a preventive strategy and in the management of the type 2 diabetes, which increases with age. Various studies have examined the use of certain antioxidants, either as single supplements or in combination, as a disease-prevention strategy in high-risk subjects, and as adjunct therapy in type 2 diabetes. In this section, we will review the literature for the effects on glycemic control of the various antioxidant supplementation regimens that have been employed in these studies in human subjects.

23.4.1 Vitamin E

Epidemiological studies indicate that low vitamin E intake is a risk factor for the development of type 2 diabetes, and the use of vitamin E for prevention and as adjunct therapy in the management of the disease is of significant interest [5,18,19]. As illustrated in Table 23.1, one of three earlier studies in humans had failed to show any beneficial effect of vitamin E supplementation on glycemic control [58–60]. However, it is noteworthy that the study by Sharma et al. [58], which was only for a short duration of 4 weeks, used a vitamin E dose that is less than half of the dose used in the other two studies, whose durations were 3 months or more. Furthermore, the effect of the low-dose vitamin E supplementation on blood glucose was examined only after normal blood glucose control had been achieved. In other words, the patients enrolled in the study had reduced oxidative stress and normal blood glucose levels prior to the study, leaving no room for additional improvement [58].

TABLE 23.1

Effect of Vitamin E Supplementation on Blood Glucose

References	Study Design	Dose	Duration	Result
[58]	30 diabetic patients 15 healthy controls	400 IU/day	4 weeks	No effect
[59]	Placebo-controlled, double-blind, crossover study with 35 elderly patients	900 IU/day	3 months	Reduction in plasma glucose
[60]	Placebo-controlled,15 patients and 10 healthy controls	900 IU/day	4 months	Reduction of glucose AUC in glucose tolerance tests of healthy and diabetic patients
[61]	Placebo-controlled 40 patients on metformin	800 IU/day + vitamin C 1,000 mg/day	3 months	Improved fasting blood sugar, HOMA-IR, and QISCI compared to placebo controls

AUC, area under the curve; HOMA-IR, homeostasis model assessment-insulin resistance; QISCI, quantitative insulin sensitivity check index.

A recent study has examined the effect of vitamin E supplementation on glycemic control in type 2 diabetic patients on metformin treatment. In this study, 40 type 2 diabetic male patients aged 40–60 years on metformin (500 mg twice daily) treatment were randomly divided into four groups, with each group receiving an additional one of the following twice-daily oral supplements for 90days: placebo, vitamin C (500 mg), vitamin E (400 mg), and vitamin C (500 mg) plus vitamin E (400 mg). As shown in Table 23.1, it was found that, in the patients receiving vitamin C and/or vitamin E, fasting blood sugar, hemoglobin A1c (HbA1c), lipid profile, insulin, and homeostasis model assessment-insulin resistance (HOMA-IR), GSH and quantitative insulin sensitivity check index (QISCI) improved significantly when compared to the control group receiving placebo [61]. This study thus provides strong support for the use of vitamin E or vitamin C as adjuvant therapy in the management of patients with type 2 diabetes.

23.4.2 VITAMIN C

Some investigators have also examined the effect of vitamin C supplementation on insulin secretion and insulin action. In some studies, vitamin C supplementation was provided by systemic infusion in the dose range of 500–2,000 mg, and it was observed that this vitamin enhanced glucose disposal by enhancing insulin sensitivity without affecting insulin secretion [62–64]. Another study was performed using a randomized, double-blind, crossover design, and supplementation was done by oral ingestion of vitamin C (2,000 mg/day), which was compared to magnesium supplementation (600 mg/day) for 3 months. It was found that vitamin C caused a reduction in fasting plasma glucose and HbA1c levels, which were not affected by magnesium supplementation [65]. These observations are consistent with the recent study by El-Aal et al., which showed the same benefits of vitamin C supplementation on glycemic control in type 2 diabetic patients [61].

23.4.3 BETA-CAROTENE

A large-scale, long-term study has been performed with β-carotene [66]. In the study, a total of 22,071 healthy US male physicians aged 40–84 years were enrolled in a randomized, double-blind, placebo-controlled trial from 1982 to 1995. Of those, 10,756 subjects were randomly assigned to receive β-carotene (50 mg on alternate days), and 10,712 received a placebo. At the end of the follow-up period (mean duration, 12 years), the incidence of type 2 diabetes did not differ between the two groups. Thus, in this study of apparently healthy men, supplementation with β-carotene had no effect on the risk of development of type 2 diabetes [66]. Perhaps it is pertinent to point out that the dose of β-carotene used in this trial is significantly below the revised recommended upper intake for this supplement [67]. Therefore, it is probably advisable to exercise caution in using this observation to determine whether β-carotene has any role in the prevention and treatment of type 2 diabetes.

23.4.4 GLUTATHIONE

GSH, a tripeptide molecule that plays an important role in cellular metabolism and protects against oxidative stress [68,69], has been studied as an antioxidant supplement in type 2 diabetes. In two studies by the same group of investigators, GSH supplementation was performed by systemic infusion in the dose range of 10–15 mg/min for 120 minutes, using normal saline infusion for control. In one study, it was found that GSH enhanced glucose-stimulated insulin secretion in aged individuals with impaired glucose tolerance, but not in normal control subjects [70]. In the other study, the investigators observed that, while GSH only enhanced insulin secretion in diabetic patients, it increased nonoxidative glucose disposal in both healthy and diabetic individuals [71]. In another study by a different group of investigators, GSH was infused at the rate of 1.35 g/m^2/h for 1 hour in 10 healthy and 10 diabetic individuals, and the data were compared to saline infusion in the same experimental subjects. It was found that GSH enhanced glucose uptake assessed by the euglycemic clamp technique [72], consistent with the observations by Paolisso et al. [71]. However, studies with the GSH pro-drug, N-acetylcysteine (NAC) [73], have reported that its supplementation in type 2 diabetic patients had either no effect or worsened glucose tolerance [74,75].

23.4.5 ALPHA-LIPOIC ACID

α-Lipoic acid is a disulfide compound that is produced in small quantities in cells and normally functions as a coenzyme in the pyruvate dehydrogenase and α-ketoglutarate dehydrogenase enzyme complexes of the tricarboxylic acid cycle, but has antioxidant properties in pharmacological doses [76]. In patients with type 2 diabetes, it has been reported that, while intravenous infusion of α-lipoic acid significantly enhanced insulin-mediated glucose disposal, oral supplementation had only marginal effects [76], thus suggesting that the issue here may be bioavailability through the oral route. This view is consistent with a study that showed no beneficial effect on glycemic control in patients who received 600 mg α-lipoic acid orally per day for 3 months [77]. Some investigators have suggested that bioavailability of oral supplements may be enhanced if taken with meals. Indeed, it has been shown that daily meal supplementation with α-lipoic acid (600 mg), L-camosin (165 mg), zinc (7.5 mg), and vitamin B complex improved glycemic control, lipid profile, and antioxidant stress markers [78].

23.4.6 COENZYME Q$_{10}$

Coenzyme Q$_{10}$ (CoQ$_{10}$), also called *ubiquinone*, is an isoprenoid derivative that is involved in the mitochondrial electron transport chain, where it accepts and donates electrons, thereby functioning as an antioxidant. Based on observations that CoQ$_{10}$ deficiency is associated with type 2 diabetes, two groups of investigators had earlier examined the effect of CoQ$_{10}$ supplementation on metabolic control in individuals afflicted with the disease. In one small study, 23 patients were enrolled in a randomized 6-month double-blind, placebo-controlled trial in which one group received 100 mg CoQ$_{10}$ twice per day, and another received a placebo. CoQ$_{10}$ supplementation caused a more than threefold rise in serum concentrations but did not affect glycemic control in the diabetic patients [79]. In the other study, using a randomized, placebo-controlled 2×2 factorial design, 74 individuals with uncomplicated type 2 diabetes and dyslipidemia were assigned to receive either an oral dose of 100 mg twice per day or a placebo for 12 weeks. The CoQ$_{10}$ supplementation also resulted in a threefold increase of the supplement in plasma concentrations, which was accompanied by an improvement in glycemic control, as apparent in significant reductions in plasma HbA1c levels [80].

TABLE 23.2

Effect of Supplementation with Coenzyme Q_{10} on Blood Glucose

References	Study Design	Dose	Duration	Result
[79]	Randomized, placebo-controlled, double-blind study with 23 patients	200 mg/day	6 months	No effect on glycemic control
[80]	Randomized, placebo-controlled, 2 × 2 factorial designed study with 74 patients	200 mg/day	3 months	Improved glycemic control (HbA1c) in contrast to placebo
[81]	Small study with 9 patients	200 mg/day	3 months	Improved glycemic control in contrast to placebo
[82]	Randomized, double-blind, placebo-controlled study with 64 patients	200 mg/day	3 months	Improved glycemic control in contrast to placebo
[83]	Placebo-controlled study with 40 patients	150 mg/day	3 months	Improved fasting blood sugar and HbA1c levels compared to placebo controls

The reason for the discrepancy between these two observations on the effect of the same dose of CoQ_{10} supplementation on glycemic control is unclear.

As shown in Table 23.2, three more recent studies have examined the effect of 200 mg CoQ_{10} daily supplementation on glycemic control with type 2 diabetes. In one small study, nine patients (three males and six females) on conventional medication were assigned to receive an oral dose of 200 mg CoQ_{10} daily for 12 weeks, which resulted in significant improvements in HbA1c levels in these patients [81]. In another study, which was a randomized, double-blind, placebo-controlled trial, 64 subjects with type 2 diabetes were randomly assigned to receive either 200 mg CoQ_{10} or placebo daily for 12 weeks. It was found that HbA1c levels decreased in the CoQ_{10}-treated group with no change in the placebo group, indicating a positive effect on glycemic control [82]. The third study was also a randomized, placebo-controlled study, in which 50 patients with type 2 diabetes were randomly assigned to receive either 150 mg CoQ_{10} or placebo daily for 12 weeks. Of the 40 patients who completed the study, it was found that fasting plasma glucose and HbA1c levels were significantly lower when compared to the placebo group, again demonstrating the beneficial effect of CoQ_{10} supplementation on glycemic control [83].

23.4.7 TRACE ELEMENTS

Blood glucose regulation is dependent upon normal glucose metabolism, which, in turn, is regulated by chains of reactions catalyzed by enzymes. Some enzymes require no chemical groups other than their amino residues for activity, and others require an additional chemical component referred to as a *cofactor*. The cofactor may be either one or more inorganic ions or a complex organic or metal-lorganic molecule called a *coenzyme*. Certain enzymes require both a coenzyme and one or more metal ions for activity. These metal ions are usually transition metals, which are obtained from the diet in small (micrograms and milligrams) amounts, hence the term *trace elements*. As already mentioned, some of these elements are present in the cells and tissues as cofactors of certain antioxidant enzymes, such as zinc in superoxide dismutase (SOD) and selenium in glutathione peroxidase (GPx). As transition metals, the trace elements have antioxidant potential, and the effect of supplementation with certain trace elements on glycemic control has been examined in diabetic patients.

23.4.7.1 Chromium

A number of investigators have examined the effect of chromium (Cr) supplementation on glycemic control in type 2 diabetes. In earlier studies, one group examined 180 individuals being treated for type 2 diabetes who were randomly assigned to receive either a placebo, 100 µg, as chromium picolinate twice per day, or 500 µg Cr twice per day. During the period of supplementation, the patients continued to take their normal medications and were instructed not to change their dietary patterns and lifestyle. It was found that HbA1c levels improved significantly after 2 months in the group receiving 1000 µg Cr per day and were lower in both Cr-supplemented groups after 4 months when compared to the placebo group. There was also significant improvement in fasting plasma glucose levels in the Cr-supplemented groups [84]. In another study, Anderson et al. examined the effects of Cr and zinc (Zn) supplementation in adult Tunisian subjects with type 2 diabetes whose plasma HbA$_{1c}$ levels were above 7.5% [30]. The subjects were supplemented for 6 months with 30 mg per day of Zn as zinc gluconate or 400 µg per day Cr as chromium pidolate, or a combination of both Zn and Cr supplements, or a placebo. In this study, supplementation had no effect on HbA1c levels or glucose homeostasis, although it reduced lipid peroxide levels in each of the supplementation groups [30]. It is not clear why these two studies by the same group of investigators produced different results in terms of the effect of Cr supplementation on glycemic control. The observation of a lack of effect of Zn supplementation on glycemic control is consistent with that made in another study that examined the effects of Zn supplementation in Tunisians with type 2 diabetes [36].

In another study, one group of investigators examined the effects of Cr supplementation in euglycemic subjects and in those with type 2 diabetes. The study subjects consisted of a group with plasma HbA1c levels below 6%, a mildly hyperglycemic group with HbA1c levels in the range of 6.8%–8.5%, and a severely hyperglycemic group with HbA1c levels above 8.5%. Each group was divided into two random subgroups, which were supplemented daily with either 1,000 µg Cr as yeast Cr (III) or a placebo. The investigators found that, although supplementation reduced oxidative stress, it had no effect on glycemic control in any of the three groups when compared to a placebo [26]. Another group of investigators studied 39 subjects (18 males and 21 females) with type 2 diabetes (mean age = 73 years) in rehabilitation after stroke or hip fracture. A control group of additional 39 diabetic patients were included in the study. Along with standard treatment for diabetes, the test group received 200 µg of Cr twice daily for 3 weeks. All study participants received a diet of approximately 1,500 kcal/day. The Cr supplementation resulted in significant differences in the fasting blood level of glucose compared to the baseline, and the HbA1c also improved significantly from 8.2% to 7.6% [85].

Furthermore, in another study, 100 patients with type 2 diabetes were enrolled in a randomized, placebo-controlled trial with chromium dinicocysteinate (CDNC) supplementation in which the patients were assigned to one of three groups. One group received a placebo, another group received 400 µg per day chromium picolinate (CP), and the third group received CDNC (400 µg/day). Although there was a significant decrease in insulin resistance at 3 months and in the levels of protein oxidation and tumor necrosis factor-alpha (TNF-α) in the CDNC-supplemented cohort compared to baseline, there was no statistically significant change in these markers in the CP-supplemented group compared to baseline. Also, insulin levels significantly decreased in subjects receiving CDNC but not CP. There was no significant impact of supplementation on HbA1c or glucose levels in either of the groups. Thus, this study highlights the importance of the chromium supplementation formula in demonstrating efficacy of Cr supplementation in diabetic patients [86].

Chromium nicotinate has been also been examined as a Cr supplementation formula in another study in which 56 individuals with type 2 diabetes were randomized in a double-blind, placebo-controlled clinical trial of three groups. One group received a placebo (NCO), another group received 50 µg (NC50), and the third group received 200 µg (NC100) daily for 90 days. This study failed to show any improvements in glucose homeostasis or anthropometry in the patients supplemented with chromium nicotinate at either dose in the trial [87]. Most recently, the long-term benefit of whole wheat bread supplemented with Cr (WWCrB) in type 2 diabetic patients has

TABLE 23.3

Effect of Chromium Supplementation on Blood Glucose

Reference #	Study Design	Dose	Duration	Result
26	Placebo-controlled (Total 63 patients)	1000 µg/day	6 months	No effect on glycemic control but reduction in oxidative stress
30	Placebo-controlled	400 µg/day + 30 mg Zn/day	6 months	No effect on glycemic control but reduced peroxide levels
85	Placebo-controlled with caloric restriction (Total 78 patients)	400 µg/day	3 weeks	Improved glycemic control (HbA1c) in contrast to placebo
86	Randomized placebo- controlled study with 100 patients	400 µg/day either as PC or CDNC	3 months	Improved glycemic control with CDNC but not PC
87	Randomized Double-blind Placebo-controlled Study with 56 subjects	50–200 µg/day Chromium nicotinate	3 months	No effect on glycemic control in any group
88	Randomized Study 30 patients	WWCrB or Plain Wheat Bread	3 months	Improved HbA1c levels and HOMA-IR

PC = picolinate

CDNC = chromium dinicocysteinate

WWCrB = Whole Wheat Bread supplemented with chromium

HbA1c = Hemoglobin A1c

HOMA-IR = Homeostasis Model Assessment–Insulin Resistance

been studied. Thirty patients were equally divided into two groups (n = 15/group) and randomly assigned to receive either the WWCrB or the plain wheat bread (WWB) for 12 weeks. At the end of the study, it was found that plasma glucose, insulin, and HbA1c levels were significantly lower in the WWCrB group, with improved HOMA-IR compared to the control group receiving WWB [88]. These data are also consistent with the notion that the modality of delivery of Cr during supplementation is important to eliciting benefit in glycemic control of patients afflicted with type 2 diabetes. Table 23.3 represents the summary of results of the research on Cr supplementation in type 2 diabetic patients.

23.4.8   PHYTOCHEMICALS

Herbal preparations have emerged as part of the armamentarium of adjuvant therapy to enhance glycemic control in diabetic patients [89]. Several classes of phytochemicals have now been examined for their putative effects on glycemic control when used as adjuvant therapy in diabetic patients.

23.4.8.1   Resveratrol

Two studies have examined the effect of resveratrol at different doses and durations of treatment. In one study, 14 patients with diet-controlled type 2 diabetes received resveratrol (500 mg twice daily) or a placebo over two 5-week intervention periods with a 5-week washout period in between in a double-blind, randomized, crossover design. The data from this study led to the conclusion that, in patients with diet-controlled type 2 diabetes, the 5 weeks of twice-daily 500 mg-resveratrol supplementation had no effect on glycemic control, gastric emptying, body weight, or energy intake [90]. In the other study, 62 patients with type 2 diabetes were enrolled in a prospective, open-label, randomized, controlled trial of control and intervention groups. The control group received only oral hypoglycemic agents, whereas the intervention group received resveratrol (250 mg/d) along with their oral hypoglycemic agents for a period of 3 months. It was found that this oral supplementation of resveratrol for 3 months resulted in significant improvements in HbA1c and other parameters of the metabolic syndrome in the diabetic patients. Thus, the lower dose of resveratrol over an extended period of supplementation was positively effective in glycemic control in these patients [91].

23.4.8.2 Seaweeds

Seaweeds are frequently consumed in some parts of the world and are rich in nonstarch polysaccharides (dietary fiber), proteins, minerals, and vitamins. They have low lipid content and provide few calories, and have the potential to interfere with the bioavailability of other dietary components. As their polysaccharides cannot be entirely digested by human intestinal enzymes, they are considered to be a source of dietary fiber, which differs in composition, chemical structure, physicochemical properties, and biological effects [92]. Since seaweeds appear to be resistant to oxidative damage in their structural components (polyunsaturated fatty acids) and are stable during storage, there has arisen an interest in examining their use as protective antioxidative systems. Thus, one study has examined the effect of seaweed supplementation on blood glucose levels and lipid profile, along with antioxidant enzyme activities, in patients with type 2 diabetes.

Nine men and 11 women with type 2 diabetes were selected according to specific criteria that included management by diet control and oral hypoglycemic agents. The study participants were randomized into either a control group or a seaweed supplementation group. Pills with equal parts of dry, powdered sea tangle and sea mustard were provided to the seaweed supplementation group three times a day for 4 weeks. It was found that total dietary fiber intake was 2.5 times higher in subjects receiving seaweed supplementation than in the control group. In addition, fasting blood glucose levels and 2-hour postprandial blood glucose measurements and serum triglycerides were significantly decreased, while high-density lipoprotein (HDL) levels increased in the seaweed-supplementation group. Catalase and glutathione peroxidase activities with seaweed supplementation were higher than the controls, leading to the conclusion that ingestion of seaweed positively influences glycemic control, lowers blood lipids, and increases antioxidant enzyme activities [92].

23.4.8.3 Caffeine

Caffeine is a member of the class of phytochemicals called *methylxanthines*, which are abundant in coffee, tea, and dark chocolate [93]. There has been some interest in studying the effect of caffeine on chronic glucose control in type 2 diabetes. In one study, coffee drinkers (six males) with established type 2 diabetes participated in a trial with five other males completing 3 months of total caffeine abstinence. Measures of chronic glucose control, long-term (HbA1c) and short-term (1,5-anhydroglucitol [1,5-AG]), were collected at baseline and during follow-up. It was found that abstinence resulted in significant decreases in HbA1c and increases in 1,5-AG, both indicating improvements in chronic glucose control. Fasting glucose and insulin did not change, nor were changes in body weight observed [94]. This study indicates that caffeine negatively affects glycemic control and is consistent with the results of another study of the acute effect of caffeine on insulin sensitivity and glycemic control in subjects with type 2 diabetes, which reported that caffeine intake increases blood glucose levels and sustains hyperglycemia [95].

23.5   CONCLUSION

In summary, the occurrence of redox reactions in both the glycolytic and electron transport chain during oxidative phosphorylation during glucose metabolism, if not adequately regulated by antioxidants, as well as the increased production of ROS in diabetes, will cause oxidative stress that is capable of inhibiting glucose metabolism and resulting in hyperglycemia. It is therefore reasonable to suggest that oxidative stress may actually play a role, even if it is only secondary, in the pathogenesis of type 2 diabetes. This putative role constitutes a biochemical basis for the need to use antioxidants as adjunct therapy in type 2 diabetes, in order to diminish oxidative stress and thus help to control blood glucose levels in diabetic patients.

The review of the literature in this chapter clearly shows that a good number of individual antioxidant supplementation regimens can have a positive outcome for glycemic control in diabetic patients. It had previously been suggested that some degree of supplementation with certain vitamins and minerals would be worthwhile for the regulation of blood glucose levels in diabetic patients [96]. While there are still some conflicting results for some of the micronutrients popularly used as adjunct therapy in type 2 diabetes, the data from studies with vitamins C, vitamin E, and CoQ$_{10}$ appear to show consistently that they have beneficial effects on glycemic control in the patients using either of these individual or combined antioxidant micronutrients at appropriate doses over a period of 3 months, as shown in Tables 23.1 and 23.2. With some micronutrients, such as chromium, the efficacy appears to be critically dependent on the modality of supplement formula used. However, there is currently no standardized antioxidant regimen for use as adjunct therapy in the management of diabetes. Based on the natural biochemical chain of interactions of micronutrient and enzymatic antioxidants in the defense against oxidative stress [68], for future studies, it is prudent to suggest that an appropriate approach to designing a regimen is to use a formula consisting of relevant trace elements and vitamins. It is noteworthy that, for therapeutic use, individual doses of the constituents of such a formula must exceed the RDA levels, for any efficacy to be observed. In this chapter, the importance of the modality of formulation of the antioxidant for use as an effective supplement on glycemic control has been highlighted.

We have also reviewed the emerging role of phytochemicals in blood glucose regulation in diabetic patients. In particular, we have noted the adverse effect of caffeine, a common constituent of routine beverages, on glycemic control in diabetic patients. Thus, additional studies involving appropriate antioxidant regimens examined in this review as candidates for use as adjunct therapy for glycemic control in type 2 diabetes are required. Such studies should also determine the optimum duration of supplementation necessary for beneficial outcome on glycemic control. It is conceivable that long-term use of an optimum antioxidant regimen involving effective doses of relevant vitamins and trace elements as adjunct therapy may help to regulate blood glucose in type 2 diabetes. However, it is always recommended that patients using supplements of antioxidant formulations as adjunct therapy in the management of diabetes do so under the supervision of their physicians.

REFERENCES

1. Opara EC. Role of oxidative stress in the etiology of Type 2 diabetes and the effect of antioxidant supplementation on glycemic control. *J Investig Med* 52: 19–23, 2004.
2. Robertson RP, Harmon J, Tran POT, Poitout V. β-Cell glucose toxicity, lipotoxicity, and chronic oxidative stress in Type 2 diabetes. *Diabetes* 53 (Suppl.1): S119–S124, 2004.
3. Ford ES, Mokdad AH, Giles WH, Brown DW. The metabolic syndrome and antioxidant concentrations. Findings from the Third National Health and Nutrition Examination Survey. *Diabetes* 52: 2346–2352, 2003.
4. Hoeldtke RD, Bryner KD, McNeil DR, Warehime SS, Van Dyke K, Hobbs G. Oxidative stress and insulin requirements in patients with recent-onset Type 1 diabetes. *J Clin Endocrinol Metab* 88: 1624–1628, 2003.
5. Opara EC. Oxidative stress, micronutrients, diabetes mellitus and its complications. *J Royal Soc Health* 2002; 122: 28–34.
6. Evans JL, Goldfine ID, Maddux BA, Grodsky GM. Oxidative stress and stress-activated signaling pathways: Unifying hypothesis of Type 2 diabetes. *Endocr Rev* 23: 599–622, 2002.
7. West IC. Radicals and oxidative stress in diabetes. *Diabet Med* 17: 171–180, 2000.

8. Strain JJ. Disturbances of micronutrient and antioxidant status in diabetes. *Proc Nutr Soc* 50: 591–604, 1991.

9. Oberley LW. Free radicals and diabetes. *Free Rad Biol Med* 5: 113–124, 1988.

10. Baynes JW, Thorpe SR. Role of oxidative stress in diabetic complications: A new perspective on an old paradigm. *Diabetes* 48: 1–9, 1999.

11. Kedziora-Kornatowska KZ, Luciak M, Blaszczyk J, Pawlak W. Lipid peroxidation and activities of antioxidant enzymes in erythrocytes of patients with non-insulin dependent diabetes with or without diabetic nephropathy. *Nephrol Dial Transplant* 13: 2829–2832, 1998.

12. Koya D, King GL: Protein Kinase C activation and the development of diabetic complications. *Diabetes* 47: 859–866, 1998.

13. Ceriello A, Bortolotti N, Pirisi M, Crescentini A, Tonutti L, Motz E, Giacomello R, Stel G, Taboga C. Total antioxidant capacity predicts thrombosis-prone status in NIDDM patients. *Diabetes Care* 10: 1589–1593, 1997.

14. Maxwell SR, Thomason H, Sandler D, LeGuen C, Baxter MA, Thorpe GH, Jones AF, Barnett AH. Poor glycemic control is associated with reduced serum free radical scavenging (antioxidant) activity in non-insulin-dependent diabetes mellitus. *Ann Clin Biochem* 34: 638–644, 1997.

15. Maxwell SR, Thomason H, Sandler D, LeGuen C, Baxter MA, Thorpe GH, Jones AF, Barnett AH. Antioxidant status in patients with uncomplicated insulin-dependent and non-insulin-dependent diabetes mellitus. *Eur J Clin Invest* 27: 484–490, 1997.

16. Aragno M, Matrocola R, Catalano MG, Brignardello E, Danni O, Boccuzzi G. Oxidative stress impairs skeletal muscle repair in diabetic rats. *Diabetes* 53: 1082–1088, 2004.

17. Bruce CR, Carey AL, Hawley JA, Febbraio MA. Intramuscular heat shock protein 72 and heme oxygenase-1 mRNA are reduced in patients with Type 2 diabetes. Evidence of that insulin resistance is associated with a disturbed antioxidant defense mechanism. *Diabetes* 52: 2338–2345, 2003.

18. Halliwell B. Vitamin E and the treatment and prevention of diabetes: A case for a controlled clinical trial. *Singapore Med J* 43: 479–484, 2002.

19. Ruhe RC, McDonald RB. Use of antioxidant nutrients in the prevention and treatment of type 2 diabetes. *J Am Coll Nutr* 20: 363S-369S, 2001.

20. Paolisso G, Giugliano D. Oxidative stress and insulin action: Is there a relationship? *Diabetologia* 39: 357–363, 1996.

21. Opara EC, Abdel-Rahman E, Soliman S, Kamel WA, Souka S, Lowe JE, Abdel-Aleem S. Depletion of total antioxidant capacity in type 2 diabetes. *Metabolism* 48: 1414–1417, 1999.

22. Aguirre F, Martin I, Grinspon D, Ruiz M, Hager A, De Paoli T, Ihlo J, Farach HA, Poole Jr. CP. Oxidative damage, plasma antioxidant capacity, and glycemic control in elderly NIDDM patients. *Free Rad Biol Med* 24: 580–585, 1998.

23. Ceriello A, Bortolotti N, Falleti E, Taboga C, Tonutti L, Crescentini A, Motz E, Lizzio S, Russo A, Bartoli E. Total radical-trapping antioxidant parameter in NIDDM patients. *Diabetes Care* 20: 194–197, 1997.

24. Caimi G, Carollo C, Lo Presti R. Diabetes mellitus: Oxidative stress and wine. *Curr Med Res Opin* 19: 581–586, 2003.

25. Leinonen J, Rantalaiho V, Lehtimaki T, Koivula T, Wirta O, Pasternack A, Alho H. The association between total antioxidant potential of plasma and the presence of coronary heart disease and renal dysfunction in patients with NIDDM. *Free Radc Res* 29: 273–281, 1998.

26. Cheng HH, Lai MH, Hou WC, Huang CL. Antioxidant effects of chromium supplementation with diabetes mellitus and euglycemic subjects. *J Agric Food Chem* 52: 1385–1389, 2004.

27. Faure P. Protective effects of antioxidant micronutrients (vitamin E, zinc and selenium) in Type 2 diabetes mellitus. *Clin Chem Lab Med* 41: 995–998, 2003.

28. Skrha J, Prazny M, Hilgertova J, Weiserova H. Serum alpha-tocopherol and ascorbic acid concentrations in Type 1 and type 2 diabetic patients with and without angiopathy. *Clin Chim Acta* 329: 103–108, 2003.

29. Seghrouchni I, Drai J, Bannier E, Riviere J, Calmard P, Garcia I, Orgiazzi J, Revol A. Oxidative stress parameters in Type 1, Type 2 and insulin-treated Type 2 diabetes mellitus. *Clin Chim Acta* 321: 89–96, 2002.

30. Anderson RA, Roussel A-M, Zouari N, Mahjoub S, Matheau J-M, Kerkeni A. Potential antioxidant effects of zinc and chromium supplementation in people with Type 2 diabetes. *J Am Coll Nutr* 2001; 20: 212–218.

31. Polidori MC, Mecocci P, Stahl W, Parente B, Cecchetti R, Cherubini A, Cao P, Sies H, Senin U. Plasma levels of lipophilic antioxidants in very old patients with Type 2 diabetes. *Diabetes/Metabolism Res Rev* 16: 15–19, 2000.

32. Thompson KH, Godin DV. Micronutrients and antioxidants in the progression of diabetes. *Nutr Res* 15: 1377–1410, 1995.

33. Galvan AQ, Muscelli E, Catalano C, Natali A, Sanna G, Masoni A, Bernadini B, Barsacchi R, Ferrannini E. Insulin decreases circulating vitamin E levels in humans. *Metabolism* 45: 998–1003, 1996.

34. Ylonen K, Alfthan G, Groop L, Saloranta C, Aro A, Virtanen SM. Dietary intakes and plasma concentrations of carotenoids and tocopherols in relation to glucose metabolism in subjects at high risk of Type 2 diabetes: The Botnia Dietary Study. *Am J Clin Nutr* 77: 1434–1441, 2003.

35. Reunanen A, Knekt P, Aaran RK, Aromaa A. Serum antioxidants and risk of non-insulin dependent diabetes mellitus. *Eur J Clin Nutr* 52: 89–93, 1998.

36. Roussel AM, Kerkeni A, Zouari N, Mahjoub S, Matheau JM, Anderson RA. Antioxidant effects of zinc supplementation in Tunisians with type 2 diabetes mellitus. *J Am Coll Nutr* 22: 316–321, 2003.

37. Hartnett ME, Stratton RD, Browne RW, Rosner BA, Lanham RJ, Armstrong D. Serum markers of oxidative stress and severity of diabetic retinopathy. *Diabetes Care* 23: 234–240, 2000.

38. Nourooz-Zadeh J, Tajaddini-Sarmadi J, McCarthy S, Betteridge DJ. Elevated levels of authentic plasma hydroperoxides in NIDDM. *Diabetes* 44: 1054–1058, 1995.

39. Niskanen LK, Salonen JT, Nyyssonen K, Uusitupa MIJ. Plasma lipid peroxidation and hyperglycemia: A connection through hyperinsulinemia. *Diabet Med* 12: 802–808, 1995.

40. Abdella N, Al Awadi F, Salman A, Armstrong D. Thiobarbituric acid test as a measure of lipid peroxidation in Arab patients with NIDDM. *Diabetes Res* 15: 173–177, 1990.

41. Peerapatdit T, Patchanans N, Likidlilid A, Poldee S, Sriratanasathavorn C. Plasma lipid peroxidation and antioxidiant nutrients in type 2 diabetic patients. *J Med Assoc Thai* 89(Suppl 5): S147–S155, 2006.

42. Collier A, Rumley A, Rumley AG, Paterson JR, Leach JP, Lowe GDO, Small M. Free radical activity and hemostatic factors in NIDDM patients with and without microalbuminuria. *Diabetes* 41: 909–913, 1992.

43. Morrow JD, Roberts LJ. The isoprostanes: Unique bioactive products of lipid peroxidation. *Prog Lipid Res* 36: 1–21, 1997.

44. Sampson MJ, Gopaul N, Davies IR, Hughes DA, Carrier MJ. Plasma F2 isoprostanes: Direct evidence of increased free radical damage during acute hyperglycemia in type 2 diabetes. *Diabetes Care* 25: 537–541, 2002.

45. Sozmen EY, Sozmen B, Delen Y, Onat T. Catalase/superoxide dismutase (SOD) and catalase/paraoxonase (PON) ratios may implicate poor glycemic control. *Arch Med Res* 32: 283–287, 2001.

46. Ceriello A, dello Russo P, Amstad P, Cerutti P. High glucose induces antioxidant enzymes in human endothelial cells in culture. Evidence linking hyperglycemia and oxidative stress. *Diabetes* 45: 471–477, 1996.

47. Lehninger AL, Nelson DL, Cox MM (editors). *Principles of Biochemistry*. 2nd ed., New York, Worth Publishers, 1993.

48. Janero DR, Hreniuk D, Sharif HM. Hydroproxide-induced oxidative stress impairs heart muscle cell carbohydrate metabolism. *Am J Physiol* 266 (Cell Physiol.35): C179–C188, 1994.

49. Hyslop PA, Hinshaw DB, Halsey Jr. WA, Schraufstatter IU, Spragg RG, Jackson JH, Cochrane CG. Mechanisms of oxidant-mediated cell injury. *J Biol Chem* 263: 1665–1675, 1987.

50. Wahl MA, Koopman I, Ammon HPT. Oxidative stress causes depolarization and calcium uptake in the rat insulinoma cell RINm5F. *Exp Clin Endocrinol Diabetes* 106: 173–177, 1998.

51. Opara EC, Garfinkel M, Hubbard VS, Burch WM, Akwari OE. Effect of fatty acids on insulin release: Role of chain length and degree of unsaturation. *Am J Physiol* 266 (Endocrinol Metab 29): E635–E639, 1994.

52. Gavin JR 3rd, Roth J, Neville DM, De Meyts P, Buell DN. Insulin-dependent regulation of insulin receptor concentrations: A direct demonstration in cell culture. *Proc Natl Acad Sci* 71: 84–88, 1974.

53. DeFronzo RA. Lilly lecture 1987. The triumvirate: Beta cell, muscle, liver. A collision responsible for NIDDM. *Diabetes* 37: 667–687, 1988.

54. Randle PJ, Hales CN, Garland PB, Newsholme EA. The glucose-fatty acid cycle: Its role in insulin sensitivity and the metabolic disturbances of diabetes mellitus. *Lancet* 1: 785–789, 1963.

55. McGarry JD. What if Minkowski had been ageusic? An alternative angle on diabetes. *Science* 258: 766–770, 1992.

56. Davegårdh C, García-Calzón S, Bacos K, Ling C. DNA methylation in the pathogenesis of type 2 diabetes in humans. *Mol Metab* pii: S2212-8778(17)31102-X, 2018. doi:10.1016/j.molmet.2018.01.022. [Epub ahead of print].

57. Dabhi B, Mistry KN. Oxidative stress and its association with TNF-α-308 G/C and IL-1α-889 C/T gene polymorphisms in patients with diabetes and diabetic nephropathy. *Gene* 562(2): 197–202, 2015.

58. Sharma A, Kharb S, Chugh SN, Kakkar R, Singh GP. Evaluation of oxidative stress before and after control of glycemia and after vitamin E supplementation in diabetic patients. *Metabolism* 49: 160–162, 2000.

59. Paolisso G, D'Amore A, Galzerano D, Balbi V, Giugliano D, Varriccio M, D'Onofrio F. Daily vitamin E supplements improve metabolic control but not insulin secretion in elderly type 2 diabetic patients. *Diabetes Care* 1433–1437, 1993.

60. Paolisso G, D'Amore A, Giugliano D, Ceriello A, Varricchio M, D'Onofrio F. Pharmacologic doses of vitamin E improve insulin action in healthy subjects and non-insulin-dependent diabetic patients. *Am J Clin Nutr* 57: 650–656, 1993.

61. El-Aal AA, El-Ghffar EAA, Ghali AA, Zughbur MR, Sirdah MM. The effect of vitamin C and/or E supplementations on type 2 diabetic adult males under metformin treatment: A single-blinded randomized controlled clinical trial. *Diabetes Metab Syndr* pii: S1871-4021(18)30043-2, 2018. doi:10.1016/j. dsx.2018.03.013. [Epub ahead of print].

62. Paolisso G, D'Amore, Balbi V, Volpe C, Galzerano D, Giugliano D, Sgambato S, Varricchio M, D'Onofrio F. Plasma vitamin C affects glucose homeostasis in healthy subjects and in non-insulin-dependent diabetics. *Am J Physiol* 266(Endocrinol. Metab.29): E261–E268, 1994.

63. Hirashima O, Kawano H, Motoyama T, Hirai N, Ohgushi M, Kugiyama K, Ogawa H, Yasue H. Improvement of endothelial function and insulin sensitivity with vitamin C in patients with coronary spastic angina. *J Am Coll Cardiol* 35: 1860–1866, 2000.

64. Hirai N, Kawano H, Hirashima O, Motoyama T, Motoyama Y, Sakamoto T, Kugiyama K, Ogawa H, Nakao K, Yasue H. Insulin resistance and endothelial dysfunction in smokers: Effects of vitamin C. *Am J Physiol Heart Circ Physiol* 279: H1172–H1178, 2000.

65. Eriksson J, Kohvakka A. Magnesium and ascorbic acid supplementation in diabetes mellitus. *Ann Nutr Metab* 39: 217–223, 1995.

66. Liu S, Ajani U, Chae C, Hennekens C, Buring JE, Manson JE. Long-term beta carotene supplementation and risk of Type 2 diabetes mellitus: A randomized controlled trial. *JAMA* 282: 1073–1075, 1995.

67. National Academy of Sciences. *Report on Dietary Reference Intakes for Antioxidants*. April 12, 2000. Washington, DC: National Academy Press.

68. Machlin LJ, Bendich A. Free radical tissue damage: Protective role of antioxidant nutrients. *FASEB J* 1: 441–445, 1987.

69. White AC, Thannickal VJ, Fanburg BL. Glutathione deficiency in human disease. *J Nutr Biochem* 5: 218–226, 1994.

70. Paolisso G, Giugliano D, Pizza G, Tesauro P, Varricchio M, D'Onofrio F. Glutathione infusion potentiates glucose-induced insulin secretion in aged patients with impaired glucose tolerance. *Diabetes Care* 15: 1–7, 1992.

71. Paolisso G, Di Maro G, Pizza G, D'Amore A, Sgambato S, Tesauro P, Varricchio M, D'Onofrio F. Plasma GSH/GSSG affects glucose homeostasis in healthy subjects and non-insulin-dependent diabetics. *Am J Physiol* 263(Endocrinol. Metab.26): E435–E440, 1992.

72. Mattia GD, Bravi MC, Laurenti O, Cassone-Faldetta M, Armiento A, Ferri C, Balsano F. Influence of reduced glutathione infusion on glucose metabolism in patients with non-insulin dependent diabetes mellitus. *Metabolism* 47: 993–997, 1998.

73. Gamage AM, Lee KO, Gan YH. Effect of oral N-acetyl cysteine supplementation in type 2 diabetic patients on intracellular glutathione content and innate immune responses to Burkholderia pseudomallei. *Microbes Infect* 16(8): 661–671, 2014.

74. Hildebrandt W, Hamann A, Krakowski-Roosen H, et al. Effect of thiol antioxidant on body fat and insulin reactivity. *J Mol Med* (Berl) 82(5): 336–344, 2004.

75. Ozkilic AC, Cengiz M, Ozaydin A, Cobanoglu A, Kanigur G. The role of N-acetylcysteine treatment on anti-oxidative status in patients with type II diabetes mellitus. *J Basic Clin Physiol Pharmacol* 17(4): 245–254, 2006.

76. Evans JL, Goldfine ID. Alpha-lipoic acid: A multifunctional antioxidant that improves insulin sensitivity in patients with Type 2 diabetes. *Diabetes Technol Ther* 2: 401–413, 2000.

77. Borcea V, Nourooz-Zadeh J, Wolff SP. Alpha-Lipoic acid decreases oxidative stress even in diabetic patients with poor glycemic control and albuminuria. *Free Radic Biol Med* 26(11–12): 1495–500, 1999.

78. Derosa G, D'Angelo A, Romano D, Maffioli P. A Clinical trial about a food supplement containing α-Lipoic acid on oxidative stress markers in type 2 diabetic patients. *Int J Mol Sci* 17(11). pii: E1802, 2016.

79. Eriksson JG, Forsen TJ, Mortensen SA, Rohde M. The effect of coenzyme Q_{10} administration on metabolic control in patients with Type 2 diabetes mellitus. *Biofactors* 9: 315–318, 1999.
80. Hodgson JM, Watts GF, Playford DA, Burke V, Croft KD. Coenzyme Q_{10} improves blood pressure and glycemic control: A controlled trial in subjects with type 2 diabetes. *Eur J Clin Nutr* 56: 1137–1142, 2002.
81. Mezawa M, Takemoto M, Onishi S, et al. The reduced form of coenzyme Q10 improves glycemic control in patients with type 2 diabetes: An open label pilot study. *Biofactors* 38(6): 416–421, 2012.
82. Kolahdouz Mohammadi R, Hosseinzadeh-Attar MJ, Eshraghian MR, Nakhjavani M, Khorami E, Esteghamati A. The effect of coenzyme Q10 supplementation on metabolic status of type 2 diabetic patients. *Minerva Gastroenterol Dietol* 2013;59(2): 231–236.
83. Zahedi H, Eghtesadi S, Seifirad S, Rezaee N, Shidfar F, Heydari I, Golestan B, Jazayeri S. Effects of CoQ10 supplementation on lipid profiles and Glycemic control in patients with type 2 diabetes: A randomized, double blind, placebo-controlled trial. *J Diabetes Metab Disord* 2014 25;13: 81.
84. Anderson RA, Cheng N, Bryden N, Polansky MM, Cheng N, Chi J. Elevated intakes of supplemental chromium improves glucose and insulin variables in individuals with Type 2 diabetes. *Diabetes* 46: 1786–1791, 1997.
85. Rabinovitz H, Friedensohn A, Leibovitz A, Gabay G, Rocas C, Habot B. Effect of chromium supplementation on blood glucose and lipid levels in type 2 diabetes mellitus elderly patients. *Int J Vitam Nutr Res* 74(3): 178–182, 2004.
86. Jain SK, Kahlon G, Morehead L. Effect of chromium dinicocysteinate supplementation on circulating levels of insulin, TNF-α, oxidative stress, and insulin resistance in type 2 diabetic subjects: Randomized, double-blind, placebo-controlled study. *Mol Nutr Food Res* ;56(8): 1333–1341, 2012.
87. Guimarães MM, Carvalho AC, Silva MS. Effect of chromium supplementation on the glucose homeostasis and anthropometry of type 2 diabetic patients: Double blind, randomized clinical trial: Chromium, glucose homeostasis and anthropometry. *J Trace Elem Med Biol* 36: 65–72, 2016.
88. Yanni AE, Stamataki NS, Konstantopoulos P, et al. Controlling type-2 diabetes by inclusion of Cr-enriched yeast bread in the daily dietary pattern: A randomized clinical trial. *Eur J Nutr* 57(1): 259–267, 2018.
89. Triggiani V, Resta F, Guastamacchia E, Sabbà C, Licchelli B, Ghiyasaldin S, Tafaro E. Role of antioxidants, essential fatty acids, carnitine, vitamins, phytochemicals and trace elements in the treatment of diabetes mellitus and its chronic complications. *Endocr Metab Immune Disord Drug Targets* 6(1): 77–93, 2006.
90. Thazhath SS, Wu T, Bound MJ, et al. Administration of resveratrol for 5 wk has no effect on glucagon-like peptide 1 secretion, gastric emptying, or glycemic control in type 2 diabetes: A randomized controlled trial. *Am J Clin Nutr* 103(1): 66–70, 2016.
91. Bhatt JK, Thomas S, Nanjan MJ. Resveratrol supplementation improves glycemic control in type 2 diabetes mellitus. *Diabetes Metab Syndr* 11 Suppl 2:S631–S635, 2017.
92. Kim MS, Kim JY, Choi WH, Lee SS. Effects of seaweed supplementation on blood glucose concentration, lipid profile, and antioxidant enzyme activities in patients with type 2 diabetes mellitus. *Nutr Res Pract* 2(2): 62–67, 2008.
93. Camandola S, Plick N, Mattson MP. Impact of coffee and cacao purine metabolites on neuroplasticity and neurodegenerative disease. *Neurochem Res* 2018. doi:10.1007/s11064-018-2492-0. [Epub ahead of print].
94. Lane JD, Lane AJ, Surwit RS, Kuhn CM, Feinglos MN. Pilot study of caffeine abstinence for control of chronic glucose in type 2 diabetes. *J Caffeine Res* 24;2(1): 45–47, 2012.
95. Dewar L, Heuberger R. The effect of acute caffeine intake on insulin sensitivity and glycemic control in people with diabetes. *Diabetes Metab Syndr* 11 Suppl 2:S631–S635, 2017.
96. Baker DE, Campbell RK. Vitamin and mineral supplementation in patients with diabetes mellitus. *Diabetes Educ* 18: 420–427, 1992.

24 Management of Diabetic Gastroparesis

Kenneth L. Koch and Khalil N. Bitar

CONTENTS

24.1   INTRODUCTION

Gastroparesis (GP) is defined as a delay in the emptying of ingested food in the absence of mechanical obstruction of the stomach or duodenum [1]. When GP afflicts patients with type 1 diabetes mellitus (T1DM) or type 2 diabetes mellitus (T2DM), the consequences are particularly severe. Symptoms associated with GP, such as early satiety, prolonged fullness, nausea, and vomiting of undigested food, not only reduce the quality of life but also compound difficulties in controlling blood glucose levels. In patients with diabetes complicated by GP, ingested food is not emptied in a predictable time period; thus, the nutrient absorption anticipated by the patient and physician is not the reality. Consequently, the selected dose and timing of insulin therapy to control postprandial glucose may be inappropriate and lead to large excursions in glycemia.

In many patients with GP, erratic postprandial glucose levels result in swings from hypoglycemia to severe hyperglycemia and even ketoacidosis [2]. Hyperglycemia itself elicits gastric dysrhythmias and slows gastric emptying [3,4]. Patients with GP frequently are seen in emergency rooms for low glucose, severe hyperglycemia, and/or ketoacidosis. The physician must identify those diabetic patients with GP in order to properly manage alternative dietary and drug approaches to improve symptoms and nutrition. In this chapter the epidemiology, gastric pathophysiology, and diet, drug, and device approaches to the management of diabetic GP are reviewed.

24.2   EPIDEMIOLOGY

The prevalence of GP in DM varies widely depending on the medical setting. In tertiary centers, up to 40% of patients with T1DM have GP [5]. On the other hand, surveys in Olmsted County, Minnesota, indicated the GP prevalence was 5% in T1DM and 1% in T2DM [6]. An analysis of more than 40 million electronic medical records indicated the prevalence of diabetic GP is less than 5% [7]. Thus, GP in diabetes may not be so common, but it has a large negative impact on the lifestyle of afflicted patients and increases very intensively the use of hospital resources by these patients. In a recent study of a community-based cohort of 1,142 subjects with T2DM, almost 6% of European Americans and 7% of African Americans had moderate to severe symptoms associated with GP [8]. Compared with T2DM, T1DM patients with GP are younger and thinner, and tend to have more severe delays in gastric emptying [9]. Although good control of glycemia prevents or delays many of the chronic complications of T1DM [10], the effect of good glucose control on the onset or progression of GP in DM is unknown. Mortality is increased in diabetic patients when they develop GP and is usually related to cardiovascular events.

24.3   NORMAL GASTRIC NEUROMUSCULAR ACTIVITY AFTER INGESTION OF MEALS

The normal stomach performs a series of complex neuromuscular activities in response to the ingestion of solid foods [11]. First, the fundus relaxes to accommodate the volume of ingested food (Figure 24.1). Normal fundic relaxation requires an intact vagus nerve and is mediated by enteric neurons containing nitric oxide. The relaxation of the fundus allows food to be accommodated without excess stretch on the fundic walls.

Secondly, the corpus and antrum produce recurrent peristaltic waves that mix or triturate the ingested solids into fine particles termed *chyme*. The mixing and emptying of food from the stomach is altered by the nature of the constituents (carbohydrate, protein, and fat) and the fiber and indigestible food components. Carbohydrates are emptied faster than proteins, which are emptied faster than fats and fiber [12]. Emptying of chyme begins when the ingested solid foods are sufficiently triturated. The peristaltic waves occur every 20 seconds, or three cycles per minute, and each peristaltic wave empties aliquots of chyme (fine nutrient particles in suspension) through the

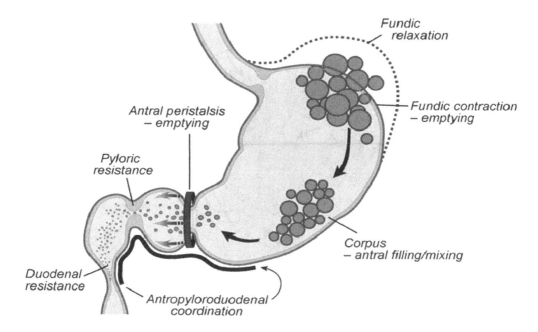

FIGURE 24.1 Gastric neuromuscular responses to the ingestion of solid food. The fundus, corpus, antrum, pylorus, and duodenum are shown. The fundus relaxes to accommodate the ingested solid food. The fundus presses the food into the corpus antrum, the "mixing chamber" of the stomach. Recurrent peristaltic waves triturate the solids into 1- to 2-mm particles (termed *chyme*), which are emptied from the antrum through the pylorus into the duodenum. Liquids are also emptied with recurrent peristaltic waves according to caloric content and viscosity. Gastric emptying of liquids and solids requires antral-pyloro-duodenal coordination. (Modified from Koch, K.L., et al. *Gastroenterology*, 144, S926–S927, 2013.)

pylorus into the duodenum (Figure 24.1). In the normal condition, the number of calories emptied per minute is very consistent at approximately 5 calories per minute in humans [13]. Finally, normal postprandial neuromuscular activity is associated with a sense of comfortable fullness. In contrast, the ingestion of food elicits early satiety, nausea, vomiting, and epigastric discomfort or pain in diabetic patients with GP.

24.4 PATHOPHYSIOLOGY OF DIABETIC GASTROPARESIS

Full-thickness biopsies of the gastric corpus from patients with T1DM and T2DM and GP indicate the disease is primarily a disease of gastric enteric neurons and interstitial cells of Cajal (ICC) [14,15]. Interestingly, these enteric neurons are surrounded by an immune infiltrate composed primarily of type 2 macrophages, suggesting a role for the immune system. ICCs are specialized cells that are crucial for maintaining gastric slow waves or pacesetter potentials that are needed for the normal three-cycle-per-minute (cpm) gastric peristaltic waves. The loss of ICCs is associated with loss of the normal three-cpm gastric pacemaker rhythm. Gastric dysrhythmias develop when ICCs are depleted and result in delayed gastric emptying of ingested food.

The pathophysiological alterations in stomach neuromuscular function in GP are illustrated in Figure 24.2 and include (1) impaired fundic relaxation due to abnormal vagal-induced relaxation of the fundus and dysfunction of the ICCs, which also serve as fundic stretch receptors [16,17], (2) depletion of ICCs in the corpus and antrum that leads to gastric dysrhythmias (e.g., tachygastria, bradygastria, and mixed gastric dysrhythmias) and loss of the normal three-cpm gastric myoelectrical rhythm [16–20], resulting in weak and ineffective contractions for mixing and emptying (e.g., hypomotility), and (3) pyloric sphincter dysfunction, such as pylorospasm, that interferes with

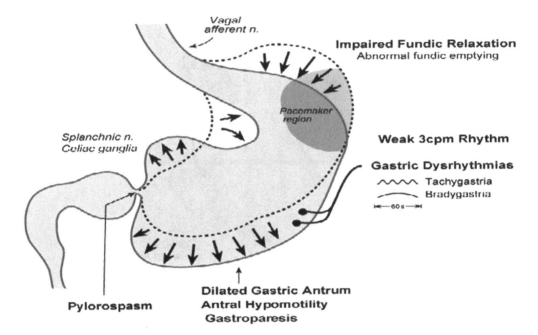

FIGURE 24.2 Neuromuscular disorders of the stomach in diabetic gastroparesis (GP). The fundus fails to relax normally to accommodate food. The gastric electrical rhythm is abnormal due to the loss of interstitial cells of Cajal (ICCs), resulting in weak or absent three-cpm activity and tachygastria and bradygastria. The antrum may dilate and antral contractions are weak and uncoordinated, all of which leads to delayed gastric emptying. In a subset of patients with GP, three-cpm myoelectrical activity is present, but GP occurs because of pyloric dysfunction. Abnormalities of vagal afferent nerve or splanchnic nerve innervation may also be present in patients with diabetic GP. (Modified from Koch, K.L., et al., *Gastroenterology*, 144, S926–S927, 2013.)

gastric emptying. In almost 25% of patients with diabetic GP, pylorospasm (failure of pyloric relaxation in coordination with antral peristaltic waves) results in GP [21,22].

24.5   CLINICAL PRESENTATION OF DIABETIC GASTROPARESIS

Symptoms associated with diabetic GP are nonspecific and include early satiety, prolonged fullness, bloating, nausea, vomiting, and abdominal discomfort and pain. Approximately 20% of patients develop these symptoms acutely. Nausea is the most bothersome and predominant symptom in diabetic patients with GP. Vomitus frequently contains previously ingested solid food. Prolonged stomach fullness and vague epigastric discomfort are common. Symptoms are similar in patients with T1DM and T2DM, although T2DM patients tend to have more fullness and bloating [23]. In a minority of GP patients (20%), abdominal pain is the predominant symptom. The symptoms of GP may be episodic with periods of severe nausea and vomiting; the intensity of the latter frequently requires emergency room visits and/or hospitalization. Nausea and vomiting plus hyperglycemia leads to dehydration, hypovolemia, alterations in serum electrolytes, altered pH balance due to loss of HCl and volume contraction sometimes combined with full-blown diabetic ketoacidosis (DKA).

Physical examination may be normal or reveal obesity or undernutrition, retinopathy, neuropathy, or signs of vitamin deficiency (cheilosis). Obesity in patients with T2DM is a risk factor for GP. Abdominal examination may reveal abdominal distention and a succession splash. Standard laboratory studies are usually normal. Hemoglobin A1c levels have a wide range and do not correlate with severity of GP [25]. TSH levels and fasting cortisol should be measured to screen for Addison's disease and hypothyroidism. Vitamin D levels are frequently low.

24.6 DIAGNOSTIC TESTS FOR GASTROPARESIS

If the physician is suspicious GP is present, then clinical tests should be ordered to confirm the diagnosis so new diet or drug therapies can be confidently initiated. The standard test to confirm GP is the nuclear medicine gastric emptying test using a solid test meal and 1-minute sampling at each postprandial hour for a total of 4 hours [26]. An upper endoscopy to rule out esophagitis, peptic ulcer disease, or mechanical obstruction must be performed to rule out these treatable diseases. Also, an increased risk of bacterial overgrowth of the small intestine has been reported, which requires a targeted therapy [27]. Prior to performing the gastric emptying test, it is important to stop medications that delay gastric emptying for at least 5 days. Those medications include narcotics, anticholinergic agents, glucagon-like polypeptide (GLP)-1 analogues, and amylin analogues. Markedly elevated blood sugar levels also delay gastric emptying. Thus, blood glucose levels should be less than 270 mg/dl before the gastric emptying test meal, which consists of a 257-calorie EggBeaters sandwich. Other tests of gastric emptying are the wireless capsule motility test, which measures intraluminal pH and pressure [28]. The capsule is swallowed during ingestion of a nutrient bar; no further food intake is allowed for 5 hours. A sudden change from an acid pH to a neutral or alkaline pH indicates exit of the capsule from the stomach into the duodenum. If the capsule does not empty from the stomach into the duodenum in 5 hours, then delayed gastric emptying is confirmed [28]. A breath test for measuring gastric emptying is also now available. C^{13}-labeled spirulina in a muffin is ingested, and breath samples are obtained every hour for 4 hours to indirectly determine the rate of emptying of the meal [29].

Electrogastrography is the method to record gastric myoelectrical activity (GMA) before and after a noncaloric water load test. In response to the water load, the GMA may be the normal 3-cpm rhythm or a gastric dysrhythmia, such as tachygastria, bradygastria, or mixed gastric dysrhythmias [30].

24.7 MANAGEMENT OF PATIENTS WITH DIABETIC GASTROPARESIS

24.7.1 DIETARY MANAGEMENT

The American Diabetes Association (ADA)–recommended diet for patients with diabetes is to eat a certain total number of calories per day but also to increase consumption of salads, fresh raw fruits, and fresh raw vegetables [31]. These raw fruits and vegetables are filling and have a low glycemic index but are the most difficult foods for the gastroparetic stomach to triturate and empty. Thus, these foods often induce nausea, early satiety, abdominal discomfort, and vomiting.

Most patients with GP learn to alter their diets because they identify what foods increase or decrease their nausea. Others, however, continue to consume foods rich in fat and fiber. Patients are coached that fatty or fried foods delay gastric emptying and fibrous foods are the most difficult foods for a weak stomach to mill and empty. Patients with diabetic GP may not appreciate that salads with lettuce, carrots, and other fresh, fibrous vegetables are difficult foods for the stomach to mill and empty. These foods are standard ADA diet recommendations for diabetic patients with normal gastric emptying, but are very difficult foods for the diabetic patients with GP [11,32]. The fruits, vegetables, and beans are choices that require much more gastric work to empty (compared with other choices) and often evoke early satiety, prolonged fullness, and nausea and vomiting. Patients with GP may also form phytobezoars, masses of fibrous food that are retained in the fundus or corpus, because the weak stomach cannot empty these foods. Foods known to form bezoars include coconuts, berries, apples, sauerkraut, figs, legumes, oranges, and potato peels [33,34]. Thus, patients need to be advised that these and any fibrous, pulpy foods are to be avoided.

Many patients with GP and chronic nausea and vomiting may gain weight; others lose weight. More than 45% of patients with GP are overweight or obese [35]. The postprandial symptoms and weight changes may result in frustration and depression. The patients who are overweight often feel their nausea and vomiting symptoms are met with skepticism by doctors. Social interactions and the enjoyment of eating food disappear.

24.7.1.1 The Gastroparesis Diet

The patient, physician, and dietitian need to understand the key gastric neuromuscular abnormalities in the gastroparetic stomach. When patients with GP understand the reasons to eat smaller volumes of select foods, they often find they can achieve their nutritional goals *and* reduce the postprandial nausea and noxious fullness that lead to vomiting episodes [36]. Patients learn a three-step diet, and the choice of step depends on the intensity of their nausea and fullness symptoms throughout the day [36]. For example, if a patient is having a difficult day with frequent vomiting, then he or she should choose only liquids, such as Gatorade™, bouillon, or ginger ale that day (see Table 24.1, Step 1). The patient is coached to consume at least 1 to 1.5 liters of an electrolyte solution in small quantities (60–90 ml per hour) on such a day to prevent dehydration and to avoid a visit to the hospital for intravenous hydration. The patient understands gastric accommodation may be impaired and learns that, by taking small sips of electrolyte-containing liquids every hour, the nausea and vomiting symptoms and dehydration can be limited.

Citrus juices and highly sweetened beverages are to be avoided because they are acidic and may irritate gastritis or esophagitis if present and thereby worsen nausea. Carbonated beverages or sodas are avoided because release of carbon dioxide may increase gastric distension and result in bloating, fullness, or heartburn. Peppermint, chocolate, fat, and caffeine decrease lower esophageal sphincter pressure and may increase heartburn. A chewable vitamin should be taken to maintain vitamin levels. Some patients may tolerate clear liquid caloric supplements such as Ensure Clear™, Boost Breeze™, or Enlive™ during step 1. Weight should be monitored twice a week at home. If weight is trending downward, then nutritional supplements described in step 2 below should be added. Overall, the goal of step 1 is to consume enough electrolyte solutions to maintain hydration and avoid increasing postprandial nausea and vomiting. If the step 1 diet is tolerated and nausea and vomiting decreased, then patients can decide to move to step 2.

TABLE 24.1
Diet for Nausea and Vomiting in Patients with Diabetic Gastroparesis

Diet	Goal	Avoid
Step 1: Sports Drinks and Bouillon		
For severe nausea and vomiting: Small volumes of salty liquids, with some caloric content to avoid volume depletion. Chewable multiple vitamin each day	1,000–1,500 ml/day in multiple servings (e.g., twelve 120-ml servings over 12–14 hr). Patient can sip 30–60 ml at a time to reach approximately 120 ml/hr	Citrus drinks of all kinds; highly sweetened drinks
Step 2: Soups and Smoothies		
If step 1 is tolerated: Soup with noodles or rice and crackers. Smoothies with low-fat dairy. Peanut butter, cheese, and crackers in small amounts, caramels or other chewy confections. Ingest above foods in at least 6 small-volume meals/day. Chewable multiple vitamin each day	Approximately 1,500 calories/ day to avoid volume depletion and maintain weight (often more realistic than weight gain)	Creamy, milk-based liquids
Step 3: Starches, Chicken, Fish		
If step 2 is tolerated: Noodles, pastas, potatoes (mashed or baked), rice, baked chicken breast, fish (all easily mixed and emptied by the stomach). Ingest solids in at least 6 small-volume meals/day. Chewable multiple vitamin each day	Common foods that patient finds interesting and satisfying and that provoke minimal nausea/ vomiting symptoms	Fatty foods that delay gastric emptying; red meats and fresh vegetables that require considerable trituration; pulpy, fibrous foods that promote formation of bezoars

The step 2 phase is nutrition in liquid form as provided by soups and smoothies. Step 2 foods include, for example, chicken noodle soup, chicken and rice soup, and small amounts of cheese, crackers, peanut butter, or soft caramels or soft chewy fruit candies require little trituration before emptying. Milk-based liquids that contain fat are often not tolerated, but the patient may try almond milk, soy milk, or Lactaid milk. Some patients have lactose intolerance, and lactose-free milk products or almond or soy milk products are appropriate for them. The goal of step 2 is for the patient to consume at least 1,500 calories in six or more meals or snacks of small volume in order to maintain or gain weight while selecting foods that consider dysfunction in gastric accommodation and peristalsis. Protein and calorie intake goals can be achieved with step 2 if the patient adds protein supplements like soy or whey and uses complete vitamin products.

In addition to soups, the patient may try smoothies with soy milk, Lactaid™ milk, or almond milk products, and vegetables and fruits blenderized into very small particles. Liquid caloric meals can be tasty, require less gastric work to empty than solid foods, and may elicit few postprandial symptoms. Patients are reminded that the supine position may contribute to delayed emptying, since ingested nutrients pool in the fundus. Thus, patients are encouraged to remain sitting up after even small-volume meals for at least 1 hour. Patients with GP may consider elevating the head of the bed onto 6- to 8-inch blocks to prevent regurgitation and gastroesophageal reflux when sleeping. Thus, the goal of step 2 is to find liquid nutritional foods that are tasty, provide calories to maintain weight, and evoke minimal postprandial symptoms. If patients tolerate the step 2 phase, and nausea and vomiting are controlled, then they can advance to step 3.

Step 3 emphasizes solid foods that are low in fat and fiber because these foods delay gastric emptying. Thus, step 3 includes foods such as rice, pasta, and potatoes. Mashed potatoes would be a choice example for patients to appreciate as a food that requires almost no milling and is easy for their weak stomach to mix and empty. The starches have a high glycemic index, but patients with GP usually cannot tolerate large volumes of these foods. Small portions (e.g., 3–4 ounces) of broiled, baked, or grilled lean meats such as chicken, turkey, or fish may be tolerated if diced or chewed thoroughly. Other solid foods recommended in small portions include canned fruit in its own juice, applesauce, or cooked, fork-tender vegetables. Puddings and yogurts are also semisolid foods that require little milling and elicit less postprandial symptoms.

A recent study showed that meals comprised of small particles reduced upper gastrointestinal symptoms in patients with diabetic GP [37]. This randomized, controlled trial showed that a diet with small-particle foods was associated with improved upper gastrointestinal symptoms associated with GP in patients with diabetes mellitus compared with the standard ADA diet [37]. Nausea/vomiting, postprandial fullness, early satiety, and bloating improved significantly in the small-particle-size meal group. The meals were small-volume and low in fat and fiber content and were consumed four to five times a day [37]. The diet is similar to the step-three diet suggestions shown in Table 24.1.

The 3-step diet for patients with nausea and vomiting is low in protein and fat and therefore is not a "complete diet." Almost 32% of patients with GP have diets deficient in calories, vitamins, and minerals; unfortunately, only one-third of these patients were taking multivitamins on a daily basis [35]. Patients with idiopathic GP were more likely to have diets with deficiencies in vitamins B_6, vitamin K, and iron and less likely to have seen a dietitian compared with patients with diabetic GP. Baseline vitamin levels such as vitamin D, iron panel, zinc, vitamin B12, and folate should be obtained, and vitamins or minerals that are deficient should be treated. Laboratory tests should be repeated 3–6 months later to assure repletion. A chewable multivitamin should be added to the daily diet regimen for all patients with GP. The chewable vitamin should say "complete" on the label. Some of the gummy vitamins lack certain vitamins and minerals. A dietitian should be consulted for additional advice in regards to diets for GP.

24.7.1.2 Enteral Nutrition

GP presents a number of challenges for patients to consume adequate calories and balance fat, protein, vitamin, and mineral requirements. Enteral nutrition support may be indicated when patients have severe, persistent symptoms of nausea and vomiting or early satiety or fullness that regularly inhibits adequate oral intake. If patients experience significant weight loss of 5%–10% of body weight over 3–6 months, frequent hospitalizations with intractable nausea and vomiting, inability to maintain adequate calorie intake, and evidence of protein-calorie malnutrition (low albumin or prealbumin, hair loss, brittle nails, or vitamin and mineral deficiencies), then enteral support is the next step in nutritional management. The guidelines for the identification of patients at nutritional risk are body mass index (BMI) less than 20 kg/m^2 and unintentional weight loss of 5%–10% over 3–6 months [33,38]. Unintentional weight loss is one of the most important parameters to assess, regardless of the patient's overall appearance. Enteral nutrition support is preferred over total parental nutrition (TPN), because line infections and sepsis are avoided and expenses are fewer. Enteral feeding also provides physiological delivery of nutrients into the small bowel, enhances glucose control, and utilizes the gut. TPN is rarely necessary for patients with GP and should be reserved for those who have had small bowel resections or small bowel motility abnormalities, or who failed enteral therapy [38].

A trial of nasojejunal feeding prior to placement of permanent enteral access is recommended for 2–4 weeks to determine if enteral feeding is tolerated. However, these tubes can migrate back into the stomach, which may require multiple tube placements and X-rays to confirm placement. If enteral feeding results in minimal gastrointestinal symptoms and some weight gain, then proceeding to surgical jejunostomy is reasonable for long-term enteral feeding. A percutaneous endoscopic gastrostomy tube with a jejunal extension (PEG-J) is not recommended for long-term enteral feeding because GP patients frequently vomit and the J-tube extension reverts to the stomach. Therefore, a feeding jejunostomy tube, which bypasses the gastroparetic stomach, is a much more dependable access to the small bowel for predictable enteral nutrition.

24.8   GLUCOSE MANAGEMENT IN PATIENTS WITH DIABETIC GASTROPARESIS

Glucose control in the patient with diabetic GP can be extremely difficult both in the outpatient and inpatient environments. Ultimately, glucose control is dictated to a great extent by the relationship between glycemia and gastric emptying [39], whereby hyperglycemia further delays gastric emptying rates. Thus, GP affects the expected rate of nutrient emptying and absorption and subsequently oftentimes results in unpredictable glucose excursions.

The delayed rate of gastric emptying of ingested nutrients may be unappreciated by the patient or physician. Thus, on a day-to-day basis, gastric emptying is not predictable and regular ingestion of meals is then compromised by episodic nausea and vomiting. Vomiting reduces absorption of anticipated calories. Liquid nutrients and solid foods may be retained in the stomach much longer than expected by the patient or by the treating physician. Thus, unexplained postprandial hypoglycemia and/or hyperglycemia are a distinctive feature of patients with diabetes and GP due to the mismatch of insulin absorption and the slow and frequently erratic entry of nutrients into the duodenum and small intestine.

24.8.1   GLUCOSE MANAGEMENT WITH PHARMACOLOGICAL AGENTS IN PATIENTS WITH DIABETIC GASTROPARESIS

Patients with T1DM require insulin replacement, as do most (if not all) of the patients with T2DM and GP. In diabetic patients with GP, oral medications [40] may not empty from the stomach for hours, resulting in erratic pharmacokinetics and pharmacodynamics. The sulfonylureas are associated with protracted hypoglycemia in these patients. The GLP-1 incretins slow stomach emptying and are associated with nausea and vomiting themselves and hence are not recommended [41]. While inhibitors of the enzyme dipeptidyl peptidase-4 (DPP4) do not have much effect on slowing gastric emptying [42], their efficacy depend upon good insulin reserve, and most patients with T2DM and GP have had long-duration diabetes and likely have severely decreased capacity to secrete insulin. In addition, no clinical trials have been published on the safety or efficacy of the use of these agents in diabetic GP.

The current approach to insulin administration in GP is based on the basal-bolus model, which is easier to model with pumps rather than multiple shots [43]. A standard assumption of meal bolus is that gastric emptying of the ingested meal in the diabetic patient is completed within 4 hours and intestinal absorption of nutrients is completed within 4–6 hours. The administration of meal-time insulin is "timed" to match anticipated nutrient absorption. This is problematic for patients with GP because the onset and duration of the small intestinal absorption phase is critically dependent on the rate of gastric emptying. Besides the slow emptying of the stomach, the day-to-day variability in gastric emptying of common foods is unknown.

Continuous insulin infusion (pump) for managing glycemia in patients with diabetes and GP has been recommended [44,45]. Our recent study showed that intense glucose control with insulin pump and continuous glucose monitoring (CGM) in patients with diabetic GP resulted in significant reductions in upper GI symptoms associated with GP and a 1.1% decrease in HbA1c [46]. If insurance coverage and costs are an unsurmountable obstacle, then multiple daily insulin injections are the next best option. Monitoring of glycemia for insulin adjustment is preferably established with a system based on finger sticks augmented with CGM. The estimated initial dose of basal insulin can be calculated using a formula of 0.3 units/kg/day for a T2DM patient and 0.15 units/kg/day for someone with T1DM. Traditional adjustment of the basal insulin is based on the glycemia measured before breakfast, which assumes postabsorptive state (some 11–14 hours after last meal). In patients with diabetic GP, however, the postabsorptive state is not so easy to define, because gastric emptying may be delayed all day and an unknown amount of food (from accumulated breakfast, lunch, and/or dinner) is emptied during the night. Thus, the prebreakfast glycemia may not reflect real basal glycemia but ongoing postprandial glycemic excursions. More details regarding an approach to insulin pump therapy with CGM in patients with GP are reviewed in [47].

24.9 PROKINETIC DRUGS FOR PATIENTS WITH DIABETIC GASTROPARESIS

Prokinetic drugs increase the rate of gastric emptying. Currently, the only prokinetic drugs available to treat GP are metoclopramide (Reglan) and erythromycin (Table 24.2). Metoclopramide is a dopamine$_2$ receptor antagonist, a 5HT$_3$ receptor antagonist, and an acetylcholinesterase inhibitor [48]. Gastric emptying is increased by metoclopramide, but the drug also crosses the blood-brain barrier and causes a variety of central nervous symptoms, ranging from nervousness to Parkinson's disease and irreversible tardive dyskinesia. Erythromycin is a macrolide antibiotic that stimulates motilin receptors and contractions in the corpus and antrum, which increases the rate of gastric emptying [49].

Unfortunately, many drugs designed to improve the rate of gastric emptying have not improved the symptoms associated with GP. Studies of prokinetic drugs and gastric stimulation have shown that the rate of gastric emptying does not correlate with the symptoms associated with GP [50]. Domperidone is a dopamine$_2$ antagonist that does not cross the blood-brain barrier, improves nausea and gastric dysrhythmias, and improves the rates of gastric emptying in some patients with diabetic GP [51]. Domperidone is not available in the United States, except through a special US Food and

TABLE 24.2
Prokinetic Drugs for Patients with Diabetic Gastroparesis

Agent	Mechanism	Dose
Metoclopramide	Dopamine D$_2$ receptor antagonist, 5HT$_4$ agonist, acetylcholinesterase inhibitor	10 mg TID
Erythromycin	Motilin receptor agonist	250 mg TID
Physiostigmine	Acetylcholinesterase inhibitor	30–60 mg TID
Relamorelin	Ghrelin receptor agonist	Investigational drug

TABLE 24.3
Antinausea Medications for Patients with Diabetic Gastroparesis

Agent	Mechanism	Dose
Ondansetron	5HT$_3$ receptor antagonist	4–8 mg PO
Promethazine	Histamine$_1$ receptor antagonist	25 mg PO
Aprepitant	Neurokinin (NK)$_1$-receptor antagonist	25 mg PO
Tetrahydrocannabinol	Cannabinoid receptors	5 mg BID PO
Lorazepam	Benzodiazepines	1 mg TID PO
Mirtazapine	Atypical antidepressant	5 mg BID PO

Drug Administration (FDA) program. The ghrelin-agonist relamorelin (Allergan) is in phase III trials for patients with vomiting and T1DM or T2DM and GP [52]. The stimulation of ghrelin appears to increase the rate of gastric emptying and reduce vomiting.

24.10   ANTINAUSEA DRUGS FOR PATIENTS WITH DIABETIC GASTROPARESIS

The quality of life for patients with GP is extremely poor due to constant nausea and episodic vomiting. These symptoms may lead to dehydration, which requires frequent emergency room visits or hospitalizations. Table 24.3 lists a number of drugs that are used empirically to treat nausea for patients with GP. At the present time, there is no way to predict which medication will decrease nausea in an individual patient. Each drug may be tried to see if nausea and vomiting improve. These drugs have not been specifically approved for use in patients who have symptoms associated with diabetic GP. In unremitting nausea and vomiting, normal weight cannot be maintained, and jejunostomy feeding tubes for enteral nutrition or TPN may be needed in a minority of patients to support nutrition.

24.11   PYLORIC THERAPIES (BOTULINUM TOXIN INJECTION, SURGICAL MYOTOMY) AND GASTRIC ELECTRICAL STIMULATION FOR PATIENTS WITH DIABETIC GASTROPARESIS

A subset of patients with GP have normal three-cpm GMA (rather than gastric dysrhythmias). These discordant findings suggest pyloric sphincter dysfunction, because the numbers of ICCs are normal if three-cpm GMA is present. This pattern of GP plus normal three-cpm GMA was also reported in GP due to pyloric stenosis [53]. Diagnostic tools for diagnosing pyloric dysfunction include endoscopy to exclude pyloric stenosis and intraluminal pressure or compliance measures. Compliance abnormalities of the pyloric sphincter were reported in almost 40% of patients with GP [54]. Treatment of suspected pylorospasm with injections of botulinum toxin into the pylorus resulted in no better symptom improvement than placebo in patients with GP [55], but these patients were not classified by GMA. On the other hand, 73% of patients with idiopathic GP and normal three-cpm myoelectrical activity (functional obstructive GP) who underwent pyloric treatment with botulinum toxin A or balloon dilation had improvement in symptoms [56]. Gastric electrical stimulation is provided by a stimulator device attached to electrodes placed on the serosa of the stomach to relieve nausea and vomiting. This treatment in uncontrolled trials relieves nausea and vomiting in diabetic patients with GP [57,58].

24.12   INPATIENT MANAGEMENT OF THE PATIENT WITH DIABETES AND GASTROPARESIS

The main reasons for patients with DM and GP to be hospitalized are (1) acute exacerbations of GP symptoms (nausea, vomiting, pain) that lead to dehydration and hypovolemia, (2) severe hyperglycemia with ketoacidosis and symptoms that resemble acute exacerbation of GP, (3) severe hypoglycemia, and (4) combinations of 1, 2, and 3. There are no clinical trials to define the best treatment approaches for inpatient or outpatient treatment of patients with diabetes and GP. The initial treatment in the hospital is restoration of volume status, correction of electrolyte imbalances, and stabilization of glucose with an insulin drip to treat hyperglycemia or DKA or dextrose infusion for hypoglycemia. After hemodynamic stabilization, the three-step diet approach can be used to begin *per os* intake. Step 1 (Table 24.1) is aimed at maintaining hydration with oral fluids. Patients are encouraged to sip small volumes (e.g., 2 oz every 30–60 minutes) of liquids with sugar and electrolytes (may be accomplished with commercially available sports drinks) and bouillon throughout the day. As nausea and vomiting improve with hydration, the patient may then advance to steps 2 and 3, as outlined in Table 24.1 [9].

24.13 REGENERATIVE MEDICINE TREATMENTS FOR DIABETIC GASTROPARESIS

The gastrointestinal tract is a hollow organ composed of mucosal, muscular, and neural components along with supporting cells, including ICCs and endothelial cells. The mucosa is surrounded by circular and longitudinal smooth muscle layers that promote the mechanical breakdown and propulsion of food within the GI tract, through coordinated contraction and relaxation events termed *peristalsis*. The neural component of the GI tract, the enteric nervous system (ENS), is an independent division of the peripheral nervous system responsible for regulating gut functions including motility, secretion and absorption [59]. To date, approximately 10–15 subtypes of myenteric and 4–5 subtypes of submucosal neurons have been identified, including excitatory and inhibitory motor neurons, interneurons, intrinsic primary afferent neurons (IPANs), and secretomotor and vasodilator neurons [60].

Coordination of smooth muscle activity, together with propulsion and expulsion across sphincteric barriers, requires slow waves. Slow waves coordinate smooth muscle contraction by combining action potentials propagated by ICCs that also form gap junctions with neurons and smooth muscle cells (SMC). Thus, ICC and SMC are electrically coupled. Electrical coupling combines ICC slow wave with smooth muscle potential to result in a larger combined potential that results in coordinated contractions. The slow wave rhythm is dependent on the activity of Ano1 (calcium activated chloride channel) in the ICC cells. Therefore, the slow wave dictates the maximum frequency of contractions. In humans, the slow wave frequency is three cpm in the stomach and 10–12 cpm in the small intestine.

Diabetic (and idiopathic) GP is a particularly challenging disease. Depletions of ICC and/or enteric neurons have been associated with diabetic GP. Histological analysis shows patients may be missing one or both cell types [61]. It is estimated that at least 50% of T1DM and 30% of T2DM patients develop GP. The loss of ICCs or enteric neurons in GP opens the door to "specialized medicine" with specific new therapeutic avenues. That is, bioengineered tissues or cell therapy approaches could replenish the neural and/or ICC population in abnormal stomach or pyloric sphincter areas to restore normal neuromuscular function.

24.13.1 CELLULAR REPLACEMENT THERAPIES FOR GASTROINTESTINAL MOTILITY DISORDERS

Advances in regenerative medicine and cellular replacement therapies for gastrointestinal neuromuscular disorders are rapidly progressing. Successful cellular replacement therapies include (1) identifying a viable stem/progenitor cell source, (2) optimizing delivery methods, (3) developing techniques for in vitro propagation, expansion, and differentiation of these cells, and (4) ensuring survival, integration, and functioning of implanted cells. Thus far, researchers have identified autologous and heterologous neural stem/progenitor cells from embryonic and adult sources that can be expanded and differentiated in vitro, tested delivery methods, and begun to develop methods that enhance survival of implanted cells [62–67].

24.13.1.1 Sources of Enteric Nerve Cells for Implantation in the Gut

Use of embryonic stem cells (ESCs) for enteric neural cell replacement has demonstrated limited success because these cells failed to maintain neuronal differentiation when transplanted in vivo [68,69].

Furthermore, the use of ESCs in humans is associated with a number of drawbacks, including immune rejection and tumor formation, along with ethical considerations.

The central nervous system (CNS) presents another source of stem and progenitor cells that can be used to repopulate the ENS. Stem cells derived from the CNS of mouse embryos restored inhibitory motor neurons and gastric emptying in mouse models of GP [70], and CNS-derived stem cells transplanted into aganglionic rat rectums restored both cholinergic and nitrergic population of enteric neurons and rectoanal inhibitory reflex (RAIR) [71]. However, the cells used in these studies were isolated from the embryonic CNS, and translation into humans would pose huge technical and ethical challenges, and the concern of immune rejection would remain.

More reliable cell sources for both ENS and ICC transplantation are those derived from the gastrointestinal tract. The ability to easily access and isolate enteric neural progenitor cells (ENPCs) and ICCs from the gut makes this cell source much more attractive. Isolation of neural progenitor cells from the gut was initiated more than a decade ago, at which time it was shown that these cells could repopulate neural cells in aganglionated organ cultures [72,73]. ENPCs can be isolated from full-thickness samples of patients with Hirschsprung's disease and healthy individuals [74]. ENPCs can also be isolated from biopsies harvested during routine endoscopic procedures, thereby minimizing the discomfort and risk for the patients. Furthermore, these ENPCs have been shown to migrate, integrate, and differentiate upon implantation [75].

Much work needs to be done to improve the survival and functioning of regenerated neurons and ICCs following implantation. The benefits of using ENPCs derived from autologous sources are numerous, including no risk of immune rejection, safe and efficient cell harvest, and no ethical considerations.

24.13.1.2 Delivery Methods for Regenerated, Bioengineered Neural, and Interstitial Cajal Cells into the Gut

Delivery of bioengineered cells into the gut is not a trivial task and must be properly addressed in order to ensure survival and integration of the transplanted cells or tissue. Routinely performed and minimally invasive procedures, such as endoscopy and laparotomy, may be amenable techniques for cell delivery. Several studies have demonstrated the feasibility of transplanting ENPCs and CNS-derived stem cells via laparotomies [76]. Integration of neural cells was observed following transplantation through laparotomies, and gastric emptying was increased in a mouse model of GP [77]. Direct injection of cells into the gastrointestinal tract is the most common technique used, but a major disadvantage is the inability of cells to migrate a significant distance away from the injection site. This disadvantage could be turned into an advantage, since it presents the opportunity to inject two cell types, either neural progenitor cells or ICC in adjacent locations, to achieve beneficial effects of colocalization of two cell types.

Delivery methods that have yet to be thoroughly investigated in vivo include the transplantation of extracellular matrix (ECM) gels seeded with neural/ICC cells or bio-electro spraying of neural cells/ICC cells, which could increase the area of affected gut to be treated. The use of an endoscope for cell delivery would have many advantages in that it is minimally invasive, well-established technology. Indeed, the collection of ENPCs using an endoscope has already been performed and cell sheets have been administered via endoscopes to treat ulcerations in a canine model [78]. However, standard procedures must be developed in order to successfully and reproducibly administer cells using this method.

24.13.1.3 Methods to Enhance Migration, Survival, Differentiation and Integration of Enteric Neural Interstitial Cajal Cells for Transplantation

Successful isolation and culture of ENPCs has been possible for more than 10 years, but the migration of unstimulated transplanted ENPCs is limited to a couple of millimeters [79]. The isolation of ICCs is routine in our lab, and the co-culture of ICCs with neural progenitor cells and ICCs is a routine ex vivo procedure.

Prolonged survival of cells after transplantation into the gut is another necessary step for successful cell replacement therapy. Methods to increase antiapoptotic signaling, such as addition of small molecules, may be preferable to the use of gene therapy due to the hazards associated with gene therapy. The use of small molecules to inhibit pro-apoptotic factor caspase-3 has been shown to improve survival of neural stem cells transplanted into the pylorus of mice [80]. Pretreatment of cells with caspase inhibitors may be a good approach to enhance survival following in vivo transplantation.

In order to effectively restore function to the aganglionic gut, transplanted neural progenitor cells must not only migrate and survive, but also differentiate into neurons and become further specialized to release specific neurotransmitters. To restore motility, both excitatory motor neurons that promote smooth muscle cell contraction and inhibitory neurons to promote relaxation must be present. The ECM and smooth muscle cell–derived factors are critical mediators of enteric neural subset activation. The selective differentiation of neurons is stimulated by ECM proteins laminin, collagen I, and collagen IV in two-dimensional co-culture methods with ENPCs and SMCs [81]. Furthermore, the specific expression of excitatory neurons that express choline acetyltransferase (ChAT) and of inhibitory motor neurons that express neuronal nitric oxide synthase (nNOS) are stimulated by collagen I and collagen IV, respectively, in three-dimensional gels.

24.13.2 IMPLANTATION OF A FUNCTIONAL REPLACEMENT PYLORUS SPHINCTER FOR GASTROPARESIS

As described earlier, a subset of patients with GP has neuromuscular dysfunction of the pyloric sphincter that accounts for delayed gastric emptying. Thus, tissue or cellular therapy is a regenerative medicine treatment option. The implantation of a bioengineered internal anal sphincter has proven to be a success in large animal studies [82]. Implanting a bioengineered pylorus to treat a subset of GP patients with a deficient pylorus is a possibility.

We have bioengineered innervated human pylorus constructs [83] utilizing autologous human pyloric sphincter SMCs and human ENPCs. SMCs and ENPCs were co-cultured in dual-layered hydrogels and formed concentrically aligned pylorus constructs. Innervated human pylorus constructs were characterized through biochemical and physiologic assays to assess the phenotype and functionality of SMCs and neurons. SMCs within bioengineered human pylorus constructs displayed a tonic contractile phenotype and maintained circumferential alignment. Neural differentiation within bioengineered constructs was verified by positive expression of βIII-tubulin, nNOS, and ChAT. Bioengineered innervated human pylorus constructs generated a robust spontaneous basal tone and contracted in response to potassium chloride (KCl). Contraction in response to exogenous neurotransmitter acetylcholine (ACh) and relaxation in response to vasoactive intestinal peptide (VIP) and electrical field stimulation (EFS) were also observed. Neural network integrity was demonstrated by inhibition of EFS-induced relaxation in the presence of a neurotoxin or nNOS inhibitors. Partial inhibition of ACh-induced contraction and VIP-induced relaxation following neurotoxin treatment was observed. These studies provide a proof of concept for bioengineering functional innervated human pyloric sphincter constructs to be used as functional replacement organs.

To our knowledge, this is the first demonstration of bioengineering a human pylorus construct with autologous cells that is innervated with functional differentiated neurons. These constructs (1) maintained smooth muscle alignment and phenotype, (2) expressed mature excitatory and inhibitory neurons, and (3) exhibited spontaneous basal tone and responded to physiological stimuli. Bioengineered innervated human pyloric sphincter constructs have the potential for (1) use as physiologically relevant models to investigate human pyloric sphincter disorders, and (2) use as functional replacement organs for patients with pyloric dysfunction and GP.

24.14 CONCLUSIONS

GP is a complication of chronic T1DM and T2DM. Symptoms associated with GP are nonspecific and include early satiety, prolonged postprandial fullness, bloating, nausea, vomiting, and abdominal pain. ICCs are depleted, and gastric enteric neurons are abnormal in GP, suggesting the disease is a neuropathy affecting control of gastric smooth muscle relaxation and contraction and a Cajalopathy affecting gastric electrical rhythm. A subset of patients with diabetic GP has normal three-cpm GMA, reflecting pyloric sphincter dysfunction that results in functional obstructive GP.

GP delays gastric emptying of food and hence retards entry of nutrients from the small intestine into the bloodstream. As a consequence of the latter, there is oftentimes a mismatch of peak insulin levels and postprandial glycemia. Thus, GP increases the risk of large swings to hypo- and hyperglycemia. Current management should focus first on dietary changes/counseling and careful insulin administration to maintain appropriate glycemia goals.

Prokinetic and antinausea agents should be considered, as well as referral or consultation with a gastroenterologist interested in GP. Identifying patients with GP and three-cpm GMA, the obstructive subtype, is important because therapy is directed to the pylorus in these patients.

New prokinetic agents and gastric electrical stimulation are treatment options for selected patients. Future therapies will include regenerative medicine approaches such as bioengineered enteric nerves and ICCs or pyloric sphincter constructs that will be implanted to restore neuromuscular function of the corpus antrum or pylorus for patients with diabetic GP.

DISCLOSURE OF CONFLICT OF INTEREST

K. Koch, MD - no conflicts of interest

K. Bitar, PhD - no conflicts of interest

REFERENCES

1. Camilleri M, Parkman H, Shafi M, et al. Clinical guideline: Management of gastroparesis. *Am J Gastroenterol* 2013;108:18–37.
2. Koch KL. Diabetic gastropathy: Gastric neuromuscular dysfunction in diabetes mellitus. A review of symptoms, pathophysiology, and treatment. *Dig Dis Sci* 1999;44:1061–1075.
3. Hasler WL, Soudah HC, Dulai G, Owyang C. Mediation of hyperglycemia-evoked gastric slow-wave dysrhythmias by endogenous prostaglandins. *Gastroenterology* 1995;108:726–736.
4. Fraser R, Horowitz M, Maddox A, et al. Hyperglycemia slows gastric emptying in type 1 diabetes mellitus. *Diabetologia* 1990;33:675–680.
5. Bharucha AE. Epidemiology and natural history of gastroparesis. *Gastroenterol Clin North Am* 2015;44:9.
6. Jung, HK, Choung RS, Locke GR, Schleck CD, Zinsmeister AR, Szarka, LA, Mullan B, and Talley NJ. The incidence, prevalence, and outcomes of patients with gastroparesis in Olmsted County, Minnesota, from 1996 to 2006. *Gastroenterology* 2009;136;4:1225–1233.
7. Syed A, Calles-Escandon J, Wolfe M. Epidemiology of gastroparesis with and without diabetes in a large cohort from 340 USA hospitals. *Gastroenterology* 2015;146S.
8. Brown L, Bowden D, Freedman B, Hsu F-C, Xu J, Koch K. Symptoms associated with gastroparesis in community-based patients with type 2 diabetes mellitus. *Gastroenterology* 2017;152;5:S517.
9. Koch KL, Hasler WL, et al. for the Gastroparesis clinical research consortium. Contrasting gastroparesis in type 1 (T1DM) vs. type 2 (T2DM) diabetes: Clinical course after 48 weeks of follow-up and relation to comorbidities and health resource utilization. *Gastroenterology* 2013;144:S926–S927.
10. The Diabetes Control and Complications Trial Research Group. The effect of intensive diabetes therapy on measures of autonomic nervous system function in the diabetes control and complications Trial (DCCT). *Diabetologia* 1998;4:416–423.
11. Koch KL. Gastric neuromuscular function and neuromuscular disorders. In *Sleisenger and Fordtran's Gastrointestinal and Liver Disease: Pathophysiology/Diagnosis/Management.* (Eds.), Feldman M, Friedman LS, Brandt LJ. Elsevier, Philadelphia, PA, 2015;811–838.

12. Camilleri M. Integrated upper gastrointestinal response to food intake. *Gastroenterology* 2006;131:640–658.

13. Moran TH, Wirth JB, Schwartz GJ, et al. Interactions between gastric volume and duodenal nutrients in the control of liquid gastric emptying. *Am J Physiol* 1999;276:R997–R1002.

14. Ordog T. Interstitial cells of Cajal in diabetic gastroenteropathy. *Neurogastroenterol Motil* 2008;20:8–18.

15. Farrugia G, Lurken MS, Bernard CE, Faussone-Pellegrini MS, Smyrk TC, Parkman HP, Abell TL, et al. Cellular changes in diabetic and idiopathic gastroparesis. *Gastroenterology* 2011;140:1575–1585.

16. Rayner CK, Verhagen MA, Hebbard GG, et al. Proximal gastric compliance and perception of distension in type 1 diabetes mellitus: Effects of hyperglycemia. *Am J Gastroenterology* 2000;95:1175–1183.

17. Won KJ, Sanders KM, Ward SM. Interstitial cells of Cajal mediate mechanosensitive responses in the stomach. *Proc Natl Acad Sci U S A* 2005;102:14913–14918.

18. He C-L, Soffer EE, Ferris CD, et al. Loss of interstitial cells of Cajal and inhibitory innervation in insulin-dependent diabetes. *Gastroenterology* 2001;121:427–434.

19. O'Grady G, Angeli T, Du P, Lahr C, Lammers WJ, Windsor JA, Abell TL, Farrugia G, Pullan AJ, Cheng LK. Abnormal initiation and conduction of slow wave activity in gastroparesis defined by a high resolution electrical mapping. *Gastroenterology* 2012;143:589–598.

20. Lin Z, Sarosiek I, Forster J, et al. Association of the status of interstitial cells of Cajal and electrogastrogram parameters, gastric emptying, and symptoms in patients with gastroparesis. *Neurogastroenterol Motil* 2010;22:56–61.

21. Mearin F, Camilleri M, Malagelada JR. Pyloric dysfunction in diabetics with recurrent nausea and vomiting. *Gastroenterology* 1986;90:1919–1925.

22. Brzana RJ, Bingaman S, Koch KL. Gastric myoelectrical activity in patients with gastric outlet obstruction and idiopathic gastroparesis. *Am J Gastroenterol* 1998;93:1083–1089.

23. Parkman HP, Yates K, Hasler WL, et al. Similarities and differences between diabetic and idiopathic gastroparesis. *Clin Gastroenterol Hepatol* 2011;9:1056–1064.

24. Dickman R, Kislov J, Boaz M, et al. Prevalence of symptoms suggestive of gastroparesis in a cohort of patients with diabetes mellitus. *J Diab Comp* 2013;27:376–379.

25. Reddy S, Ramsubeik K, Vega KJ, Federico J, Palacia C. Do HbA1c levels correlate with delayed gastric emptying in diabetic patients? *J Neurogastroenterol Motil* 2010;16:414–417.

26. Tougas G, Eaker EY, Abell TL, et al. Assessment of gastric emptying using a low fat meal: Establishment of international control values. *Am J Gastroenterol* 2000;95:1456–1462.

27. George NS, et al. Small intestinal overgrowth in gastroparesis. *Dig Dis Sci* 2014:59;645–652.

28. Kuo B, McCallum RW, Koch KL, et al. Comparison of gastric emptying of a nondigestible capsule to a radio-labelled meal in healthy and gastroparetic subjects. *Aliment Pharmacol Ther* 2008;27:186–196.

29. Szarka LA, Camilleri M, Vella A, Burton D, Baxter K, Simonson J, Zinsmeister AR. A stable isotope breath test with a standard meal for abnormal gastric emptying of solids in the clinic and in research. *Clin Gastro Hepatol* 2008;6:635–643.

30. Koch KL, Hong S-P, Xu L. Reproducibility of gastric myoelectrical activity and the water load test in patients with dysmotility-like dyspepsia symptoms and in control subjects. *J Clin Gastroenterol* 2000;31(2):125–129.

31. American Diabetes Association. Clinical practice guidelines 2014. *Diabetes Care* 2014;37:S28–S30.

32. Sadiva A. Nutritional therapy for the management of diabetic gastroparesis: Clinical review. *Diabetes Metab Syndr Obes* 2012;5:329–335.

33. Parrish CR, Pastors JG. Nutritional management of gastroparesis in people with diabetes. *Diabetes Spectr* 2007;209: 231–234.

34. Institute of Medicine. 2005. *Dietary Reference Intakes for Energy, Carbohydrate, Fiber, Fat, Fatty Acids, Cholesterol, Protein, and Amino Acids.* Washington, DC: National Academy Press. (Food and Nutrition Board, Institute of Medicine, National Academies).

35. Parkman HP, et al. Dietary intake and nutritional deficiencies in patients with diabetic or idiopathic gastroparesis. *Gastroenterology* 2011;141:486–498.

36. Koch KL. Review article: Clinical approaches to unexplained nausea and vomiting. *Adv Gastroenterol Hepatol Clin Nutr* 1998;3:163–178.

37. Olausson EA, Störsrud S, Grundin H, Isaksson M, Attvall S, Simrén M. A small particle size diet reduces upper gastrointestinal symptoms in patients with diabetic gastroparesis: A randomized controlled trial. *Am J Gastroenterol* 2014;109:375–385.

38. Parrish CR, Yoshida CM. Nutrition intervention for the patient with gastroparesis: An update. Nutritional issues in gastroenterology, series #30. *Pract Gastroenterol* 2005: 29–66.

39. Marahe C, et al. Relationship between gastric emptying, postprandial glycemia and incretin hormones. *Diabetes Car* 2013;36:1396–1405.

40. Bolen S, Feldman L, Vassy J, et al. Systematic review: Comparative effectiveness and safety of oral medications for type 2 diabetes mellitus. *Ann Intern Med* 2007;147:386–399.

41. Amori RE, Lau J, Pittas AG. Efficacy and safety of incretin therapy in type 2 diabetes: Systematic review and meta-analysis. *JAMA* 2007;298(2):194–206.

42. Stevens J, et al. The effect of sitagliptin on gastric emptying in healthy humans: A randomized controlled study. *Aliment Pharmacol Ther* 2012;36:379–390.

43. Jeitler K, Horvath K, Berghold A, et al. Continuous subcutaneous insulin infusion versus multiple daily insulin injections in patients with diabetes mellitus: Systematic review and meta-analysis. *Diabetologia* 2008;51:941–951.

44. Sharma D, Morrison G, Joseph F, et al. The role of continuous subcutaneous insulin infusion therapy in patients with diabetic gastroparesis. *Diabetologia* 2011;54:2768–2770.

45. Calles-Escandon J, Hasler WL, Koch KL, et al. Continuous blood glucose patterns in diabetic patients with gastroparesis: Baseline findings from the GpCRC GLUMIT-DG study. *Gastroenterology* 2014;146:S616.

46. Calles-Escandon J, Van Natta M, Koch KL, Hasler W, et al. On behalf of the NIH Gastroparesis consortium. Pilot study of the safety, feasibility, and efficacy of continuous glucose monitoring (CGM) and insulin pump therapy in diabetic gastroparesis (GLUMIT-DG): A multicenter, longitudinal trial by the NIDDK Gastroparesis Clinical Consortium (GpCRC). *Gastroenterology* 2015;146:S295.

47. Koch KL, Calles-Escandón J. diabetic gastroparesis. *Gastroenterol Clin North Am* 2015;44(1):39–57.

48. Lata PF, Pigarelli DL. Chronic metoclopramide therapy for diabetic gastroparesis. *Ann Pharmacother* 2003;37:122–1226.

49. Rayner CK, Su YC, Doran SM, et al. The relation between symptom improvement and gastric emptying in the treatment of diabetic and idiopathic gastroparesis. *Am J Gastroenterology* 2013;108:1382–1391.

50. Janssen P, Harris MS, Jones M, Masaoka T, et al. The relation between symptom improvement and gastric emptying in the treatment of diabetic and idiopathic gastroparesis. *Am J Gastroenterology* 2013;108(9):1382–1391.

51. Koch KL, Stern RM, Stewart WR, et al. Gastric emptying and gastric myoelectrical activity in patients with symptomatic diabetic gastroparesis: Effect of long-term domperidone treatment. *Am J Gastroenterol* 1989;84:1069–1075.

52. Camilleri M, McCallum RW, Tack J, Spence SC, Gottesdiener K, Fiedorek FT. Efficacy and safety of relamorelin in diabetics with symptoms of gastroparesis: A randomized, placebo-controlled study. *Gastroenterology* 2017; 153;5:1240–1250.

53. Brzana RJ, Bingaman S, Koch KL. Gastric myoelectrical activity in patients with gastric outlet obstruction and idiopathic gastroparesis. *Am J Gastroenterol* 1998;93:1083–1089.

54. Snape WJ, Lin MS, Agarwal N, Shaw RE. Evaluation of the pylorus with concurrent intraluminal pressure and EndoFLIP in patients with nausea and vomiting. *Neurogastroenterol Motil* 2016;28:758–764.

55. Friedenberg FK, Palit A, Parkman HP, et al. Botulinum toxin A for the treatment of delayed gastric emptying. *Am J Gastroenterol* 2008;103:416–423.

56. Wellington J, Scott B, Kundu S, Stuart P, Koch KL. Effect of endoscopic pyloric therapies for patients with nausea and vomiting and functional obstructive gastroparesis. *Auton Neurosci* 2017;202:56–61.

57. McCallum RW, Snape W, Brody F, et al. Gastric electrical stimulation with enterra improves symptoms from diabetic gastroparesis in a prospective study. *Clin Gastroenterol Hepatol* 2010;8:947–954.

58. McLin VA, Henning SJ, Jamrich M. The role of the visceral mesoderm in the development of the gastrointestinal tract. *Gastroenterology* 2009;136:2074–2091.

59. Burns AJ, Thapar N. Neural stem cell therapies for enteric nervous system disorders. *Nat Rev Gastroenterol Hepatol* 2014;11:317–328.

60. Hao MM, Young HM. Development of enteric neuron diversity. *J Cell Mol Med* 2009;13:1193–1210.

61. Grover M, Farrugia G, Lurken MS, Bernard CE, Faussone-Pellegrini MS, Smyrk TC, Parkman HP et al., NIDDK gastroparesis clinical research consortium. Cellular changes in diabetic and idiopathic gastroparesis. *Gastroenterology* 2011;140:1575–1585.

62. Bitar KN, Zakhem E. Tissue engineering and regenerative medicine as applied to the gastrointestinal tract. *Curr Opin Biotechnol* 2013;24:909–915.

63. Gilmont RR, Raghavan S, Somara S, Bitar KN. Bioengineering of physiologically functional intrinsically innervated human internal anal sphincter constructs. *Tissue Eng Part A* 2014;20:1603–1611.

64. Hashish M, Raghavan S, Somara S, Gilmont RR, Miyasaka E, Bitar KN, et al. Surgical implantation of a bioengineered internal anal sphincter. *J Pediatr Surg* 2010;45:52–58.

65. Raghavan S, Gilmont RR, Miyasaka EA, Somara S, Srinivasan S, Teitelbaum DH, et al. Successful implantation of bioengineered, intrinsically innervated, human internal anal sphincter. *Gastroenterology* 2011;141:310–319.
66. Raghavan S, Miyasaka EA, Gilmont RR, Somara S, Teitelbaum DH, Bitar KN. Perianal implantation of bioengineered human internal anal sphincter constructs intrinsically innervated with human neural progenitor cells. *Surgery* 2013;155:668–674.
67. Zakhem E, Raghavan S, Bitar KN. Neo-innervation of a bioengineered intestinal smooth muscle construct around chitosan scaffold. *Biomaterials* 2014;35:1882–1889.
68. Sasselli V, Micci MA, Kahrig KM, Pasricha PJ. Evaluation of ES-derived neural progenitors as a potential source for cell replacement therapy in the gut. *BMC Gastroenterol* 2012;12:81.
69. Kawaguchi J, Nichols J, Gierl MS, Faial T, Smith A. Isolation and propagation of enteric neural crest progenitor cells from mouse embryonic stem cells and embryos. *Development* 2010;137:693–704.
70. Micci, MA, Kahrig KM, Simmons RS, Sarna SK, Espejo-Navarro MR, Pasricha PJ. Neural stem cell transplantation in the stomach rescues gastric function in neuronal nitric oxide synthase-deficient mice. *Gastroenterology* 2005;129:1817–1824.
71. Dong YL, Liu W, Gao YM, Wu RD, Zhang YH, Wang HF, et al. Neural stem cell transplantation rescues rectum function in the aganglionic rat. *Transplant Proc* 2008;40:3646–3652.
72. Natarajan D, Grigoriou M, Marcos-Gutierrez CV, Atkins C, Pachnis V. Multipotential progenitors of the mammalian enteric nervous system capable of colonising aganglionic bowel in organ culture. *Development* 1999;126:157–168.
73. Morrison SJ, White PM, Zock C, Anderson DJ. Prospective identification, isolation by flow cytometry, and in vivo self-renewal of multipotent mammalian neural crest stem cells. *Cell* 1999;96:737–749.
74. Metzger M, Caldwell C, Barlow AJ, Burns AJ, Thapar N. Enteric nervous system stem cells derived from human gut mucosa for the treatment of aganglionic gut disorders. *Gastroenterology* 2009;136:2214–2225 e1–e3.
75. Hotta R, Stamp LA, Foong JP, McConnell SN, Bergner AJ, Anderson AB, et al. Transplanted progenitors generate functional enteric neurons in the postnatal colon. *J Clin Invest* 2013;123:1182–1191.
76. Liu MT, Kuan YH, Wang J, Hen R, Gershon MD. 5-HT4 receptor-mediated neuroprotection and neurogenesis in the enteric nervous system of adult mice. *J Neurosci* 2009;29:9683–9699.
77. Micci MA, Kahrig KM, Simmons RS, Sarna SK, Espejo-Navarro MR, Pasricha PJ. Neural stem cell transplantation in the stomach rescues gastric function in neuronal nitric oxide synthase-deficient mice. *Gastroenterology* 2005;129:1817–1824.
78. Ohki T, Yamato M, Murakami D, Takagi R, Yang J, Namiki H, et al. Treatment of esophageal ulcerations using endoscopic transplantation of tissue-engineered autologous oral mucosal epithelial cell sheets in a canine model. *Gut* 2006;55:1704–1710.
79. Metzger M, Caldwell C, Barlow AJ, Burns AJ, Thapar N. Enteric nervous system stem cells derived from human gut mucosa for the treatment of aganglionic gut disorders. *Gastroenterology* 2009;136:2214–2225 e1–3.
80. Micci MA, Pattillo MT, Kahrig KM, Pasricha PJ. Caspase inhibition increases survival of neural stem cells in the gastrointestinal tract. *Neurogastroenterol Motil* 2005;17:557–564.
81. Raghavan S, Gilmont RR, Bitar KN. Neuroglial differentiation of adult enteric neuronal progenitor cells as a function of extracellular matrix composition. *Biomaterials* 2013;34:6649–6658.
82. Bohl JL, Zakhem E, Bitar KN. Successful treatment of passive fecal incontinence in an animal model using engineered biosphincters: A 3-month follow-up study. *Stem Cells Transl Med* 2017;6:1795–1802.
83. Rego SL, Zakhem E, Orlando G, Bitar KN. Bioengineered human pyloric sphincters using autologous smooth muscle and neural progenitor cells. *Tissue Eng Part A* 2016;22:151–160.

Index

Note: Page numbers in italic and bold refer to figures and tables respectively.

Printed in the United States
by Baker & Taylor Publisher Services